THE GREAT AMERICAN GUIDE TO DIET AND HEALTH

Edited by
SUSAN OSBORN

McGraw-Hill Book Company

New York St. Louis San Francisco Auckland Bogotá Guatemala
Hamburg Johannesburg Lisbon London Madrid Mexico Montreal
New Delhi Panama Paris San Juan São Paulo Singapore
Sydney Tokyo Toronto

1234567890 SMSM 8765432

ISBN 0-07-069072-3 {PBK}
0-07-069074-X {HC}

Library of Congress Cataloging in Publication Data

Main entry under title:
The Great American guide to diet and health.
1. Nutrition. 2. Food. 3. Diet. 4. Health.
I. Osborn, Susan.
TX353.G678 641 82-15175
ISBN 0-07-069074-X AACR2
ISBN 0-07-069072-3 (pbk.)

Book designed by and original illustrations by David M. Nehila

THE GREAT AMERICAN GUIDE TO DIET AND HEALTH

CONTENTS

DIET AND NUTRITION

Part 1

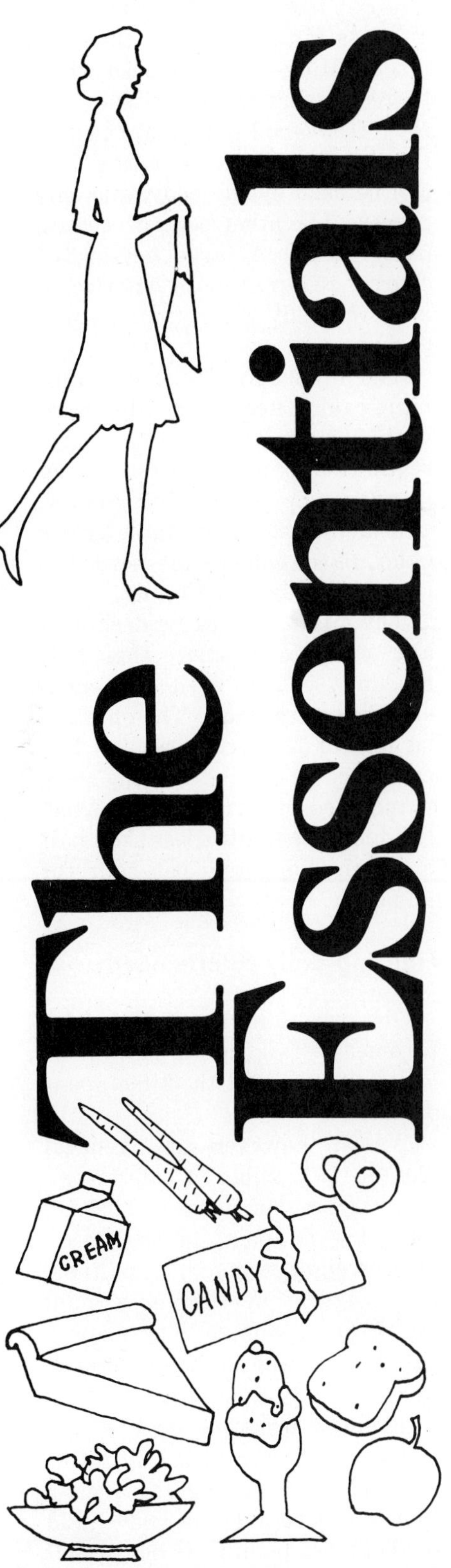

Food and Your Weight

Food is the source of energy for the body.

We need this energy just to keep alive—for continuous body functions, such as breathing, the beating of the heart, the maintenance of muscle tone. We need it for carrying out all work and leisure activities. Children and youth need it for growth.

When the foods we eat provide more energy than is needed to meet the demands of the body, the extra energy is stored in the body as fat. If we furnish the body regularly with too much food, we gain weight.

If the foods we eat provide less energy than is needed, the body uses stored fat. If all reserve fatty tissues are used up and we continue to give the body a short supply of food, the body uses its other tissues for energy.

The unit used to measure food energy is the calorie. We commonly use the term "calories" to mean food energy—as we use "miles" to mean distance, "pounds" to mean weight, or "hours" to mean time.

YOUR WEIGHT

How much should an adult weigh? In general, the weight that is desirable for you when you are in your midtwenties is considered the best weight for later years, too.

You can get an idea of what your desirable weight might be by using the weight table.

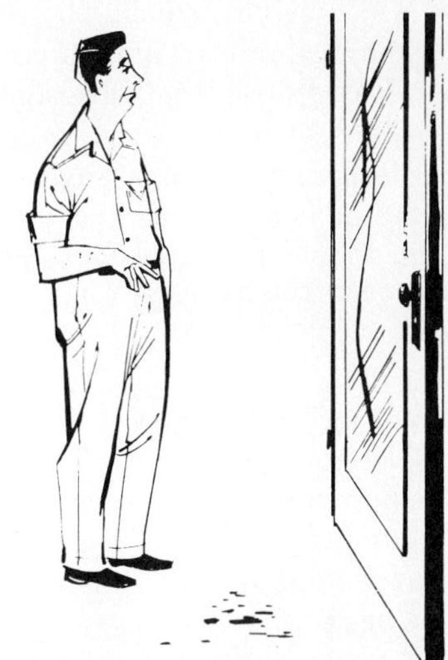

To use the table, first find in the left-hand column your height, without shoes. If you have a small frame, your weight should proba-

Weights of Persons 20 to 30 Years Old

Height (without shoes)	Weight (without clothing)		
	Low	Average	High
	Pounds	Pounds	Pounds
Men			
5 feet 3 inches	118	129	141
5 feet 4 inches	122	133	145
5 feet 5 inches	126	137	149
5 feet 6 inches	130	142	155
5 feet 7 inches	134	147	161
5 feet 8 inches	139	151	166
5 feet 9 inches	143	155	170
5 feet 10 inches	147	159	174
5 feet 11 inches	150	163	178
6 feet	154	167	183
6 feet 1 inch	158	171	188
6 feet 2 inches	162	175	192
6 feet 3 inches	165	178	195
Women			
5 feet	100	109	118
5 feet 1 inch	104	112	121
5 feet 2 inches	107	115	125
5 feet 3 inches	110	118	128
5 feet 4 inches	113	122	132
5 feet 5 inches	116	125	135
5 feet 6 inches	120	129	139
5 feet 7 inches	123	132	142
5 feet 8 inches	126	136	146
5 feet 9 inches	130	140	151
5 feet 10 inches	133	144	156
5 feet 11 inches	137	148	161
6 feet	141	152	166

bly be no lower than the weight in the "low" column and no higher than the weight given in the "average" column. If you have a large frame, use the "average" and "high" columns to determine your desirable weight range. If your frame is about average, your weight should probably be somewhere near the average for your height.

DAILY CALORIE NEED

The number of calories used by the body each day to maintain present weight is called the daily calorie need.

Of this, part is the minimum calorie need for basal metabolism —calories spent to keep the body functioning. The remainder is the number of calories spent by the body in carrying out various work and leisure activities.

Minimum calorie need

The amount of energy required to keep the body functioning is influenced by body composition and size, and by age.

Generally, men have a higher minimum calorie need than women because they have a greater proportion of lean (or muscle) tissue and less fat and because they are larger. More energy is used when there is more muscle tissue; energy from food is transformed in the muscle tissues to energy that can be used by the body, and this process, like other body processes, uses energy. A large person, of course, requires more calories to keep the body going than a small person.

The influence of age on minimum calorie need is usually linked with periods of growth. Calorie requirements are greatest during infancy, adolescence, pregnancy, and lactation. As an adult grows older, fewer calories are needed to keep the body functioning.

The minimum calorie need usually accounts for more than half the daily calorie need of a moderately active adult. The share is larger for less active adults. Energy used by the body during sleep is included in this minimum need. It amounts to a little less than half a calorie per pound per hour for an adult.

Figuring daily calorie need

One way to find our daily calorie need is to keep an account of our activities and the time spent on each.

We can, however, get a general idea of the number of calories we use by a simpler method. That is: Take the midpoint of the desirable weight range; multiply this figure by 18 for a man, by 16 for a woman. The answer will be the approximate number of calories used daily by an adult of average activity.

To illustrate: The desirable weight for a woman 5 feet 5 inches tall of average body build is about 125 pounds. If her activities are average, she will use about 125 × 16, or about 2,000 calories per day.

If you are vigorously active, your calorie needs will be much higher than the number of calories you get by this simple method.

If you are relatively inactive—or an older adult—you probably will need fewer calories than calculated by this method. Older adults also are likely to be less active.

The Key to Weight Control

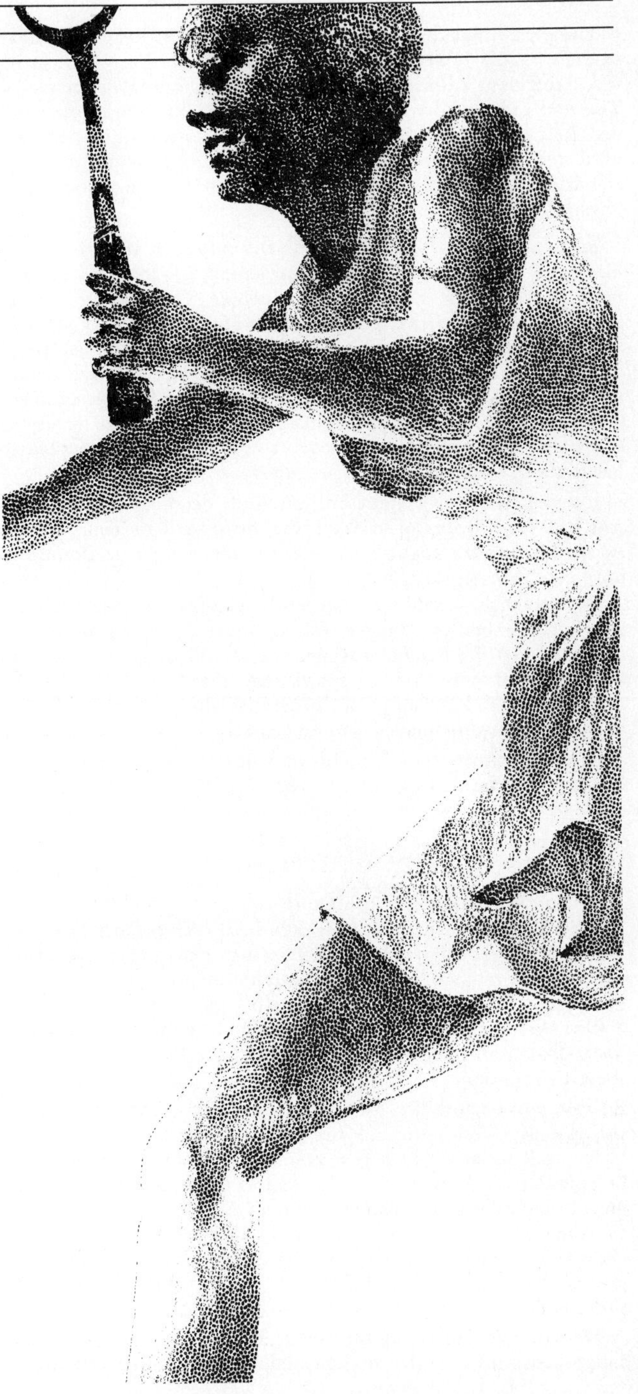

The key to effective weight control is keeping energy intake (food) and activity energy output (physical activity) in balance. This is true at all ages for both sexes. When the calories consumed in food equal those used to meet the body's needs, weight will remain about the same. When one eats more than this amount, one will put on fat unless physical activity is increased proportionately.

For years physicians have talked about the varying caloric needs of differing occupations and physical recreations. Yet in their attempts to lose excess fat, weight-watchers have often concentrated on counting the calories in their diets and have neglected the role of exercise. For those who are too fat, increasing physical activity can be just as important as decreasing food intake.

Weight depends not only on how many calories are taken in during the day, but also on how many are used up in physical activity. The overly fat person who merely cuts down his intake of food to lose weight will make slow progress since the number of calories needed to maintain the body is much smaller than most people think.

In fact, lack of exercise has been cited as the most important cause of the "creeping" obesity found in modern mechanized societies. Few occupations now require vigorous physical activity. Although there is more time available for recreation, many persons fail to fill this gap by choosing leisure time activities that give them exercise. Even among those who do exercise, their activity is often neither vigorous nor sustained.

Authorities point out that adding 30 minutes per day of moderate exercise to one's schedule can result in a loss of about 25 pounds in one year, assuming food consumption remains constant. To put it another way—just one extra slice of bread a day—or a soft drink—or any other food item that contains about 100 calories—can add up to 10 extra pounds in a year if the amount of physical activity is not increased accordingly.

Recent studies seem to indicate that lack of physical activity is more often the cause of overweight than is overeating. These studies have compared the food intake and activity patterns of obese persons with those of normal weight. Several age levels—teen-age, adults, and older persons—have been studied. In each instance, the findings showed that the obese people did not consume any more calories than their normal-weighted age-mates, but that they were very much less active.

The person who has a trim figure and wants to keep it should exercise regularly and eat a balanced, nutritious diet which provides sufficient calories to make up for the energy expended. The thin individual who wishes to gain weight should exercise regularly and increase the number of calories he consumes until the desired weight is reached. The overweight person should decrease the food intake and step up the amount of physical activity.

Most people will exercise regularly only if it brings enjoyment and satisfaction. Walking, gardening, cycling, and swimming provide these values for some people. The lifetime sports such as tennis, bowling, golfing, badminton and archery satisfy the needs of many others and establish desirable exercise patterns that can be enjoyed by people of all ages. Active team sports such as basketball, volleyball or softball furnish similar benefits for still others, particularly the younger age groups. Calisthenics or weight training are a bore to some, but a pleasure to those who practice them regularly.

Jogging has nearly eight million adult devotees in America and has the advantage of requiring little skill or equipment. Accessibility on a regular basis is an important consideration in selecting an activity.

The exercise should be sufficiently vigorous to use up the required number of calories, and to some degree, it must be sustained. To the extent possible, one should meet one's needs for regular activity through sports and other forms of physical recreation that are enjoyable; otherwise the activity is likely to be abandoned or played only irregularly.

Exercising once a week yields only sore muscles; pick activities that can be done regularly. They needn't be the same ones every day; in fact variety adds spice to an exercise schedule.

WEIGHT CONTROL FALLACIES

Two basic fallacies have been widely held with respect to exercise and weight control. The first is that a great deal of time and effort is required to use up enough calories to affect weight materially. The second is that exercise increases the appetite and so will increase, not decrease, weight. Scientific experiments on animals and man have demonstrated the falsity of both of these assumptions.

Energy expenditure in exercise. If activity is not increased eating only a few more calories per day than are utilized can have a telling effect in a few years, since small gains tend to be cumulative. A woman would need to eat an average of only 96 calories a day more than she expends to gain 50 pounds from the time of her marriage to the arrival of her third child five years later. Had she added only 25 minutes of brisk walking to her daily activities, this weight gain would have been prevented.

The average adult man will burn up 2,400 to 4,500 calories a day depending on the amount and kind of exercise he gets. Active persons such as laborers, soldiers in the field and athletes may consume as many as 6,000 calories a day and yet not gain weight. This is a fact that has been well-known for many years.

In an experiment a few years ago, a group of university students increased their daily food intake (from 3,000 calories daily to 6,000) without gaining weight. This was accomplished merely by stepping up the amount of exercise they did each day.

The cost in calories of different types of exercise has been established and is shown in the chart that is part of this booklet. The number of calories expended depends on how strenuously these activities are undertaken.

The figures on energy expenditure through various activities are probably underestimates. They are usually derived by measuring the amount of oxygen consumed during a specific bout of exercise and then computing the equivalent number of calories burned. However, the effects of exercise continue after the actual time in which the exercise is performed. Body processes have been stepped-up and only gradually are lowered; this takes energy—sometimes for long periods after the exercise is stopped.

Energy expended is also affected by body weight since in those activities where the individual has to move his own weight, energy costs are increased for the heavier person and decreased for the lighter. To illustrate, a person walking 3 mph, weighing 100 pounds, will burn as few as 50 calories in 15 minutes, while someone weighing 200 pounds would use up as many as 80 calories in the same length of time.

Remember that although it takes an hour's jogging to use up 900 calories, one does not have to do it all in one stretch; a half-hour, for example, uses up 450 calories. It is a fact that one must walk 35 miles at lose one pound of fat but the 35 miles need not be walked at one time.

Walking an additional mile each day for 35 days also will take off that pound. This means one can lose 10 pounds in one year by walking an extra mile a day—providing, of course,

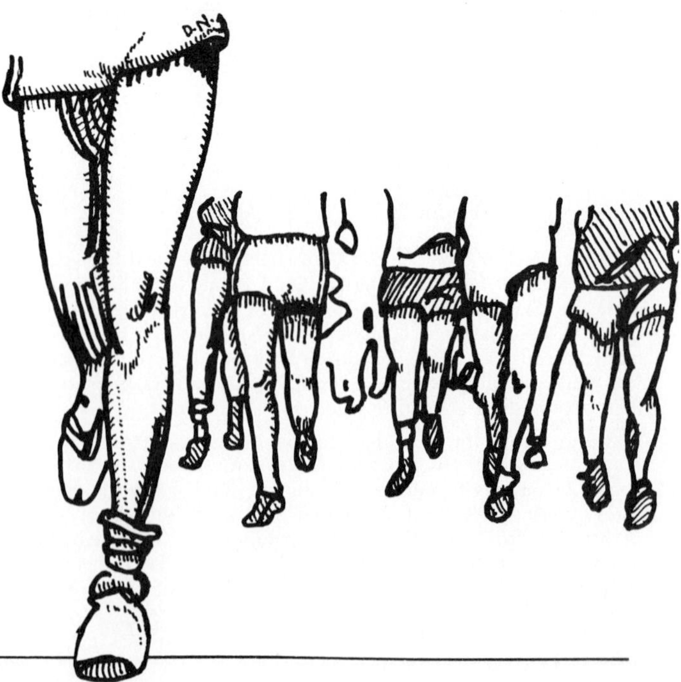

that food intake and other physical activity remain the same. This really isn't an impractical amount of time or effort and to lose more or faster one needs only to increase the extent of activity.

Appetite and exercise. The idea that increased physical activity is useless as a means of losing weight because it always increases the appetite is equally fallacious.

It is true that a lean person in good condition may eat more following increased activity, but his exercise will burn up the extra calories he consumes. But the obese—the overly fat person—does not react the same way to exercise. Only when he exercises to excess will his appetite increase. Because he has large stores of fat, moderate exercise does not stimulate his appetite. This difference between the response to exercise of fat and lean people is important.

Laboratory tests on experimental animals have borne this out. When their exercise was moderate food intake did not increase. In one experiment animals exercised one hour a day ate a smaller amount of food than those exercised less than an hour a day or not at all! On the other hand when the animals were exercised vigorously over longer periods they ate more, but the extra activity kept their weight constant.

In other experiments, when the animals' activity was decreased, they continued to eat the same amount of food and became obese.

Similarly, a study of overweight adults showed that the start of their obesity corresponded with their decline in activity. Although their activity decreased, their appetites didn't. This is a common observation. When people finish school and go to work (especially if the job is a sedentary one), they tend to exercise less, but through habit, eat as much as ever. Before long they are obese.

ADVANTAGES OF EXERCISE

If weight control can be achieved either through dieting or exercise, wouldn't it be simpler to concentrate on dieting and not worry about exercise? Remarkable claims are made for a variety of so-called crash or very restricted diets.

Some crash diets do achieve noticeable weight loss in a short time. Much of this may be due to a loss of body water, however, and such a loss is quickly restored when a normal food and liquid intake is resumed. Those dieters who fail to realize that fat is lost very slowly became discouraged and conclude that it is impossible for them to lose weight.

Furthermore, extreme diets carried out for an extended period, if they are not well-balanced and under medical supervision, may create nutritional problems. This is especially true among teen-age girls who may attempt self-prescribed diets to improve their figures and only make themselves ill by causing deficiencies of essential food substances. Recent studies indicate that weight reduction through near starvation may be at the expense of valuable body tissues rather than reduction of fat.

The person who gives proper attention to exercise derives benefits in addition to weight control and does not create nutritional problems for himself. Muscles which may have been weak and sagging become strong and firm. Feelings of listlessness and fatigue are replaced by sensations of alertness and energy. Sleep is better and more restful. With proper guidance, body posture can be improved, which, in addition to reduction of body fat and toning up the muscles, creates a more pleasing body profile.

Moreover, exercise can be fun, provide recreation, and offer opportunity for companionship. The exhilaration and emotional release of participating in sports or other activities are a boon to good mental, as well as physical health. Pent-up anxieties and frustrations seem to disappear as one concentrates on knocking over pins, returning a serve, or sinking a putt. Cutting the lawn, weeding the garden, or taking a brisk walk can be good tonics for both mind and body.

The man or woman who takes regular exercise will maintain a better state of physical fitness, will keep active longer, and is more apt to be resistant to the degenerative diseases of middle and later life, especially diseases of the heart and of the blood vessels.

IMPORTANCE OF DIET

This book emphasizes the role of exercise in weight control because its value has only recently been given attention. Many booklets and articles on weight control have stressed diet but have not recognized the dual role of exercise. This emphasis on exercise here should not minimize the need for proper nutrition in keeping fit and in maintaining a desirable weight. Both are valuable.

So remember, increasing exercise doesn't give license also to increase one's diet! Step up the exercise, but keep the diet well-balanced, the calorie intake the same—or a little less—for the best long-range results.

The reader is advised to choose his daily food requirements from the Basic Four—(1) Milk Group (2) Meat Group (3) Vegetable-Fruit Group (4) Bread-Cereal Group. Doing so he can follow a low calorie diet and yet make sure that his body receives the needed nutrients.

EXERCISE AND MODERN LIVING

What kind of exercise does a given person need? Health authorities recommend regular activity that utilizes many parts of the body. The activity should be vigorous enough to tax the power of the muscles and should be done long enough and strenuously enough to produce a sense of healthful fatigue.

The exercise also should be suited to age, and physical condition. It is wise to consult the personal physician before launching into a program of increased physical activity. Some persons have conditions that could be aggravated by the wrong kind of exercise.

One thing is certain. Most people do not get enough exercise in their ordinary routines. All of the advances of modern technology—from electric can openers to power steering—have made life easier, more comfortable, and much less demanding physically. Yet human bodies need activity. This requires a definite plan—and purposeful pursuit of that plan.

There are four main approaches to being adequately active:

1. A regular exercise schedule
2. Supplementary physical recreation
3. Stepped-up ordinary physical activity
4. Physical activity in the day's occupation

Each of these outlets for participating is important in keeping fit and in burning calories. The sum total activities for a day or a week should be sufficient and balanced.

Regular Exercise Schedule. Each individual should commit himself to a planned program of exercise and stick with it. This means setting aside 30 minutes to an hour a day about five times per week for physical activity. This schedule of exercise should be thought of as being as essential as a proper diet.

An exercise program should be balanced just as a diet should be balanced. Some parts should be designed primarily to exercise the heart and lungs in a way that will develop endurance. Brisk walking, jogging, and swimming relatively long distances are good for this purpose.

Other parts of the program should be directed toward the improvement of strength, agility, flexibility, balance, and muscle tone.

Make this a personal keep-fit program. Start easily. Keep a record of what is done and how many times it is done. Gradually increase the amount of exercise until a reasonably good level is reached.

Of course, alternatives can be employed. If one can enroll in a keep-fit program at the Y, or the school, or the recreation center, or the club, the home routine can be skipped on the meeting days. On those days when there is no class, the do-it-yourself program can be followed. Those fortunate enough to have the time and facilities for sports should by all means take part.

One should swim when he can but should really swim; sunbathing doesn't use up many calories. A vigorous game of handball, or tennis, or badminton will meet activity needs for that day. Golf is fine if one walks fast between strokes—for eighteen holes—but not if he rides a cart. Likewise continuous, individual or dual bowling is more beneficial than interrupted team bowling. Hunting, snow skiing, skin diving, bicycling, water skiing, canoeing, hiking are all good for that day—that is, if one gets at least the equivalent in exercise of what he would otherwise do in his home exercise program.

Many people who engage in sports can do so only occasionally on weekends or in season. However, a home exercise program can help maintain good condition so that when one has the opportunity to engage in sports, he will not become stiff, sore, or overtired.

A person may follow the new program for several days and yet find no difference showing on the bathroom scale. Adjustments in metabolism take place and it may be some time before any reduction in weight can be seen.

When one exercises regularly some flabby tissue is changed to muscle. Muscle tissue takes much less space, hence a trimmer figure results even though weight may not drop markedly.

Supplementary Recreation. Most people, especially those who wish to lose weight, should supplement the scheduled exercise with additional physical recreation. Gardening on weekends, a pleasant walk, bird watching, bowling in the office league, a family outing or fishing trip, an evening of social dancing, the square dance club's regular sessions; these and many more such activities provide recreational benefits and a bit of exercise as well. These should be looked upon as an extra bonus in the weight-watcher's campaign.

Stepped-Up Daily Activities. To a scheduled program and supplementary recreation add a little more action each day. Walk to the neighborhood grocery instead of using the car. Park several blocks from the office and walk the rest of the way. Walk up a flight or more of stairs instead of using the elevator; start with a few steps and gradually increase. Stand

ENERGY EXPENDITURE BY A 150 POUND PERSON IN VARIOUS ACTIVITIES *

Activity	*Gross Energy Cost-Cal per hr.*
A. Rest and Light Activity	**50–200**
Lying down or sleeping	80
Sitting	100
Driving an automobile	120
Standing	140
Domestic work	180
B. Moderate Activity	**200–350**
Bicycling (5½ mph)	210
Walking (2½ mph)	210
Gardening	220
Canoeing (2½ mph)	230
Golf	250
Lawn mowing (power mower)	250
Bowling	270
Lawn mowing (hand mower)	270
Fencing	300
Rowboating (2½ mph)	300
Swimming (¼ mph)	300
Walking (3¾ mph)	300
Badminton	350
Horseback riding (trotting)	350
Square dancing	350
Volleyball	350
Roller skating	350
C. Vigorous Activity	**over 350**
Table tennis	360
Ditch digging (hand shovel)	400
Ice skating (10 mph)	400
Wood chopping or sawing	400
Tennis	420
Water skiing	480
Hill climbing (100 ft. per hr.)	490
Skiing (10 mph)	600
Squash and handball	600
Cycling (13 mph)	660
Scull rowing (race)	840
Running (10 mph)	900

**The standards represent a compromise between those proposed by the British Medical Association (1950), Christensen (1953) and Wells, Balke, and Van Fossan (1956). Where available, actual measured values have been used; for other values a "best guess" was made.*

†Prepared by Robert E. Johnson, M.D., Ph.D., and colleagues, Department of Physiology and Biophysics, University of Illinois, August, 1967.

up to put on and remove stockings and shoes; most people neglect to use their sense of balance. Get off the chair to get what is needed. Bend, stoop, stretch, squat, reach, move, lift, carry.

In today's sedentary world, people need to re-direct their whole approach to movement. Look for opportunities to use the body. Time-saving devices and gadgets that eliminate drudgery are boons to mankind, but when they substitute increasingly for physical activity they can demand a high cost in health and fitness.

These little bits of action, while not taxing, are cumulative in their good effects. A few calories used up by walking, going up steps, bending or otherwise moving can add up to a fair-sized total in the course of the day. And the contribution they make to muscle tone, flexibility, and balance are also significant.

The Day's Occupation. The amount of activity involved in one's job also is important. The suggestions above on daily activities of living apply also to on-the-job opportunities for exercise.

Within reason, one should look for ways of increasing his activity. It is a matter of outlook. Instead of considering an extra little walk, or trip to the files, or an errand downstairs as an annoyance, look upon it as an added fitness boost.

Nutritive Value of Foods

A glass of milk...a slice of cooked meat...an apple...a slice of bread... What food values does each contain? How much cooked meat will a pound of raw meat yield? How much daily protein is recommended for a healthy 14-year-old boy?

Ready answers to questions like those are helpful to homemakers who need the information to plan nutritionally adequate diets and to nutritionists, dietitians, physicians, and other consumers.

EXPLANATION OF THE TABLES

Some helpful volume and weight equivalents are shown in table 1.

Table 1.—Equivalents by Volume and Weight

Volume

Level measure	*Equivalent*
1 gallon (3.786 liters; 3,786 milliliters)	4 quarts
1 quart (0.946 liter; 946 milliliters)	4 cups
1 cup (237 milliliters)	8 fluid ounces ½ pint 16 tablespoons
2 tablespoons (30 milliliters)	1 fluid ounce
1 tablespoon (15 milliliters)	3 teaspoons
1 pound regular butter or margarine	4 sticks 2 cups
1 pound whipped butter or margarine	6 sticks Two 8-ounce containers 3 cups

Weight

Avoirdupois weight	*Equivalent*
1 pound (16 ounces)	453.6 grams
1 ounce	28.35 grams
3½ ounces	100 grams

Nutritive Value of Foods (Table 2)

Table 2 shows the food values in 730 foods commonly used.

Foods listed.—Foods are grouped under the following main headings:

- Dairy products
- Eggs
- Fats and oils
- Fish, shellfish, meat, and poultry
- Fruits and fruit products
- Grain products
- Legumes (dry), nuts, and seeds
- Sugars and sweets
- Vegetables and vegetable products
- Miscellaneous items

Most of the foods listed are in ready-to-eat form. Some are basic products widely used in food preparation, such as flour, fat, and cornmeal.

The weight in grams for an approximate measure of each food is shown. A footnote indicates if inedible parts are included in the description and the weight. For example, item 246 is half a grapefruit with peel having a weight of 241 grams. A footnote to this item explains that the 241 grams include the weight of the peel.

The approximate measure shown for each food is in cups, ounces, pounds, some other well-known unit, or a piece of certain size. The cup measure refers to the standard measuring cup of 8 fluid ounces or one-half liquid pint. The ounce refers to one-sixteenth of a pound avoirdupois, unless fluid ounce is indicated. The weight of a fluid ounce varies according to the food measured.

Food values.—Table 2 also shows values for protein, fat, total saturated fatty acids, two unsaturated fatty acids (oleic acid and linoleic acid), total carbohydrates, four minerals (calcium, iron, phosphorus, and potassium), and five vitamins (vitamin A, thiamin, riboflavin, niacin, and ascorbic acid or vitamin C). Food energy is in calories. The calorie is the unit of measurement for the energy furnished the body by protein, fat, and carbohydrate.

Those values can be used to compare kinds and amounts of nutrients in different foods. They sometimes can be used to compare different forms of the same food.

Water content is included because the percentage of moisture present is needed for identification and comparison of many food items.

The values for food energy (calories) and nutrients shown in table 2 are the amounts present in the edible part of the item, that is, in only that portion customarily eaten—corn without cob, meat without bone, potatoes without skin, European-type grapes without seeds. If additional parts are eaten—the potato skin, for example—amounts of some nutrients obtained will be somewhat greater than those shown.

Values for thiamin, riboflavin, and niacin in white flours and white bread and rolls are based on the increased enrichment levels put into effect for those products by the Food and Drug Administration in 1974. Iron values for those products and the values for enriched cornmeals, pastas, farina, and rice (except riboflavin) represent the minimum levels of enrichment promulgated under the Federal Food, Drug, and Cosmetic Act of 1955. Riboflavin values of rice are for unenriched rice, as the levels for added riboflavin have not been approved. Thiamin, riboflavin, and niacin values for products prepared with white flours represent the use of flours enriched at the 1974 levels and iron at the 1955 levels. Enriched flour is predominately used in home-prepared and commercially prepared baked goods.

Fatty acid values are given for dairy products, eggs, meats, some grain products, nuts, and soups. The values are based on comprehensive research by USDA to update and extend tables for fatty acid content for foods.

Niacin values are for preformed niacin occurring naturally in foods. The values do not include additional niacin that the body may form from tryptophan, an essential amino acid in the protein of most foods. Among the better sources of tryptophan are milk, meats, eggs, legumes, and nuts.

Values have been calculated from the ingredients in typical recipes for many of the prepared items such as biscuits, corn muffins, macaroni and cheese, custard, and many dessert-type items.

Values for toast and cooked vegetables are without fat added, either during preparation or at the table. Some destruction of vitamins, especially ascorbic acid, may occur when vegetables are cut or shredded. Since such losses are variable, no deduction has been made.

For meat, values are for meat cooked and drained of the drippings. For many cuts, two sets of values are shown: meat including fat and meat from which the fat has been removed either in the kitchen or on the plate.

A variety of manufactured items—some of the milk products, ready-to-eat breakfast cereals, imitation cream products, fruit drinks, and various mixes—are included in table 2. Frequently those foods are fortified with one or more nutrients. If nutrients are added, this information is on the label. Values shown here for those foods are usually based on products from several manufacturers and may differ somewhat from the values provided by any one source.

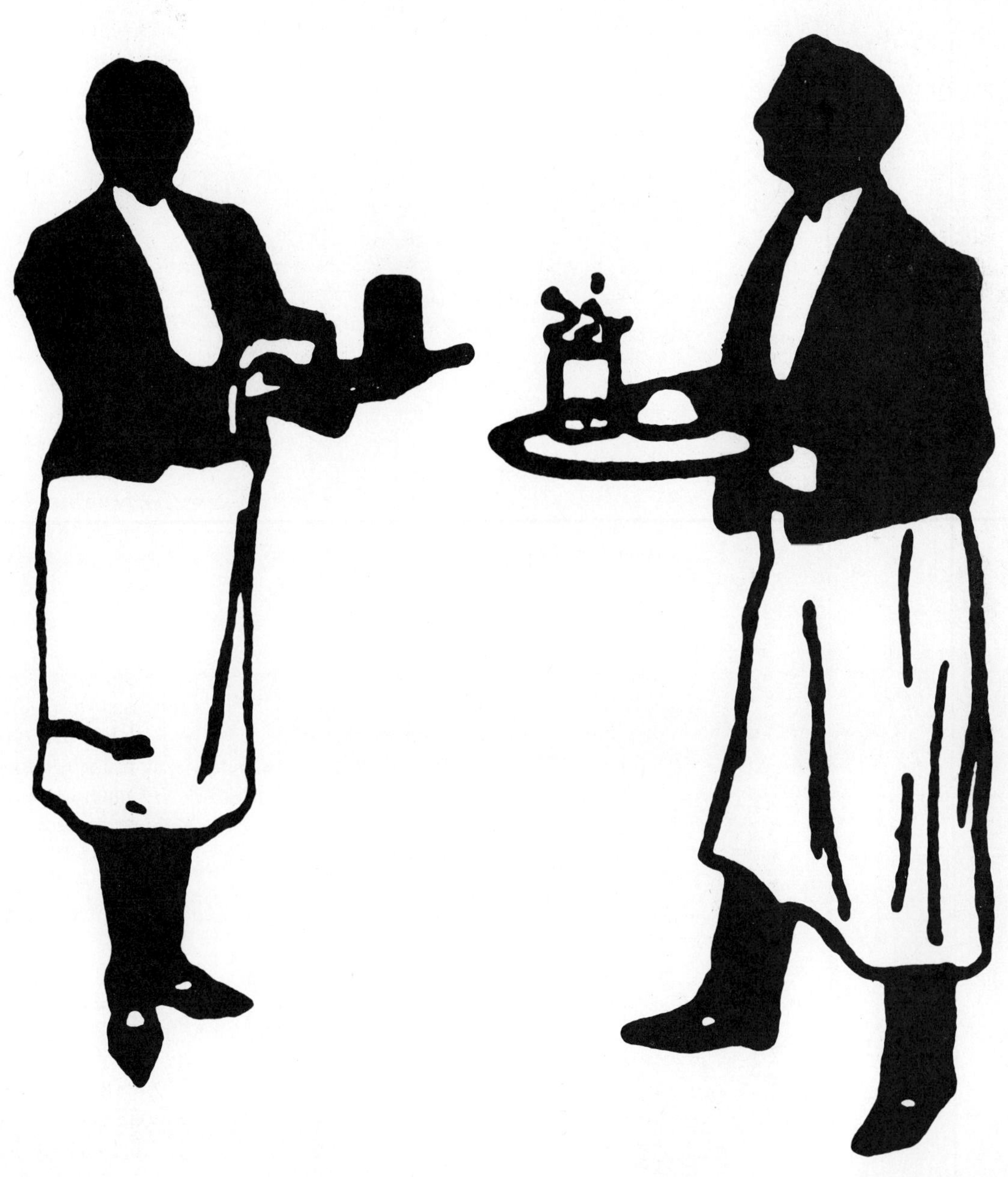

TABLE 2.—NUTRITIVE VALUES OF THE EDIBLE PART OF FOODS

(Dashes (—) denote lack of reliable data for a constituent believed to be present in measurable amount)

Item No.	Foods, approximate measures, units, and weight (edible part unless footnotes indicate otherwise)			Water	Food energy	Protein	Fat	Fatty Acids: Saturated (total)	Fatty Acids: Unsaturated: Oleic	Fatty Acids: Unsaturated: Linoleic	Carbohydrate	Calcium	Phosphorus	Iron	Potassium	Vitamin A value	Thiamin	Riboflavin	Niacin	Ascorbic acid
(A)	(B)			(C)	(D)	(E)	(F)	(G)	(H)	(I)	(J)	(K)	(L)	(M)	(N)	(O)	(P)	(Q)	(R)	(S)
			Grams	Percent	Calories	Grams	Grams	Grams	Grams	Grams	Grams	Milligrams	Milligrams	Milligrams	Milligrams	International units	Milligrams	Milligrams	Milligrams	Milligrams
	DAIRY PRODUCTS (CHEESE, CREAM, IMITATION CREAM, MILK; RELATED PRODUCTS)																			
	Butter. See Fats, oils; related products, items 103-108.																			
	Cheese:																			
	Natural:																			
1	Blue	1 oz	28	42	100	6	8	5.3	1.9	0.2	1	150	110	0.1	73	200	0.01	0.11	0.3	0
2	Camembert (3 wedges per 4-oz container).	1 wedge	38	52	115	8	9	5.8	2.2	.2	Trace	147	132	.1	71	350	.01	.19	.2	0
	Cheddar:																			
3	Cut pieces	1 oz	28	37	115	7	9	6.1	2.1	.2	Trace	204	145	.2	28	300	.01	.11	Trace	0
4		1 cu in	17.2	37	70	4	6	3.7	1.3	.1	Trace	124	88	.1	17	180	Trace	.06	Trace	0
5	Shredded	1 cup	113	37	455	28	37	24.2	8.5	.7	1	815	579	.8	111	1,200	.03	.42	.1	0
	Cottage (curd not pressed down):																			
	Creamed (cottage cheese, 4% fat):																			
6	Large curd	1 cup	225	79	235	28	10	6.4	2.4	.2	6	135	297	.3	190	370	.05	.37	.3	Trace
7	Small curd	1 cup	210	79	220	26	9	6.0	2.2	.2	6	126	277	.3	177	340	.04	.34	.3	Trace
8	Low fat (2%)	1 cup	226	79	205	31	4	2.8	1.0	.1	8	155	340	.4	217	160	.05	.42	.3	Trace
9	Low fat (1%)	1 cup	226	82	165	28	2	1.5	.5	.1	6	138	302	.3	193	80	.05	.37	.3	Trace
10	Uncreamed (cottage cheese dry curd, less than 1/2% fat).	1 cup	145	80	125	25	1	.4	.1	Trace	3	46	151	.3	47	40	.04	.21	.2	0
11	Cream	1 oz	28	54	100	2	10	6.2	2.4	.2	1	23	30	.3	34	400	Trace	.06	Trace	0
	Mozzarella, made with—																			
12	Whole milk	1 oz	28	48	90	6	7	4.4	1.7	.2	1	163	117	.1	21	260	Trace	.08	Trace	0
13	Part skim milk	1 oz	28	49	80	8	5	3.1	1.2	.1	1	207	149	.1	27	180	.01	.10	Trace	0
	Parmesan, grated:																			
14	Cup, not pressed down	1 cup	100	18	455	42	30	19.1	7.7	.3	4	1,376	807	1.0	107	700	.05	.39	.3	0
15	Tablespoon	1 tbsp	5	18	25	2	2	1.0	.4	Trace	Trace	69	40	Trace	5	40	Trace	.02	Trace	0
16	Ounce	1 oz	28	18	130	12	9	5.4	2.2	.1	1	390	229	.3	30	200	.01	.11	.1	0
17	Provolone	1 oz	28	41	100	7	8	4.8	1.7	.1	1	214	141	.1	39	230	.01	.09	Trace	0
	Ricotta, made with—																			
18	Whole milk	1 cup	246	72	430	28	32	20.4	7.1	.7	7	509	389	.9	257	1,210	.03	.48	.3	0
19	Part skim milk	1 cup	246	74	340	28	19	12.1	4.7	.5	13	669	449	1.1	308	1,060	.05	.46	.2	0
20	Romano	1 oz	28	31	110	9	8	—	—	—	1	302	215	—	—	160	—	.11	Trace	0
21	Swiss	1 oz	28	37	105	8	8	5.0	1.7	.2	1	272	171	Trace	31	240	.01	.10	Trace	0
	Pasteurized process cheese:																			
22	American	1 oz	28	39	105	6	9	5.6	2.1	.2	Trace	174	211	.1	46	340	.01	.10	Trace	0
23	Swiss	1 oz	28	42	95	7	7	4.5	1.7	.1	1	219	216	.2	61	230	Trace	.08	Trace	0
24	Pasteurized process cheese food, American.	1 oz	28	43	95	6	7	4.4	1.7	.1	2	163	130	.2	79	260	.01	.13	Trace	0
25	Pasteurized process cheese spread, American.	1 oz	28	48	80	5	6	3.8	1.5	.1	2	159	202	.1	69	220	.01	.12	Trace	0
	Cream, sweet:																			
26	Half-and-half (cream and milk)	1 cup	242	81	315	7	28	17.3	7.0	.6	10	254	230	.2	314	260	.08	.36	.2	2
27		1 tbsp	15	81	20	Trace	2	1.1	.4	Trace	1	16	14	Trace	19	20	.01	.02	Trace	Trace
28	Light, coffee, or table	1 cup	240	74	470	6	46	28.8	11.7	1.0	9	231	192	.1	292	1,730	.08	.36	.1	2
29		1 tbsp	15	74	30	Trace	3	1.8	.7	.1	1	14	12	Trace	18	110	Trace	.02	Trace	Trace

(A)	(B)			(C)	(D)	(E)	(F)	(G)	(H)	(I)	(J)	(K)	(L)	(M)	(N)	(O)	(P)	(Q)	(R)	(S)
	Whipping, unwhipped (volume about double when whipped):																			
30	Light	1 cup	239	64	700	5	74	46.2	18.3	1.5	7	166	146	0.1	231	2.690	0.06	0.30	0.1	1
31		1 tbsp	15	64	45	Trace	5	2.9	1.1	.1	Trace	10	9	Trace	15	170	Trace	.02	Trace	Trace
32	Heavy	1 cup	238	58	820	5	88	54.8	22.2	2.0	7	154	149	.1	179	3,500	.05	.26	.1	1
33		1 tbsp	15	58	80	Trace	6	3.5	1.4	.1	Trace	10	9	Trace	11	220	Trace	.02	Trace	Trace
34	Whipped topping, (pressurized)	1 cup	60	61	155	2	13	8.3	3.4	.3	7	61	54	Trace	88	550	.02	.04	Trace	0
35		1 tbsp	3	61	10	Trace	1	.4	.2	Trace	Trace	3	3	Trace	4	30	Trace	Trace	Trace	0
36	Cream, sour	1 cup	230	71	495	7	48	30.0	12.1	1.1	10	268	195	.1	331	1,820	.08	.34	.2	2
37		1 tbsp	12	71	25	Trace	3	1.6	.6	.1	1	14	10	Trace	17	90	Trace	.02	Trace	Trace
	Cream products, imitation (made with vegetable fat):																			
	Sweet:																			
	Creamers:																			
38	Liquid (frozen)	1 cup	245	77	335	2	24	22.8	.3	Trace	28	23	157	.1	467	[1]220	0	0	0	0
39		1 tbsp	15	77	20	Trace	1	1.4	Trace	0	2	1	10	Trace	29	[1]10	0	0	0	0
40	Powdered	1 cup	94	2	515	5	33	30.6	.9	Trace	52	21	397	.1	763	[1]190	0	[1].16	0	0
41		1 tsp	2	2	10	Trace	1	.7	Trace	0	1	Trace	8	Trace	16	[1]Trace	0	[1]Trace	0	0
	Whipped topping:																			
42	Frozen	1 cup	75	50	240	1	19	16.3	1.0	.2	17	5	6	.1	14	[1]650	0	0	0	0
43		1 tbsp	4	50	15	Trace	1	.9	.1	Trace	1	Trace	Trace	Trace	1	[1]30	0	0	0	0
44	Powdered, made with whole milk.	1 cup	80	67	150	3	10	8.5	.6	.1	13	72	69	Trace	121	[1]290	.02	.09	Trace	1
45		1 tbsp	4	67	10	Trace	Trace	.4	Trace	Trace	1	4	3	Trace	6	[1]10	Trace	Trace	Trace	Trace
46	Pressurized	1 cup	70	60	185	1	16	13.2	1.4	.2	11	4	13	Trace	13	[1]330	0	0	0	0
47		1 tbsp	4	60	10	Trace	1	.8	.1	Trace	1	Trace	1	Trace	1	[1]20	0	0	0	0
48	Sour dressing (imitation sour cream) made with nonfat dry milk.	1 cup	235	75	415	8	39	31.2	4.4	1.1	11	266	205	.1	380	[1]20	.09	.38	.2	2
49		1 tbsp	12	75	20	Trace	2	1.6	.2	.1	1	14	10	Trace	19	[1]Trace	.01	.02	Trace	Trace
	Ice cream. See Milk desserts, frozen (items 75-80).																			
	Ice milk. See Milk desserts, frozen (items 81-83).																			
	Milk:																			
	Fluid:																			
50	Whole (3.3% fat)	1 cup	244	88	150	8	8	5.1	2.1	.2	11	291	228	.1	370	[2]310	.09	.40	.2	2
	Lowfat (2%):																			
51	No milk solids added	1 cup	244	89	120	8	5	2.9	1.2	.1	12	297	232	.1	377	500	.10	.40	.2	2
	Milk solids added:																			
52	Label claim less than 10 g of protein per cup.	1 cup	245	89	125	9	5	2.9	1.2	.1	12	313	245	.1	397	500	.10	.42	.2	2
53	Label claim 10 or more grams of protein per cup (protein fortified).	1 cup	246	88	135	10	5	3.0	1.2	.1	14	352	276	.1	447	500	.11	.48	.2	3
	Lowfat (1%):																			
54	No milk solids added	1 cup	244	90	100	8	3	1.6	.7	.1	12	300	235	.1	381	500	.10	.41	.2	2
	Milk solids added:																			
55	Label claim less than 10 g of protein per cup.	1 cup	245	90	105	9	2	1.5	.6	.1	12	313	245	.1	397	500	.10	.42	.2	2
56	Label claim 10 or more grams of protein per cup (protein fortified).	1 cup	246	89	120	10	3	1.8	.7	.1	14	349	273	.1	444	500	.11	.47	.2	3
	Nonfat (skim):																			
57	No milk solids added	1 cup	245	91	85	8	Trace	.3	.1	Trace	12	302	247	.1	406	500	.09	.34	.2	2

[1]Vitamin A value is largely from beta-carotene used for coloring. Riboflavin value for items 40-41 apply to products with added riboflavin.
[2]Applies to product without added vitamin A. With added vitamin A, value is 500 International Units (I.U.).

TABLE 2.— NUTRITIVE VALUES OF THE EDIBLE PART OF FOODS - Continued

(Dashes (—) denote lack of reliable data for a constituent believed to be present in measurable amount)

Item No. (A)	Foods, approximate measures, units, and weight (edible part unless footnotes indicate otherwise) (B)			Water (C)	Food energy (D)	Protein (E)	Fat (F)	Fatty Acids: Saturated (total) (G)	Fatty Acids: Unsaturated: Oleic (H)	Fatty Acids: Unsaturated: Linoleic (I)	Carbohydrate (J)	Calcium (K)	Phosphorus (L)	Iron (M)	Potassium (N)	Vitamin A value (O)	Thiamin (P)	Riboflavin (Q)	Niacin (R)	Ascorbic acid (S)
			Grams	Percent	Calories	Grams	Grams	Grams	Grams	Grams	Grams	Milligrams	Milligrams	Milligrams	Milligrams	International units	Milligrams	Milligrams	Milligrams	Milligrams
	DAIRY PRODUCTS (CHEESE, CREAM, IMITATION CREAM, MILK; RELATED PRODUCTS)—Con.																			
	Milk—Continued																			
	Fluid—Continued																			
	Nonfat (skim)—Continued																			
	Milk solids added:																			
58	Label claim less than 10 g of protein per cup.	1 cup	245	90	90	9	1	0.4	0.1	Trace	12	316	255	0.1	418	500	0.10	0.43	0.2	2
59	Label claim 10 or more grams of protein per cup (protein fortified).	1 cup	246	89	100	10	1	.4	.1	Trace	14	352	275	.1	446	500	.11	.48	.2	3
60	Buttermilk	1 cup	245	90	100	8	2	1.3	.5	Trace	12	285	219	.1	371	[3]80	.08	.38	.1	2
	Canned:																			
	Evaporated, unsweetened:																			
61	Whole milk	1 cup	252	74	340	17	19	11.6	5.3	0.4	25	657	510	.5	764	[3]610	.12	.80	.5	5
62	Skim milk	1 cup	255	79	200	19	1	.3	.1	Trace	29	738	497	.7	845	[4]1,000	.11	.79	.4	3
63	Sweetened, condensed	1 cup	306	27	980	24	27	16.8	6.7	.7	166	868	775	.6	1,136	[3]1,000	.28	1.27	.6	8
	Dried:																			
64	Buttermilk	1 cup	120	3	465	41	7	4.3	1.7	.2	59	1,421	1,119	.4	1,910	[3]260	.47	1.90	1.1	7
	Nonfat instant:																			
65	Envelope, net wt., 3.2 oz[5]	1 envelope	91	4	325	32	1	.4	.1	Trace	47	1,120	896	.3	1,552	[6]2,160	.38	1.59	.8	5
66	Cup[7]	1 cup	68	4	245	24	Trace	.3	.1	Trace	35	837	670	.2	1,160	[6]1,610	.28	1.19	.6	4
	Milk beverages:																			
	Chocolate milk (commercial):																			
67	Regular	1 cup	250	82	210	8	8	5.3	2.2	.2	26	280	251	.6	417	[3]300	.09	.41	.3	2
68	Lowfat (2%)	1 cup	250	84	180	8	5	3.1	1.3	.1	26	284	254	.6	422	500	.10	.42	.3	2
69	Lowfat (1%)	1 cup	250	85	160	8	3	1.5	.7	.1	26	287	257	.6	426	500	.10	.40	.2	2
70	Eggnog (commercial)	1 cup	254	74	340	10	19	11.3	5.0	.6	34	330	278	.5	420	890	.09	.48	.3	4
	Malted milk, home-prepared with 1 cup of whole milk and 2 to 3 heaping tsp of malted milk powder (about 3/4 oz):																			
71	Chocolate	1 cup of milk plus 3/4 oz of powder.	265	81	235	9	9	5.5	—	—	29	304	265	.5	500	330	.14	.43	.7	2
72	Natural	1 cup of milk plus 3/4 oz of powder.	265	81	235	11	10	6.0	—	—	27	347	307	.3	529	380	.20	.54	1.3	2
	Shakes, thick:[8]																			
73	Chocolate, container, net wt., 10.6 oz.	1 container	300	72	355	9	8	5.0	2.0	.2	63	396	378	.9	672	260	.14	.67	.4	0
74	Vanilla, container, net wt., 11 oz.	1 container	313	74	350	12	9	5.9	2.4	.2	56	457	361	.3	572	360	.09	.61	.5	0
	Milk desserts, frozen:																			
	Ice cream:																			
	Regular (about 11% fat):																			
75	Hardened	1/2 gal	1,064	61	2,155	38	115	71.3	28.8	2.6	254	1,406	1,075	1.0	2,052	4,340	.42	2.63	1.1	6
76		1 cup	133	61	270	5	14	8.9	3.6	.3	32	176	134	.1	257	540	.05	.33	.1	1
77		3-fl oz container	50	61	100	2	5	3.4	1.4	.1	12	66	51	Trace	96	200	.02	.12	.1	Trace
78	Soft serve (frozen custard)	1 cup	173	60	375	7	23	13.5	5.9	.6	38	236	199	.4	338	790	.08	.45	.2	1
79	Rich (about 16% fat), hardened.	1/2 gal	1,188	59	2,805	33	190	118.3	47.8	4.3	256	1,213	927	.8	1,771	7,200	.36	2.27	.9	5
80		1 cup	148	59	350	4	24	14.7	6.0	.5	32	151	115	.1	221	900	.04	.28	.1	1
	Ice milk:																			
81	Hardened (about 4.3% fat)	1/2 gal	1,048	69	1,470	41	45	28.1	11.3	1.0	232	1,409	1,035	1.5	2,117	1,710	.61	2.78	.9	6
82		1 cup	131	69	185	5	6	3.5	1.4	.1	29	176	129	.1	265	210	.08	.35	.1	1

(A)	(B)			(C)	(D)	(E)	(F)	(G)	(H)	(I)	(J)	(K)	(L)	(M)	(N)	(O)	(P)	(Q)	(R)	(S)
83	Soft serve (about 2.6% fat)	1 cup	175	70	225	8	5	2.9	1.2	0.1	38	274	202	0.3	412	180	0.12	0.54	0.2	1
84	Sherbet (about 2% fat)	1/2 gal	1,542	66	2,160	17	31	19.0	7.7	.7	469	827	594	2.5	1,585	1,480	.26	.71	1.0	31
85		1 cup	193	66	270	2	4	2.4	1.0	.1	59	103	74	.3	198	190	.03	.09	.1	4
	Milk desserts, other:																			
86	Custard, baked	1 cup	265	77	305	14	15	6.8	5.4	.7	29	297	310	1.1	387	930	.11	.50	.3	1
	Puddings:																			
	From home recipe:																			
	Starch base:																			
87	Chocolate	1 cup	260	66	385	8	12	7.6	3.3	.3	67	250	255	1.3	445	390	.05	.36	.3	1
88	Vanilla (blancmange)	1 cup	255	76	285	9	10	6.2	2.5	.2	41	298	232	Trace	352	410	.08	.41	.3	2
89	Tapioca cream	1 cup	165	72	220	8	8	4.1	2.5	.5	28	173	180	.7	223	480	.07	.30	.2	2
	From mix (chocolate) and milk:																			
90	Regular (cooked)	1 cup	260	70	320	9	8	4.3	2.6	.2	59	265	247	.8	354	340	.05	.39	.3	2
91	Instant	1 cup	260	69	325	8	7	3.6	2.2	.3	63	374	237	1.3	335	340	.08	.39	.3	2
	Yogurt:																			
	With added milk solids:																			
	Made with lowfat milk:																			
92	Fruit-flavored[9]	1 container, net wt., 8 oz	227	75	230	10	3	1.8	.6	.1	42	343	269	.2	439	[10]120	.08	.40	.2	1
93	Plain	1 container, net wt., 8 oz	227	85	145	12	4	2.3	.8	.1	16	415	326	.2	531	[10]150	.10	.49	.3	2
94	Made with nonfat milk	1 container, net wt., 8 oz	227	85	125	13	Trace	.3	.1	Trace	17	452	355	.2	579	[10]20	.11	.53	.3	2
	Without added milk solids:																			
95	Made with whole milk	1 container, net wt., 8 oz	227	88	140	8	7	4.8	1.7	.1	11	274	215	.1	351	280	.07	.32	.2	1
	EGGS																			
	Eggs, large (24 oz per dozen):																			
	Raw:																			
96	Whole, without shell	1 egg	50	75	80	6	6	1.7	2.0	.6	1	28	90	1.0	65	260	.04	.15	Trace	0
97	White	1 white	33	88	15	3	Trace	0	0	0	Trace	4	4	Trace	45	0	Trace	.09	Trace	0
98	Yolk	1 yolk	17	49	65	3	6	1.7	2.1	.6	Trace	26	86	.9	15	310	.04	.07	Trace	0
	Cooked:																			
99	Fried in butter	1 egg	46	72	85	5	6	2.4	2.2	.6	1	26	80	.9	58	290	.03	.13	Trace	0
100	Hard-cooked, shell removed	1 egg	50	75	80	6	6	1.7	2.0	.6	1	28	90	1.0	65	260	.04	.14	Trace	0
101	Poached	1 egg	50	74	80	6	6	1.7	2.0	.6	1	28	90	1.0	65	260	.04	.13	Trace	0
102	Scrambled (milk added) in butter. Also omelet.	1 egg	64	76	95	6	7	2.8	2.3	.6	1	47	97	.9	85	310	.04	.16	Trace	0
	FATS, OILS; RELATED PRODUCTS																			
	Butter:																			
	Regular (1 brick or 4 sticks per lb):																			
103	Stick (1/2 cup)	1 stick	113	16	815	1	92	57.3	23.1	2.1	Trace	27	26	.2	29	[11]3,470	.01	.04	Trace	0
104	Tablespoon (about 1/8 stick).	1 tbsp	14	16	100	Trace	12	7.2	2.9	.3	Trace	3	3	Trace	4	[11]430	Trace	Trace	Trace	0
105	Pat (1 in square, 1/3 in high; 90 per lb).	1 pat	5	16	35	Trace	4	2.5	1.0	.1	Trace	1	1	Trace	1	[11]150	Trace	Trace	Trace	0
	Whipped (6 sticks or two 8-oz containers per lb).																			
106	Stick (1/2 cup)	1 stick	76	16	540	1	61	38.2	15.4	1.4	Trace	18	17	.1	20	[11]2,310	Trace	.03	Trace	0
107	Tablespoon (about 1/8 stick).	1 tbsp	9	16	65	Trace	8	4.7	1.9	.2	Trace	2	2	Trace	2	[11]290	Trace	Trace	Trace	0
108	Pat (1 1/4 in square, 1/3 in high; 120 per lb).	1 pat	4	16	25	Trace	3	1.9	.8	.1	Trace	1	1	Trace	1	[11]120	0	Trace	Trace	0

[3]Applies to product without vitamin A added.
[4]Applies to product with added vitamin A. Without added vitamin A, value is 20 International Units (I.U.).
[5]Yields 1 qt of fluid milk when reconstituted according to package directions.
[6]Applies to product with added vitamin A.
[7]Weight applies to product with label claim of 1 1/3 cups equal 3.2 oz.
[8]Applies to products made from thick shake mixes and that do not contain added ice cream. Products made from milk shake mixes are higher in fat and usually contain added ice cream.
[9]Content of fat, vitamin A, and carbohydrate varies. Consult the label when precise values are needed for special diets.
[10]Applies to product made with milk containing no added vitamin A.
[11]Based on year-round average.

TABLE 2.—NUTRITIVE VALUES OF THE EDIBLE PART OF FOODS - Continued

(Dashes (—) denote lack of reliable data for a constituent believed to be present in measurable amount)

Item No. (A)	Foods, approximate measures, units, and weight (edible part unless footnotes indicate otherwise) (B)			Water (C)	Food energy (D)	Protein (E)	Fat (F)	Fatty Acids: Saturated (total) (G)	Fatty Acids: Unsaturated: Oleic (H)	Fatty Acids: Unsaturated: Linoleic (I)	Carbohydrate (J)	Calcium (K)	Phosphorus (L)	Iron (M)	Potassium (N)	Vitamin A value (O)	Thiamin (P)	Riboflavin (Q)	Niacin (R)	Ascorbic acid (S)
			Grams	Percent	Calories	Grams	Grams	Grams	Grams	Grams	Grams	Milligrams	Milligrams	Milligrams	Milligrams	International units	Milligrams	Milligrams	Milligrams	Milligrams
	FATS, OILS; RELATED PRODUCTS—Con.																			
109	Fats, cooking (vegetable shortenings).	1 cup	200	0	1,770	0	200	48.8	88.2	48.4	0	0	0	0	0	—	0	0	0	0
110		1 tbsp	13	0	110	0	13	3.2	5.7	3.1	0	0	0	0	0	—	0	0	0	0
111	Lard	1 cup	205	0	1,850	0	205	81.0	83.8	20.5	0	0	0	0	0	0	0	0	0	0
112		1 tbsp	13	0	115	0	13	5.1	5.3	1.3	0	0	0	0	0	0	0	0	0	0
	Margarine:																			
	Regular (1 brick or 4 sticks per lb):																			
113	Stick (1/2 cup)	1 stick	113	16	815	1	92	16.7	42.9	24.9	Trace	27	26	.2	29	[12]3,750	.01	.04	Trace	0
114	Tablespoon (about 1/8 stick)	1 tbsp	14	16	100	Trace	12	2.1	5.3	3.1	Trace	3	3	Trace	4	[12]470	Trace	Trace	Trace	0
115	Pat (1 in square, 1/3 in high; 90 per lb).	1 pat	5	16	35	Trace	4	.7	1.9	1.1	Trace	1	1	Trace	1	[12]170	Trace	Trace	Trace	0
116	Soft, two 8-oz containers per lb.	1 container	227	16	1,635	1	184	32.5	71.5	65.4	Trace	53	52	.4	59	[12]7,500	.01	.08	.1	0
117		1 tbsp	14	16	100	Trace	12	2.0	4.5	4.1	Trace	3	3	Trace	4	[12]470	Trace	Trace	Trace	0
	Whipped (6 sticks per lb):																			
118	Stick (1/2 cup)	1 stick	76	16	545	Trace	61	11.2	28.7	16.7	Trace	18	17	.1	20	[12]2,500	Trace	.03	Trace	0
119	Tablespoon (about 1/8 stick)	1 tbsp	9	16	70	Trace	8	1.4	3.6	2.1	Trace	2	2	Trace	2	[12]310	Trace	Trace	Trace	0
	Oils, salad or cooking:																			
120	Corn	1 cup	218	0	1,925	0	218	27.7	53.6	125.1	0	0	0	0	0	—	0	0	0	0
121		1 tbsp	14	0	120	0	14	1.7	3.3	7.8	0	0	0	0	0	—	0	0	0	0
122	Olive	1 cup	216	0	1,910	0	216	30.7	154.4	17.7	0	0	0	0	0	—	0	0	0	0
123		1 tbsp	14	0	120	0	14	1.9	9.7	1.1	0	0	0	0	0	—	0	0	0	0
124	Peanut	1 cup	216	0	1,910	0	216	37.4	98.5	67.0	0	0	0	0	0	—	0	0	0	0
125		1 tbsp	14	0	120	0	14	2.3	6.2	4.2	0	0	0	0	0	—	0	0	0	0
126	Safflower	1 cup	218	0	1,925	0	218	20.5	25.9	159.8	0	0	0	0	0	—	0	0	0	0
127		1 tbsp	14	0	120	0	14	1.3	1.6	10.0	0	0	0	0	0	—	0	0	0	0
128	Soybean oil, hydrogenated (partially hardened).	1 cup	218	0	1,925	0	218	31.8	93.1	75.6	0	0	0	0	0	—	0	0	0	0
129		1 tbsp	14	0	120	0	14	2.0	5.8	4.7	0	0	0	0	0	—	0	0	0	0
130	Soybean-cottonseed oil blend, hydrogenated.	1 cup	218	0	1,925	0	218	38.2	63.0	99.6	0	0	0	0	0	—	0	0	0	0
131		1 tbsp	14	0	120	0	14	2.4	3.9	6.2	0	0	0	0	0	—	0	0	0	0
	Salad dressings:																			
	Commercial:																			
	Blue cheese:																			
132	Regular	1 tbsp	15	32	75	1	8	1.6	1.7	3.8	1	12	11	Trace	6	30	Trace	.02	Trace	Trace
133	Low calorie (5 Cal per tsp)	1 tbsp	16	84	10	Trace	1	.5	.3	Trace	1	10	8	Trace	5	30	Trace	.01	Trace	Trace
	French:																			
134	Regular	1 tbsp	16	39	65	Trace	6	1.1	1.3	3.2	3	2	2	.1	13	—	—	—	—	—
135	Low calorie (5 Cal per tsp)	1 tbsp	16	77	15	Trace	1	.1	.1	.4	2	2	2	.1	13	—	—	—	—	—
	Italian:																			
136	Regular	1 tbsp	15	28	85	Trace	9	1.6	1.9	4.7	1	2	1	Trace	2	Trace	Trace	Trace	Trace	—
137	Low calorie (2 Cal per tsp)	1 tbsp	15	90	10	Trace	1	.1	.1	.4	Trace	Trace	1	Trace	2	Trace	Trace	Trace	Trace	—
138	Mayonnaise	1 tbsp	14	15	100	Trace	11	2.0	2.4	5.6	Trace	3	4	.1	5	40	Trace	.01	Trace	—
	Mayonnaise type:																			
139	Regular	1 tbsp	15	41	65	Trace	6	1.1	1.4	3.2	2	2	4	Trace	1	30	Trace	Trace	Trace	—
140	Low calorie (8 Cal per tsp)	1 tbsp	16	81	20	Trace	2	.4	.4	1.0	2	3	4	Trace	1	40	Trace	Trace	Trace	—
141	Tartar sauce, regular	1 tbsp	14	34	75	Trace	8	1.5	1.8	4.1	1	3	4	.1	11	30	Trace	Trace	Trace	Trace
	Thousand Island:																			
142	Regular	1 tbsp	16	32	80	Trace	8	1.4	1.7	4.0	2	2	3	.1	18	50	Trace	Trace	Trace	Trace
143	Low calorie (10 Cal per tsp)	1 tbsp	15	68	25	Trace	2	.4	.4	1.0	2	2	3	.1	17	50	Trace	Trace	Trace	Trace
	From home recipe:																			
144	Cooked type[13]	1 tbsp	16	68	25	1	2	.5	.6	.3	2	14	15	.1	19	80	.01	.03	Trace	Trace

(A)	(B)			(C)	(D)	(E)	(F)	(G)	(H)	(I)	(J)	(K)	(L)	(M)	(N)	(O)	(P)	(Q)	(R)	(S)
	FISH, SHELLFISH, MEAT, POULTRY; RELATED PRODUCTS																			
	Fish and shellfish:																			
145	Bluefish, baked with butter or margarine.	3 oz	85	68	135	22	4	—	—	—	0	25	244	0.6	—	40	0.09	0.08	1.6	—
	Clams:																			
146	Raw, meat only	3 oz	85	82	65	11	1	—	—	—	2	59	138	5.2	154	90	.08	.15	1.1	8
147	Canned, solids and liquid	3 oz	85	86	45	7	1	0.2	Trace	Trace	2	47	116	3.5	119	—	.01	.09	.9	—
148	Crabmeat (white or king), canned, not pressed down.	1 cup	135	77	135	24	3	.6	0.4	0.1	1	61	246	1.1	149	—	.11	.11	2.6	—
149	Fish sticks, breaded, cooked, frozen (stick, 4 by 1 by 1/2 in).	1 fish stick or 1 oz	28	66	50	5	3	—	—	—	2	3	47	.1	—	0	.01	.02	.5	—
150	Haddock, breaded, fried[14]	3 oz	85	66	140	17	5	1.4	2.2	1.2	.5	34	210	1.0	296	—	.03	.06	2.7	2
151	Ocean perch, breaded, fried[14]	1 fillet	85	59	195	16	11	2.7	4.4	2.3	6	28	192	1.1	242	—	.10	.10	1.6	—
152	Oysters, raw, meat only (13-19 medium Selects).	1 cup	240	85	160	20	4	1.3	.2	.1	8	226	343	13.2	290	740	.34	.43	6.0	—
153	Salmon, pink, canned, solids and liquid.	3 oz	85	71	120	17	5	.9	.8	.1	0	[15]167	243	.7	307	60	.03	.16	6.8	—
154	Sardines, Atlantic, canned in oil, drained solids.	3 oz	85	62	175	20	9	3.0	2.5	.5	0	372	424	2.5	502	190	.02	.17	4.6	—
155	Scallops, frozen, breaded, fried, reheated.	6 scallops	90	60	175	16	8	—	—	—	9	—	—	—	—	—	—	—	—	—
156	Shad, baked with butter or margarine, bacon.	3 oz	85	64	170	20	10	—	—	—	0	20	266	.5	320	30	.11	.22	7.3	—
	Shrimp:																			
157	Canned meat	3 oz	85	70	100	21	1	.1	.1	Trace	1	98	224	2.6	104	50	.01	.03	1.5	—
158	French fried[16]	3 oz	85	57	190	17	9	2.3	3.7	2.0	9	61	162	1.7	195	—	.03	.07	2.3	—
159	Tuna, canned in oil, drained solids.	3 oz	85	61	170	24	7	1.7	1.7	.7	0	7	199	1.6	—	70	.04	.10	10.1	—
160	Tuna salad[17]	1 cup	205	70	350	30	22	4.3	6.3	6.7	7	41	291	2.7	—	590	.08	.23	10.3	2
	Meat and meat products:																			
161	Bacon, (20 slices per lb, raw), broiled or fried, crisp.	2 slices	15	8	85	4	8	2.5	3.7	.7	Trace	2	34	.5	35	0	.08	.05	.8	—
	Beef,[18] cooked:																			
	Cuts braised, simmered or pot roasted:																			
162	Lean and fat (piece, 2 1/2 by 2 1/2 by 3/4 in).	3 oz	85	53	245	23	16	6.8	6.5	.4	0	10	114	2.9	184	30	.04	.18	3.6	—
163	Lean only from item 162	2.5 oz	72	62	140	22	5	2.1	1.8	.2	0	10	108	2.7	176	10	.04	.17	3.3	—
	Ground beef, broiled:																			
164	Lean with 10% fat	3 oz or patty 3 by 5/8 in	85	60	185	23	10	4.0	3.9	.3	0	10	196	3.0	261	20	.08	.20	5.1	—
165	Lean with 21% fat	2.9 oz or patty 3 by 5/8 in	82	54	235	20	17	7.0	6.7	.4	0	9	159	2.6	221	30	.07	.17	4.4	—
	Roast, oven cooked, no liquid added:																			
	Relatively fat, such as rib:																			
166	Lean and fat (2 pieces, 4 1/8 by 2 1/4 by 1/4 in).	3 oz	85	40	375	17	33	14.0	13.6	.8	0	8	158	2.2	189	70	.05	.13	3.1	—
167	Lean only from item 166	1.8 oz	51	57	125	14	7	3.0	2.5	.3	0	6	131	1.8	161	10	.04	.11	2.6	—
	Relatively lean, such as heel of round:																			
168	Lean and fat (2 pieces, 4 1/8 by 2 1/4 by 1/4 in).	3 oz	85	62	165	25	7	2.8	2.7	.2	0	11	208	3.2	279	10	.06	.19	4.5	—

[12] Based on average vitamin A content of fortified margarine. Federal specifications for fortified margarine require a minimum of 15,000 International Units (I.U.) of vitamin A per pound.
[13] Fatty acid values apply to product made with regular-type margarine.
[14] Dipped in egg, milk or water, and breadcrumbs; fried in vegetable shortening.
[15] If bones are discarded, value for calcium will be greatly reduced.
[16] Dipped in egg, breadcrumbs, and flour or batter.
[17] Prepared with tuna, celery, salad dressing (mayonnaise type), pickle, onion, and egg.
[18] Outer layer of fat on the cut was removed to within approximately 1/2 in of the lean. Deposits of fat within the cut were not removed.

TABLE 2.— NUTRITIVE VALUES OF THE EDIBLE PART OF FOODS · Continued

(Dashes (—) denote lack of reliable data for a constituent believed to be present in measurable amount)

Item No. (A)	Foods, approximate measures, units, and weight (edible part unless footnotes indicate otherwise) (B)			Water (C)	Food energy (D)	Protein (E)	Fat (F)	Fatty Acids: Saturated (total) (G)	Fatty Acids: Unsaturated: Oleic (H)	Fatty Acids: Unsaturated: Linoleic (I)	Carbohydrate (J)	Calcium (K)	Phosphorus (L)	Iron (M)	Potassium (N)	Vitamin A value (O)	Thiamin (P)	Riboflavin (Q)	Niacin (R)	Ascorbic acid (S)
			Grams	Percent	Calories	Grams	Grams	Grams	Grams	Grams	Grams	Milligrams	Milligrams	Milligrams	Milligrams	International units	Milligrams	Milligrams	Milligrams	Milligrams
	FISH, SHELLFISH, MEAT, POULTRY; RELATED PRODUCTS—Con.																			
	Meat and meat products—Continued																			
	Beef,[18] cooked—Continued																			
	Roast, oven cooked, no liquid added—Continued																			
	Relatively lean such as heel of round—Continued																			
169	Lean only from item 168	2.8 oz	78	65	125	24	3	1.2	1.0	0.1	0	10	199	3.0	268	Trace	0.06	0.18	4.3	—
	Steak:																			
	Relatively fat—sirloin, broiled:																			
170	Lean and fat (piece, 2 1/2 by 2 1/2 by 3/4 in).	3 oz	85	44	330	20	27	11.3	11.1	.6	0	9	162	2.5	220	50	.05	.15	4.0	—
171	Lean only from item 170	2.0 oz	56	59	115	18	4	1.8	1.6	.2	0	7	146	2.2	202	10	.05	.14	3.6	—
	Relatively lean—round, braised:																			
172	Lean and fat (piece, 4 1/8 by 2 1/4 by 1/2 in).	3 oz	85	55	220	24	13	5.5	5.2	.4	0	10	213	3.0	272	20	.07	.19	4.8	—
173	Lean only from item 172	2.4 oz	68	61	130	21	4	1.7	1.5	.2	0	9	182	2.5	238	10	.05	.16	4.1	—
	Beef, canned:																			
174	Corned beef	3 oz	85	59	185	22	10	4.9	4.5	.2	0	17	90	3.7	—	—	.01	.20	2.9	—
175	Corned beef hash	1 cup	220	67	400	19	25	11.9	10.9	.5	24	29	147	4.4	440	—	.02	.20	4.6	—
176	Beef, dried, chipped	2 1/2-oz jar	71	48	145	24	4	2.1	2.0	.1	0	14	287	3.6	142	—	.05	.23	2.7	0
177	Beef and vegetable stew	1 cup	245	82	220	16	11	4.9	4.5	.2	15	29	184	2.9	613	2,400	.15	.17	4.7	17
178	Beef potpie (home recipe), baked[19] (piece, 1/3 of 9-in diam. pie).	1 piece	210	55	515	21	30	7.9	12.8	6.7	39	29	149	3.8	334	1,720	.30	.30	5.5	6
179	Chili con carne with beans, canned.	1 cup	255	72	340	19	16	7.5	6.8	.3	31	82	321	4.3	594	150	.08	.18	3.3	—
180	Chop suey with beef and pork (home recipe).	1 cup	250	75	300	26	17	8.5	6.2	.7	13	60	248	4.8	425	600	.28	.38	5.0	33
181	Heart, beef, lean, braised	3 oz	85	61	160	27	5	1.5	1.1	.6	1	5	154	5.0	197	20	.21	1.04	6.5	1
	Lamb, cooked:																			
	Chop, rib (cut 3 per lb with bone), broiled:																			
182	Lean and fat	3.1 oz	89	43	360	18	32	14.8	12.1	1.2	0	8	139	1.0	200	—	.11	.19	4.1	—
183	Lean only from item 182	2 oz	57	60	120	16	6	2.5	2.1	.2	0	6	121	1.1	174	—	.09	.15	3.4	—
	Leg, roasted:																			
184	Lean and fat (2 pieces, 4 1/8 by 2 1/4 by 1/4 in).	3 oz	85	54	235	22	16	7.3	6.0	.6	0	9	177	1.4	241	—	.13	.23	4.7	—
185	Lean only from item 184	2.5 oz	71	62	130	20	5	2.1	1.8	.2	0	9	169	1.4	227	—	.12	.21	4.4	—
	Shoulder, roasted:																			
186	Lean and fat (3 pieces, 2 1/2 by 2 1/2 by 1/4 in).	3 oz	85	50	285	18	23	10.8	8.8	.9	0	9	146	1.0	206	—	.11	.20	4.0	—
187	Lean only from item 186	2.3 oz	64	61	130	17	6	3.6	2.3	.2	0	8	140	1.0	193	—	.10	.18	3.7	—
188	Liver, beef, fried[20] (slice, 6 1/2 by 2 3/8 by 3/8 in).	3 oz	85	56	195	22	9	2.5	3.5	.9	5	9	405	7.5	323	[21]45,390	.22	3.56	14.0	23
	Pork, cured, cooked:																			
189	Ham, light cure, lean and fat, roasted (2 pieces, 4 1/8 by 2 1/4 by 1/4 in).[22]	3 oz	85	54	245	18	19	6.8	7.9	1.7	0	8	146	2.2	199	0	.40	.15	3.1	—
	Luncheon meat:																			
190	Boiled ham, slice (8 per 8-oz pkg.).	1 oz	28	59	65	5	5	1.7	2.0	.4	0	3	47	.8	—	0	.12	.04	.7	—
	Canned, spiced or unspiced:																			
191	Slice, approx. 3 by 2 by 1/2 in.	1 slice	60	55	175	9	15	5.4	6.7	1.0	1	5	65	1.3	133	0	.19	.13	1.8	—

(A)	(B)			(C)	(D)	(E)	(F)	(G)	(H)	(I)	(J)	(K)	(L)	(M)	(N)	(O)	(P)	(Q)	(R)	(S)
	Pork, fresh,[18] cooked:																			
	Chop, loin (cut 3 per lb with bone), broiled:																			
192	Lean and fat	2.7 oz	78	42	305	19	25	8.9	10.4	2.2	0	9	209	2.7	216	0	0.75	0.22	4.5	—
193	Lean only from item 192	2 oz	56	53	150	17	9	3.1	3.6	.8	0	7	181	2.2	192	0	.63	.18	3.8	—
	Roast, oven cooked, no liquid added:																			
194	Lean and fat (piece, 2 1/2 by 2 1/2 by 3/4 in).	3 oz	85	46	310	21	24	8.7	10.2	2.2	0	9	218	2.7	233	0	.78	.22	4.8	—
195	Lean only from item 194	2.4 oz	68	55	175	20	10	3.5	4.1	.8	0	9	211	2.6	224	0	.73	.21	4.4	—
	Shoulder cut, simmered:																			
196	Lean and fat (3 pieces, 2 1/2 by 2 1/2 by 1/4 in).	3 oz	85	46	320	20	26	9.3	10.9	2.3	0	9	118	2.6	158	0	.46	.21	4.1	—
197	Lean only from item 196	2.2 oz	63	60	135	18	6	2.2	2.6	.6	0	8	111	2.3	146	0	.42	.19	3.7	—
	Sausages (see also Luncheon meat (items 190-191)):																			
198	Bologna, slice (8 per 8-oz pkg.).	1 slice	28	56	85	3	8	3.0	3.4	.5	Trace	2	36	.5	65	—	.05	.06	.7	—
199	Braunschweiger, slice (6 per 6-oz pkg.).	1 slice	28	53	90	4	8	2.6	3.4	.8	1	3	69	1.7	—	1,850	.05	.41	2.3	—
200	Brown and serve (10-11 per 8-oz pkg.), browned.	1 link	17	40	70	3	6	2.3	2.8	.7	Trace	—	—	—	—	—	—	—	—	—
201	Deviled ham, canned	1 tbsp	13	51	45	2	4	1.5	1.8	.4	0	1	12	.3	—	0	.02	.01	.2	—
202	Frankfurter (8 per 1-lb pkg.), cooked (reheated).	1 frankfurter	56	57	170	7	15	5.6	6.5	1.2	1	3	57	.8	—	—	.08	.11	1.4	—
203	Meat, potted (beef, chicken, turkey), canned.	1 tbsp	13	61	30	2	2	—	—	—	0	—	—	—	—	—	Trace	.03	.2	—
204	Pork link (16 per 1-lb pkg.), cooked.	1 link	13	35	60	2	6	2.1	2.4	.5	Trace	1	21	.3	35	0	.10	.04	.5	—
	Salami:																			
205	Dry type, slice (12 per 4-oz pkg.).	1 slice	10	30	45	2	4	1.6	1.6	.1	Trace	1	28	.4	—	—	.04	.03	.5	—
206	Cooked type, slice (8 per 8-oz pkg.).	1 slice	28	51	90	5	7	3.1	3.0	.2	Trace	3	57	.7	—	—	.07	.07	1.2	—
207	Vienna sausage (7 per 4-oz can).	1 sausage	16	63	40	2	3	1.2	1.4	.2	Trace	1	24	.3	—	—	.01	.02	.4	—
	Veal, medium fat, cooked, bone removed:																			
208	Cutlet (4 1/8 by 2 1/4 by 1/2 in), braised or broiled.	3 oz	85	60	185	23	9	4.0	3.4	.4	0	9	196	2.7	258	—	.06	.21	4.6	—
209	Rib (2 pieces, 4 1/8 by 2 1/4 by 1/4 in), roasted.	3 oz	85	55	230	23	14	6.1	5.1	.6	0	10	211	2.9	259	—	.11	.26	6.6	—
	Poultry and poultry products:																			
	Chicken, cooked:																			
210	Breast, fried,[23] bones removed, 1/2 breast (3.3 oz with bones).	2.8 oz	79	58	160	26	5	1.4	1.8	1.1	1	9	218	1.3	—	70	.04	.17	11.6	—
211	Drumstick, fried,[23] bones removed (2 oz with bones).	1.3 oz	38	55	90	12	4	1.1	1.3	.9	Trace	6	89	.9	—	50	.03	.15	2.7	—
212	Half broiler, broiled, bones removed (10.4 oz with bones).	6.2 oz	176	71	240	42	7	2.2	2.5	1.3	0	16	355	3.0	483	160	.09	.34	15.5	—
213	Chicken, canned, boneless	3 oz	85	65	170	18	10	3.2	3.8	2.0	0	18	210	1.3	117	200	.03	.11	3.7	3
214	Chicken a la king, cooked (home recipe).	1 cup	245	68	470	27	34	12.7	14.3	3.3	12	127	358	2.5	404	1,130	.10	.42	5.4	12
215	Chicken and noodles, cooked (home recipe).	1 cup	240	71	365	22	18	5.9	7.1	3.5	26	26	247	2.2	149	430	.05	.17	4.3	Trace

[18]Outer layer of fat on the cut was removed to within approximately 1/2 in of the lean. Deposits of fat within the cut were not removed.
[19]Crust made with vegetable shortening and enriched flour.
[20]Regular-type margarine used.
[21]Value varies widely.
[22]About one-fourth of the outer layer of fat on the cut was removed. Deposits of fat within the cut were not removed.
[23]Vegetable shortening used.

TABLE 2.– NUTRITIVE VALUES OF THE EDIBLE PART OF FOODS - Continued

(Dashes (—) denote lack of reliable data for a constituent believed to be present in measurable amount)

Item No. (A)	Foods, approximate measures, units, and weight (edible part unless footnotes indicate otherwise) (B)			Water (C)	Food energy (D)	Protein (E)	Fat (F)	Fatty Acids: Saturated (total) (G)	Fatty Acids: Unsaturated: Oleic (H)	Fatty Acids: Unsaturated: Linoleic (I)	Carbohydrate (J)	Calcium (K)	Phosphorus (L)	Iron (M)	Potassium (N)	Vitamin A value (O)	Thiamin (P)	Riboflavin (Q)	Niacin (R)	Ascorbic acid (S)
			Grams	Percent	Calories	Grams	Grams	Grams	Grams	Grams	Grams	Milligrams	Milligrams	Milligrams	Milligrams	International units	Milligrams	Milligrams	Milligrams	Milligrams
	FISH, SHELLFISH, MEAT, POULTRY; RELATED PRODUCTS—Con.																			
	Poultry and poultry products—Continued																			
	Chicken chow mein:																			
216	Canned	1 cup	250	89	95	7	Trace	—	—	—	18	45	35	1.3	418	150	0.05	0.10	1.0	13
217	From home recipe	1 cup	250	78	255	31	10	2.4	3.4	3.1	10	58	293	2.5	473	280	.08	.23	4.3	10
218	Chicken potpie (home recipe), baked, [19] piece (1/3 or 9-in diam. pie).	1 piece	232	57	545	23	31	11.3	10.9	5.6	42	70	232	3.0	343	3,090	.34	.31	5.5	5
	Turkey, roasted, flesh without skin:																			
219	Dark meat, piece, 2 1/2 by 1 5/8 by 1/4 in.	4 pieces	85	61	175	26	7	2.1	1.5	1.5	0	—	—	2.0	338	—	.03	.20	3.6	—
220	Light meat, piece, 4 by 2 by 1/4 in.	2 pieces	85	62	150	28	3	.9	.6	.7	0	—	—	1.0	349	—	.04	.12	9.4	—
	Light and dark meat:																			
221	Chopped or diced	1 cup	140	61	265	44	9	2.5	1.7	1.8	0	11	351	2.5	514	—	.07	.25	10.8	—
222	Pieces (1 slice white meat, 4 by 2 by 1/4 in with 2 slices dark meat, 2 1/2 by 1 5/8 by 1/4 in).	3 pieces	85	61	160	27	5	1.5	1.0	1.1	0	7	213	1.5	312	—	.04	.15	6.5	—
	FRUITS AND FRUIT PRODUCTS																			
	Apples, raw, unpeeled, without cores:																			
223	2 3/4-in diam. (about 3 per lb with cores).	1 apple	138	84	80	Trace	1	—	—	—	20	10	14	.4	152	120	.04	.03	.1	6
224	3 1/4 in diam. (about 2 per lb with cores).	1 apple	212	84	125	Trace	1	—	—	—	31	15	21	.6	233	190	.06	.04	.2	8
225	Applejuice, bottled or canned[24]	1 cup	248	88	120	Trace	Trace	—	—	—	30	15	22	1.5	250	—	.02	.05	.2	[25]2
	Applesauce, canned:																			
226	Sweetened	1 cup	255	76	230	1	Trace	—	—	—	61	10	13	1.3	166	100	.05	.03	.1	[25]3
227	Unsweetened	1 cup	244	89	100	Trace	Trace	—	—	—	26	10	12	1.2	190	100	.05	.02	.1	[25]2
	Apricots:																			
228	Raw, without pits (about 12 per lb with pits).	3 apricots	107	85	55	1	Trace	—	—	—	14	18	25	.5	301	2,890	.03	.04	.6	11
229	Canned in heavy sirup (halves and sirup).	1 cup	258	77	220	2	Trace	—	—	—	57	28	39	.8	604	4,490	.05	.05	1.0	10
	Dried:																			
230	Uncooked (28 large or 37 medium halves per cup).	1 cup	130	25	340	7	1	—	—	—	86	87	140	7.2	1,273	14,170	.01	.21	4.3	16
231	Cooked, unsweetened, fruit and liquid.	1 cup	250	76	215	4	1	—	—	—	54	55	88	4.5	795	7,500	.01	.13	2.5	8
232	Apricot nectar, canned	1 cup	251	85	145	1	Trace	—	—	—	37	23	30	.5	379	2,380	.03	.03	.5	[26]36
	Avocados, raw, whole, without skins and seeds:																			
233	California, mid- and late-winter (with skin and seed, 3 1/8-in diam.; wt., 10 oz).	1 avocado	216	74	370	5	37	5.5	22.0	3.7	13	22	91	1.3	1,303	630	.24	.43	3.5	30
234	Florida, late summer and fall (with skin and seed, 3 5/8-in diam.; wt., 1 lb).	1 avocado	304	78	390	4	33	6.7	15.7	5.3	27	30	128	1.8	1,836	880	.33	.61	4.9	43
235	Banana without peel (about 2.6 per lb with peel).	1 banana	119	76	100	1	Trace	—	—	—	26	10	31	.8	440	230	.06	.07	.8	12
236	Banana flakes	1 tbsp	6	3	20	Trace	Trace	—	—	—	5	2	6	.2	92	50	.01	.01	.2	Trace

(A)	(B)			(C)	(D)	(E)	(F)	(G)	(H)	(I)	(J)	(K)	(L)	(M)	(N)	(O)	(P)	(Q)	(R)	(S)
237	Blackberries, raw-----------------	1 cup----------------------	144	85	85	2	1	—	—	—	19	46	27	1.3	245	290	0.04	0.06	0.6	30
238	Blueberries, raw------------------	1 cup----------------------	145	83	90	1	1	—	—	—	22	22	19	1.5	117	150	.04	.09	.7	20
	Cantaloup. See Muskmelons (item 271).																			
	Cherries:																			
239	Sour (tart), red, pitted, canned, water pack.	1 cup----------------------	244	88	105	2	Trace	—	—	—	26	37	32	.7	317	1,660	.07	.05	.5	12
240	Sweet, raw, without pits and stems.	10 cherries----------------	68	80	45	1	Trace	—	—	—	12	15	13	.3	129	70	.03	.04	.3	7
241	Cranberry juice cocktail, bottled, sweetened.	1 cup----------------------	253	83	165	Trace	Trace	—	—	—	42	13	8	.8	25	Trace	.03	.03	.1	[27]81
242	Cranberry sauce, sweetened, canned, strained.	1 cup----------------------	277	62	405	Trace	1	—	—	—	104	17	11	.6	83	60	.03	.03	.1	6
	Dates:																			
243	Whole, without pits-------------	10 dates-------------------	80	23	220	2	Trace	—	—	—	58	47	50	2.4	518	40	.07	.08	1.8	0
244	Chopped-------------------------	1 cup----------------------	178	23	490	4	1	—	—	—	130	105	112	5.3	1,153	90	.16	.18	3.9	0
245	Fruit cocktail, canned, in heavy sirup.	1 cup----------------------	255	80	195	1	Trace	—	—	—	50	23	31	1.0	411	360	.05	.03	1.0	5
	Grapefruit:																			
	Raw, medium, 3 3/4-in diam. (about 1 lb 1 oz):																			
246	Pink or red------------------	1/2 grapefruit with peel[28]	241	89	50	1	Trace	—	—	—	13	20	20	.5	166	540	.05	.02	.2	44
247	White------------------------	1/2 grapefruit with peel[28]	241	89	45	1	Trace	—	—	—	12	19	19	.5	159	10	.05	.02	.2	44
248	Canned, sections with sirup-----	1 cup----------------------	254	81	180	2	Trace	—	—	—	45	33	36	.8	343	30	.08	.05	.5	76
	Grapefruit juice:																			
249	Raw, pink, red, or white--------	1 cup----------------------	246	90	95	1	Trace	—	—	—	23	22	37	.5	399	([29])	.10	.05	.5	93
	Canned, white:																			
250	Unsweetened------------------	1 cup----------------------	247	89	100	1	Trace	—	—	—	24	20	35	1.0	400	20	.07	.05	.5	84
251	Sweetened--------------------	1 cup----------------------	250	86	135	1	Trace	—	—	—	32	20	35	1.0	405	30	.08	.05	.5	78
	Frozen, concentrate, unsweetened:																			
252	Undiluted, 6-fl oz can--------	1 can----------------------	207	62	300	4	1	—	—	—	72	70	124	.8	1,250	60	.29	.12	1.4	286
253	Diluted with 3 parts water by volume.	1 cup----------------------	247	89	100	1	Trace	—	—	—	24	25	42	.2	420	20	.10	.04	.5	96
254	Dehydrated crystals, prepared with water (1 lb yields about 1 gal).	1 cup----------------------	247	90	100	1	Trace	—	—	—	24	22	40	.2	412	20	.10	.05	.5	91
	Grapes, European type (adherent skin), raw:																			
255	Thompson Seedless---------------	10 grapes------------------	50	81	35	Trace	Trace	—	—	—	9	6	10	.2	87	50	.03	.02	.2	2
256	Tokay and Emperor, seeded types-	10 grapes[30]----------------	60	81	40	Trace	Trace	—	—	—	10	7	11	.2	99	60	.03	.02	.2	2
	Grapejuice:																			
257	Canned or bottled---------------	1 cup----------------------	253	83	165	1	Trace	—	—	—	42	28	30	.8	293	—	.10	.05	.5	[25]Trace
	Frozen concentrate, sweetened:																			
258	Undiluted, 6-fl oz can--------	1 can----------------------	216	53	395	1	Trace	—	—	—	100	22	32	.9	255	40	.13	.22	1.5	[31]32
259	Diluted with 3 parts water by volume.	1 cup----------------------	250	86	135	1	Trace	—	—	—	33	8	10	.3	85	10	.05	.08	.5	[31]10
260	Grape drink, canned-------------	1 cup----------------------	250	86	135	Trace	Trace	—	—	—	35	8	10	.3	88	—	[32].03	[32].03	.3	([32])
261	Lemon, raw, size 165, without peel and seeds (about 4 per lb with peels and seeds).	1 lemon--------------------	74	90	20	1	Trace	—	—	—	6	19	12	.4	102	10	.03	.01	.1	39
	Lemon juice:																			
262	Raw-----------------------------	1 cup----------------------	244	91	60	1	Trace	—	—	—	20	17	24	.5	344	50	.07	.02	.2	112
263	Canned, or bottled, unsweetened-	1 cup----------------------	244	92	55	1	Trace	—	—	—	19	17	24	.5	344	50	.07	.02	.2	102
264	Frozen, single strength, unsweetened, 6-fl oz can.	1 can----------------------	183	92	40	1	Trace	—	—	—	13	13	16	.5	258	40	.05	.02	.2	81
	Lemonade concentrate, frozen:																			
265	Undiluted, 6-fl oz can----------	1 can----------------------	219	49	425	Trace	Trace	—	—	—	112	9	13	.4	153	40	.05	.06	.7	66
266	Diluted with 4 1/3 parts water by volume.	1 cup----------------------	248	89	105	Trace	Trace	—	—	—	28	2	3	.1	40	10	.01	.02	.2	17

[19]Crust made with vegetable shortening and enriched flour.
[24]Also applies to pasteurized apple cider.
[25]Applies to product without added ascorbic acid. For value of product with added ascorbic acid, refer to label.
[26]Based on product with label claim of 45% of U.S. RDA in 6 fl oz.
[27]Based on product with label claim of 100% of U.S. RDA in 6 fl oz.
[28]Weight includes peel and membranes between sections. Without these parts, the weight of the edible portion is 123 g for item 246 and 118 g for item 247.
[29]For white-fleshed varieties, value is about 20 International Units (I.U.) per cup; for red-fleshed varieties, 1,080 I.U.
[30]Weight includes seeds. Without seeds, weight of the edible portion is 57 g.
[31]Applies to product without added ascorbic acid. With added ascorbic acid, based on claim that 6 fl oz of reconstituted juice contain 45% or 50% of the U.S. RDA, value in milligrams is 108 or 120 for a 6-fl oz can (item 258), 36 or 40 for 1 cup of diluted juice (item 259).
[32]For products with added thiamin and riboflavin but without added ascorbic acid, values in milligrams would be 0.60 for thiamin, 0.80 for riboflavin, and trace for ascorbic acid. For products with only ascorbic acid added, value varies with the brand. Consult the label.

TABLE 2.— NUTRITIVE VALUES OF THE EDIBLE PART OF FOODS - Continued

(Dashes (—) denote lack of reliable data for a constituent believed to be present in measurable amount)

Item No. (A)	Foods, approximate measures, units, and weight (edible part unless footnotes indicate otherwise) (B)			Water (C)	Food energy (D)	Protein (E)	Fat (F)	Fatty Acids: Saturated (total) (G)	Fatty Acids: Unsaturated: Oleic (H)	Fatty Acids: Unsaturated: Linoleic (I)	Carbohydrate (J)	Calcium (K)	Phosphorus (L)	Iron (M)	Potassium (N)	Vitamin A value (O)	Thiamin (P)	Riboflavin (Q)	Niacin (R)	Ascorbic acid (S)
			Grams	Percent	Calories	Grams	Grams	Grams	Grams	Grams	Grams	Milligrams	Milligrams	Milligrams	Milligrams	International units	Milligrams	Milligrams	Milligrams	Milligrams
	FRUITS AND FRUIT PRODUCTS—Con.																			
	Limeade concentrate, frozen:																			
267	Undiluted, 6-fl oz can----------	1 can---------------------	218	50	410	Trace	Trace	—	—	—	108	11	13	0.2	129	Trace	0.02	0.02	0.2	26
268	Diluted with 4 1/3 parts water by volume.	1 cup---------------------	247	89	100	Trace	Trace	—	—	—	27	3	3	Trace	32	Trace	Trace	Trace	Trace	6
	Limejuice:																			
269	Raw----------------------------	1 cup---------------------	246	90	65	1	Trace	—	—	—	22	22	27	.5	256	20	.05	.02	.2	79
270	Canned, unsweetened-------------	1 cup---------------------	246	90	65	1	Trace	—	—	—	22	22	27	.5	256	20	.05	.02	.2	52
	Muskmelons, raw, with rind, without seed cavity:																			
271	Cantaloup, orange-fleshed (with rind and seed cavity, 5-in diam., 2 1/3 lb).	1/2 melon with rind[33]-----	477	91	80	2	Trace	—	—	—	20	38	44	1.1	682	9,240	.11	.08	1.6	90
272	Honeydew (with rind and seed cavity, 6 1/2-in diam., 5 1/4 lb).	1/10 melon with rind[33]----	226	91	50	1	Trace	—	—	—	11	21	24	.6	374	60	.06	.04	.9	34
	Oranges, all commercial varieties, raw:																			
273	Whole, 2 5/8-in diam., without peel and seeds (about 2 1/2 per lb with peel and seeds).	1 orange------------------	131	86	65	1	Trace	—	—	—	16	54	26	.5	263	260	.13	.05	.5	66
274	Sections without membranes------	1 cup---------------------	180	86	90	2	Trace	—	—	—	22	74	36	.7	360	360	.18	.07	.7	90
	Orange juice:																			
275	Raw, all varieties--------------	1 cup---------------------	248	88	110	2	Trace	—	—	—	26	27	42	.5	496	500	.22	.07	1.0	124
276	Canned, unsweetened-------------	1 cup---------------------	249	87	120	2	Trace	—	—	—	28	25	45	1.0	496	500	.17	.05	.7	100
	Frozen concentrate:																			
277	Undiluted, 6-fl oz can--------	1 can---------------------	213	55	360	5	Trace	—	—	—	87	75	126	.9	1,500	1,620	.68	.11	2.8	360
278	Diluted with 3 parts water by volume.	1 cup---------------------	249	87	120	2	Trace	—	—	—	29	25	42	.2	503	540	.23	.03	.9	120
279	Dehydrated crystals, prepared with water (1 lb yields about 1 gal).	1 cup---------------------	248	88	115	1	Trace	—	—	—	27	25	40	.5	518	500	.20	.07	1.0	109
	Orange and grapefruit juice:																			
	Frozen concentrate:																			
280	Undiluted, 6-fl oz can--------	1 can---------------------	210	59	330	4	1	—	—	—	78	61	99	.8	1,308	800	.48	.06	2.3	302
281	Diluted with 3 parts water by volume.	1 cup---------------------	248	88	110	1	Trace	—	—	—	26	20	32	.2	439	270	.15	.02	.7	102
282	Papayas, raw, 1/2-in cubes--------	1 cup---------------------	140	89	55	1	Trace	—	—	—	14	28	22	.4	328	2,450	.06	.06	.4	78
	Peaches:																			
	Raw:																			
283	Whole, 2 1/2-in diam., peeled, pitted (about 4 per lb with peels and pits).	1 peach-------------------	100	89	40	1	Trace	—	—	—	10	9	19	.5	202	[34]1,330	.02	.05	1.0	7
284	Sliced------------------------	1 cup---------------------	170	89	65	1	Trace	—	—	—	16	15	32	.9	343	[34]2,260	.03	.09	1.7	12
	Canned, yellow-fleshed, solids and liquid (halves or slices):																			
285	Sirup pack--------------------	1 cup---------------------	256	79	200	1	Trace	—	—	—	51	10	31	.8	333	1,100	.03	.05	1.5	8
286	Water pack--------------------	1 cup---------------------	244	91	75	1	Trace	—	—	—	20	10	32	.7	334	1,100	.02	.07	1.5	7
	Dried:																			
287	Uncooked----------------------	1 cup---------------------	160	25	420	5	1	—	—	—	109	77	187	9.6	1,520	6,240	.02	.30	8.5	29
288	Cooked, unsweetened, halves and juice.	1 cup---------------------	250	77	205	3	1	—	—	—	54	38	93	4.8	743	3,050	.01	.15	3.8	5

(A)	(B)			(C)	(D)	(E)	(F)	(G)	(H)	(I)	(J)	(K)	(L)	(M)	(N)	(O)	(P)	(Q)	(R)	(S)
	Frozen, sliced, sweetened:																			
289	10-oz container	1 container	284	77	250	1	Trace	—	—	—	64	11	37	1.4	352	1,850	0.03	0.11	2.0	[35]116
290	Cup	1 cup	250	77	220	1	Trace	—	—	—	57	10	33	1.3	310	1,630	.03	.10	1.8	[35]103
	Pears:																			
	Raw, with skin, cored:																			
291	Bartlett, 2 1/2-in diam. (about 2 1/2 per lb with cores and stems).	1 pear	164	83	100	1	1	—	—	—	25	13	18	.5	213	30	.03	.07	.2	7
292	Bosc, 2 1/2-in diam. (about 3 per lb with cores and stems).	1 pear	141	83	85	1	1	—	—	—	22	11	16	.4	83	30	.03	.06	.1	6
293	D'Anjou, 3-in diam. (about 2 per lb with cores and stems).	1 pear	200	83	120	1	1	—	—	—	31	16	22	.6	260	40	.04	.08	.2	8
294	Canned, solids and liquid, sirup pack, heavy (halves or slices).	1 cup	255	80	195	1	1	—	—	—	50	13	18	.5	214	10	.03	.05	.3	3
	Pineapple:																			
295	Raw, diced	1 cup	155	85	80	1	Trace	—	—	—	21	26	12	.8	226	110	.14	.05	.3	26
	Canned, heavy sirup pack, solids and liquid:																			
296	Crushed, chunks, tidbits	1 cup	255	80	190	1	Trace	—	—	—	49	28	13	.8	245	130	.20	.05	.5	18
	Slices and liquid:																			
297	Large	1 slice; 2 1/4 tbsp liquid.	105	80	80	Trace	Trace	—	—	—	20	12	5	.3	101	50	.08	.02	.2	7
298	Medium	1 slice; 1 1/4 tbsp liquid.	58	80	45	Trace	Trace	—	—	—	11	6	3	.2	56	30	.05	.01	.1	4
299	Pineapple juice, unsweetened, canned.	1 cup	250	86	140	1	Trace	—	—	—	34	38	23	.8	373	130	.13	.05	.5	[27]80
	Plums:																			
	Raw, without pits:																			
300	Japanese and hybrid (2 1/8-in diam., about 6 1/2 per lb with pits).	1 plum	66	87	30	Trace	Trace	—	—	—	8	8	12	.3	112	160	.02	.02	.3	4
301	Prune-type (1 1/2-in diam., about 15 per lb with pits).	1 plum	28	79	20	Trace	Trace	—	—	—	6	3	5	.1	48	80	.01	.01	.1	1
	Canned, heavy sirup pack (Italian prunes), with pits and liquid:																			
302	Cup	1 cup[36]	272	77	215	1	Trace	—	—	—	56	23	26	2.3	367	3,130	.05	.05	1.0	5
303	Portion	3 plums; 2 3/4 tbsp liquid.[36]	140	77	110	1	Trace	—	—	—	29	12	13	1.2	189	1,610	.03	.03	.5	3
	Prunes, dried, "softenized," with pits:																			
304	Uncooked	4 extra large or 5 large prunes.[36]	49	28	110	1	Trace	—	—	—	29	22	34	1.7	298	690	.04	.07	.7	1
305	Cooked, unsweetened, all sizes, fruit and liquid.	1 cup[36]	250	66	255	2	1	—	—	—	67	51	79	3.8	695	1,590	.07	.15	1.5	2
306	Prune juice, canned or bottled	1 cup	256	80	195	1	Trace	—	—	—	49	36	51	1.8	602	—	.03	.03	1.0	5
	Raisins, seedless:																			
307	Cup, not pressed down	1 cup	145	18	420	4	Trace	—	—	—	112	90	146	5.1	1,106	30	.16	.12	.7	1
308	Packet, 1/2 oz (1 1/2 tbsp)	1 packet	14	18	40	Trace	Trace	—	—	—	11	9	14	.5	107	Trace	.02	.01	.1	Trace
	Raspberries, red:																			
309	Raw, capped, whole	1 cup	123	84	70	1	1	—	—	—	17	27	27	1.1	207	160	.04	.11	1.1	31
310	Frozen, sweetened, 10-oz container	1 container	284	74	280	2	1	—	—	—	70	37	48	1.7	284	200	.06	.17	1.7	60
	Rhubarb, cooked, added sugar:																			
311	From raw	1 cup	270	63	380	1	Trace	—	—	—	97	211	41	1.6	548	220	.05	.14	.8	16
312	From frozen, sweetened	1 cup	270	63	385	1	1	—	—	—	98	211	32	1.9	475	190	.05	.11	.5	16

[27]Based on product with label claim of 100% of U.S. RDA in 6 fl oz.
[33]Weight includes rind. Without rind, the weight of the edible portion is 272 g for item 271 and 149 g for item 272.
[34]Represents yellow-fleshed varieties. For white-fleshed varieties, value is 50 International Units (I.U.) for 1 peach, 90 I.U. for 1 cup of slices.
[35]Value represents products with added ascorbic acid. For products without added ascorbic acid, value in milligrams is 116 for a 10-oz container, 103 for 1 cup.
[36]Weight includes pits. After removal of the pits, the weight of the edible portion is 258 g for item 302, 133 g for item 303, 43 g for item 304, and 213 g for item 305.

TABLE 2.– NUTRITIVE VALUES OF THE EDIBLE PART OF FOODS - Continued

(Dashes (—) denote lack of reliable data for a constituent believed to be present in measurable amount)

Item No.	Foods, approximate measures, units, and weight (edible part unless footnotes indicate otherwise)			Water	Food energy	Protein	Fat	Fatty Acids: Saturated (total)	Fatty Acids: Unsaturated Oleic	Fatty Acids: Unsaturated Linoleic	Carbohydrate	Calcium	Phosphorus	Iron	Potassium	Vitamin A value	Thiamin	Riboflavin	Niacin	Ascorbic acid
(A)	(B)			(C)	(D)	(E)	(F)	(G)	(H)	(I)	(J)	(K)	(L)	(M)	(N)	(O)	(P)	(Q)	(R)	(S)
			Grams	Percent	Calories	Grams	Grams	Grams	Grams	Grams	Grams	Milligrams	Milligrams	Milligrams	Milligrams	International units	Milligrams	Milligrams	Milligrams	Milligrams
	FRUITS AND FRUIT PRODUCTS—Con.																			
	Strawberries:																			
313	Raw, whole berries, capped	1 cup	149	90	55	1	1	—	—	—	13	31	31	1.5	244	90	0.04	0.10	0.9	88
	Frozen, sweetened:																			
314	Sliced, 10-oz container	1 container	284	71	310	1	1	—	—	—	79	40	48	2.0	318	90	.06	.17	1.4	151
315	Whole, 1-lb container (about 1 3/4 cups).	1 container	454	76	415	2	1	—	—	—	107	59	73	2.7	472	140	.09	.27	2.3	249
316	Tangerine, raw, 2 3/8-in diam., size 176, without peel (about 4 per lb with peels and seeds).	1 tangerine	86	87	40	1	Trace	—	—	—	10	34	15	.3	108	360	.05	.02	.1	27
317	Tangerine juice, canned, sweetened.	1 cup	249	87	125	1	Trace	—	—	—	30	44	35	.5	440	1,040	.15	.05	.2	54
318	Watermelon, raw, 4 by 8 in wedge with rind and seeds (1/16 of 32 2/3-lb melon, 10 by 16 in).	1 wedge with rind and seeds[37]	926	93	110	2	1	—	—	—	27	30	43	2.1	426	2,510	.13	.13	.9	30
	GRAIN PRODUCTS																			
	Bagel, 3-in diam.:																			
319	Egg	1 bagel	55	32	165	6	2	0.5	0.9	0.8	28	9	43	1.2	41	30	.14	.10	1.2	0
320	Water	1 bagel	55	29	165	6	1	.2	.4	.6	30	8	41	1.2	42	0	.15	.11	1.4	0
321	Barley, pearled, light, uncooked	1 cup	200	11	700	16	2	.3	.2	.8	158	32	378	4.0	320	0	.24	.10	6.2	0
	Biscuits, baking powder, 2-in diam. (enriched flour, vegetable shortening):																			
322	From home recipe	1 biscuit	28	27	105	2	5	1.2	2.0	1.2	13	34	49	.4	33	Trace	.08	.08	.7	Trace
323	From mix	1 biscuit	28	29	90	2	3	.6	1.1	.7	15	19	65	.6	32	Trace	.09	.08	.8	Trace
	Breadcrumbs (enriched):[38]																			
324	Dry, grated	1 cup	100	7	390	13	5	1.0	1.6	1.4	73	122	141	3.6	152	Trace	.35	.35	4.8	Trace
	Soft. See White bread (items 349-350).																			
	Breads:																			
325	Boston brown bread, canned, slice, 3 1/4 by 1/2 in.[38]	1 slice	45	45	95	2	1	.1	.2	.2	21	41	72	.9	131	[39]0	.06	.04	.7	0
	Cracked-wheat bread (3/4 enriched wheat flour, 1/4 cracked wheat):[38]																			
326	Loaf, 1 lb	1 loaf	454	35	1,195	39	10	2.2	3.0	3.9	236	399	581	9.5	608	Trace	1.52	1.13	14.4	Trace
327	Slice (18 per loaf)	1 slice	25	35	65	2	1	.1	.2	.2	13	22	32	.5	34	Trace	.08	.06	.8	Trace
	French or vienna bread, enriched:[38]																			
328	Loaf, 1 lb	1 loaf	454	31	1,315	41	14	3.2	4.7	4.6	251	195	386	10.0	408	Trace	1.80	1.10	15.0	Trace
	Slice:																			
329	French (5 by 2 1/2 by 1 in)	1 slice	35	31	100	3	1	.2	.4	.4	19	15	30	.8	32	Trace	.14	.08	1.2	Trace
330	Vienna (4 3/4 by 4 by 1/2 in).	1 slice	25	31	75	2	1	.2	.3	.3	14	11	21	.6	23	Trace	.10	.06	.8	Trace
	Italian bread, enriched:																			
331	Loaf, 1 lb	1 loaf	454	32	1,250	41	4	.6	.3	1.5	256	77	349	10.0	336	0	1.80	1.10	15.0	0
332	Slice, 4 1/2 by 3 1/4 by 3/4 in.	1 slice	30	32	85	3	Trace	Trace	Trace	.1	17	5	23	.7	22	0	.12	.07	1.0	0
	Raisin bread, enriched:[38]																			
333	Loaf, 1 lb	1 loaf	454	35	1,190	30	13	3.0	4.7	3.9	243	322	395	10.0	1,057	Trace	1.70	1.07	10.7	Trace
334	Slice (18 per loaf)	1 slice	25	35	65	2	1	.2	.3	.2	13	18	22	.6	58	Trace	.09	.06	.6	Trace

(A)	(B)			(C)	(D)	(E)	(F)	(G)	(H)	(I)	(J)	(K)	(L)	(M)	(N)	(O)	(P)	(Q)	(R)	(S)
	Rye Bread:																			
	American, light (2/3 enriched wheat flour, 1/3 rye flour):																			
335	Loaf, 1 lb------------------	1 loaf--------------------	454	36	1,100	41	5	0.7	0.5	2.2	236	340	667	9.1	658	0	1.35	0.98	12.9	0
336	Slice (4 3/4 by 3 3/4 by 7/16 in).	1 slice-------------------	25	36	60	2	Trace	Trace	Trace	.1	13	19	37	.5	36	0	.07	.05	.7	0
	Pumpernickel (2/3 rye flour, 1/3 enriched wheat flour):																			
337	Loaf, 1 lb------------------	1 loaf--------------------	454	34	1,115	41	5	.7	.5	2.4	241	381	1,039	11.8	2,059	0	1.30	.93	8.5	0
338	Slice (5 by 4 by 3/8 in)----	1 slice-------------------	32	34	80	3	Trace	.1	Trace	.2	17	27	73	.8	145	0	.09	.07	.6	0
	White bread, enriched:[38]																			
	Soft-crumb type:																			
339	Loaf, 1 lb------------------	1 loaf--------------------	454	36	1,225	39	15	3.4	5.3	4.6	229	381	440	11.3	476	Trace	1.80	1.10	15.0	Trace
340	Slice (18 per loaf)-------	1 slice-------------------	25	36	70	2	1	.2	.3	.3	13	21	24	.6	26	Trace	.10	.06	.8	Trace
341	Slice, toasted----------	1 slice-------------------	22	25	70	2	1	.2	.3	.3	13	21	24	.6	26	Trace	.08	.06	.8	Trace
342	Slice (22 per loaf)-------	1 slice-------------------	20	36	55	2	1	.2	.2	.2	10	17	19	.5	21	Trace	.08	.05	.7	Trace
343	Slice, toasted----------	1 slice-------------------	17	25	55	2	1	.2	.2	.2	10	17	19	.5	21	Trace	.06	.05	.7	Trace
344	Loaf, 1 1/2 lb--------------	1 loaf--------------------	680	36	1,835	59	22	5.2	7.9	6.9	343	571	660	17.0	714	Trace	2.70	1.65	22.5	Trace
345	Slice (24 per loaf)-------	1 slice-------------------	28	36	75	2	1	.2	.3	.3	14	24	27	.7	29	Trace	.11	.07	.9	Trace
346	Slice, toasted----------	1 slice-------------------	24	25	75	2	1	.2	.3	.3	14	24	27	.7	29	Trace	.09	.07	.9	Trace
347	Slice (28 per loaf)-------	1 slice-------------------	24	36	65	2	1	.2	.3	.2	12	20	23	.6	25	Trace	.10	.06	.8	Trace
348	Slice, toasted----------	1 slice-------------------	21	25	65	2	1	.2	.3	.2	12	20	23	.6	25	Trace	.08	.06	.8	Trace
349	Cubes----------------------	1 cup---------------------	30	36	80	3	1	.2	.3	.3	15	25	29	.8	32	Trace	.12	.07	1.0	Trace
350	Crumbs---------------------	1 cup---------------------	45	36	120	4	1	.3	.5	.5	23	38	44	1.1	47	Trace	.18	.11	1.5	Trace
	Firm-crumb type:																			
351	Loaf, 1 lb------------------	1 loaf--------------------	454	35	1,245	41	17	3.9	5.9	5.2	228	435	463	11.3	549	Trace	1.80	1.10	15.0	Trace
352	Slice (20 per loaf)-------	1 slice-------------------	23	35	65	2	1	.2	.3	.3	12	22	23	.6	28	Trace	.09	.06	.8	Trace
353	Slice, toasted----------	1 slice-------------------	20	24	65	2	1	.2	.3	.3	12	22	23	.6	28	Trace	.07	.06	.8	Trace
354	Loaf, 2 lb------------------	1 loaf--------------------	907	35	2,495	82	34	7.7	11.8	10.4	455	871	925	22.7	1,097	Trace	3.60	2.20	30.0	Trace
355	Slice (34 per loaf)-------	1 slice-------------------	27	35	75	2	1	.2	.3	.3	14	26	28	.7	33	Trace	.11	.06	.9	Trace
356	Slice, toasted----------	1 slice-------------------	23	24	75	2	1	.2	.3	.3	14	26	28	.7	33	Trace	.09	.06	.9	Trace
	Whole-wheat bread:																			
	Soft-crumb type:[38]																			
357	Loaf, 1 lb------------------	1 loaf--------------------	454	36	1,095	41	12	2.2	2.9	4.2	224	381	1,152	13.6	1,161	Trace	1.37	.45	12.7	Trace
358	Slice (16 per loaf)-------	1 slice-------------------	28	36	65	3	1	.1	.2	.2	14	24	71	.8	72	Trace	.09	.03	.8	Trace
359	Slice, toasted----------	1 slice-------------------	24	24	65	3	1	.1	.2	.2	14	24	71	.8	72	Trace	.07	.03	.8	Trace
	Firm-crumb type:[38]																			
360	Loaf, 1 lb------------------	1 loaf--------------------	454	36	1,100	48	14	2.5	3.3	4.9	216	449	1,034	13.6	1,238	Trace	1.17	.54	12.7	Trace
361	Slice (18 per loaf)-------	1 slice-------------------	25	36	60	3	1	.1	.2	.3	12	25	57	.8	68	Trace	.06	.03	.7	Trace
362	Slice, toasted----------	1 slice-------------------	21	24	60	3	1	.1	.2	.3	12	25	57	.8	68	Trace	.05	.03	.7	Trace
	Breakfast cereals:																			
	Hot type, cooked:																			
	Corn (hominy) grits, degermed:																			
363	Enriched--------------------	1 cup---------------------	245	87	125	3	Trace	Trace	Trace	.1	27	2	25	.7	27	[40]Trace	.10	.07	1.0	0
364	Unenriched------------------	1 cup---------------------	245	87	125	3	Trace	Trace	Trace	.1	27	2	25	.2	27	[40]Trace	.05	.02	.5	0
365	Farina, quick-cooking, enriched.	1 cup---------------------	245	89	105	3	Trace	Trace	Trace	.1	22	147	[41]113	([42])	25	0	.12	.07	1.0	0
366	Oatmeal or rolled oats--------	1 cup---------------------	240	87	130	5	2	.4	.8	.9	23	22	137	1.4	146	0	.19	.05	.2	0
367	Wheat, rolled-----------------	1 cup---------------------	240	80	180	5	1	—	—	—	41	19	182	1.7	202	0	.17	.07	2.2	0
368	Wheat, whole-meal-------------	1 cup---------------------	245	88	110	4	1	—	—	—	23	17	127	1.2	118	0	.15	.05	1.5	0
	Ready-to-eat:																			
369	Bran flakes (40% bran), added sugar, salt, iron, vitamins.	1 cup---------------------	35	3	105	4	1	—	—	—	28	19	125	5.6	137	1,540	.46	.52	6.2	0
370	Bran flakes with raisins, added sugar, salt, iron, vitamins.	1 cup---------------------	50	7	145	4	1	—	—	—	40	28	146	7.9	154	[43]2,200	([44])	([44])	([44])	0

[37]Weight includes rind and seeds. Without rind and seeds, weight of the edible portion is 426 g.
[38]Made with vegetable shortening.
[39]Applies to product made with white cornmeal. With yellow cornmeal, value is 30 International Units (I.U.).
[40]Applies to white varieties. For yellow varieties, value is 150 International Units (I.U.).
[41]Applies to products that do not contain di-sodium phosphate. If di-sodium phosphate is an ingredient, value is 162 mg.
[42]Value may range from less than 1 mg to about 8 mg depending on the brand. Consult the label.
[43]Applies to product with added nutrient. Without added nutrient, value is trace.
[44]Value varies with the brand. Consult the label.

TABLE 2.— NUTRITIVE VALUES OF THE EDIBLE PART OF FOODS · Continued

(Dashes (—) denote lack of reliable data for a constituent believed to be present in measurable amount)

Item No.	Foods, approximate measures, units, and weight (edible part unless footnotes indicate otherwise)			Water	Food energy	Protein	Fat	Fatty Acids: Saturated (total)	Unsaturated: Oleic	Unsaturated: Linoleic	Carbohydrate	Calcium	Phosphorus	Iron	Potassium	Vitamin A value	Thiamin	Riboflavin	Niacin	Ascorbic acid
(A)	(B)			(C)	(D)	(E)	(F)	(G)	(H)	(I)	(J)	(K)	(L)	(M)	(N)	(O)	(P)	(Q)	(R)	(S)
	GRAIN PRODUCTS—Con.		Grams	Percent	Calories	Grams	Grams	Grams	Grams	Grams	Grams	Milligrams	Milligrams	Milligrams	Milligrams	International units	Milligrams	Milligrams	Milligrams	Milligrams
	Breakfast cereals—Continued																			
	Ready-to-eat—Continued																			
	Corn flakes:																			
371	Plain, added sugar, salt, iron, vitamins.	1 cup	25	4	95	2	Trace	—	—	—	21	([44])	9	([44])	30	([44])	([44])	([44])	([44])	[45]13
372	Sugar-coated, added salt, iron, vitamins.	1 cup	40	2	155	2	Trace	—	—	—	37	1	10	([44])	27	1,760	.53	.60	7.1	[45]21
373	Corn, oat flour, puffed, added sugar, salt, iron, vitamins.	1 cup	20	4	80	2	1	—	—	—	16	4	18	5.7	—	880	.26	.30	3.5	11
374	Corn, shredded, added sugar, salt, iron, thiamin, niacin.	1 cup	25	3	95	2	Trace	—	—	—	22	1	10	.6	—	0	.33	.05	4.4	13
375	Oats, puffed, added sugar, salt, minerals, vitamins.	1 cup	25	3	100	3	1	—	—	—	19	44	102	4.0	—	1,100	.33	.38	4.4	13
	Rice, puffed:																			
376	Plain, added iron, thiamin, niacin.	1 cup	15	4	60	1	Trace	—	—	—	13	3	14	.3	15	0	.07	.01	.7	0
377	Presweetened, added salt, iron, vitamins.	1 cup	28	3	115	1	0	—	—	—	26	3	14	([44])	43	[45]1,240	([44])	([44])	([44])	[45]15
378	Wheat flakes, added sugar, salt, iron, vitamins.	1 cup	30	4	105	3	Trace	—	—	—	24	12	83	4.8	81	1,320	.40	.45	5.3	16
	Wheat, puffed:																			
379	Plain, added iron, thiamin, niacin.	1 cup	15	3	55	2	Trace	—	—	—	12	4	48	.6	51	0	.08	.03	1.2	0
380	Presweetened, added salt, iron, vitamins.	1 cup	38	3	140	3	Trace	—	—	—	33	7	52	([44])	63	1,680	.50	.57	6.7	[45]20
381	Wheat, shredded, plain	1 oblong biscuit or 1/2 cup spoon-size biscuits.	25	7	90	2	1	—	—	—	20	11	97	.9	87	0	.06	.03	1.1	0
382	Wheat germ, without salt and sugar, toasted.	1 tbsp	6	4	25	2	1	—	—	—	3	3	70	.5	57	10	.11	.05	.3	1
383	Buckwheat flour, light, sifted	1 cup	98	12	340	6	1	0.2	0.4	0.4	78	11	86	1.0	314	0	.08	.04	.4	0
384	Bulgur, canned, seasoned	1 cup	135	56	245	8	4	—	—	—	44	27	263	1.9	151	0	.08	.05	4.1	0
	Cake icings. See Sugars and Sweets (items 532-536).																			
	Cakes made from cake mixes with enriched flour:[46]																			
	Angelfood:																			
385	Whole cake (9 3/4-in diam. tube cake).	1 cake	635	34	1,645	36	1	—	—	—	377	603	756	2.5	381	0	.37	.95	3.6	0
386	Piece, 1/12 of cake	1 piece	53	34	135	3	Trace	—	—	—	32	50	63	.2	32	0	.03	.08	.3	0
	Coffeecake:																			
387	Whole cake (7 3/4 by 5 5/8 by 1 1/4 in).	1 cake	430	30	1,385	27	41	11.7	16.3	8.8	225	262	748	6.9	469	690	.82	.91	7.7	1
388	Piece, 1/6 of cake	1 piece	72	30	230	5	7	2.0	2.7	1.5	38	44	125	1.2	78	120	.14	.15	1.3	Trace
	Cupcakes, made with egg, milk, 2 1/2-in diam.:																			
389	Without icing	1 cupcake	25	26	90	1	3	.8	1.2	.7	14	40	59	.3	21	40	.05	.05	.4	Trace
390	With chocolate icing	1 cupcake	36	22	130	2	5	2.0	1.6	.6	21	47	71	.4	42	60	.05	.06	.4	Trace
	Devil's food with chocolate icing:																			
391	Whole, 2 layer cake (8- or 9-in diam.).	1 cake	1,107	24	3,755	49	136	50.0	44.9	17.0	645	653	1,162	16.6	1,439	1,660	1.06	1.65	10.1	1
392	Piece, 1/16 of cake	1 piece	69	24	235	3	8	3.1	2.8	1.1	40	41	72	1.0	90	100	.07	.10	.6	Trace
393	Cupcake, 2 1/2-in diam	1 cupcake	35	24	120	2	4	1.6	1.4	.5	20	21	37	.5	46	50	.03	.05	.3	Trace

(A)	(B)			(C)	(D)	(E)	(F)	(G)	(H)	(I)	(J)	(K)	(L)	(M)	(N)	(O)	(P)	(Q)	(R)	(S)
	Gingerbread:																			
394	Whole cake (8-in square)-------	1 cake------------------	570	37	1,575	18	39	9.7	16.6	10.0	291	513	570	8.6	1,562	Trace	0.84	1.00	7.4	Trace
395	Piece, 1/9 of cake-------------	1 piece-----------------	63	37	175	2	4	1.1	1.8	1.1	32	57	63	.9	173	Trace	.09	.11	.8	Trace
	White, 2 layer with chocolate icing:																			
396	Whole cake (8- or 9-in diam.)--	1 cake------------------	1,140	21	4,000	44	122	48.2	46.4	20.0	716	1,129	2,041	11.4	1,322	680	1.50	1.77	12.5	2
397	Piece, 1/16 of cake------------	1 piece-----------------	71	21	250	3	8	3.0	2.9	1.2	45	70	127	.7	82	40	.09	.11	.8	Trace
	Yellow, 2 layer with chocolate icing:																			
398	Whole cake (8- or 9-in diam.)--	1 cake------------------	1,108	26	3,735	45	125	47.8	47.8	20.3	638	1,008	2,017	12.2	1,208	1,550	1.24	1.67	10.6	2
399	Piece, 1/16 of cake------------	1 piece-----------------	69	26	235	3	8	3.0	3.0	1.3	40	63	126	.8	75	100	.08	.10	.7	Trace
	Cakes made from home recipes using enriched flour:[47]																			
	Boston cream pie with custard filling:																			
400	Whole cake (8-in diam.)--------	1 cake------------------	825	35	2,490	41	78	23.0	30.1	15.2	412	553	833	8.2	[48]734	1,730	1.04	1.27	9.6	2
401	Piece, 1/12 of cake------------	1 piece-----------------	69	35	210	3	6	1.9	2.5	1.3	34	46	70	.7	[48]61	140	.09	.11	.8	Trace
	Fruitcake, dark:																			
402	Loaf, 1-lb (7 1/2 by 2 by 1 1/2 in).	1 loaf------------------	454	18	1,720	22	69	14.4	33.5	14.8	271	327	513	11.8	2,250	540	.72	.73	4.9	2
403	Slice, 1/30 of loaf------------	1 slice-----------------	15	18	55	1	2	.5	1.1	.5	9	11	17	.4	74	20	.02	.02	.2	Trace
	Plain, sheet cake:																			
	Without icing:																			
404	Whole cake (9-in square)-----	1 cake------------------	777	25	2,830	35	108	29.5	44.4	23.9	434	497	793	8.5	[48]614	1,320	1.21	1.40	10.2	2
405	Piece, 1/9 of cake----------	1 piece-----------------	86	25	315	4	12	3.3	4.9	2.6	48	55	88	.9	[48]68	150	.13	.15	1.1	Trace
	With uncooked white icing:																			
406	Whole cake (9-in square)-----	1 cake------------------	1,096	21	4,020	37	129	42.2	49.5	24.4	694	548	822	8.2	[48]669	2,190	1.22	1.47	10.2	2
407	Piece, 1/9 of cake----------	1 piece-----------------	121	21	445	4	14	4.7	5.5	2.7	77	61	91	.8	[48]74	240	.14	.16	1.1	Trace
	Pound:[49]																			
408	Loaf, 8 1/2 by 3 1/2 by 3 1/4 in.	1 loaf------------------	565	16	2,725	31	170	42.9	73.1	39.6	273	107	418	7.9	345	1,410	.90	.99	7.3	0
409	Slice, 1/17 of loaf------------	1 slice-----------------	33	16	160	2	10	2.5	4.3	2.3	16	6	24	.5	20	80	.05	.06	.4	0
	Spongecake:																			
410	Whole cake (9 3/4-in diam. tube cake).	1 cake------------------	790	32	2,345	60	45	13.1	15.8	5.7	427	237	885	13.4	687	3,560	1.10	1.64	7.4	Trace
411	Piece, 1/12 of cake------------	1 piece-----------------	66	32	195	5	4	1.1	1.3	.5	36	20	74	1.1	57	300	.09	.14	.6	Trace
	Cookies made with enriched flour:[50, 51]																			
	Brownies with nuts:																			
	Home-prepared, 1 3/4 by 1 3/4 by 7/8 in:																			
412	From home recipe------------	1 brownie---------------	20	10	95	1	6	1.5	3.0	1.2	10	8	30	.4	38	40	.04	.03	.2	Trace
413	From commercial recipe-------	1 brownie---------------	20	11	85	1	4	.9	1.4	1.3	13	9	27	.4	34	20	.03	.02	.2	Trace
414	Frozen, with chocolate icing,[52] 1 1/2 by 1 3/4 by 7/8 in.	1 brownie---------------	25	13	105	1	5	2.0	2.2	.7	15	10	31	.4	44	50	.03	.03	.2	Trace
	Chocolate chip:																			
415	Commercial, 2 1/4-in diam., 3/8 in thick.	4 cookies---------------	42	3	200	2	9	2.8	2.9	2.2	29	16	48	1.0	56	50	.10	.17	.9	Trace
416	From home recipe, 2 1/3-in diam.	4 cookies---------------	40	3	205	2	12	3.5	4.5	2.9	24	14	40	.8	47	40	.06	.06	.5	Trace
417	Fig bars, square (1 5/8 by 1 5/8 by 3/8 in) or rectangular (1 1/2 by 1 3/4 by 1/2 in).	4 cookies---------------	56	14	200	2	3	.8	1.2	.7	42	44	34	1.0	111	60	.04	.14	.9	Trace
418	Gingersnaps, 2-in diam., 1/4 in thick.	4 cookies---------------	28	3	90	2	2	.7	1.0	.6	22	20	13	.7	129	20	.08	.06	.7	0
419	Macaroons, 2 3/4-in diam., 1/4 in thick.	2 cookies---------------	38	4	180	2	9	—	—	—	25	10	32	.3	176	0	.02	.06	.2	0
420	Oatmeal with raisins, 2 5/8-in diam., 1/4 in thick.	4 cookies---------------	52	3	235	3	8	2.0	3.3	2.0	38	11	53	1.4	192	30	.15	.10	1.0	Trace

[44]Value varies with the brand. Consult the label.
[45]Applies to product with added nutrient. Without added nutrient, value is trace.
[46]Excepting angelfood cake, cakes were made from mixes containing vegetable shortening; icings, with butter.
[47]Excepting spongecake, vegetable shortening used for cake portion; butter, for icing. If butter or margarine used for cake portion, vitamin A values would be higher.
[48]Applies to product made with a sodium aluminum-sulfate type baking powder. With a low-sodium type baking powder containing potassium, value would be about twice the amount shown.
[49]Equal weights of flour, sugar, eggs, and vegetable shortening.
[50]Products are commercial unless otherwise specified.
[51]Made with enriched flour and vegetable shortening except for macaroons which do not contain flour or shortening.
[52]Icing made with butter.

TABLE 2.– NUTRITIVE VALUES OF THE EDIBLE PART OF FOODS - Continued

(Dashes (–) denote lack of reliable data for a constituent believed to be present in measurable amount)

Item No.	Foods, approximate measures, units, and weight (edible part unless footnotes indicate otherwise)			Water	Food energy	Protein	Fat	Fatty Acids: Saturated (total)	Fatty Acids: Unsaturated: Oleic	Fatty Acids: Unsaturated: Linoleic	Carbohydrate	Calcium	Phosphorus	Iron	Potassium	Vitamin A value	Thiamin	Riboflavin	Niacin	Ascorbic acid
(A)	(B)			(C)	(D)	(E)	(F)	(G)	(H)	(I)	(J)	(K)	(L)	(M)	(N)	(O)	(P)	(Q)	(R)	(S)
			Grams	Percent	Calories	Grams	Grams	Grams	Grams	Grams	Grams	Milligrams	Milligrams	Milligrams	Milligrams	International units	Milligrams	Milligrams	Milligrams	Milligrams
	GRAIN PRODUCTS—Con.																			
	Cookies made with enriched flour[50, 51]—Continued																			
421	Plain, prepared from commercial chilled dough, 2 1/2-in diam., 1/4 in thick.	4 cookies	48	5	240	2	12	3.0	5.2	2.9	31	17	35	0.6	23	30	0.10	0.08	0.9	0
422	Sandwich type (chocolate or vanilla), 1 3/4-in diam., 3/8 in thick.	4 cookies	40	2	200	2	9	2.2	3.9	2.2	28	10	96	.7	15	0	.06	.10	.7	0
423	Vanilla wafers, 1 3/4-in diam., 1/4 in thick.	10 cookies	40	3	185	2	6	—	—	—	30	16	25	.6	29	50	.10	.09	.8	0
	Cornmeal:																			
424	Whole-ground, unbolted, dry form.	1 cup	122	12	435	11	5	.5	1.0	2.5	90	24	312	2.9	346	[53]620	.46	.13	2.4	0
425	Bolted (nearly whole-grain), dry form.	1 cup	122	12	440	11	4	.5	.9	2.1	91	21	272	2.2	303	[53]590	.37	.10	2.3	0
	Degermed, enriched:																			
426	Dry form	1 cup	138	12	500	11	2	.2	.4	.9	108	8	137	4.0	166	[53]610	.61	.36	4.8	0
427	Cooked	1 cup	240	88	120	3	Trace	Trace	.1	.2	26	2	34	1.0	38	[53]140	.14	.10	1.2	0
	Degermed, unenriched:																			
428	Dry form	1 cup	138	12	500	11	2	.2	.4	.9	108	8	137	1.5	166	[53]610	.19	.07	1.4	0
429	Cooked	1 cup	240	88	120	3	Trace	Trace	.1	.2	26	2	34	.5	38	[53]140	.05	.02	.2	0
	Crackers:[38]																			
430	Graham, plain, 2 1/2-in square	2 crackers	14	6	55	1	1	.3	.5	.3	10	6	21	.5	55	0	.02	.08	.5	0
431	Rye wafers, whole-grain, 1 7/8 by 3 1/2 in.	2 wafers	13	6	45	2	Trace	—	—	—	10	7	50	.5	78	0	.04	.03	.2	0
432	Saltines, made with enriched flour.	4 crackers or 1 packet	11	4	50	1	1	.3	.5	.4	8	2	10	.5	13	0	.05	.05	.4	0
	Danish pastry (enriched flour), plain without fruit or nuts:[54]																			
433	Packaged ring, 12 oz	1 ring	340	22	1,435	25	80	24.3	31.7	16.5	155	170	371	6.1	381	1,050	.97	1.01	8.6	Trace
434	Round piece, about 4 1/4-in diam. by 1 in.	1 pastry	65	22	275	5	15	4.7	6.1	3.2	30	33	71	1.2	73	200	.18	.19	1.7	Trace
435	Ounce	1 oz	28	22	120	2	7	2.0	2.7	1.4	13	14	31	.5	32	90	.08	.08	.7	Trace
	Doughnuts, made with enriched flour:[38]																			
436	Cake type, plain, 2 1/2-in diam., 1 in high.	1 doughnut	25	24	100	1	5	1.2	2.0	1.1	13	10	48	.4	23	20	.05	.05	.4	Trace
437	Yeast-leavened, glazed, 3 3/4-in diam., 1 1/4 in high.	1 doughnut	50	26	205	3	11	3.3	5.8	3.3	22	16	33	.6	34	25	.10	.10	.8	0
	Macaroni, enriched, cooked (cut lengths, elbows, shells):																			
438	Firm stage (hot)	1 cup	130	64	190	7	1	—	—	—	39	14	85	1.4	103	0	.23	.13	1.8	0
	Tender stage:																			
439	Cold macaroni	1 cup	105	73	115	4	Trace	—	—	—	24	8	53	.9	64	0	.15	.08	1.2	0
440	Hot macaroni	1 cup	140	73	155	5	1	—	—	—	32	11	70	1.3	85	.0	.20	.11	1.5	0
	Macaroni (enriched) and cheese:																			
441	Canned[55]	1 cup	240	80	230	9	10	4.2	3.1	1.4	26	199	182	1.0	139	260	.12	.24	1.0	Trace
442	From home recipe (served hot)[56]	1 cup	200	58	430	17	22	8.9	8.8	2.9	40	362	322	1.8	240	860	.20	.40	1.8	Trace
	Muffins made with enriched flour:[38]																			
	From home recipe:																			
443	Blueberry, 2 3/8-in diam., 1 1/2 in high.	1 muffin	40	39	110	3	4	1.1	1.4	.7	17	34	53	.6	46	90	.09	.10	.7	Trace
444	Bran	1 muffin	40	35	105	3	4	1.2	1.4	.8	17	57	162	1.5	172	90	.07	.10	1.7	Trace
445	Corn (enriched degermed cornmeal and flour), 2 3/8-in diam., 1 1/2 in high.	1 muffin	40	33	125	3	4	1.2	1.6	.9	19	42	68	.7	54	[57]120	.10	.10	.7	Trace

(A)	(B)			(C)	(D)	(E)	(F)	(G)	(H)	(I)	(J)	(K)	(L)	(M)	(N)	(O)	(P)	(Q)	(R)	(S)
446	Plain, 3-in diam., 1 1/2 in high.	1 muffin	40	38	120	3	4	1.0	1.7	1.0	17	42	60	0.6	50	40	0.09	0.12	0.9	Trace
	From mix, egg, milk:																			
447	Corn, 2 3/8-in diam., 1 1/2 in high.[58]	1 muffin	40	30	130	3	4	1.2	1.7	.9	20	96	152	.6	44	[57]100	.08	.09	.7	Trace
448	Noodles (egg noodles), enriched, cooked.	1 cup	160	71	200	7	2	—	—	—	37	16	94	1.4	70	110	.22	.13	1.9	0
449	Noodles, chow mein, canned	1 cup	45	1	220	6	11	—	—	—	26	—	—	—	—	—	—	—	—	—
	Pancakes, (4-in diam.):[38]																			
450	Buckwheat, made from mix (with buckwheat and enriched flours), egg and milk added.	1 cake	27	58	55	2	2	.8	.9	.4	6	59	91	.4	66	60	.04	.05	.2	Trace
	Plain:																			
451	Made from home recipe using enriched flour.	1 cake	27	50	60	2	2	.5	.8	.5	9	27	38	.4	33	30	.06	.07	.5	Trace
452	Made from mix with enriched flour, egg and milk added.	1 cake	27	51	60	2	2	.7	.7	.3	9	58	70	.3	42	70	.04	.06	.2	Trace
	Pies, piecrust made with enriched flour, vegetable shortening (9-in diam.):																			
	Apple:																			
453	Whole	1 pie	945	48	2,420	21	105	27.0	44.5	25.2	360	76	208	6.6	756	280	1.06	.79	9.3	9
454	Sector, 1/7 of pie	1 sector	135	48	345	3	15	3.9	6.4	3.6	51	11	30	.9	108	40	.15	.11	1.3	2
	Banana cream:																			
455	Whole	1 pie	910	54	2,010	41	85	26.7	33.2	16.2	279	601	746	7.3	1,847	2,280	.77	1.51	7.0	9
456	Sector, 1/7 of pie	1 sector	130	54	285	6	12	3.8	4.7	2.3	40	86	107	1.0	264	330	.11	.22	1.0	1
	Blueberry:																			
457	Whole	1 pie	945	51	2,285	23	102	24.8	43.7	25.1	330	104	217	9.5	614	280	1.03	.80	10.0	28
458	Sector, 1/7 of pie	1 sector	135	51	325	3	15	3.5	6.2	3.6	47	15	31	1.4	88	40	.15	.11	1.4	4
	Cherry:																			
459	Whole	1 pie	945	47	2,465	25	107	28.2	45.0	25.3	363	132	236	6.6	992	4,160	1.09	.84	9.8	Trace
460	Sector, 1/7 of pie	1 sector	135	47	350	4	15	4.0	6.4	3.6	52	19	34	.9	142	590	.16	.12	1.4	Trace
	Custard:																			
461	Whole	1 pie	910	58	1,985	56	101	33.9	38.5	17.5	213	874	1,028	8.2	1,247	2,090	.79	1.92	5.6	0
462	Sector, 1/7 of pie	1 sector	130	58	285	8	14	4.8	5.5	2.5	30	125	147	1.2	178	300	.11	.27	.8	0
	Lemon meringue:																			
463	Whole	1 pie	840	47	2,140	31	86	26.1	33.8	16.4	317	118	412	6.7	420	1,430	.61	.84	5.2	25
464	Sector, 1/7 of pie	1 sector	120	47	305	4	12	3.7	4.8	2.3	45	17	59	1.0	60	200	.09	.12	.7	4
	Mince:																			
465	**Whole**	1 pie	945	43	2,560	24	109	28.0	45.9	25.2	389	265	359	13.3	1,682	20	.96	.86	9.8	9
466	**Sector, 1/7 of pie**	1 sector	135	43	365	3	16	4.0	6.6	3.6	56	38	51	1.9	240	Trace	.14	.12	1.4	1
	Peach:																			
467	**Whole**	1 pie	945	48	2,410	24	101	24.8	43.7	25.1	361	95	274	8.5	1,408	6,900	1.04	.97	14.0	28
468	**Sector, 1/7 of pie**	1 sector	135	48	345	3	14	3.5	6.2	3.6	52	14	39	1.2	201	990	.15	.14	2.0	4
	Pecan:																			
469	**Whole**	1 pie	825	20	3,450	42	189	27.8	101.0	44.2	423	388	850	25.6	1,015	1,320	1.80	.95	6.9	Trace
470	**Sector, 1/7 of pie**	1 sector	118	20	495	6	27	4.0	14.4	6.3	61	55	122	3.7	145	190	.26	.14	1.0	Trace
	Pumpkin:																			
471	Whole	1 pie	910	59	1,920	36	102	37.4	37.5	16.6	223	464	628	7.3	1,456	22,480	.78	1.27	7.0	Trace
472	Sector, 1/7 of pie	1 sector	130	59	275	5	15	5.4	5.4	2.4	32	66	90	1.0	208	3,210	.11	.18	1.0	Trace
473	Piecrust (home recipe) made with enriched flour and vegetable shortening, baked.	1 pie shell, 9-in diam.	180	15	900	11	60	14.8	26.1	14.9	79	25	90	3.1	89	0	.47	.40	5.0	0
474	Piecrust mix with enriched flour and vegetable shortening, 10-oz pkg. prepared and baked.	Piecrust for 2-crust pie, 9-in diam.	320	19	1,485	20	93	22.7	39.7	23.4	141	131	272	6.1	179	0	1.07	.79	9.9	0

[38]Made with vegetable shortening.
[50]Products are commercial unless otherwise specified.
[51]Made with enriched flour and vegetable shortening except for macaroons which do not contain flour or shortening.
[53]Applies to yellow varieties; white varieties contain only a trace.
[54]Contains vegetable shortening and butter.
[55]Made with corn oil.
[56]Made with regular margarine.
[57]Applies to product made with yellow cornmeal.
[58]Made with enriched degermed cornmeal and enriched flour.

TABLE 2.— NUTRITIVE VALUES OF THE EDIBLE PART OF FOODS - Continued

(Dashes (—) denote lack of reliable data for a constituent believed to be present in measurable amount)

Item No.	Foods, approximate measures, units, and weight (edible part unless footnotes indicate otherwise)			Water	Food energy	Protein	Fat	Fatty Acids: Saturated (total)	Fatty Acids: Unsaturated: Oleic	Fatty Acids: Unsaturated: Linoleic	Carbohydrate	Calcium	Phosphorus	Iron	Potassium	Vitamin A value	Thiamin	Riboflavin	Niacin	Ascorbic acid
(A)	(B)			(C)	(D)	(E)	(F)	(G)	(H)	(I)	(J)	(K)	(L)	(M)	(N)	(O)	(P)	(Q)	(R)	(S)
			Grams	Percent	Calories	Grams	Grams	Grams	Grams	Grams	Grams	Milligrams	Milligrams	Milligrams	Milligrams	International units	Milligrams	Milligrams	Milligrams	Milligrams
	GRAIN PRODUCTS—Con.																			
475	Pizza (cheese) baked, 4 3/4-in sector; 1/8 of 12-in diam. pie.[19]	1 sector	60	45	145	6	4	1.7	1.5	0.6	22	86	89	1.1	67	230	0.16	0.18	1.6	4
	Popcorn, popped:																			
476	Plain, large kernel	1 cup	6	4	25	1	Trace	Trace	.1	.2	5	1	17	.2	—	—	—	.01	.1	0
477	With oil (coconut) and salt added, large kernel.	1 cup	9	3	40	1	2	1.5	.2	.2	5	1	19	.2	—	—	—	.01	.2	0
478	Sugar coated	1 cup	35	4	135	2	1	.5	.2	.4	30	2	47	.5	—	—	—	.02	.4	0
	Pretzels, made with enriched flour:																			
479	Dutch, twisted, 2 3/4 by 2 5/8 in.	1 pretzel	16	5	60	2	1	—	—	—	12	4	21	.2	21	0	.05	.04	.7	0
480	Thin, twisted, 3 1/4 by 2 1/4 by 1/4 in.	10 pretzels	60	5	235	6	3	—	—	—	46	13	79	.9	78	0	.20	.15	2.5	0
481	Stick, 2 1/4 in long	10 pretzels	3	5	10	Trace	Trace	—	—	—	2	1	4	Trace	4	0	.01	.01	.1	0
	Rice, white, enriched:																			
482	Instant, ready-to-serve, hot	1 cup	165	73	180	4	Trace	Trace	Trace	Trace	40	5	31	1.3	—	0	.21	([59])	1.7	0
	Long grain:																			
483	Raw	1 cup	185	12	670	12	1	.2	.2	.2	149	44	174	5.4	170	0	.81	.06	6.5	0
484	Cooked, served hot	1 cup	205	73	225	4	Trace	.1	.1	.1	50	21	57	1.8	57	0	.23	.02	2.1	0
	Parboiled:																			
485	Raw	1 cup	185	10	685	14	1	.2	.1	.2	150	111	370	5.4	278	0	.81	.07	6.5	0
486	Cooked, served hot	1 cup	175	73	185	4	Trace	.1	.1	.1	41	33	100	1.4	75	0	.19	.02	2.1	0
	Rolls, enriched:[38]																			
	Commercial:																			
487	Brown-and-serve (12 per 12-oz pkg.), browned.	1 roll	26	27	85	2	2	.4	.7	.5	14	20	23	.5	25	Trace	.10	.06	.9	Trace
488	Cloverleaf or pan, 2 1/2-in diam., 2 in high.	1 roll	28	31	85	2	2	.4	.6	.4	15	21	24	.5	27	Trace	.11	.07	.9	Trace
489	Frankfurter and hamburger (8 per 11 1/2-oz pkg.).	1 roll	40	31	120	3	2	.5	.8	.6	21	30	34	.8	38	Trace	.16	.10	1.3	Trace
490	Hard, 3 3/4-in diam., 2 in high.	1 roll	50	25	155	5	2	.4	.6	.5	30	24	46	1.2	49	Trace	.20	.12	1.7	Trace
491	Hoagie or submarine, 11 1/2 by 3 by 2 1/2 in.	1 roll	135	31	390	12	4	.9	1.4	1.4	75	58	115	3.0	122	Trace	.54	.32	4.5	Trace
	From home recipe:																			
492	Cloverleaf, 2 1/2-in diam., 2 in high.	1 roll	35	26	120	3	3	.8	1.1	.7	20	16	36	.7	41	30	.12	.12	1.2	Trace
	Spaghetti, enriched, cooked:																			
493	Firm stage, "al dente," served hot.	1 cup	130	64	190	7	1	—	—	—	39	14	85	1.4	103	0	.23	.13	1.8	0
494	Tender stage, served hot	1 cup	140	73	155	5	1	—	—	—	32	11	70	1.3	85	0	.20	.11	1.5	0
	Spaghetti (enriched) in tomato sauce with cheese:																			
495	From home recipe	1 cup	250	77	260	9	9	2.0	5.4	.7	37	80	135	2.3	408	1,080	.25	.18	2.3	13
496	Canned	1 cup	250	80	190	6	2	.5	.3	.4	39	40	88	2.8	303	930	.35	.28	4.5	10
	Spaghetti (enriched) with meat balls and tomato sauce:																			
497	From home recipe	1 cup	248	70	330	19	12	3.3	6.3	.9	39	124	236	3.7	665	1,590	.25	.30	4.0	22
498	Canned	1 cup	250	78	260	12	10	2.2	3.3	3.9	29	53	113	3.3	245	1,000	.15	.18	2.3	5
499	Toaster pastries	1 pastry	50	12	200	3	6	—	—	—	36	[60]54	[60]67	1.9	[60]74	500	.16	.17	2.1	([60])
	Waffles, made with enriched flour, 7-in diam.:[38]																			
500	From home recipe	1 waffle	75	41	210	7	7	2.3	2.8	1.4	28	85	130	1.3	109	250	.17	.23	1.4	Trace
501	From mix, egg and milk added	1 waffle	75	42	205	7	8	2.8	2.9	1.2	27	179	257	1.0	146	170	.14	.22	.9	Trace

(A)	(B)			(C)	(D)	(E)	(F)	(G)	(H)	(I)	(J)	(K)	(L)	(M)	(N)	(O)	(P)	(Q)	(R)	(S)
	Wheat flours:																			
	All-purpose or family flour, enriched:																			
502	Sifted, spooned	1 cup	115	12	420	12	1	0.2	0.1	0.5	88	18	100	3.3	109	0	0.74	0.46	6.1	0
503	Unsifted, spooned	1 cup	125	12	455	13	1	.2	.1	.5	95	20	109	3.6	119	0	.80	.50	6.6	0
504	Cake or pastry flour, enriched, sifted, spooned.	1 cup	96	12	350	7	1	.1	.1	.3	76	16	70	2.8	91	0	.61	.38	5.1	0
505	Self-rising, enriched, unsifted, spooned.	1 cup	125	12	440	12	1	.2	.1	.5	93	331	583	3.6	—	0	.80	.50	6.6	0
506	Whole-wheat, from hard wheats, stirred.	1 cup	120	12	400	16	2	.4	.2	1.0	85	49	446	4.0	444	0	.66	.14	5.2	0
	LEGUMES (DRY), NUTS, SEEDS; RELATED PRODUCTS																			
	Almonds, shelled:																			
507	Chopped (about 130 almonds)	1 cup	130	5	775	24	70	5.6	47.7	12.8	25	304	655	6.1	1,005	0	.31	1.20	4.6	Trace
508	Slivered, not pressed down (about 115 almonds).	1 cup	115	5	690	21	62	5.0	42.2	11.3	22	269	580	5.4	889	0	.28	1.06	4.0	Trace
	Beans, dry:																			
	Common varieties as Great Northern, navy, and others:																			
	Cooked, drained:																			
509	Great Northern	1 cup	180	69	210	14	1	—	—	—	38	90	266	4.9	749	0	.25	.13	1.3	0
510	Pea (navy)	1 cup	190	69	225	15	1	—	—	—	40	95	281	5.1	790	0	.27	.13	1.3	0
	Canned, solids and liquid:																			
	White with—																			
511	Frankfurters (sliced)	1 cup	255	71	365	19	18	—	—	—	32	94	303	4.8	668	330	.18	.15	3.3	Trace
512	Pork and tomato sauce	1 cup	255	71	310	16	7	2.4	2.8	.6	48	138	235	4.6	536	330	.20	.08	1.5	5
513	Pork and sweet sauce	1 cup	255	66	385	16	12	4.3	5.0	1.1	54	161	291	5.9	—	—	.15	.10	1.3	—
514	Red kidney	1 cup	255	76	230	15	1	—	—	—	42	74	278	4.6	673	10	.13	.10	1.5	—
515	Lima, cooked, drained	1 cup	190	64	260	16	1	—	—	—	49	55	293	5.9	1,163	—	.25	.11	1.3	—
516	Blackeye peas, dry, cooked (with residual cooking liquid).	1 cup	250	80	190	13	1	—	—	—	35	43	238	3.3	573	30	.40	.10	1.0	—
517	Brazil nuts, shelled (6-8 large kernels).	1 oz	28	5	185	4	19	4.8	6.2	7.1	3	53	196	1.0	203	Trace	.27	.03	.5	—
518	Cashew nuts, roasted in oil	1 cup	140	5	785	24	64	12.9	36.8	10.2	41	53	522	5.3	650	140	.60	.35	2.5	—
	Coconut meat, fresh:																			
519	Piece, about 2 by 2 by 1/2 in	1 piece	45	51	155	2	16	14.0	.9	.3	4	6	43	.8	115	0	.02	.01	.2	1
520	Shredded or grated, not pressed down.	1 cup	80	51	275	3	28	24.8	1.6	.5	8	10	76	1.4	205	0	.04	.02	.4	2
521	Filberts (hazelnuts), chopped (about 80 kernels).	1 cup	115	6	730	14	72	5.1	55.2	7.3	19	240	388	3.9	810	—	.53	—	1.0	Trace
522	Lentils, whole, cooked	1 cup	200	72	210	16	Trace	—	—	—	39	50	238	4.2	498	40	.14	.12	1.2	0
523	Peanuts, roasted in oil, salted (whole, halves, chopped).	1 cup	144	2	840	37	72	13.7	33.0	20.7	27	107	577	3.0	971	—	.46	.19	24.8	0
524	Peanut butter	1 tbsp	16	2	95	4	8	1.5	3.7	2.3	3	9	61	.3	100	—	.02	.02	2.4	0
525	Peas, split, dry, cooked	1 cup	200	70	230	16	1	—	—	—	42	22	178	3.4	592	80	.30	.18	1.8	—
526	Pecans, chopped or pieces (about 120 large halves).	1 cup	118	3	810	11	84	7.2	50.5	20.0	17	86	341	2.8	712	150	1.01	.15	1.1	2
527	Pumpkin and squash kernels, dry, hulled.	1 cup	140	4	775	41	65	11.8	23.5	27.5	21	71	1,602	15.7	1,386	100	.34	.27	3.4	—
528	Sunflower seeds, dry, hulled	1 cup	145	5	810	35	69	8.2	13.7	43.2	29	174	1,214	10.3	1,334	70	2.84	.33	7.8	—
	Walnuts:																			
	Black:																			
529	Chopped or broken kernels	1 cup	125	3	785	26	74	6.3	13.3	45.7	19	Trace	713	7.5	575	380	.28	.14	.9	—
530	Ground (finely)	1 cup	80	3	500	16	47	4.0	8.5	29.2	12	Trace	456	4.8	368	240	.18	.09	.6	—
531	Persian or English, chopped (about 60 halves).	1 cup	120	4	780	18	77	8.4	11.8	42.2	19	119	456	3.7	540	40	.40	.16	1.1	2

[19] Crust made with vegetable shortening and enriched flour.
[38] Made with vegetable shortening.
[59] Product may or may not be enriched with riboflavin. Consult the label.
[60] Value varies with the brand. Consult the label.

TABLE 2.– NUTRITIVE VALUES OF THE EDIBLE PART OF FOODS - Continued

(Dashes (—) denote lack of reliable data for a constituent believed to be present in measurable amount)

Item No.	Foods, approximate measures, units, and weight (edible part unless footnotes indicate otherwise)			Water	Food energy	Protein	Fat	Fatty Acids: Saturated (total)	Fatty Acids: Unsaturated: Oleic	Fatty Acids: Unsaturated: Linoleic	Carbohydrate	Calcium	Phosphorus	Iron	Potassium	Vitamin A value	Thiamin	Riboflavin	Niacin	Ascorbic acid
(A)	(B)			(C)	(D)	(E)	(F)	(G)	(H)	(I)	(J)	(K)	(L)	(M)	(N)	(O)	(P)	(Q)	(R)	(S)
			Grams	Percent	Calories	Grams	Grams	Grams	Grams	Grams	Grams	Milligrams	Milligrams	Milligrams	Milligrams	International units	Milligrams	Milligrams	Milligrams	Milligrams
	SUGARS AND SWEETS																			
	Cake icings:																			
	Boiled, white:																			
532	Plain	1 cup	94	18	295	1	0	0	0	0	75	2	2	Trace	17	0	Trace	0.03	Trace	0
533	With coconut	1 cup	166	15	605	3	13	11.0	.9	Trace	124	10	50	0.8	277	0	0.02	.07	0.3	0
	Uncooked:																			
534	Chocolate made with milk and butter.	1 cup	275	14	1,035	9	38	23.4	11.7	1.0	185	165	305	3.3	536	580	.06	.28	.6	1
535	Creamy fudge from mix and water.	1 cup	245	15	830	7	16	5.1	6.7	3.1	183	96	218	2.7	238	Trace	.05	.20	.7	Trace
536	White	1 cup	319	11	1,200	2	21	12.7	5.1	.5	260	48	38	Trace	57	860	Trace	.06	Trace	Trace
	Candy:																			
537	Caramels, plain or chocolate	1 oz	28	8	115	1	3	1.6	1.1	.1	22	42	35	.4	54	Trace	.01	.05	.1	Trace
	Chocolate:																			
538	Milk, plain	1 oz	28	1	145	2	9	5.5	3.0	.3	16	65	65	.3	109	80	.02	.10	.1	Trace
539	Semisweet, small pieces (60 per oz).	1 cup or 6-oz pkg	170	1	860	7	61	36.2	19.8	1.7	97	51	255	4.4	553	30	.02	.14	.9	0
540	Chocolate-coated peanuts	1 oz	28	1	160	5	12	4.0	4.7	2.1	11	33	84	.4	143	Trace	.10	.05	2.1	Trace
541	Fondant, uncoated (mints, candy corn, other).	1 oz	28	8	105	Trace	1	.1	.3	.1	25	4	2	.3	1	0	Trace	Trace	Trace	0
542	Fudge, chocolate, plain	1 oz	28	8	115	1	3	1.3	1.4	.6	21	22	24	.3	42	Trace	.01	.03	.1	Trace
543	Gum drops	1 oz	28	12	100	Trace	Trace	—	—	—	25	2	Trace	.1	1	0	0	Trace	Trace	0
544	Hard	1 oz	28	1	110	0	Trace	—	—	—	28	6	2	.5	1	0	0	0	0	0
545	Marshmallows	1 oz	28	17	90	1	Trace	—	—	—	23	5	2	.5	2	0	0	Trace	Trace	0
	Chocolate-flavored beverage powders (about 4 heaping tsp per oz):																			
546	With nonfat dry milk	1 oz	28	2	100	5	1	.5	.3	Trace	20	167	155	.5	227	10	.04	.21	.2	1
547	Without milk	1 oz	28	1	100	1	1	.4	.2	Trace	25	9	48	.6	142	—	.01	.03	.1	0
548	Honey, strained or extracted	1 tbsp	21	17	65	Trace	0	0	0	0	17	1	1	.1	11	0	Trace	.01	.1	Trace
549	Jams and preserves	1 tbsp	20	29	55	Trace	Trace	—	—	—	14	4	2	.2	18	Trace	Trace	.01	Trace	Trace
550		1 packet	14	29	40	Trace	Trace	—	—	—	10	3	1	.1	12	Trace	Trace	Trace	Trace	Trace
551	Jellies	1 tbsp	18	29	50	Trace	Trace	—	—	—	13	4	1	.3	14	Trace	Trace	.01	Trace	1
552		1 packet	14	29	40	Trace	Trace	—	—	—	10	3	1	.2	11	Trace	Trace	Trace	Trace	1
	Sirups:																			
	Chocolate-flavored sirup or topping:																			
553	Thin type	1 fl oz or 2 tbsp	38	32	90	1	1	.5	.3	Trace	24	6	35	.6	106	Trace	.01	.03	.2	0
554	Fudge type	1 fl oz or 2 tbsp	38	25	125	2	5	3.1	1.6	.1	20	48	60	.5	107	60	.02	.08	.2	Trace
	Molasses, cane:																			
555	Light (first extraction)	1 tbsp	20	24	50	—	—	—	—	—	13	33	9	.9	183	—	.01	.01	Trace	—
556	Blackstrap (third extraction)	1 tbsp	20	24	45	—	—	—	—	—	11	137	17	3.2	585	—	.02	.04	.4	—
557	Sorghum	1 tbsp	21	23	55	—	—	—	—	—	14	35	5	2.6	—	—	—	.02	Trace	—
558	Table blends, chiefly corn, light and dark.	1 tbsp	21	24	60	0	0	0	0	0	15	9	3	.8	1	0	0	0	0	0
	Sugars:																			
559	Brown, pressed down	1 cup	220	2	820	0	0	0	0	0	212	187	42	7.5	757	0	.02	.07	.4	0
	White:																			
560	Granulated	1 cup	200	1	770	0	0	0	0	0	199	0	0	.2	6	0	0	0	0	0
561		1 tbsp	12	1	45	0	0	0	0	0	12	0	0	Trace	Trace	0	0	0	0	0
562		1 packet	6	1	23	0	0	0	0	0	6	0	0	Trace	Trace	0	0	0	0	0
563	Powdered, sifted, spooned into cup.	1 cup	100	1	385	0	0	0	0	0	100	0	0	.1	3	0	0	0	0	0

(A)	(B)			(C)	(D)	(E)	(F)	(G)	(H)	(I)	(J)	(K)	(L)	(M)	(N)	(O)	(P)	(Q)	(R)	(S)
	VEGETABLE AND VEGETABLE PRODUCTS																			
	Asparagus, green:																			
	Cooked, drained:																			
	Cuts and tips, 1 1/2- to 2-in lengths:																			
564	From raw--------------------	1 cup--------------------	145	94	30	3	Trace	—	—	—	5	30	73	0.9	265	1,310	0.23	0.26	2.0	38
565	From frozen-----------------	1 cup--------------------	180	93	40	6	Trace	—	—	—	6	40	115	2.2	396	1,530	.25	.23	1.8	41
	Spears, 1/2-in diam. at base:																			
566	From raw--------------------	4 spears-----------------	60	94	10	1	Trace	—	—	—	2	13	30	.4	110	540	.10	.11	.8	16
567	From frozen-----------------	4 spears-----------------	60	92	15	2	Trace	—	—	—	2	13	40	.7	143	470	.10	.08	.7	16
568	Canned, spears, 1/2-in diam. at base.	4 spears-----------------	80	93	15	2	Trace	—	—	—	3	15	42	1.5	133	640	.05	.08	.6	12
	Beans:																			
	Lima, immature seeds, frozen, cooked, drained:																			
569	Thick-seeded types (Fordhooks)	1 cup--------------------	170	74	170	10	Trace	—	—	—	32	34	153	2.9	724	390	.12	.09	1.7	29
570	Thin-seeded types (baby limas)	1 cup--------------------	180	69	210	13	Trace	—	—	—	40	63	227	4.7	709	400	.16	.09	2.2	22
	Snap:																			
	Green:																			
	Cooked, drained:																			
571	From raw (cuts and French style).	1 cup--------------------	125	92	30	2	Trace	—	—	—	7	63	46	.8	189	680	.09	.11	.6	15
	From frozen:																			
572	Cuts--------------------	1 cup--------------------	135	92	35	2	Trace	—	—	—	8	54	43	.9	205	780	.09	.12	.5	7
573	French style------------	1 cup--------------------	130	92	35	2	Trace	—	—	—	8	49	39	1.2	177	690	.08	.10	.4	9
574	Canned, drained solids (cuts).	1 cup--------------------	135	92	30	2	Trace	—	—	—	7	61	34	2.0	128	630	.04	.07	.4	5
	Yellow or wax:																			
	Cooked, drained:																			
575	From raw (cuts and French style).	1 cup--------------------	125	93	30	2	Trace	—	—	—	6	63	46	.8	189	290	.09	.11	.6	16
576	From frozen (cuts)--------	1 cup--------------------	135	92	35	2	Trace	—	—	—	8	47	42	.9	221	140	.09	.11	.5	8
577	Canned, drained solids (cuts).	1 cup--------------------	135	92	30	2	Trace	—	—	—	7	61	34	2.0	128	140	.04	.07	.4	7
	Beans, mature. See Beans, dry (items 509-515) and Blackeye peas, dry (item 516).																			
	Bean sprouts (mung):																			
578	Raw-------------------------	1 cup--------------------	105	89	35	4	Trace	—	—	—	7	20	67	1.4	234	20	.14	.14	.8	20
579	Cooked, drained-------------	1 cup--------------------	125	91	35	4	Trace	—	—	—	7	21	60	1.1	195	30	.11	.13	.9	8
	Beets:																			
	Cooked, drained, peeled:																			
580	Whole beets, 2-in diam.-------	2 beets------------------	100	91	30	1	Trace	—	—	—	7	14	23	.5	208	20	.03	.04	.3	6
581	Diced or sliced---------------	1 cup--------------------	170	91	55	2	Trace	—	—	—	12	24	39	.9	354	30	.05	.07	.5	10
	Canned, drained solids:																			
582	Whole beets, small-----------	1 cup--------------------	160	89	60	2	Trace	—	—	—	14	30	29	1.1	267	30	.02	.05	.2	5
583	Diced or sliced--------------	1 cup--------------------	170	89	65	2	Trace	—	—	—	15	32	31	1.2	284	30	.02	.05	.2	5
584	Beet greens, leaves and stems, cooked, drained.	1 cup--------------------	145	94	25	2	Trace	—	—	—	5	144	36	2.8	481	7,400	.10	.22	.4	22
	Blackeye peas, immature seeds, cooked and drained:																			
585	From raw--------------------	1 cup--------------------	165	72	180	13	1	—	—	—	30	40	241	3.5	625	580	.50	.18	2.3	28
586	From frozen-----------------	1 cup--------------------	170	66	220	15	1	—	—	—	40	43	286	4.8	573	290	.68	.19	2.4	15
	Broccoli, cooked, drained:																			
	From raw:																			
587	Stalk, medium size-----------	1 stalk------------------	180	91	45	6	1	—	—	—	8	158	112	1.4	481	4,500	.16	.36	1.4	162
588	Stalks cut into 1/2-in pieces-	1 cup--------------------	155	91	40	5	Trace	—	—	—	7	136	96	1.2	414	3,880	.14	.31	1.2	140
	From frozen:																			
589	Stalk, 4 1/2 to 5 in long-----	1 stalk------------------	30	91	10	1	Trace	—	—	—	1	12	17	.2	66	570	.02	.03	.2	22
590	Chopped----------------------	1 cup--------------------	185	92	50	5	1	—	—	—	9	100	104	1.3	392	4,810	.11	.22	.9	105
	Brussels sprouts, cooked, drained:																			
591	From raw, 7-8 sprouts (1 1/4- to 1 1/2-in diam.).	1 cup--------------------	155	88	55	7	1	—	—	—	10	50	112	1.7	423	810	.12	.22	1.2	135
592	From frozen-------------------	1 cup--------------------	155	89	50	5	Trace	—	—	—	10	33	95	1.2	457	880	.12	.16	.9	126

TABLE 2.— NUTRITIVE VALUES OF THE EDIBLE PART OF FOODS - Continued

(Dashes (—) denote lack of reliable data for a constituent believed to be present in measurable amount)

Item No.	Foods, approximate measures, units, and weight (edible part unless footnotes indicate otherwise)			Water	Food energy	Protein	Fat	Fatty Acids: Saturated (total)	Fatty Acids: Unsaturated Oleic	Fatty Acids: Unsaturated Linoleic	Carbohydrate	Calcium	Phosphorus	Iron	Potassium	Vitamin A value	Thiamin	Riboflavin	Niacin	Ascorbic acid
(A)	(B)			(C)	(D)	(E)	(F)	(G)	(H)	(I)	(J)	(K)	(L)	(M)	(N)	(O)	(P)	(Q)	(R)	(S)
			Grams	Percent	Calories	Grams	Grams	Grams	Grams	Grams	Grams	Milligrams	Milligrams	Milligrams	Milligrams	International units	Milligrams	Milligrams	Milligrams	Milligrams
	VEGETABLE AND VEGETABLE PRODUCTS—Con.																			
	Cabbage:																			
	Common varieties:																			
	Raw:																			
593	Coarsely shredded or sliced	1 cup	70	92	15	1	Trace	—	—	—	4	34	20	0.3	163	90	0.04	0.04	0.2	33
594	Finely shredded or chopped	1 cup	90	92	20	1	Trace	—	—	—	5	44	26	.4	210	120	.05	.05	.3	42
595	Cooked, drained	1 cup	145	94	30	2	Trace	—	—	—	6	64	29	.4	236	190	.06	.06	.4	48
596	Red, raw, coarsely shredded or sliced.	1 cup	70	90	20	1	Trace	—	—	—	5	29	25	.6	188	30	.06	.04	.3	43
597	Savoy, raw, coarsely shredded or sliced.	1 cup	70	92	15	2	Trace	—	—	—	3	47	38	.6	188	140	.04	.06	.2	39
598	Cabbage, celery (also called pe-tsai or wongbok), raw, 1-in pieces.	1 cup	75	95	10	1	Trace	—	—	—	2	32	30	.5	190	110	.04	.03	.5	19
599	Cabbage, white mustard (also called bokchoy or pakchoy), cooked, drained.	1 cup	170	95	25	2	Trace	—	—	—	4	252	56	1.0	364	5,270	.07	.14	1.2	26
	Carrots:																			
	Raw, without crowns and tips, scraped:																			
600	Whole, 7 1/2 by 1 1/8 in, or strips, 2 1/2 to 3 in long.	1 carrot or 18 strips	72	88	30	1	Trace	—	—	—	7	27	26	.5	246	7,930	.04	.04	.4	6
601	Grated	1 cup	110	88	45	1	Trace	—	—	—	11	41	40	.8	375	12,100	.07	.06	.7	9
602	Cooked (crosswise cuts), drained	1 cup	155	91	50	1	Trace	—	—	—	11	51	48	.9	344	16,280	.08	.08	.8	9
	Canned:																			
603	Sliced, drained solids	1 cup	155	91	45	1	Trace	—	—	—	10	47	34	1.1	186	23,250	.03	.05	.6	3
604	Strained or junior (baby food)	1 oz (1 3/4 to 2 tbsp)	28	92	10	Trace	Trace	—	—	—	2	7	6	.1	51	3,690	.01	.01	.1	1
	Cauliflower:																			
605	Raw, chopped	1 cup	115	91	31	3	Trace	—	—	—	6	29	64	1.3	339	70	.13	.12	.8	90
	Cooked, drained:																			
606	From raw (flower buds)	1 cup	125	93	30	3	Trace	—	—	—	5	26	53	.9	258	80	.11	.10	.8	69
607	From frozen (flowerets)	1 cup	180	94	30	3	Trace	—	—	—	6	31	68	.9	373	50	.07	.09	.7	74
	Celery, Pascal type, raw:																			
608	Stalk, large outer, 8 by 1 1/2 in, at root end.	1 stalk	40	94	5	Trace	Trace	—	—	—	2	16	11	.1	136	110	.01	.01	.1	4
609	Pieces, diced	1 cup	120	94	20	1	Trace	—	—	—	5	47	34	.4	409	320	.04	.04	.4	11
	Collards, cooked, drained:																			
610	From raw (leaves without stems)	1 cup	190	90	65	7	1	—	—	—	10	357	99	1.5	498	14,820	.21	.38	2.3	144
611	From frozen (chopped)	1 cup	170	90	50	5	1	—	—	—	10	299	87	1.7	401	11,560	.10	.24	1.0	56
	Corn, sweet:																			
	Cooked, drained:																			
612	From raw, ear 5 by 1 3/4 in	1 ear[61]	140	74	70	2	1	—	—	—	16	2	69	.5	151	[62]310	.09	.08	1.1	7
	From frozen:																			
613	Ear, 5 in long	1 ear[61]	229	73	120	4	1	—	—	—	27	4	121	1.0	291	[62]440	.18	.10	2.1	9
614	Kernels	1 cup	165	77	130	5	1	—	—	—	31	5	120	1.3	304	[62]580	.15	.10	2.5	8
	Canned:																			
615	Cream style	1 cup	256	76	210	5	2	—	—	—	51	8	143	1.5	248	[62]840	.08	.13	2.6	13
	Whole kernel:																			
616	Vacuum pack	1 cup	210	76	175	5	1	—	—	—	43	6	153	1.1	204	[62]740	.06	.13	2.3	11
617	Wet pack, drained solids	1 cup	165	76	140	4	1	—	—	—	33	8	81	.8	160	[62]580	.05	.08	1.5	7
	Cowpeas. See Blackeye peas. (Items 585-586).																			
	Cucumber slices, 1/8 in thick (large, 2 1/8-in diam.; small, 1 3/4-in diam.):																			
618	With peel	6 large or 8 small slices	28	95	5	Trace	Trace	—	—	—	1	7	8	.3	45	70	.01	.01	.1	3

(A)	(B)			(C)	(D)	(E)	(F)	(G)	(H)	(I)	(J)	(K)	(L)	(M)	(N)	(O)	(P)	(Q)	(R)	(S)
619	Without peel-------------------	6 1/2 large or 9 small pieces.	28	96	5	Trace	Trace	—	—	—	1	5	5	0.1	45	Trace	0.01	0.01	0.1	3
620	Dandelion greens, cooked, drained-	1 cup-------------------	105	90	35	2	1	—	—	—	7	147	44	1.9	244	12,290	.14	.17	—	19
621	Endive, curly (including escarole), raw, small pieces.	1 cup-------------------	50	93	10	1	Trace	—	—	—	2	41	27	.9	147	1,650	.04	.07	.3	5
	Kale, cooked, drained:																			
622	From raw (leaves without stems and midribs).	1 cup-------------------	110	88	45	5	1	—	—	—	7	206	64	1.8	243	9,130	.11	.20	1.8	102
623	From frozen (leaf style)--------	1 cup-------------------	130	91	40	4	1	—	—	—	7	157	62	1.3	251	10,660	.08	.20	.9	49
	Lettuce, raw:																			
	Butterhead, as Boston types:																			
624	Head, 5-in diam---------------	1 head[63]----------------	220	95	25	2	Trace	—	—	—	4	57	42	3.3	430	1,580	.10	.10	.5	13
625	Leaves------------------------	1 outer or 2 inner or 3 heart leaves.	15	95	Trace	Trace	Trace	—	—	—	Trace	5	4	.3	40	150	.01	.01	Trace	1
	Crisphead, as Iceberg:																			
626	Head, 6-in diam---------------	1 head[64]----------------	567	96	70	5	1	—	—	—	16	108	118	2.7	943	1,780	.32	.32	1.6	32
627	Wedge, 1/4 of head------------	1 wedge-----------------	135	96	20	1	Trace	—	—	—	4	27	30	.7	236	450	.08	.08	.4	8
628	Pieces, chopped or shredded---	1 cup-------------------	55	96	5	Trace	Trace	—	—	—	2	11	12	.3	96	180	.03	.03	.2	3
629	Looseleaf (bunching varieties including romaine or cos), chopped or shredded pieces.	1 cup-------------------	55	94	10	1	Trace	—	—	—	2	37	14	.8	145	1.050	.03	.04	.2	10
630	Mushrooms, raw, sliced or chopped-	1 cup-------------------	70	90	20	2	Trace	—	—	—	3	4	81	.6	290	Trace	.07	.32	2.9	2
631	Mustard greens, without stems and midribs, cooked, drained.	1 cup-------------------	140	93	30	3	1	—	—	—	6	193	45	2.5	308	8,120	.11	.20	.8	67
632	Okra pods, 3 by 5/8 in, cooked----	10 pods-----------------	106	91	30	2	Trace	—	—	—	6	98	43	.5	184	520	.14	.19	1.0	21
	Onions:																			
	Mature:																			
	Raw:																			
633	Chopped---------------------	1 cup-------------------	170	89	65	3	Trace	—	—	—	15	46	61	.9	267	[65]Trace	.05	.07	.3	17
634	Sliced----------------------	1 cup-------------------	115	89	45	2	Trace	—	—	—	10	31	41	.6	181	[65]Trace	.03	.05	.2	12
635	Cooked (whole or sliced), drained.	1 cup-------------------	210	92	60	3	Trace	—	—	—	14	50	61	.8	231	[65]Trace	.06	.06	.4	15
636	Young green, bulb (3/8 in diam.) and white portion of top.	6 onions----------------	30	88	15	Trace	Trace	—	—	—	3	12	12	.2	69	Trace	.02	.01	.1	8
637	Parsley, raw, chopped------------	1 tbsp------------------	4	85	Trace	Trace	Trace	—	—	—	Trace	7	2	.2	25	300	Trace	.01	Trace	6
638	Parsnips, cooked (diced or 2-in lengths).	1 cup-------------------	155	82	100	2	1	—	—	—	23	70	96	.9	587	50	.11	.12	.2	16
	Peas, green:																			
	Canned:																			
639	Whole, drained solids---------	1 cup-------------------	170	77	150	8	1	—	—	—	29	44	129	3.2	163	1,170	.15	.10	1.4	14
640	Strained (baby food)----------	1 oz (1 3/4 to 2 tbsp)--	28	86	15	1	Trace	—	—	—	3	3	18	.3	28	140	.02	.03	.3	3
641	Frozen, cooked, drained--------	1 cup-------------------	160	82	110	8	Trace	—	—	—	19	30	138	3.0	216	960	.43	.14	2.7	21
642	Peppers, hot, red, without seeds, dried (ground chili powder, added seasonings).	1 tsp-------------------	2	9	5	Trace	Trace	—	—	—	1	5	4	.3	20	1,300	Trace	.02	.2	Trace
	Peppers, sweet (about 5 per lb, whole), stem and seeds removed:																			
643	Raw----------------------------	1 pod-------------------	74	93	15	1	Trace	—	—	—	4	7	16	.5	157	310	.06	.06	.4	94
644	Cooked, boiled, drained--------	1 pod-------------------	73	95	15	1	Trace	—	—	—	3	7	12	.4	109	310	.05	.05	.4	70
	Potatoes, cooked:																			
645	Baked, peeled after baking (about 2 per lb, raw).	1 potato----------------	156	75	145	4	Trace	—	—	—	33	14	101	1.1	782	Trace	.15	.07	2.7	31
	Boiled (about 3 per lb, raw):																			
646	Peeled after boiling----------	1 potato----------------	137	80	105	3	Trace	—	—	—	23	10	72	.8	556	Trace	.12	.05	2.0	22
647	Peeled before boiling---------	1 potato----------------	135	83	90	3	Trace	—	—	—	20	8	57	.7	385	Trace	.12	.05	1.6	22
	French-fried, strip, 2 to 3 1/2 in long:																			
648	Prepared from raw------------	10 strips---------------	50	45	135	2	7	1.7	1.2	3.3	18	8	56	.7	427	Trace	.07	.04	1.6	11
649	Frozen, oven heated----------	10 strips---------------	50	53	110	2	4	1.1	.8	2.1	17	5	43	.9	326	Trace	.07	.01	1.3	11
650	Hashed brown, prepared from frozen.	1 cup-------------------	155	56	345	3	18	4.6	3.2	9.0	45	28	78	1.9	439	Trace	.11	.03	1.6	12
	Mashed, prepared from—																			
	Raw:																			
651	Milk added------------------	1 cup-------------------	210	83	135	4	2	.7	.4	Trace	27	50	103	8	548	40	.17	.11	2.1	21

[61]Weight includes cob. Without cob, weight is 77 g for item 612, 126 g for item 613.
[62]Based on yellow varieties. For white varieties, value is trace.
[63]Weight includes refuse of outer leaves and core. Without these parts, weight is 163 g.
[64]Weight includes core. Without core, weight is 539 g.
[65]Value based on white-fleshed varieties. For yellow-fleshed varieties, value in International Units (I.U.) is 70 for item 633, 50 for item 634, and 80 for item 635.

TABLE 2.— NUTRITIVE VALUES OF THE EDIBLE PART OF FOODS - Continued

(Dashes (—) denote lack of reliable data for a constituent believed to be present in measurable amount)

Item No. (A)	Foods, approximate measures, units, and weight (edible part unless footnotes indicate otherwise) (B)			Water (C)	Food energy (D)	Protein (E)	Fat (F)	Fatty Acids: Saturated (total) (G)	Fatty Acids: Unsaturated: Oleic (H)	Fatty Acids: Unsaturated: Linoleic (I)	Carbohydrate (J)	Calcium (K)	Phosphorus (L)	Iron (M)	Potassium (N)	Vitamin A value (O)	Thiamin (P)	Riboflavin (Q)	Niacin (R)	Ascorbic acid (S)
			Grams	Percent	Calories	Grams	Grams	Grams	Grams	Grams	Grams	Milligrams	Milligrams	Milligrams	Milligrams	International units	Milligrams	Milligrams	Milligrams	Milligrams
	VEGETABLE AND VEGETABLE PRODUCTS—Con.																			
	Potatoes, cooked—Continued																			
	Mashed, prepared from—Continued																			
	Raw-Continued																			
652	Milk and butter added-------	1 cup--------------------	210	80	195	4	9	5.6	2.3	0.2	26	50	101	0.8	525	360	0.17	0.11	2.1	19
653	Dehydrated flakes (without milk), water, milk, butter, and salt added.	1 cup--------------------	210	79	195	4	7	3.6	2.1	.2	30	65	99	.6	601	270	.08	.08	1.9	11
654	Potato chips, 1 3/4 by 2 1/2 in oval cross section.	10 chips----------------	20	2	115	1	8	2.1	1.4	4.0	10	8	28	.4	226	Trace	.04	.01	1.0	3
655	Potato salad, made with cooked salad dressing.	1 cup--------------------	250	76	250	7	7	2.0	2.7	1.3	41	80	160	1.5	798	350	.20	.18	2.8	28
656	Pumpkin, canned-------------------	1 cup--------------------	245	90	80	2	1	—	—	—	19	61	64	1.0	588	15,680	.07	.12	1.5	12
657	Radishes, raw (prepackaged) stem ends, rootlets cut off.	4 radishes---------------	18	95	5	Trace	Trace	—	—	—	1	5	6	.2	58	Trace	.01	.01	.1	5
658	Sauerkraut, canned, solids and liquid.	1 cup--------------------	235	93	40	2	Trace	—	—	—	9	85	42	1.2	329	120	.07	.09	.5	33
	Southern peas. See Blackeye peas (items 585-586).																			
	Spinach:																			
659	Raw, chopped--------------------	1 cup--------------------	55	91	15	2	Trace	—	—	—	2	51	28	1.7	259	4,460	.06	.11	.3	28
	Cooked, drained:																			
660	From raw-----------------------	1 cup--------------------	180	92	40	5	1	—	—	—	6	167	68	4.0	583	14,580	.13	.25	.9	50
	From frozen:																			
661	Chopped--------------------	1 cup--------------------	205	92	45	6	1	—	—	—	8	232	90	4.3	683	16,200	.14	.31	.8	39
662	Leaf-----------------------	1 cup--------------------	190	92	45	6	1	—	—	—	7	200	84	4.8	688	15,390	.15	.27	1.0	53
663	Canned, drained solids----------	1 cup--------------------	205	91	50	6	1	—	—	—	7	242	53	5.3	513	16,400	.04	.25	.6	29
	Squash, cooked:																			
664	Summer (all varieties), diced, drained.	1 cup--------------------	210	96	30	2	Trace	—	—	—	7	53	53	.8	296	820	.11	.17	1.7	21
665	Winter (all varieties), baked, mashed.	1 cup--------------------	205	81	130	4	1	—	—	—	32	57	98	1.6	945	8,610	.10	.27	1.4	27
	Sweetpotatoes:																			
	Cooked (raw, 5 by 2 in; about 2 1/2 per lb):																			
666	Baked in skin, peeled---------	1 potato-----------------	114	64	160	2	1	—	—	—	37	46	66	1.0	342	9,230	.10	.08	.8	25
667	Boiled in skin, peeled--------	1 potato-----------------	151	71	170	3	1	—	—	—	40	48	71	1.1	367	11,940	.14	.09	.9	26
668	Candied, 2 1/2 by 2-in piece----	1 piece------------------	105	60	175	1	3	2.0	.8	.1	36	39	45	.9	200	6,620	.06	.04	.4	11
	Canned:																			
669	Solid pack (mashed)-----------	1 cup--------------------	255	72	275	5	1	—	—	—	63	64	105	2.0	510	19,890	.13	.10	1.5	36
670	Vacuum pack, piece 2 3/4 by 1 in.	1 piece------------------	40	72	45	1	Trace	—	—	—	10	10	16	.3	80	3,120	.02	.02	.2	6
	Tomatoes:																			
671	Raw, 2 3/5-in diam. (3 per 12 oz pkg.).	1 tomato[66]---------------	135	94	25	1	Trace	—	—	—	6	16	33	.6	300	1,110	.07	.05	.9	[67]28
672	Canned, solids and liquid-------	1 cup--------------------	241	94	50	2	Trace	—	—	—	10	[68]14	46	1.2	523	2,170	.12	.07	1.7	41
673	Tomato catsup--------------------	1 cup--------------------	273	69	290	5	1	—	—	—	69	60	137	2.2	991	3,820	.25	.19	4.4	41
674		1 tbsp-------------------	15	69	15	Trace	Trace	—	—	—	4	3	8	.1	54	210	.01	.01	.2	2
	Tomato juice, canned:																			
675	Cup----------------------------	1 cup--------------------	243	94	45	2	Trace	—	—	—	10	17	44	2.2	552	1,940	.12	.07	1.9	39
676	Glass (6 fl oz)-----------------	1 glass------------------	182	94	35	2	Trace	—	—	—	8	13	33	1.6	413	1,460	.09	.05	1.5	29
677	Turnips, cooked, diced------------	1 cup--------------------	155	94	35	1	Trace	—	—	—	8	54	37	.6	291	Trace	.06	.08	.5	34
	Turnip greens, cooked, drained:																			
678	From raw (leaves and stems)-----	1 cup--------------------	145	94	30	3	Trace	—	—	—	5	252	49	1.5	—	8,270	.15	.33	.7	68
679	From frozen (chopped)-----------	1 cup--------------------	165	93	40	4	Trace	—	—	—	6	195	64	2.6	246	11,390	.08	.15	.7	31
680	Vegetables, mixed, frozen, cooked-	1 cup--------------------	182	83	115	6	1	—	—	—	24	46	115	2.4	348	9,010	.22	.13	2.0	15

MISCELLANEOUS ITEMS

(A)	(B)			(C)	(D)	(E)	(F)	(G)	(H)	(I)	(J)	(K)	(L)	(M)	(N)	(O)	(P)	(Q)	(R)	(S)
	Baking powders for home use:																			
	Sodium aluminum sulfate:																			
681	With monocalcium phosphate monohydrate.	1 tsp	3.0	2	5	Trace	Trace	0	0	0	1	58	87	—	5	0	0	0	0	0
682	With monocalcium phosphate monohydrate, calcium sulfate.	1 tsp	2.9	1	5	Trace	Trace	0	0	0	1	183	45	—	—	0	0	0	0	0
683	Straight phosphate	1 tsp	3.8	2	5	Trace	Trace	0	0	0	1	239	359	—	6	0	0	0	0	0
684	Low sodium	1 tsp	4.3	2	5	Trace	Trace	0	0	0	2	207	314	—	471	0	0	0	0	0
685	Barbecue sauce	1 cup	250	81	230	4	17	2.2	4.3	10.0	20	53	50	2.0	435	900	.03	.03	.8	13
	Beverages, alcoholic:																			
686	Beer	12 fl oz	360	92	150	1	0	0	0	0	14	18	108	Trace	90	—	.01	.11	2.2	—
	Gin, rum, vodka, whisky:																			
687	80-proof	1 1/2-fl oz jigger	42	67	95	—	—	0	0	0	Trace	—	—	—	1	—	—	—	—	—
688	86-proof	1 1/2-fl oz jigger	42	64	105	—	—	0	0	0	Trace	—	—	—	1	—	—	—	—	—
689	90-proof	1 1/2-fl oz jigger	42	62	110	—	—	0	0	0	Trace	—	—	—	1	—	—	—	—	—
	Wines:																			
690	Dessert	3 1/2-fl oz glass	103	77	140	Trace	0	0	0	0	8	8	—	—	77	—	.01	.02	.2	—
691	Table	3 1/2-fl oz glass	102	86	85	Trace	0	0	0	0	4	9	10	.4	94	—	Trace	.01	.1	—
	Beverages, carbonated, sweetened, nonalcoholic:																			
692	Carbonated water	12 fl oz	366	92	115	0	0	0	0	0	29	—	—	—	—	0	0	0	0	0
693	Cola type	12 fl oz	369	90	145	0	0	0	0	0	37	—	—	—	—	0	0	0	0	0
694	Fruit-flavored sodas and Tom Collins mixer.	12 fl oz	372	88	170	0	0	0	0	0	45	—	—	—	—	0	0	0	0	0
695	Ginger ale	12 fl oz	366	92	115	0	0	0	0	0	29	—	—	—	0	0	0	0	0	0
696	Root beer	12 fl oz	370	90	150	0	0	0	0	0	39	—	—	—	0	0	0	0	0	0
	Chili powder. See Peppers, hot, red (item 642).																			
	Chocolate:																			
697	Bitter or baking	1 oz	28	2	145	3	15	8.9	4.9	.4	8	22	109	1.9	235	20	.01	.07	.4	0
	Semisweet, see Candy, chocolate (item 539).																			
698	Gelatin, dry	1,7-g envelope	7	13	25	6	Trace	0	0	0	0	—	—	—	—	—	—	—	—	—
699	Gelatin dessert prepared with gelatin dessert powder and water.	1 cup	240	84	140	4	0	0	0	0	34	—	—	—	—	—	—	—	—	—
700	Mustard, prepared, yellow	1 tsp or individual serving pouch or cup.	5	80	5	Trace	Trace	—	—	—	Trace	4	4	.1	7	—	—	—	—	—
	Olives, pickled, canned:																			
701	Green	4 medium or 3 extra large or 2 giant.[69]	16	78	15	Trace	2	.2	1.2	.1	Trace	8	2	.2	7	40	—	—	—	—
702	Ripe, Mission	3 small or 2 large[69]	10	73	15	Trace	2	.2	1.2	.1	Trace	9	1	.1	2	10	Trace	Trace	—	—
	Pickles, cucumber:																			
703	Dill, medium, whole, 3 3/4 in long, 1 1/4-in diam.	1 pickle	65	93	5	Trace	Trace	—	—	—	1	17	14	.7	130	70	Trace	.01	Trace	4
704	Fresh-pack, slices 1 1/2-in diam., 1/4 in thick.	2 slices	15	79	10	Trace	Trace	—	—	—	3	5	4	.3	—	20	Trace	Trace	Trace	1
705	Sweet, gherkin, small, whole, about 2 1/2 in long, 3/4-in diam.	1 pickle	15	61	20	Trace	Trace	—	—	—	5	2	2	.2	—	10	Trace	Trace	Trace	1
706	Relish, finely chopped, sweet	1 tbsp	15	63	20	Trace	Trace	—	—	—	5	3	2	.1	—	—	—	—	—	—
	Popcorn. See items 476-478.																			
707	Popsicle, 3-fl oz size	1 popsicle	95	80	70	0	0	0	0	0	18	0	—	Trace	—	0	0	0	0	0

[66] Weight includes cores and stem ends. Without these parts, weight is 123 g.
[67] Based on year-round average. For tomatoes marketed from November through May, value is about 12 mg; from June through October, 32 mg.
[68] Applies to product without calcium salts added. Value for products with calcium salts added may be as much as 63 mg for whole tomatoes, 241 mg for cut forms.
[69] Weight includes pits. Without pits, weight is 13 g for item 701, 9 g for item 702.

TABLE 2.– NUTRITIVE VALUES OF THE EDIBLE PART OF FOODS - Continued

(Dashes (–) denote lack of reliable data for a constituent believed to be present in measurable amount)

Item No. (A)	Foods, approximate measures, units, and weight (edible part unless footnotes indicate otherwise) (B)			Water (C)	Food energy (D)	Protein (E)	Fat (F)	Fatty Acids: Saturated (total) (G)	Fatty Acids: Unsaturated: Oleic (H)	Fatty Acids: Unsaturated: Linoleic (I)	Carbohydrate (J)	Calcium (K)	Phosphorus (L)	Iron (M)	Potassium (N)	Vitamin A value (O)	Thiamin (P)	Riboflavin (Q)	Niacin (R)	Ascorbic acid (S)
			Grams	Percent	Calories	Grams	Grams	Grams	Grams	Grams	Grams	Milligrams	Milligrams	Milligrams	Milligrams	International units	Milligrams	Milligrams	Milligrams	Milligrams
	MISCELLANEOUS ITEMS–Con.																			
	Soups:																			
	Canned, condensed:																			
	Prepared with equal volume of milk:																			
708	Cream of chicken	1 cup	245	85	180	7	10	4.2	3.6	1.3	15	172	152	0.5	260	610	0.05	0.27	0.7	2
709	Cream of mushroom	1 cup	245	83	215	7	14	5.4	2.9	4.6	16	191	169	.5	279	250	.05	.34	.7	1
710	Tomato	1 cup	250	84	175	7	7	3.4	1.7	1.0	23	168	155	.8	418	1,200	.10	.25	1.3	15
	Prepared with equal volume of water:																			
711	Bean with pork	1 cup	250	84	170	8	6	1.2	1.8	2.4	22	63	128	2.3	395	650	.13	.08	1.0	3
712	Beef broth, bouillon, consomme.	1 cup	240	96	30	5	0	0	0	0	3	Trace	31	.5	130	Trace	Trace	.02	1.2	—
713	Beef noodle	1 cup	240	93	65	4	3	.6	.7	.8	7	7	48	1.0	77	50	.05	.07	1.0	Trace
714	Clam chowder, Manhattan type (with tomatoes, without milk).	1 cup	245	92	80	2	3	.5	.4	1.3	12	34	47	1.0	184	880	.02	.02	1.0	—
715	Cream of chicken	1 cup	240	92	95	3	6	1.6	2.3	1.1	8	24	34	.5	79	410	.02	.05	.5	Trace
716	Cream of mushroom	1 cup	240	90	135	2	10	2.6	1.7	4.6	10	41	50	.5	98	70	.02	.12	.7	Trace
717	Minestrone	1 cup	245	90	105	5	3	.7	.9	1.3	14	37	59	1.0	314	2,350	.07	.05	1.0	—
718	Split pea	1 cup	245	85	145	9	3	1.1	1.2	.4	21	29	149	1.5	270	440	.25	.15	1.5	1
719	Tomato	1 cup	245	91	90	2	3	.5	.5	1.0	16	15	34	.7	230	1,000	.05	.05	1.2	12
720	Vegetable beef	1 cup	245	92	80	5	2	—	—	—	10	12	49	.7	162	2,700	.05	.05	1.0	—
721	Vegetarian	1 cup	245	92	80	2	2	—	—	—	13	20	39	1.0	172	2,940	.05	.05	1.0	—
	Dehydrated:																			
722	Bouillon cube, 1/2 in	1 cube	4	4	5	1	Trace	—	—	—	Trace	—	—	—	4	—	—	—	—	—
	Mixes:																			
	Unprepared:																			
723	Onion	1 1/2-oz pkg	43	3	150	6	5	1.1	2.3	1.0	23	42	49	.6	238	30	.05	.03	.3	6
	Prepared with water:																			
724	Chicken noodle	1 cup	240	95	55	2	1	—	—	—	8	7	19	.2	19	50	.07	.05	.5	Trace
725	Onion	1 cup	240	96	35	1	1	—	—	—	6	10	12	.2	58	Trace	Trace	Trace	Trace	2
726	Tomato vegetable with noodles.	1 cup	240	93	65	1	1	—	—	—	12	7	19	.2	29	480	.05	.02	.5	5
727	Vinegar, cider	1 tbsp	15	94	Trace	Trace	0	0	0	0	1	1	1	.1	15	—	—	—	—	—
728	White sauce, medium, with enriched flour.	1 cup	250	73	405	10	31	19.3	7.8	.8	22	288	233	.5	348	1,150	.12	.43	.7	2
	Yeast:																			
729	Baker's, dry, active	1 pkg	7	5	20	3	Trace	—	—	—	3	3	90	1.1	140	Trace	.16	.38	2.6	Trace
730	Brewer's, dry	1 tbsp	8	5	25	3	Trace	—	—	—	3	[70]17	140	1.4	152	Trace	1.25	.34	3.0	Trace

[70]Value may vary from 6 to 60 mg.

FOOD AND NUTRITION BOARD, NATIONAL ACADEMY OF SCIENCES–NATIONAL RESEARCH COUNCIL
RECOMMENDED DAILY DIETARY ALLOWANCES,[a] Revised 1980

Designed for the maintenance of good nutrition of practically all healthy people in the U.S.A.

							Fat-Soluble Vitamins			Water-Soluble Vitamins							Minerals					
	Age	Weight		Height		Protein	Vitamin A	Vitamin D	Vitamin E	Vitamin C	Thiamin	Riboflavin	Niacin	Vitamin B-6	Folacin[f]	Vitamin B-12	Calcium	Phosphorus	Magnesium	Iron	Zinc	Iodine
	(years)	(kg)	(lb)	(cm)	(in)	(g)	(μg RE)[b]	(μg)[c]	(mg α-TE)[d]	(mg)	(mg)	(mg)	(mg NE)[e]	(mg)	(μg)	(μg)	(mg)	(mg)	(mg)	(mg)	(mg)	(μg)
Infants	0.0–0.5	6	13	60	24	kg × 2.2	420	10	3	35	0.3	0.4	6	0.3	30	0.5[g]	360	240	50	10	3	40
	0.5–1.0	9	20	71	28	kg × 2.0	400	10	4	35	0.5	0.6	8	0.6	45	1.5	540	360	70	15	5	50
Children	1–3	13	29	90	35	23	400	10	5	45	0.7	0.8	9	0.9	100	2.0	800	800	150	15	10	70
	4–6	20	44	112	44	30	500	10	6	45	0.9	1.0	11	1.3	200	2.5	800	800	200	10	10	90
	7–10	28	62	132	52	34	700	10	7	45	1.2	1.4	16	1.6	300	3.0	800	800	250	10	10	120
Males	11–14	45	99	157	62	45	1000	10	8	50	1.4	1.6	18	1.8	400	3.0	1200	1200	350	18	15	150
	15–18	66	145	176	69	56	1000	10	10	60	1.4	1.7	18	2.0	400	3.0	1200	1200	400	18	15	150
	19–22	70	154	177	70	56	1000	7.5	10	60	1.5	1.7	19	2.2	400	3.0	800	800	350	10	15	150
	23–50	70	154	178	70	56	1000	5	10	60	1.4	1.6	18	2.2	400	3.0	800	800	350	10	15	150
	51+	70	154	178	70	56	1000	5	10	60	1.2	1.4	16	2.2	400	3.0	800	800	350	10	15	150
Females	11–14	46	101	157	62	46	800	10	8	50	1.1	1.3	15	1.8	400	3.0	1200	1200	300	18	15	150
	15–18	55	120	163	64	46	800	10	8	60	1.1	1.3	14	2.0	400	3.0	1200	1200	300	18	15	150
	19–22	55	120	163	64	44	800	7.5	8	60	1.1	1.3	14	2.0	400	3.0	800	800	300	18	15	150
	23–50	55	120	163	64	44	800	5	8	60	1.0	1.2	13	2.0	400	3.0	800	800	300	18	15	150
	51+	55	120	163	64	44	800	5	8	60	1.0	1.2	13	2.0	400	3.0	800	800	300	10	15	150
Pregnant						+30	+200	+5	+2	+20	+0.4	+0.3	+2	+0.6	+400	+1.0	+400	+400	+150	*h*	+5	+25
Lactating						+20	+400	+5	+3	+40	+0.5	+0.5	+5	+0.5	+100	+1.0	+400	+400	+150	*h*	+10	+50

[a] The allowances are intended to provide for individual variations among most normal persons as they live in the United States under usual environmental stresses. Diets should be based on a variety of common foods in order to provide other nutrients for which human requirements have been less well defined. See text for detailed discussion of allowances and of nutrients not tabulated. See Table 1 for weights and heights by individual year of age. See Table 3 for suggested average energy intakes.

[b] Retinol equivalents. 1 retinol equivalent = 1 μg retinol or 6 μg β carotene. See text for calculation of vitamin A activity of diets as retinol equivalents.

[c] As cholecalciferol. 10 μg cholecalciferol = 400 IU of vitamin D.

[d] α-tocopherol equivalents. 1 mg *d*-α tocopherol = 1 α-TE. See text for variation in allowances and calculation of vitamin E activity of the diet as α-tocopherol equivalents.

[e] 1 NE (niacin equivalent) is equal to 1 mg of niacin or 60 mg of dietary tryptophan.

[f] The folacin allowances refer to dietary sources as determined by *Lactobacillus casei* assay after treatment with enzymes (conjugases) to make polyglutamyl forms of the vitamin available to the test organism.

[g] The recommended dietary allowance for vitamin B-12 in infants is based on average concentration of the vitamin in human milk. The allowances after weaning are based on energy intake (as recommended by the American Academy of Pediatrics) and consideration of other factors, such as intestinal absorption; see text.

[h] The increased requirement during pregnancy cannot be met by the iron content of habitual American diets nor by the existing iron stores of many women; therefore the use of 30–60 mg of supplemental iron is recommended. Iron needs during lactation are not substantially different from those of nonpregnant women, but continued supplementation of the mother for 2–3 months after parturition is advisable in order to replenish stores depleted by pregnancy.

Food sources of additional nutrients

Vitamins

Vitamin B_6

Bananas

Whole-grain cereals

Chicken

Dry legumes

Most dark-green leafy vegetables

Most fish and shellfish

Muscle meats, liver and kidney

Peanuts, walnuts, filberts, and peanut butter

Potatoes and sweetpotatoes

Prunes and raisins

Yeast

Vitamin B_{12}

(present in foods of animal origin only)

Kidney

Liver

Meat

Milk

Most cheese

Most fish

Shellfish

Whole egg and egg yolk

Vitamin D

Vitamin D milks

Egg yolk

Saltwater fish

Liver

Vitamin E

Vegetable oils

Margarine

Whole-grain cereals

Peanuts

Folacin

Liver

Dark-green vegetables

Dry beans

Peanuts

Wheat germ

Minerals

Iodine

Iodized salt

Seafood

Magnesium

Bananas

Whole-grain cereals

Dry beans

Milk

Most dark-green vegetables

Nuts

Peanuts and peanut butter

Zinc

Shellfish

Meat

Poultry

Cheese

Whole-grain cereals

Dry beans

Cocoa

Nuts

Conserving Nutritive Values in Foods

The great variety of foods available today makes it possible for the homemaker to select foods that provide the vitamins, minerals, protein, and other food nutrients needed for the good health of her family.

This calls attention to some of the important nutrients in foods that are affected by different practices of handling and preparation and suggests ways in which these nutrients can best be conserved in the home.

Such information affords guidelines for meal planning and preparation that will assure overall adequacy of the diet while allowing for individual preferences in the selection of foods and the form in which they are served.

Foods differ in their content of the nutrients known to be essential in nutrition. Some foods are very rich sources of one nutrient, and supply only small amounts of others; some foods are valuable sources of many nutrients.

Nutrients in foods vary greatly in their stability. Some nutrients, such as carbohydrate, are not affected to any great extent by ordinary handling. Other nutrients, such as vitamin C (ascorbic acid), are readily lost from some foods, although stable in others. Vitamin C is soluble in water; air and heat hasten its loss.

Because vitamin C is more easily destroyed than other food values, conservation of vitamin C is often used as an index to the retention of other nutrients. Measures that protect vitamin C usually protect other nutrients. Many improvements in ways of handling and processing fruits and vegetables have resulted from vitamin C research.

Fortunately some of the most important sources of vitamin C—citrus fruits and tomatoes—retain this nutrient very well.

VEGETABLES

Vegetables — fresh, frozen or canned — provide a year-round source of vitamins C and A. They also provide several valuable minerals, particularly calcium and iron. *To conserve food values and flavor, trim, store, and cook vegetables with care.*

Trimming

Fresh vegetables usually need some trimming, peeling, or scraping before they are cooked or served to remove damaged leaves, bruised spots, skins and inedible parts.

Different parts of the plant differ in nutrient content. For example, the leafy parts of collard greens, turnip greens, and kale have much more vitamin A value than the stems or midribs. If the fibrous

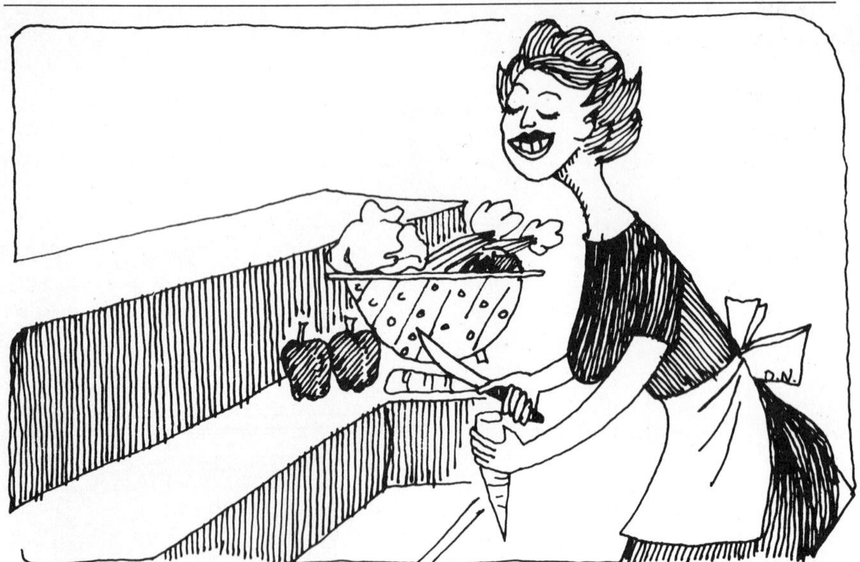

stems and midribs are removed, little loss of nutrients occurs. Such trimming is worthwhile if it makes the nutritious parts of these vegetables more acceptable to the family.

Outer green leaves of lettuce are coarser than the inner, tender leaves, but have higher calcium, iron, and vitamin A value. Use the outer leaves whenever possible.

In trimming cabbage, keep in mind that the core, as well as the leaves, is high in vitamin C.

Broccoli leaves have much higher vitamin A value than the stalks or flower buds. If broccoli leaves are tender when you get them home, plan to eat them; keep them cool and moist until you can use them.

Losses of vitamins A and C occur when vegetable tissues are bruised. To prevent bruising use a sharp blade when trimming, cutting, or shredding fresh vegetables.

Storing

Proper storage of fresh vegetables helps conserve their original food values. The length of time raw vegetables are stored, as well as storage temperature and humidity, affects retention of their nutrients.

Vegetables such as *kale, spinach, broccoli, turnip greens, chard, and salad greens* need to be refrigerated promptly in the vegetable crisper or in moisture-proof bags. They keep their nutrients best at near-freezing temperature and at high humidity.

Cabbage—a more stable source of vitamin C than most leafy vegetables—should not be allowed to dry out. If it is to be held at home for a few days, it should be wrapped or put in the vegetable crisper of the refrigerator, where the humidity is high. Stored in this way, cabbage holds its vitamin C well.

Green peas and green lima beans hold their nutrients better if left in their pods until ready to use. If shelled, put them into plastic bags before storing in the refrigerator.

Tomatoes bought or picked before they turn red keep their nutrients best if they are ripened out of the sun at temperatures from 60° to 75° F. Do not ripen tomatoes on a hot window sill or in the refrigerator. The bright-red color does not develop when the (ripening) temperature goes above 85° for very long. Tomatoes become soft and watery and subject to decay if ripened in the refrigerator.

Ripe, firm tomatoes, held in the refrigerator or at a cool room temperature for several days, do not lose much vitamin C. When they become overripe, the loss of vitamin C is increased.

Carrots, sweetpotatoes, potatoes, and other roots and tubers retain their most important food values reasonably well if they are kept cool and moist enough to prevent withering.

Cooking

Methods

One of the best methods of cooking vegetables to conserve maximum food values is to cook them only until tender in just enough water to prevent scorching. Use a pan with a tight-fitting lid. Covering the pan helps prevent the escape of steam and vapor so that vegetables can be cooked quickly in a small amount of water.

The amount of water used in cooking vegetables is of major importance in preventing loss of water-soluble nutrients, such as vitamin C, the B vitamins, and some of the minerals. The smaller the amount of water used in cooking, the more food value retained in the cooked vegetable.

If the amount of water used in cooking cabbage equals about one-third the amount of cabbage, 90 percent of the vitamin C will be retained. If a larger amount of water is used—for instance, four times as much water as cabbage—the retention of vitamin C drops to less than 50 percent.

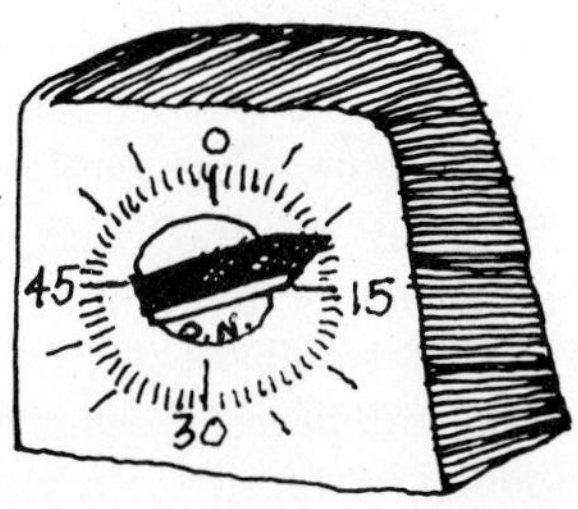

So-called "waterless" cooking refers to cooking vegetables with only the water that remains on the vegetables after rinsing and the juice extracted from the vegetables. This method does not permit quick cooking, however, and conserves nutritive values no better than cooking vegetables quickly in a small amount of water.

Boiling root and tuber vegetables (carrots, sweetpotatoes, potatoes) in their skins retains more vitamins and minerals than cooking these vegetables pared and cut.

Tests show that potatoes boiled whole in their skins retain practically all of their vitamin C, thiamin, and other nutrients.

Baking potatoes and sweetpotatoes whole in their skins also conserves the nutritive values of these vegetables well.

Panning is a quick way of cooking vegetables in a covered frying pan with a small amount of fat or meat drippings. This is a good method for conserving the nutrients in succulent vegetables, such as cabbage, summer squash, kale, and collards.

Steaming under pressure in a pressure saucepan is a quick and satisfactory method of vegetable cookery—particularly for potatoes, turnips, and carrots—if the cooking period is carefully timed. This is also a practical way to cook the dry legumes, such as dry peas, beans, and lima beans. Prolonged cooking under pressure often results in loss of food value.

Equipment

Expensive equipment is not essential for cooking vegetables or other foods to conserve their nutrients. A utensil that has a lid that fits tightly and is heavy enough to prevent the escape of vapor and steam is suitable for cooking with a minimum amount of added water.

The kind of material (aluminum,

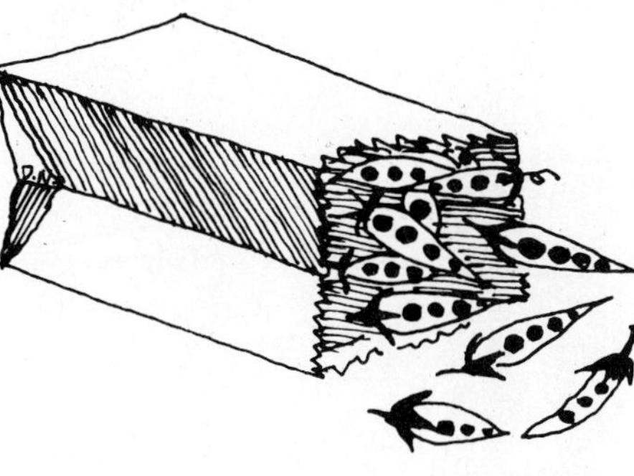

enamel, glass, stainless steel) of which modern cooking utensils are made is not important in conserving the nutritive values of the foods cooked in them. In the old-style copper utensil, the copper was in direct contact with food and hastened the oxidation of vitamin C. This, however, does not apply to modern pans with copper-plated bottoms because the inside cooking surface is made of another metal.

Holding and Reheating

To save time you may like to cook enough food for later meals, but this saving is at the expense of nutrients. Holding and reheating cooked vegetables cause additional losses of nutrients, particularly of vitamin C.

Vitamin C losses in cooked vegetables increase with the length of time they are held. They have about three-fourths as much vitamin C after 1 day in the refrigerator as when freshly cooked; about two-thirds as much after 2 days.

Cooked vegetables reheated after 2 or 3 days in the refrigerator can be depended on for only one-third to one-half as much vitamin C as when freshly prepared.

These losses need not cause concern if your meals include other, more dependable sources of vitamin C each day.

FRUITS AND FRUIT JUICES

Many kinds of fruit once considered luxuries now are eaten regularly. Some are mainstay sources of vitamin C and a few are good sources of vitamin A value. Fruits, and the juices made from them, also supply small amounts of other vitamins, and some calcium and iron.

Fruits are low in sodium, which makes them especially desirable for persons on low-sodium diets.

Vitamin A value varies from fruit to fruit. Fruits high in vitamin A value include apricots, yellow-fleshed peaches, cantaloups of

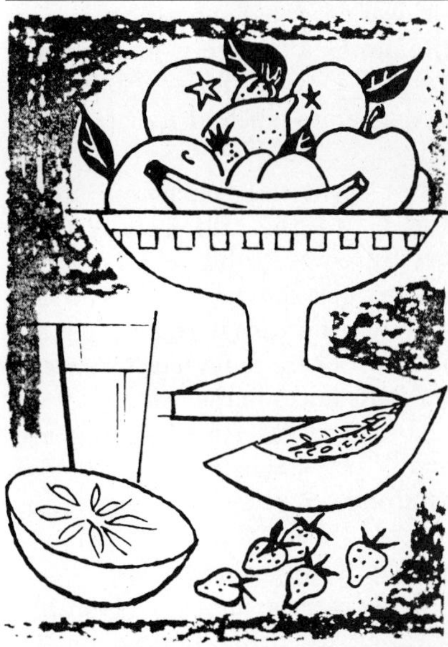

the deeply colored varieties, mangoes, and papayas.

Of the commonly used fruits and fruit juices, those of the citrus family — oranges, grapefruit, lemons, limes, and tangerines—are highest in vitamin C. Guava, a popular fruit in Hawaii, is also a rich source of vitamin C.

Fortunately vitamin C is well retained in *citrus fruits and juices.* Citrus fruits and their juices are canned or frozen with very little loss of vitamin C.

Whole citrus fruits keep their nutrients well several days at room temperature or slightly cooler (60° to 70° F.).

Fresh oranges lose edible material — and therefore nutritive value—when they are squeezed and the juice strained. The edible yield of an orange as strained juice is only about two-thirds to three-fourths that of the orange eaten by sections.

Orange juice, whether freshly squeezed, canned, or reconstituted from frozen concentrate, can be held in the refrigerator for several days before any vitamin C is lost. A few hours outside the refrigerator does not cause any serious loss in vitamin C, although it may impair flavor. Orange juice changes in flavor before much of its vitamin C is lost.

For practical purposes, foods stored in the refrigerator are usually covered, but a lid on the orange juice container makes no important difference in retaining vitamin C. There is no harm in keeping fruit juices in the can.

Unlike citrus fruits, *berries* are highly perishable and need careful handling to conserve their nutrients. They lose vitamin C quickly if capped or bruised.

Strawberries compare favorably with citrus fruits in vitamin C. About two-thirds of a cup of ripe strawberries fills an adult's daily need for vitamin C.

CANNED FOODS

Canning, one of the most familiar forms of food preservation, has made an important contribution to the variety, quality, and safety of our food supply. Some loss of vitamins in the canning process is to be expected. Losses, however, have been reduced considerably by improved processing techniques.

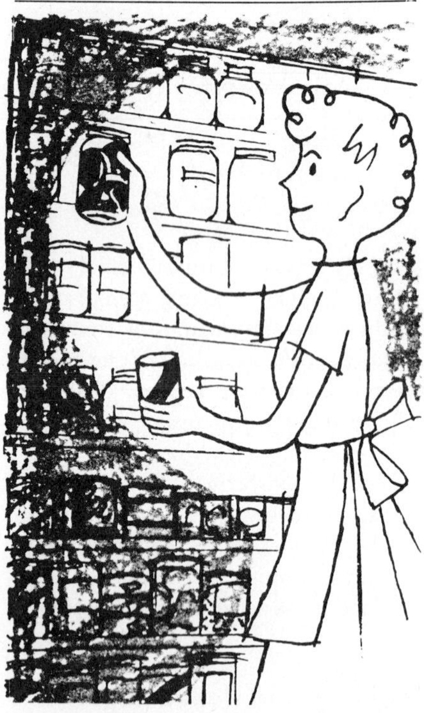

Keeping canned foods in a cool, dry place and limiting the length of time they are in storage are essential factors in conserving the nutrients in canned foods. In general, the longer the storage period and the higher the storage temperature, the greater the loss of nutrients.

Effects of Storage

Canned Fruits and Vegetables

Vitamins are retained best when canned foods are kept in a cool place. Only small losses of vitamin C, about 10 percent, occur when these foods are stored for a year at 65° F. When the temperature is 80°, losses may reach 25 percent in a year.

Canned citrus juices hold vitamin C especially well.

Carotene, a precursor of vitamin A, is well retained in canned fruits and vegetables. Losses average only about 10 percent in a year when cans are stored at 80° F. Canned tomato juice, a particularly stable, year-round source of carotene, shows no loss of this nutrient.

Thiamin in canned fruits and vegetables is well retained when stored for 1 year at 65° F. When stored at 80° for 1 year, losses may increase to 15 percent in canned fruits, and to 25 percent in canned vegetables.

Canned Meats

Some thiamin is lost from canned meats in storage. Pork luncheon meat, for example, may lose about 20 percent of its thiamin by the end of 3 months and 30 percent by the end of 6 months when it is stored at 70° F. Losses accelerate at higher temperatures.

Riboflavin, another B vitamin supplied by meat, is not affected by ordinary storage temperatures.

Nutrients in Liquids

To get the full nutritive value from canned vegetables, serve any liquid in the can or jar along with the vegetables or make use of the liquid in some other way, such as in gravy or adding it to soup.

Usually the drained solids in canned vegetables make up about two-thirds of the total contents of the cans. Soon after canning, the water-soluble nutrients in the vegetable distribute themselves evenly throughout the solids and the liquid. The solids thus contain about two-thirds of the soluble nutrients, and the other third is in the liquid.

FROZEN FOODS

Freezing offers a good way of retaining the nutrients and the eating quality of food. There is little loss of vitamin C in freezing fruits. In vegetables the amount of vitamin C is reduced during the blanching process before freezing. There is also a small loss of other water-soluble vitamins and some minerals when the blanching is done in water.

When properly packaged, frozen meat, poultry, and fish compare favorably with fresh products in food value.

An essential requirement in maintaining the food value and quality of home-frozen or purchased frozen foods is a storage temperature of 0° F. or lower.

If your home freezer or the freezing compartment of your refrigerator cannot be maintained at 0° F. or lower, it is important to realize that food stored will not hold its best nutritive value and highest quality. It may be desirable to buy frozen foods in small quantities and replenish your supply frequently.

Storage of frozen foods at too high a temperature hastens vitamin C loss. The loss increases with time. Even at 0° F., some losses occur. Stored at 0° for a year, frozen beans, broccoli, cauliflower, and spinach would lose from one-third to three-fourths of their vitamin C. At higher temperatures, the losses would be greater.

Frozen concentrated orange juice, however, holds its vitamin C content remarkably well even at freezing temperature (32° F.).

Thawing and refreezing of frozen foods should be avoided because of the adverse effect on nutrient content and flavor and the possibility of spoilage.

MEAT, POULTRY, AND FISH

Meat, poultry, and fish are normally the most expensive foods on your grocery list. They are the main dishes about which most homemakers plan their meals.

From this food group come protein of high quality, fat, minerals, and valuable vitamins.

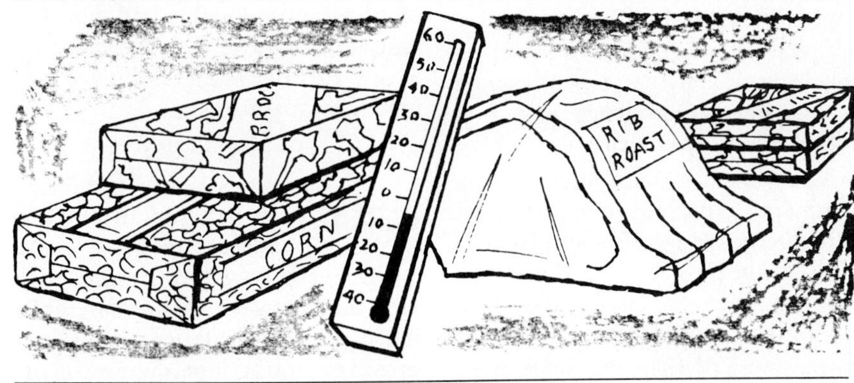

Liver, in particular, is rich in many nutrients. It contains protein, B vitamins, and minerals; it is an excellent source of vitamin A, and also provides some vitamin C.

Among the meats, pork is an exceptionally good source of thiamin.

The price paid per pound of meat is not necessarily a measure of its nutritive value. The cheaper cuts and grades of lean meat can be just as full of food value as the higher-priced steaks and chops. The protein in one is just as valuable as in the other. The main difference is that cheaper cuts require greater skill in cooking and seasoning.

Nutrients in Drippings

To get the full nutritive value from any meat, you should conserve the water-soluble B vitamins.

Meat drippings contain some of these B vitamins. Included are the drippings from thawing frozen meat, the drippings from cooking meat, and the juices released in slicing meat.

When meats and poultry are stewed, some of the B vitamins transfer into the meat stock or broth. Meat stock or broth can be used in nourishing soups or used as a part of the liquid in escalloped or creamed dishes.

After broiling, frying, and roasting meats and poultry, you may wish to skim off fat that rises to the top of pan drippings and use the remaining drippings in savory gravies or pour them directly over the meat when it is served. In this way, you recover some of the water-soluble B vitamins and extend the flavor of the meat.

Cooking Losses

Meats shrink in weight and volume as they cook. Much of the change is water, which evaporates or goes into the drippings. Some fat also is in the drippings.

The protein value of meat is not destroyed by cooking, and only small amounts of it go into the drippings.

Even when meats and poultry are stewed in large amounts of water, not more than 10 percent of the protein passes from meat to broth.

Some thiamin and vitamin B_6 are lost in cooking; riboflavin and niacin are less susceptible to loss in cooking.

Roasting beef to the rare stage conserves more thiamin than cooking it to the well-done stage.

MILK

To best conserve the valuable nutrients and good flavor of milk, keep it cold, covered, and away from strong light.

Milk is one of the best sources of calcium and the B vitamin, riboflavin. The protein it supplies rates high. Dietary studies in the United States indicate that milk and milk products provide about two-thirds of the total calcium, nearly half of the riboflavin, and more than a fifth of the protein in our diets.

Calcium, protein, and vitamin A are stable and well retained in milk. The total loss of riboflavin in milk from the time of production until it is served can be kept low with proper handling.

Milk has about the same calcium and protein value whether you drink it as whole, skim, or reconstituted from nonfat dry milk or evaporated milk.

Whole milk and cream are reliable sources of vitamin A. Skim milk, fresh or powdered, has nearly all the fat removed from it, and has little vitamin A value unless it is fortified. A glass of fresh skim milk or reconstituted nonfat dry milk has only about half the calories of a glass of whole milk.

Cottage cheese is made from skim milk and has a lower calorie value than cheeses made from whole milk. Cheeses made from cream or whole milk have a much higher content of fat and vitamin A than cheese made from skim milk.

Pasteurization of raw milk, a necessary health safeguard, does not destroy the principal nutrients in milk and milk products—the calcium, protein, riboflavin, and vitamin A.

Riboflavin, an important nutrient in milk, is subject to reduction by exposure to direct sunlight, daylight, or artificial light. However, it is well protected by present methods of handling milk from the farm to the consumer.

EGGS

Eggs have an established place in family meals—both by themselves and in cooked products. Like meat and milk, eggs supply high-quality protein. Two eggs have about as much protein as 2 ounces of cooked hamburger. One large egg furnishes about 80 calories.

Egg yolk is a rich source of iron, a mineral important in building red blood cells. Eggs also supply vitamin A and riboflavin.

When properly stored and cooked, both shell eggs and dried egg retain most of their nutrients well.

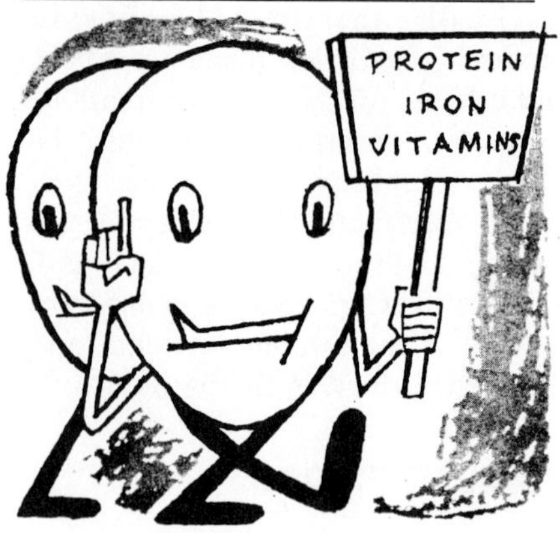

Shell eggs keep in the refrigerator or in cold storage without serious loss of nutritive value.

Cooking losses in eggs are not high, probably because the cooking period is short and the temperatures fairly low. The protein and vitamin A values are well retained. Riboflavin is well retained when eggs are cooked in the shell, but small losses may occur with other methods of cookery. Thiamin losses are small also, usually not more than 15 percent.

When dried egg is properly stored (tightly covered in the refrigerator), it has practically the same nutritive value as shell eggs. Dehydration does not reduce the protein, vitamin A, or riboflavin values.

Stored at ordinary room temperatures, dried egg loses about a third of its vitamin A value in 6 months, and about two-thirds in 9 months. The rate of loss accelerates at higher temperatures.

CEREALS

The cereals—wheat, corn, rye, rice, and oats—come to your table in a myriad of food items, including breakfast foods, hominy, breads of all kinds, macaroni and noodle products, puddings, pastries, cakes, and cookies.

Cereals are nutritional bargains. They are economical sources of food energy, protein, minerals, and the B vitamins.

The amount of vitamins and minerals your family gets from a cereal or a cereal product depends on how much remains after milling, what nutrients are added, and on how you prepare it for eating.

Whole Grain, Enriched or Restored

Whole-grain forms of cereals retain the germ and outer layers of the grain where the B vitamins and minerals are concentrated.

Whole-grain products generally available on the market include: Whole-wheat flour, sometimes called graham flour; brown rice, dark rye flour, whole-ground cornmeal, and rolled oats or oatmeal, and bread and other products made from them. Milling whole cereal grains into refined products removes all or part of the germ and a considerable amount of the outer layers.

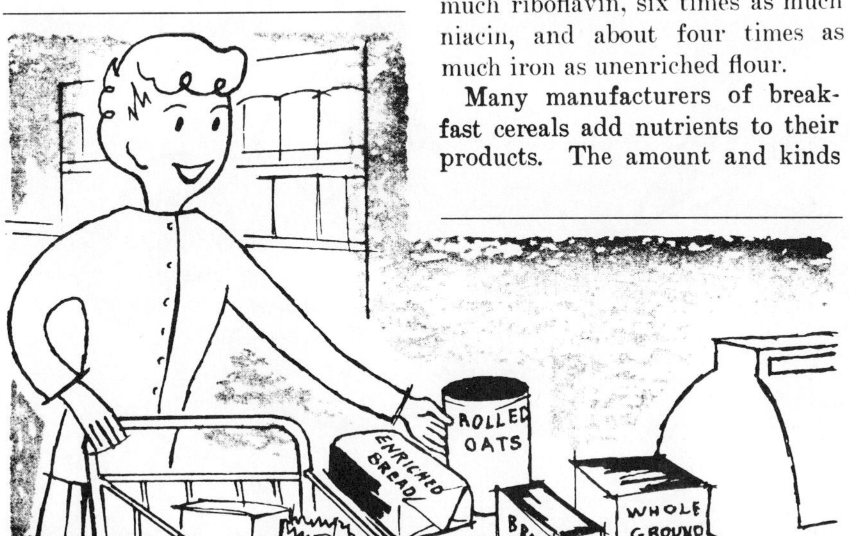

Most consumers prefer white bread and other products made of refined cereal grains. Some of the milling losses are offset through enrichment of certain staple cereal products.

Enriched cereals are milled cereals to which the B vitamins—thiamin, riboflavin, and niacin—and iron have been added within the limits specified by the Federal standard of enrichment. Provision is made for the optional addition of one other nutrient, calcium.

Federal standards for enrichment have been established for certain wheat flours, bread, rolls and buns, farina, cornmeal, corn grits, macaroni and noodle products, and rice.

Enriched flour has about ten times as much thiamin, eight times as much riboflavin, six times as much niacin, and about four times as much iron as unenriched flour.

Many manufacturers of breakfast cereals add nutrients to their products. The amount and kinds of nutrients added vary widely since there are no Federal standards for the addition of nutrients to these products.

A comparison of the nutritive values of different forms of rice shows that *parboiled rice* is intermediate in food value between *highly-milled, polished rice* and brown rice. *Brown rice* is the unprocessed kernel with the hull removed; from a nutritional standpoint, it is considered a whole grain.

Cooking Losses

Cooking cereals in excessive quantities of water, draining off the cooking water, and rinsing afterward waste nutrients.

Some persons persist in washing rice before cooking. This is an unnecessary step because today's packaged rice has already been cleaned. Moreover, washing is nutritionally expensive. Washing rice once before cooking can cause a thiamin loss of 25 percent in regular white rice, and a loss of 10 percent in brown or parboiled rice. This loss may be important in diets of persons who eat a great deal of rice.

You may have noticed these directions on some rice packages: "To retain vitamins, do not rinse before or drain after cooking."

The nutrients in rice are well retained if rice is cooked in just enough water to be absorbed during the cooking period.

Cooking causes little loss of nutrients from ready-to-cook breakfast foods, such as rolled oats, rolled wheat, hominy grits, cracked wheat, farina, and others. Many of the breakfast cereals on the market are precooked and require only seconds to prepare.

Baking, one of the popular ways of cooking cereal products, permits good retention of thiamin. You can conserve thiamin by—

- Baking the product only until the crust is light brown.
- Limiting the surface area exposed to heat. For example, less thiamin is lost when cornbread batter is baked in a pan rather than as sticks.

Toasting causes additional loss of thiamin. However, the thicker the slice of bread and the lighter the finished product, the smaller is the loss of thiamin.

One comparison showed a toasting loss to be only half as great in a thick slice as in a thin slice.

Riboflavin, another B vitamin in cereals, is not greatly affected by heat but is sensitive to light. Experimental studies of riboflavin loss in commercially baked bread indicate that heavy wax paper or other translucent covering protects the riboflavin in bread very well.

BE VITAMIN-WISE WHEN YOU SELECT VEGETABLES

- In general, freshly harvested vegetables have more vitamins than those held in storage.
- Make full use of vine-ripened tomatoes in summer when they are plentiful and inexpensive. Tomatoes vine ripened out-of-doors in summer sunlight have twice as much vitamin C as tomatoes grown in greenhouses in winter.
- You get several times as much vitamin A value from bright-orange, mature carrots as from pale-colored, young ones. Even so, young carrots are a good source of vitamin A; choose them if you prefer.
- Choose deep-orange sweetpotatoes for maximum vitamin A value.
- Among the vegetables, turnip greens, kale, and collards are good sources of riboflavin as well as of vitamins A and C. Lima beans, peas, and young cowpeas, including black-eye peas, contribute appreciable amounts of thiamin and protein.
- Peppers are high in vitamins A and C.
- The dark-green leafy vegetables are richer in nutrients, particularly vitamin A, calcium, and iron, than light-green vegetables.
- Leaf lettuce has more vitamin A value than pale-green head lettuce. The dark-green, outer leaves of head lettuce are much higher in vitamin A value than the inner leaves. For maximum food value, look for dark-green lettuce.
- Potatoes, although not rich in vitamin C, are a good source of this nutrient when eaten regularly.
- If the tops of beets are attached and still tender when you buy them, cook them—they are rich in vitamin A value.

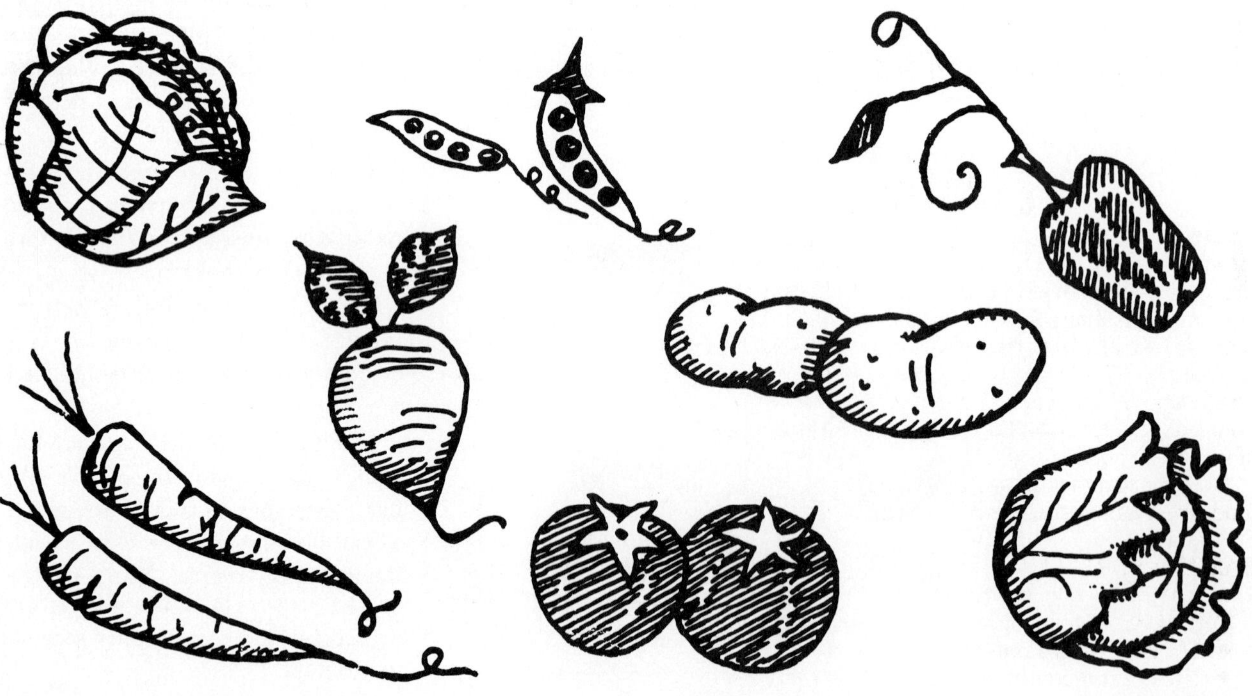

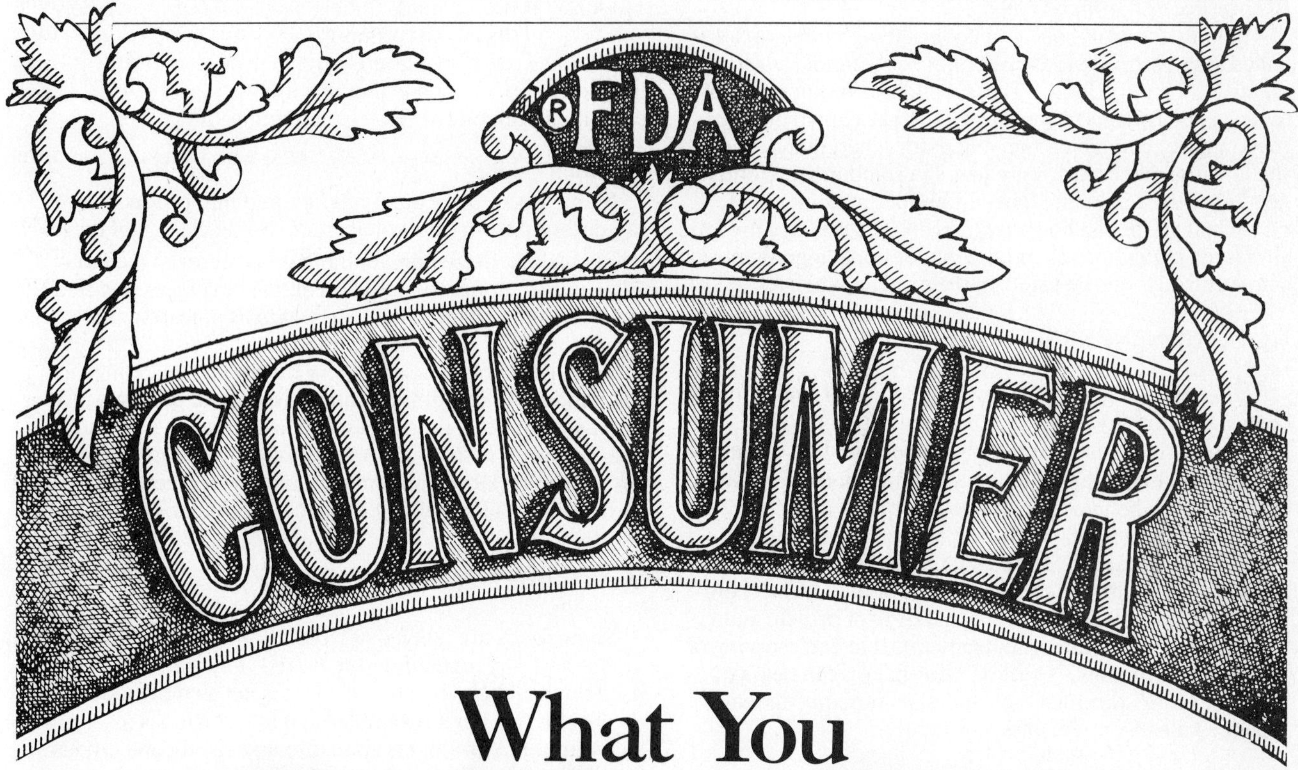

What You Should Know About Food Labels and Food Additives

Labels

Food labels provide a great deal of information that can help consumers find out more about what they're getting in the products they buy. Some of this information is required by FDA to be shown on the label; some is included on the label at the option of the manufacturer or processor. Some of the information on food labels may be in the form of symbols or codes or dates.

Here's a rundown of the information most often found on food labels along with a brief explanation of what it means.

BASIC INFORMATION

Certain information must be on all food labels:

- The name of the product.
- The net contents or net weight. The net weight on canned food includes the liquid in which the product is packed, such as water in canned vegetables and syrup in canned fruit.
- The name and place of business of the manufacturer, packer, or distributor.

List of Ingredients

On most foods, the ingredients must be listed on the label. The ingredient present in the largest amount, by weight, must be listed first, followed in descending order of weight by the other ingredients. Any additives used in the product must be listed, but colors and flavors do not have to be listed by name. The list of ingredients may simply say "artificial color" or "artificial flavor" or "natural flavor." If the flavors are artificial, this fact must be stated. Butter, cheese, and ice cream, however, are not required to state the presence of artificial color.

The only foods not required to list all ingredients are so-called standardized foods. FDA has set "standards of identity" for some foods. These standards require that all foods called by a particular name (such as catsup or mayonnaise) contain certain mandatory ingredients. Under the law, the mandatory ingredients in standardized foods need not be listed on the label. Manufacturers may add optional ingredients, however, and FDA is revising the food standards regulations to require that optional ingredients in standardized foods be listed on the product label.

NUTRITION INFORMATION

Under FDA regulations, any food to which a nutrient has been added, or any food for which a nutritional claim is made, must have the nutritional content listed on the label. In addition, many manufacturers put nutrition information on products when not required to do so.

Nutrition labels tell you how many calories and how much protein, carbohydrate, and fat are in a serving of the product. They also tell the percentage of the U.S. Recommended Daily Allowances (U.S. RDA's) of protein and seven important vitamins and minerals that each serving of the product contains. Nutrition information can help you shop for more nutritious food and plan more nutritionally balanced meals for you and your family.

How to Read Nutrition Labels

Nutrition information is given on a per serving basis. The label tells the size of a serving (for example: one cup, two ounces, 1 tablespoon), the number of servings in the container, the number of calories per serving, and the amounts in grams of protein, carbohydrate, and fat per serving.

Protein is listed twice on the label: in grams and as a percentage of the U.S. Recommended Daily Allowance.

Seven vitamins and minerals must be shown, in a specific order. The listing of 12 other vitamins and minerals, and of cholesterol, fatty acid, and sodium content is optional.

What U.S. RDA Means

The U.S. Recommended Daily Allowances (U.S. RDA's) are the approximate amounts of protein, vitamins, and minerals that an adult should eat every day to keep healthy. Nutrition labels list the U.S. RDA by percentage. For example, the label may state that one serving of the food contains 35 percent of the Recommended Daily Allowance of vitamin A and 25 percent of the Recommended Daily Allowance of iron. The total amount of food an individual eats in a day should supply the U.S. Recommended Daily Allowance of all essential nutrients.

A Key to Metric Units

Nutrition labels show amounts in grams rather than ounces, because grams are a smaller unit of measurement and many food components are present in very small amounts. Here is a guide to help you read nutrition labels:

1 pound (lb.) = 454 grams (g)
1 ounce (oz.) = 28 grams (g)
1 gram (g) = 1,000 milligrams (mg)
1 milligram (mg) = 1,000 micrograms (mcg)

Nutrition Quality

Many foods today are manufactured into products that are different from traditional foods. Some classes of these foods include frozen dinners; breakfast cereals; meal replacements; noncarbonated breakfast beverages fortified with vitamin C; and main dishes such as macaroni and cheese, pizzas, stews, and casseroles.

FDA is establishing voluntary nutritional guidelines for such foods, so consumers can be assured of getting a proper level and range of nutrients when using them. A product that complies with an FDA nutritional quality guideline may include on its label a statement that it meets the U.S. nutritional quality guideline for that particular class of food.

WHAT "IMITATION" MEANS

Some foods are labeled as "imitations" of other foods. Under an FDA regulation, the word "imitation" must be used on the label when the product is not as nutritious as the product which it resembles and for which it is a substitute. If a product is similar to an existing one, and is just as nutritious, a new name can be given to it rather than calling it "imitation." For example, eggless products which are nutritionally equivalent to eggs have been given names such as Eggbeaters and Scramblers.

COMMON OR USUAL NAME

Some foods may look from the label as though they are one thing and actually be another. To prevent deception of consumers, FDA has ruled that such foods must have a "common or usual" name which gives the consumer accurate information about what is in the package or container.

For example, a beverage that looks like orange juice but actually contains very little orange juice must use a name such as "diluted orange juice drink." The product also may be required to state on the label the percentage of the characterizing ingredient it contains. In this case, the common or usual name might be "diluted orange juice beverage, contains 10 percent orange juice."

A noncarbonated beverage that appears to contain a fruit or vegetable juice but does not contain any juice must state on the label that it contains no fruit or vegetable juice.

Another special labeling requirement concerns packaged foods in which the main ingredient or component of a recipe is not included, as in the case of some "main dishes" or "dinners." On such foods, the common or usual name consists of the following:

• The common name of each ingredient in descending order by weight—for example, "noodles and tomato sauce."

• Identification of the food to be prepared from the package—for example, "for preparation of chicken casserole."

• A statement of ingredients that must be added to complete the recipe—for example, "you must add chicken to complete the recipe."

GRADES

Some food products carry a grade on the label, such as "U.S. Grade A." Grades are set by the U.S. Department of Agriculture, based on the quality levels inherent in a product—its taste, texture, and appearance. U.S. Department of Agriculture grades are not based on nutritional content.

Milk and milk products in most States carry a "Grade A" label. This grade is based on FDA recommended sanitary standards for the production and processing of milk and milk products, which are regulated by the States. The grade is not based on nutritional values. However, FDA has established standards for milk which require certain levels of vitamins A and D when these vitamins are added to milk.

OPEN DATING

To help consumers obtain food that is fresh and wholesome, many manufacturers date their product. Open dating, as this practice often is called, is not regulated by FDA, but the following information may be helpful to you.

Four kinds of open dating are commonly used. To benefit from open dating, the consumer needs to know what kind of dating is used on the individual product and what it means.

Pack Date—This is the day the food was manufactured or processed or packaged. In other words, it tells how old the food is when you buy it. The importance of this information to consumers depends on how quickly the particular food normally spoils. Most canned and packaged foods have a long shelf life when stored under dry, cool conditions.

Pull or Sell Date—This is the last date the product should be sold, assuming it has been stored and handled properly. The pull date allows for some storage time in the home refrigerator. Cold cuts, ice cream, milk, and refrigerated fresh dough products are examples of foods with pull dates.

Expiration Date—This is the last date the food should be eaten or used. Baby formula and yeast are examples of products that may carry expiration dates.

Freshness Date—This is similar to the expiration date but may allow for normal home storage. Some bakery products that have a freshness date are sold at a reduced price for a short time after the expiration date.

CODE DATING

Many companies use code dating on products that have a long "shelf life". This is usually for the company's information, rather than for the consumer's benefit. The code gives the manufacturer and the store precise information about where and when the product was packaged, so if a recall should be required for any reason the product can be identified quickly and withdrawn from the market.

UNIVERSAL PRODUCT CODE

Many food labels now include a small block of parallel lines of various widths, with accompanying numbers. This is the Universal Product Code (UPC). The code on a label is unique to that product. Some stores are equipped with computerized checkout equipment that can read the code and automatically ring up the sale. In addition to making it possible for stores to automate part of their checkout work, the UPC, when used in conjunction with a computer, also can function as an automated inventory system. The computer can tell management how much of a specific item is on hand, how fast it is being sold, and when and how much to order.

SYMBOLS ON FOOD LABELS

The symbol "R" on a label signifies that the trademark used on the label is registered with the U.S. Patent Office.

The symbol "C" indicates that the literary and artistic content of the label is protected against infringement under the copyright laws of the United States. Copies of such labels have been filed with the Copyright Office of the Library of Congress.

The symbol which consists of the letter "U" inside the letter "O" is one whose use is authorized by the Union of Orthodox Jewish Congregations of America, more familiarly known as the Orthodox Union, for use of foods which comply with Jewish dietary laws. Detailed information regarding the significance and use of this symbol may be obtained from the headquarters of that organization at 116 E. 27th St., New York, New York 10016.

The symbol which consists of the letter "K" inside the letter "O" is used to indicate that the food is "Kosher," that is, it complies with the Jewish dietary laws, and its processing has been under the direction of a rabbi.

None of the symbols referred to above are required by, or are under the authority of, any of the Acts enforced by the Food and Drug Administration.

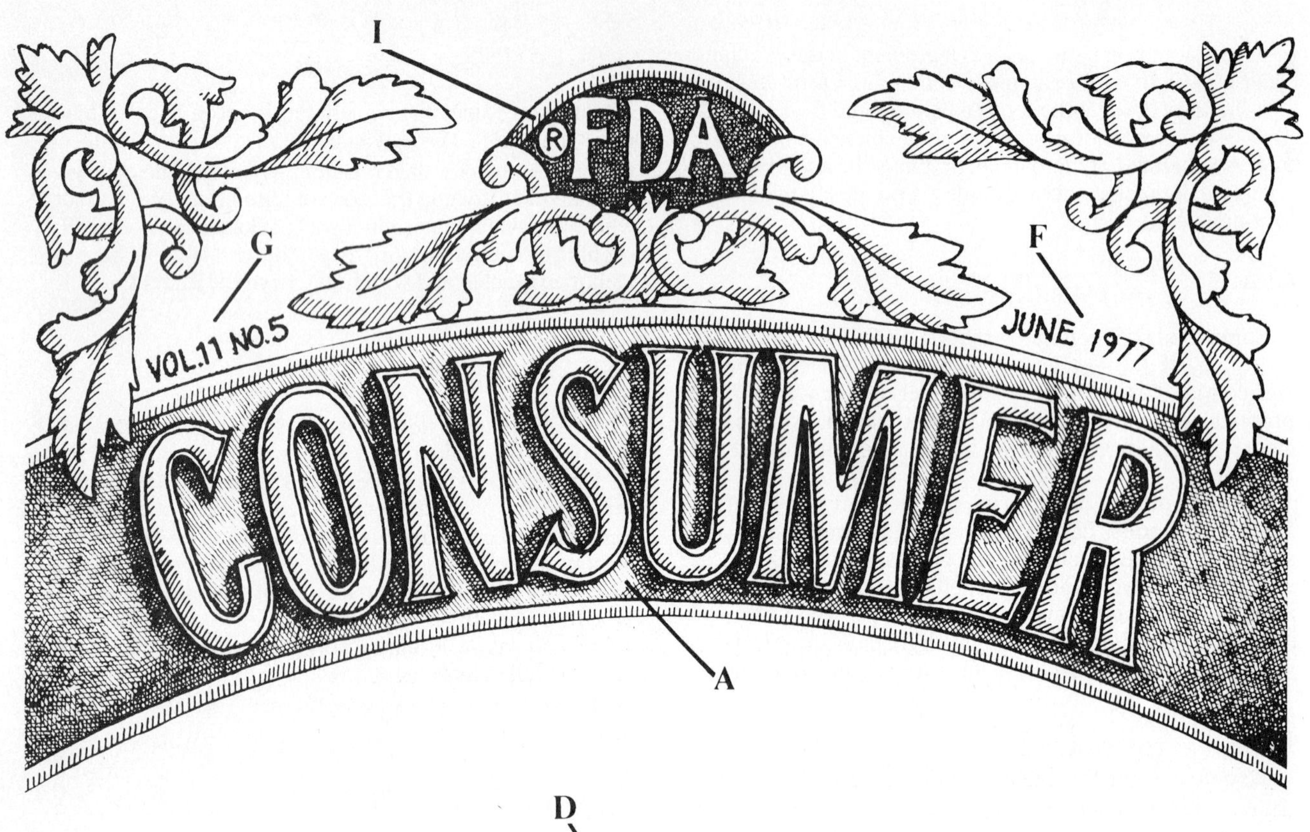

D

INGREDIENTS

FOOD ADDITIVES: DOUBLE CHECK ON SAFETY
RISK ASSESSMENT AND CONSUMER PROTECTION
A CONSUMER'S GUIDE TO FOOD LABELS
KEEPING TABS ON PRODUCT INJURIES
INFORMING WOMEN ABOUT IUD'S
UPDATE AND CONSUMER FORUM

B **NET WT. 40 PAGES GRADE A** E

C

U.S. DEPARTMENT OF HEALTH, EDUCATION, AND WELFARE
Public Health Service Food and Drug Administration
5600 Fishers Lane Rockville, Md. 20857

C 410 11 4 3 0 02010 11 4 4

H

A. *The name of the product must be on all food labels.*

B. *The net contents or net weight must be on all food labels.*

C. *The name and place of business of the manufacturer, packer or distributor must be on all food labels.*

D. *On most foods, the ingredients must be listed on the label.*

E. *Some food products carry a grade on the label.*

F. *To help consumers obtain fresh and wholesome food, many manufacturers open date their product.*

G. *Many companies use code dating on products that have a long "shelf life".*

H. *Many food labels now include a small block of parallel lines of various widths with accompanying numbers for computerized check-outs and inventories.*

I. *The symbol "®" on a label signifies that the trademark used on the label is registered with the U.S. Patent Office.*

Additives

Food additives are so much a part of the American way of eating today that most of us would find it difficult to put together a meal that did not include them.

Take a typical lunch, for example: sandwich, instant soup, gelatin dessert, and a cola drink. The bread has been fortified with vitamins and also contains an additive to keep it fresh. The margarine has been colored pale yellow—or, if you use salad dressing, it has been made with emulsifiers to keep it from "separating." The luncheon meat contains nitrite; the soup, an additive to keep it from becoming rancid; the gelatin, red coloring to make it pretty. Finally, the cola to wash it all down: without coloring, flavoring, sweeteners, or artificial carbonation, the pause that refreshes is nothing more than plain water!

No wonder many Americans have become concerned. Additives seem to be in everything we eat. Are all these substances good for us? Do they serve a useful purpose, or do they just make money for the food industry?

To help you clarify your own thinking on these questions, let's explore how our present situation came about, and what choices we have.

Food additives are not something new. Humans probably have been tinkering with food since the first caveman killed his first wild boar. Salt was used probably even before recorded history to preserve meat and fish. Herbs and spices have been treasured over the years solely for their capacity to add pizzazz to foods, not to mention their function in a less technological age as a preservative.

Changing lifestyles in this century have resulted in more additives than former generations could have imagined. As Americans moved from farms to cities, there was a need for foods that could be mass produced, distributed over considerable distances, and stored for long periods. The exodus of women from the home into the outside workplace created a demand for more pre-prepared convenience foods. Greater sophistication increased demand for year-round supplies of seasonal products. Greater buying power gave industry a bigger market to please. So today we have a wider variety of foods available—and more additives in all foods—than had ever been known in the past.

The fact that additives are in foods does not please everyone. Many contend that some additives are often dangerous or at least "unnecessary chemicals." The critics note that some additives can cause allergic reactions in some people.

Unnecessary Chemicals was the title of an article in the March 1978 issue of ENVIRONMENT magazine in which the author contended that "many hazardous chemicals (in food and other products) provide consumers with trivial or no benefits at all . . .". The writer, Anita Johnson, an attorney for the Environmental Defense Fund, believes that women shoppers don't want many of the additives. She cited a March 1976 Gallup poll done for REDBOOK magazine, which "found that 59 percent of the women surveyed said they favored banning food additives used only to improve the appearance of food even if there was no positive evidence of harm."

However, food processors apparently think otherwise and their sales figures would seem to back their thinking. Moreover, the Nation's laws on the subject are designed not to question use of additives but to assure that they are as safe as possible.

By broadest definition, a food additive is any substance that becomes part of a food product when added either directly or indirectly. Today, some 2,800 substances are intentionally added to foods to produce a desired effect. As many as 10,000 other compounds or combinations of compounds find their way into various foods during processing, packaging, or storage. Examples of these unintentional additives include infinitesimal residues of pesticides used to treat crops, minute amounts of drugs fed to animals, and chemical substances that migrate from plastic packaging materials.

An additive is intentionally used in foods for one or more of these four purposes:

• *To maintain or improve nutritional value.* Many foods are fortified with vitamins and minerals that might otherwise be lacking in a person's diet or that have been destroyed or lost in processing. Common nutritional additives include vitamin D in milk, vitamin A in margarine, vitamin C in fruit drinks, and iodine in table salt. Breads and cereals are enriched with B vitamins lost or destroyed during milling and processing of grains. Such fortification has helped eradicate once-prevalent deficiency diseases, such as rickets, scurvy, pellagra, and goiter.

• *To maintain freshness.* Foods last as long as they do on the shelf or in the refrigerator because of additives that retard spoilage, preserve natural color and flavor, and keep fats and oils from turning rancid. Preservatives such as sodium nitrates and nitrites, for example, protect cured meats, fish, and poultry from contamination by the bacterially produced toxin responsible for botulism, a food poisoning illness. Ascorbic acid (vitamin C) keeps uncooked peaches from turning brown. Antioxidants, such as BHA (butylated hydroxyanisole) or BHT (butylated hydroxytoluene), help prevent changes in color, flavor, or texture that occur when foods are exposed to air.

• *To help in processing or preparation.* A wide variety of compounds are used to give body and texture to foods, evenly distribute particles of one liquid in another, affect cooking or baking results, control acidity or alkalinity, retain moisture, and prevent caking or lumping. Chemicals called emulsifiers give such products as peanut butter and mayonnaise a consistent texture and prevent them from separating into an oily layer at the top of the jar and a dry layer at the bottom. Thickeners create smoothness and prevent ice crystals from forming in frozen foods such as ice cream. Humectants are used to keep moisture in foods like shredded coconut. Leavening agents such as yeasts and baking powder are essential to make baked goods rise.

• *To make food more appealing.* The most widely used additives are those intended to make food look and taste better. These include coloring agents, natural and synthetic flavors, flavor enhancers such as MSG (monosodium glutamate), and sweeteners. The characteristic flavor of strawberry ice cream, for example, may come from real strawberries, or it may come from a chemical flavoring. Because consumers associate strawberries with a reddish color, strawberry ice cream is tinted pink. These uses are the most controversial; industry says the public prefers foods that are colored and flavored while many consumers and consumer advocates believe too many colors and flavors are used.

By far the most widely used additives are sugar, salt, and corn syrup. These three, plus such other substances as citric acid (found in oranges and lemons), baking soda, vegetable colors, mustard, and pepper, account for more than 98 percent, by weight, of all food additives used in this country.

Food additives also are more strictly regulated now than at any other time in history. Despite our nostalgia for the good old days, eating was not especially safe at the turn of the century when it was difficult to protect foods from spoiling and when manufacturers freely used pigments containing such toxic metals as lead, copper, and arsenic to color candy, pickles, and other foods; created "strawberry" jam with only coloring, flavoring, and grass seed; or stretched ground black pepper with bits of charcoal.

The 1906 Food and Drugs Act and the more comprehensive Food, Drug, and Cosmetic Act of 1938 gave the Government authority to remove adulterated and obviously poisonous foods from the market. But it wasn't until the Food Additives Amendment was enacted in 1958 and the Color Additive Amendments in 1960 that the Nation had laws specifically regulating food additives. In those amendments, the lawmakers shifted the burden from the Government to prove a food additive unsafe to the manufacturer to prove it safe. The amendments authorized FDA to regulate additives only on the basis of safety. The Agency has no power to limit the number of additives approved or to judge whether a particular food color, thickener, or sweetener is really needed.

In an approval process that may take up to several years, manufacturers first must subject a proposed new additive to a battery of chemical tests to determine whether it does what is intended and to make sure it can be analyzed and measured in the finished food product. Then the additive must be fed in large doses over an extended period to at least two kinds of animals, usually rodents and dogs. These feeding studies are designed to determine whether the substance causes cancer, birth defects, or other injury to the animals.

Manufacturers submit the results of all these tests to FDA, and if they indicate the additive is safe, the Agency establishes regulations for how it can be used in food. A basic rule is a 100-fold margin of safety for anything added to food. This means that the manufacturer may use only 1/100th the maximum amount of an additive that has been found *not* to produce any harmful effects in test animals. A special provision of the 1958 and 1960 amendments, the so-called Delaney Clause, states that a substance shown to cause cancer in man or animal may not be added to food in *any* amount.

Under the Food Additives Amendment two major categories of additives are exempt from the testing and approval process. The first is a group of some 700 substances "generally recognized as safe" (GRAS) by qualified experts. The idea behind what has come to be known as the GRAS List was to free FDA and manufacturers from being required to prove the safety of substances already considered harmless because of past extensive use with no known harmful effect. Their efforts, it was felt, would be better spent on new additives and on those compounds about which less is known.

Also exempt from testing were "prior sanctioned substances," those that had been approved before 1958 for use in food by either FDA or the U.S. Department of Agriculture. Some prior sanctioned substances also were included on the GRAS List.

These lists of exemptions are not, however, engraved in stone. As testing methods and scientific understanding of toxicology improve, new evidence and questions may arise about the safety of old standbys. To make sure these substances are judged by the latest scientific standards, FDA is reviewing all categories of food additives.

A review of 450 natural and synthetic substances on the GRAS List was begun in 1971 and continues. It includes a search of world medical and scientific literature back to 1920 for information regarding the safety of each compound. When data turn up suggesting that an additive is unsafe, further testing by the Agency may take it off the market or require manufacturers to conduct additional studies. For example, FDA is proposing that manufacturers sponsor further study of BHT, a preservative that was both prior sanctioned and a member of the GRAS List, because of evidence that it causes liver damage in rats.

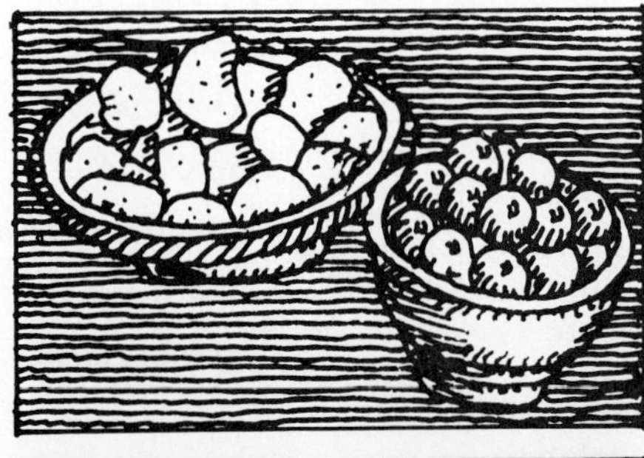

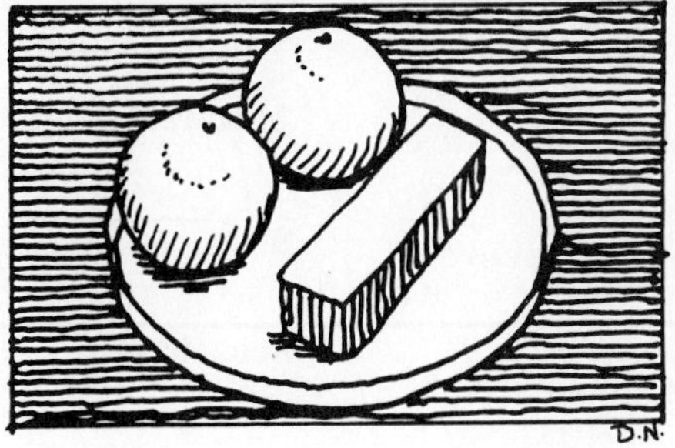

FDA also is undertaking a similar review of 2,100 flavoring agents, including those approved since 1958, prior sanctioned substances, and other agents that for some reason failed to make the original GRAS List.

The 1960 Color Additive Amendments subject coloring agents used in foods, drugs, and cosmetics to rigorous premarket testing. Colors in use when the amendment was passed were placed on a provisional approval list pending further investigation or confirmation of their safety. Nearly 200 colors have been on the provisional approval list at one time or another. But over the years about 80 have been dropped from the list because manufacturers were no longer interested in marketing them or, in some cases, because they were found to be unsafe. In 1976, for example, FDA banned Red No. 2, then the most widely used red coloring agent, because tests in test animals could not resolve whether it caused cancer or not. Currently 31 colors are fully approved for use in foods; three others are on the provisional list awaiting results of animal feeding studies.

Faced with a confusing tangle of regulations and reviews, consumers may feel that they are helpless in exerting any control over what goes into their food. In fact, the consumer wields the greatest power of all—the power of the marketplace. Anyone concerned about food additives should take the following steps:

- *Become informed.* Start by reading labels to find out what is in the foods you buy. The names of additives must be included in the list of ingredients, although the law permits colors and flavors to be described in general terms like "artificially flavored" or "artificially colored." Learn what the various additives do and decide which ones are of most concern to you. If you have questions, contact the consumer affairs officer at your nearest FDA office, listed in the telephone directory under U.S. Department of Health, Education, and Welfare. Or write to the manufacturer.
- *Exercise your right to choose.* Once you are informed, you can select foods on the basis of which characteristics—convenience, appeal, storage time—mean the most to you. You might want to continue buying bread with sodium propionate if you know it prevents mold, but you may not want to buy cookies that are artificially colored. It's your choice.
- *Make your views known.* Let manufacturers and your representatives in Congress know what you want and don't want in your food.

Food additives, like most things in life, involve a trade-off. Scientists will never be able to guarantee that anything added to food is absolutely safe. Ultimately, it is up to the consumer to decide what degree of risk is an acceptable price to pay for foods that keep well and are appealing, nutritious, convenient, and readily available year-round.

Additives Index:

An alphabetical list of some substances commonly added to foods

KEY DEFINITIONS

◆ **Maintain/Improve Nutritional Quality**
Nutrients: enrich (replace vitamins and minerals lost in processing) or fortify (add nutrients that may be lacking in the diet).

● **Maintain Product Quality**
Preservatives (Antimicrobials): prevent food spoilage from bacteria, molds, fungi, and yeast; extend shelf life; or protect natural color/flavor.

Antioxidants: delay/prevent rancidity or enzymatic browning.

■ **Aid in Processing or Preparation**
Emulsifiers: help to distribute evenly tiny particles of one liquid into another; improve homogeneity, consistency, stability, texture.

Stabilizers, Thickeners, Texturizers: impart body, improve consistency or texture; stabilize emulsions; affect "mouthfeel" of food.

Leavening Agents: affect cooking results—texture and volume.

pH Control Agents: change/maintain acidity or alkalinity.

Humectants: cause moisture retention.

Maturing and Bleaching Agents, Dough Conditioners: accelerate the aging process; improve baking qualities.

Anti-Caking Agents: prevent caking, lumping, or clustering of a finely powdered or crystalline substance.

▲ **Affect Appeal Characteristics**
Flavor Enhancers: supplement, magnify, or modify the original taste and/or aroma of food without imparting a characteristic flavor of its own.

Flavors: heighten natural flavor; restore flavors lost in processing.

Colors: give desired, appetizing, or characteristic color to food.

Sweeteners: make the aroma or taste of food more agreeable or pleasurable.

Key to Abbreviations:

stabil-thick-tex = stabilizers-thickeners-texturizers

leavening = leavening agents

pH control = pH control agents

mat-bleach-condit = maturing and bleaching agents, dough conditioners

anti-caking = anti-caking agents

A

Acetic acid	■ pH control
Acetone peroxide	■ mat-bleach-condit
Adipic acid	■ pH control
Ammonium alginate	■ stabil-thick-tex
Annatto extract	▲ color
Arabinogalactan	■ stabil-thick-tex
Ascorbic acid	◆ nutrient ● preservative ● antioxidant
Azodicarbonamide	■ mat-bleach-condit

B

Benzoic acid	● preservative
Benzoyl peroxide	■ mat-bleach-condit
Beta-apo-8′ carotenal	▲ color
Beta carotene	◆ nutrient color
BHA (butylated hydroxyanisole)	● antioxidant
BHT (butylated hydroxytoluene)	● antioxidant
Butylparaben	● preservative

C

Calcium alginate	■ stabil-thick-tex
Calcium bromate	■ mat-bleach-condit
Calcium lactate	● preservative
Calcium phosphate	■ leavening
Calcium propionate	● preservative

Calcium silicate	■ anti-caking
Calcium sorbate	● preservative
Canthaxanthin	▲ color
Caramel	▲ color
Carob bean gum	■ stabil-thick-tex
Carrageenan	■ emulsifier ■ stabil-thick-tex
Carrot oil	▲ color
Cellulose	■ stabil-thick-tex
Citric acid	● preservative ● antioxidant ■ pH control
Citrus Red No. 2	▲ color
Cochineal extract	▲ color
Corn endosperm	▲ color
Corn syrup	▲ sweetener

D

Dehydrated beets	▲ color
Dextrose	▲ sweetener
Diglycerides	■ emulsifier
Dioctyl sodium sulfosuccinate	■ emulsifier
Disodium guanylate	▲ flavor enhancer
Disodium inosinate	▲ flavor enhancer
Dried algae meal	▲ color

E

EDTA (ethylenediamine-tetraacetic acid)	● antioxidant

F

FD&C Colors:	
Blue No. 1	▲ color
Red No. 3	▲ color
Red No. 40	▲ color
Yellow No. 5	▲ color
Fructose	▲ sweetener

G

Gelatin	■ stabil-thick-tex
Glucose	▲ sweetener
Glycerine	■ humectant
Glycerol monostearate	■ humectant
Grape skin extract	▲ color
Guar gum	■ stabil-thick-tex
Gum arabic	■ stabil-thick-tex
Gum ghatti	■ stabil-thick-tex

H

Heptylparaben	● preservative
Hydrogen peroxide	■ mat-bleach-condit
Hydrolyzed vegetable protein	▲ flavor enhancer

I

Invert sugar	▲ sweetener
Iodine	◆ nutrient
Iron	◆ nutrient
Iron-ammonium citrate	■ anti-caking
Iron oxide	▲ color

K

Karaya gum	■ stabil-thick-tex

L

Lactic acid	■ pH control ● preservative
Larch gum	■ stabil-thick-tex
Lecithin	■ emulsifier
Locust bean gum	■ stabil-thick-tex

M

Mannitol	▲ sweetener ■ anti-caking ■ stabil-thick-tex

Methylparaben	● preservative
Modified food starch	■ stabil-thick-tex
Monoglycerides	■ emulsifier
MSG (monosodium glutamate)	▲ flavor enhancer

N

Niacinamide	◆ nutrient

P

Paprika (and oleoresin)	▲ flavor ▲ color
Pectin	■ stabil-thick-tex
Phosphates	■ pH control
Phosphoric acid	■ pH control
Polysorbates	■ emulsifiers
Potassium alginate	■ stabil-thick-tex
Potassium bromate	■ mat-bleach-condit
Potassium iodide	◆ nutrient
Potassium propionate	● preservative
Potassium sorbate	● preservative
Propionic acid	● preservative
Propyl gallate	● antioxidant
Propylene glycol	■ stabil-thick-tex ■ humectant
Propylparaben	● preservative

R

Riboflavin	◆ nutrient ▲ color

S

Saccharin	▲ sweetener
Saffron	▲ color
Silicon dioxide	■ anti-caking
Sodium acetate	■ pH control
Sodium alginate	■ stabil-thick-tex
Sodium aluminum sulfate	■ leavening
Sodium benzoate	● preservative
Sodium bicarbonate	■ leavening
Sodium calcium alginate	■ stabil-thick-tex
Sodium citrate	■ pH control
Sodium diacetate	● preservative
Sodium erythorbate	● preservative
Sodium nitrate	● preservative
Sodium nitrite	● preservative
Sodium propionate	● preservative
Sodium sorbate	● preservative
Sodium stearyl fumarate	■ mat-bleach-condit
Sorbic acid	● preservative
Sorbitan monostearate	■ emulsifier
Sorbitol	■ humectant ▲ sweetener
Spices	▲ flavor
Sucrose (table sugar)	▲ sweetener

T

Tagetes (Aztec Marigold)	▲ color
Tartaric acid	■ pH control
TBHQ (tertiary butyl hydroquinone)	● antioxidant
Thiamine	◆ nutrient
Titanium dioxide	▲ color
Toasted, partially defatted cooked cottonseed flour	▲ color
Tocopherols (vitamin E)	◆ nutrient ● antioxidant
Tragacanth gum	■ stabil-thick-tex
Turmeric (oleoresin)	▲ flavor ▲ color

U

Ultramarine blue	▲ color

V

Vanilla, vanillin	▲ flavor
Vitamin A	◆ nutrient
Vitamin C (ascorbic acid)	◆ nutrient ● preservative ● antioxidant
Vitamin D (D_2, D_3)	◆ nutrient
Vitamin E (tocopherols)	◆ nutrient

Y

Yeast-malt sprout extract	▲ flavor enhancer
Yellow prussiate of soda	■ anti-caking

Fact or Fancy: Vitamins and Health Foods

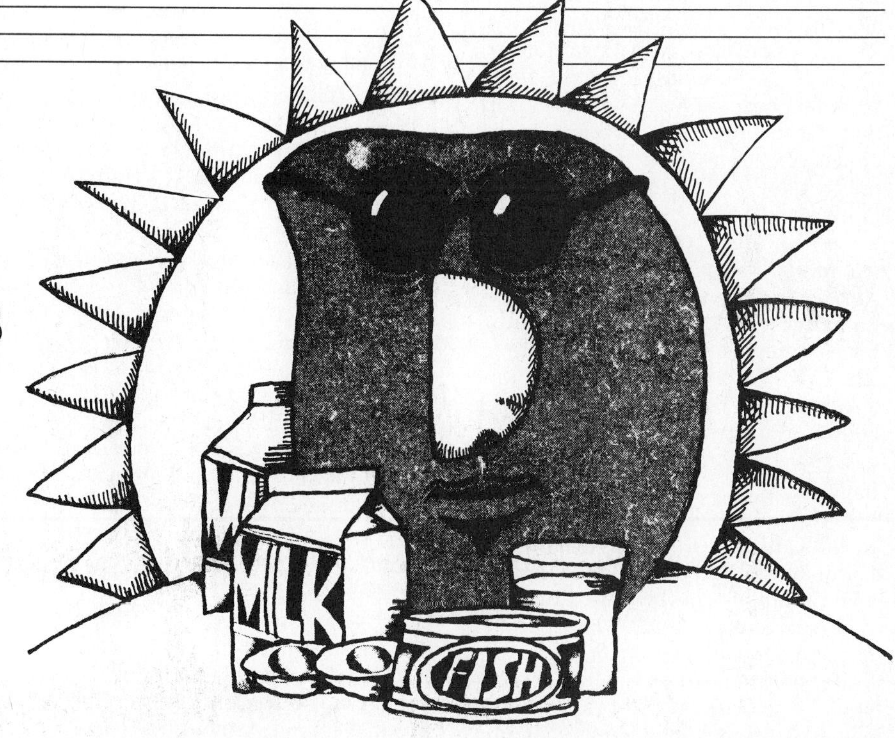

Vitamins are organic compounds necessary in small amounts in the diet for the normal growth and maintenance of life of animals, including man.

They do not provide energy, nor do they construct or build any part of the body. They are needed for transforming foods into energy and body maintenance. There are 13 or more of them, and if any is missing a deficiency disease becomes apparent.

Vitamins are similar because they are made of the same elements—carbon, hydrogen, oxygen, and sometimes nitrogen. (Vitamin B_{12} also contains cobalt.) They are different in that their elements are arranged differently, and each vitamin performs one or more specific functions in the body.

In the early 1900's scientists thought that three compounds were needed in the diet to prevent beriberi, pellagra, and scurvy. Those compounds originally were believed to belong to a class of chemical compounds called amines and were named from the Latin *vita*, or life, plus amine—vitamine. Later, the "e" was dropped when it was found that not all of the substances were amines.

At first, no one knew what they were chemically, and they were identified by letters. Later, what was thought to be one vitamin turned out to be many, and numbers were added; the Vitamin B complex is the best example.

Then some were found unnecessary for human needs and were removed from the list, which accounts for some of the gaps in the numbers. For example, B_8, adenylic acid; B_{13}, orotic acid; and B_{15}, pangamic acid. Others, originally designated differently, were found to be the same. For example, vitamins H, M, S, W, and X were all shown to be biotin; vitamin G became vitamin B_2 (riboflavin); and vitamin Y became vitamin B_6 (pyridoxine, pyridoxal, and pyridoxamine). Vitamin M seems to have been used for three different vitamins—folic acid, pantothenic acid, and biotin. The present trend is to eliminate the confusion by using the chemical names.

Extremely sensitive methods of measuring the potency or quantity of vitamins have been developed because they are present in foods only in very small amounts. Some vitamins are measured in I.U.'s (international units), which is a measure of biological activity. This is necessary because these vitamins have several natural forms that have different activities on an equal weight basis. The others are expressed by weight in micrograms or milligrams.

To illustrate the small amounts needed by the human body, let's start with an ounce, which is 28.3 grams. A milligram is 1/1000 of a gram, and a microgram is 1/1000 of a milligram. The U.S. Recommended Daily Allowance (U.S. RDA) of vitamin B_{12} for an adult is 6 micrograms a day. Just one ounce of this vitamin could supply the daily needs of 4,724,921 people!

Getting enough vitamins is essential to life, although the body has no nutritional use for excess vitamins and some vitamins can be stored only for relatively short periods. Many people, nevertheless, believe in being on the "safe side" and thus take extra vitamins. However, a well-balanced diet will usually meet all the body's vitamin needs.

So-called average or normal eaters probably never need supplemental vitamins, although many think they do. Vitamin deficiency diseases are rarely seen in the U.S. population. People *known* to have deficient diets require supplemental vitamins, as do those recovering from certain illnesses or vitamin deficiencies.

People who are interested in nutrition and good health should become familiar with the initials U.S. RDA. "United States Recommended Daily Allowances" were adopted by FDA for use in nutrition labeling and special dietary foods. They are the highest amounts of vitamins, minerals, and proteins that are needed by most people each day.

The accompanying table lists the U.S. RDA's for vitamins used in nutrition labeling of foods, including foods that are also vitamin supplements. The table is not complete because it lists only vitamins. The complete table of U.S. RDA's also includes specific minerals and protein.

Vitamin A—Retinol

Vitamin A is an oil soluble vitamin like D, E, and K, and is stored in the liver. (Generally, oil soluble vitamins can be stored for long periods—even indefinitely—in the body. Water soluble vitamins are retained for short periods, if at all.) This vitamin is necessary for new cell growth and healthy tissues and is essential for vision in dim light. Besides resulting in reduced ability to see in dim light (night blindness), high sensitivity to light, and other eye maladies, vitamin A deficiency can cause dry, rough skin that may become more susceptible to infection.

Children and young people who have been given large doses of vitamin A have developed an increased pressure inside the skull that mimics symptoms of a brain tumor so convincingly that in several cases hospital personnel made preparations for surgery before the high intake of vitamin A was discovered. Carotene, a form of Vitamin A that occurs in plants is, on the other hand, practically nontoxic.

Vitamin A activity is found in foods in two forms: carotene, a yellow pigment in green and yellow vegetables and yellow fruits that the human body converts to vitamin A, and vitamin A itself, formed from carotene by other animals and stored in certain food tissues such as liver, eggs, and milk.

Vitamin B_1—Thiamin

This vitamin is water soluble, as are all in the B complex. Thiamin is required for normal digestion, growth, fertility, lactation, the normal functioning of nerve tissue, and carbohydrate metabolism.

Vitamin B_1 deficiency causes beriberi, a dysfunctioning of the nervous system. Other deficiency problems are loss of appetite, body swelling (edema), heart problems, nausea, vomiting, and spastic muscle contractions throughout the body.

Thiamin is abundant in pork, soybeans, beans, peas, nuts, and in enriched and whole-grain breads and cereals.

Vitamin B_2—Riboflavin

Riboflavin helps the body obtain energy from carbohydrates and protein substances. A deficiency causes lip sores and cracks, as well as dimness of vision. This vitamin is abundant in leafy vegetables, enriched and whole-grain breads, liver, cheese, lean meats, milk, and eggs.

Niacin

Niacin is necessary for the healthy condition of all tissue cells. A deficiency causes pellagra, which was once, next to rickets, the most common deficiency disease in the United States. Pellagra is characterized by rough skin, mouth sores, diarrhea, and mental disorders.

Niacin is one of the most stable of the vitamins, the most easily obtained, and the cheapest. The most abundant natural sources are liver, lean meats, peas, beans, enriched and whole-grain cereal products, and fish.

Pantothenic Acid

Pantothenic acid is needed to support a variety of body functions, including proper growth and maintenance. A deficiency principally causes headache, fatigue, poor muscle coordination, nausea, and cramps.

Pantothenic acid is abundant in liver, eggs, white potatoes, sweet potatoes, peas, whole grains (particularly wheat), and peanuts.

Folic Acid (Folacin)

Folic acid helps the body to manufacture red blood cells and is essential in normal metabolism which is, basically, the conversion of food to energy. A deficiency causes a type of anemia.

The most abundant sources are liver, navy beans, and dark green leafy vegetables. Other good sources are: nuts, fresh oranges, and whole wheat products.

Vitamin B_6—Pyridoxine—Pyridoxal—Pyridoxamine

Vitamin B_6 has three forms but all are used by the body in the same way.

This vitamin is involved mostly in the utilization of protein. As with other vitamins, B_6 is essential for the proper growth and maintenance of body functions. Deficiency symptoms include mouth soreness, dizziness, nausea, and weight loss, and sometimes severe nervous disturbances.

Pyridoxine is found abundantly in liver, whole-grain cereals, potatoes, red meats, green vegetables, and yellow corn.

Vitamin B_{12}—Cyanocobalamin

Vitamin B_{12} is necessary for the normal development of red blood cells, and the functioning of all cells, particularly in the bone marrow, nervous system, and intestines.

A deficiency causes pernicious anemia, and if the deficiency is prolonged, a degeneration of the spinal cord occurs.

Abundant sources are: organ meats, lean meats, fish, milk, eggs, and shellfish. B_{12} is not present to any measurable degree in plants, which means that strict vegetarians should supplement their diets with this vitamin.

Biotin

Once called vitamin H, biotin is now the sole descriptive term for this vitamin, which is actually a member of the B complex. It is important in the metabolism of carbohydrates, proteins, and fats

Most deficiency symptoms involve mild skin disorders, some anemia, depression, sleeplessness, and muscle pain. A deficiency is extremely rare and this is probably because the bacteria in the intestinal tract produces biotin so that more is excreted than was consumed in the diet.

Abundant dietary sources include eggs, milk, and meats. *Raw* egg white contains a factor that destroys biotin.

Vitamin C—Ascorbic Acid

This least stable of the vitamins promotes growth and tissue repair, including the healing of wounds. It aids in tooth formation and bone formation. When used as a food additive, vitamin C acts as a preservative.

Lack of this vitamin causes scurvy, one of the oldest diseases known to man. The signs of scurvy include: lassitude, weakness, bleeding, loss of weight, and irritability. An early sign is bleeding of the gums and ease of bruising. Long before the 16th century, American Indians knew that scurvy could be cured by a tea made with spruce or pine needles.

Abundant sources are turnip greens, green pepper, kale, broccoli, mustard greens, citrus fruits, strawberries, currants, tomatoes, and

United States Recommended Daily Allowances

	Unit	Infants (0-12 mo.)	Children under 4 yrs.	Adults and children 4 or more yrs.	Pregnant or lactating women
Vitamin A	IU	1500	2500	5000	8000
Vitamin D	IU	400	400	400	400
Vitamin E	IU	5	10	30	30
Vitamin C	mg	35	40	60	60
Folacin	mg	0.1	0.2	0.4	0.8
Thiamine (B_1)	mg	0.5	0.7	1.5	1.7
Riboflavin (B_2)	mg	0.6	0.8	1.7	2.0
Niacin	mg	8	9	20	20
Vitamin B_6	mg	0.4	0.7	2	2.5
Vitamin B_{12}	mcg	2	3	6	8
Biotin	mg	0.05	0.15	0.3	0.3
Pantothenic acid	mg	3	5	10	10

IU = International unit
mg = milligram
mcg = microgram

The U.S. RDA system was developed by FDA for its nutrition labeling and dietary supplement programs. This table for use in the labeling of dietary supplements lists only vitamin requirements.

other vegetables. You can get all the vitamin C your body needs by eating a daily 3- to 4-ounce serving of any of the foods named.

Vitamin D—Calciferol

This vitamin also exists in several forms. The most common (and equally effective) are ergocalciferol—vitamin D_2, and cholicalciferol—vitamin D_3. The D_2 is a plant source: the D_3 comes from animal sources.

Vitamin D aids in the absorption of calcium and phosphorus in bone formation. To accomplish its work, the body—through the liver and the kidneys—converts the vitamin to a hormone-like material.

Vitamin D deficiency causes rickets. The obvious signs are skeleton deformation—bowed legs, deformed spine, "potbelly" appearance, and sometimes flat feet and stunting of growth.

Too much vitamin D can cause nausea, weight loss, weakness, excessive urination, and the more serious conditions of hypertension and calcification of soft tissues, including the blood vessels and kidneys. Bone deformities and multiple fractures are also common. In fact, many of the symptoms from an excess of vitamin D are remarkably similar to those caused by a deficiency.

Abundant sources are canned and fresh fish (particularly the salt water varieties), egg yolk, and the vitamin D-fortified foods such as milk and margarine. People who spend part of their time in the sun with exposure of the skin need no other source of vitamin D, since it is formed in the skin by the ultraviolet rays. Foods fortified with vitamin D are intended mainly for infants and the elderly who lack exposure to sunlight. The daily requirement is very small and excess amounts above that are stored in the body.

Vitamin K

There are several natural forms of vitamin K, which are essential to cause clotting of the blood. One type, K_1, occurs in plants. Another, K_2, is formed by bacteria in the intestinal tract. Yet a third is found in some animals and birds. The synthetic vitamin K, menadione, because of the potential for harm involved in its use, is dispensed only by prescription. Phyloquinone, K_1, may be used in dietary supplements up to a level of 100 micrograms per recommended daily quantity.

A deficiency causes hemorrhage and liver injury. Vitamin K is found in spinach, lettuce, kale, cabbage, cauliflower, liver, and egg yolk.

Vitamin E—The Tocopherols

Vitamin E in humans acts as an antioxidant that helps to prevent oxygen from destroying other substances. In other words, vitamin E is a preservative, protecting the activity of other compounds such as vitamin A. No clinical effects have been associated with very low intake of this vitamin in man. A rather rare form of anemia is premature infants, however, responds to vitamin E medication. A diet high in polyunsaturated fat requires a small increase in dietary vitamin E to prevent oxidation of this rather unstable form of fat.

Abundant sources are vegetable oils, beans, eggs, whole grains (the germ), liver, fruits, and vegetables.

Vitamin E is one of the most talked about vitamins, and to some extent the exaggerated and unsubstantiated claims made for vitamin E result from a combination of hope and misinterpretation.

The Committee on Nutritional Misinformation of the National Academy of Sciences has issued a report on vitamin E. Three statements are quoted here:

"Surveys of the U.S. population indicate that adequate amounts of vitamin E are supplied by the usual diet."

"Careful studies over a period of years attempting to relate these (test animal) symptoms to vitamin E deficiency in human beings have been unproductive."

"Self-medication with vitamin E in the hope that a more or less serious ***condition will be alleviated may indeed be hazardous, especially when appropriate diagnosis and treatment may thereby be delayed or avoided."***

Most of us view scientific knowledge with awe, and we are quite justified, considering the scientific achievements of our age. Misconceptions about vitamins and their proper functions are understandable; no primer would be complete that fails to clear up some of these misconceptions:

Myth: ***Organic or natural vitamins are nutritionally superior to synthetic vitamins.***

Fact: *Synthetic vitamins, manufactured in the laboratory, are identical to the natural vitamins found in foods. The body cannot tell the difference and gets the same benefits from either source. Statements to the effect that "Nature cannot be imitated" and "Natural vitamins have the essence of life" are without meaning.*

Myth: ***Vitamins give you "pep" and "energy."***

Fact: *Vitamins yield no calories. They, of themselves, provide no extra pep or vitality beyond normal expectations, nor an unusual level of well-being.*

Myth: ***The more vitamins the better.***

Fact: *Taking excess vitamins is a complete waste, both in money and effect. In fact, as noted, excess amounts of some vitamins can be harmful.*

Myth: ***You cannot get enough vitamins from the conventional foods you eat.***

Fact: *Anyone who eats a reasona-*

bly varied diet of whole food, should normally never need supplemental vitamins.

The abundant sources listed give some idea of how difficult it is to be undernourished from lack of vitamins.

Each of the following is not only an abundant source of one or more vitamins, but also contains important amounts of most of the rest of the nutrients:

Liver; eggs, cheese; fortified margarine; butter; whole milk; fortified milk; fish; egg yolk; yellow vegetables; green leafy vegetables; yellow fruits; beans; peas; nuts; whole-grain foods; red meats; lean meats; pork; shellfish; fresh vegetables; white potatoes; sweet potatoes; yellow corn; rice; strawberries; currants; citrus fruits and juices; tomatoes and juices; other fruits, juices, and berries; canned and fresh herring; salmon; tuna; lettuce; fresh oranges; cabbage; spinach; cauliflower; and vegetable oils of several kinds.

Even though the widely seen and identified vitamin deficiency diseases of 30 years ago have all but disappeared, the American consumer is approached from all sides with misinformation about the almost universal "need" for supplements of vitamins.

Is there really a need? Each person can answer this only after examining his or her regular diet and learning what vitamins can and cannot do.

Health Foods

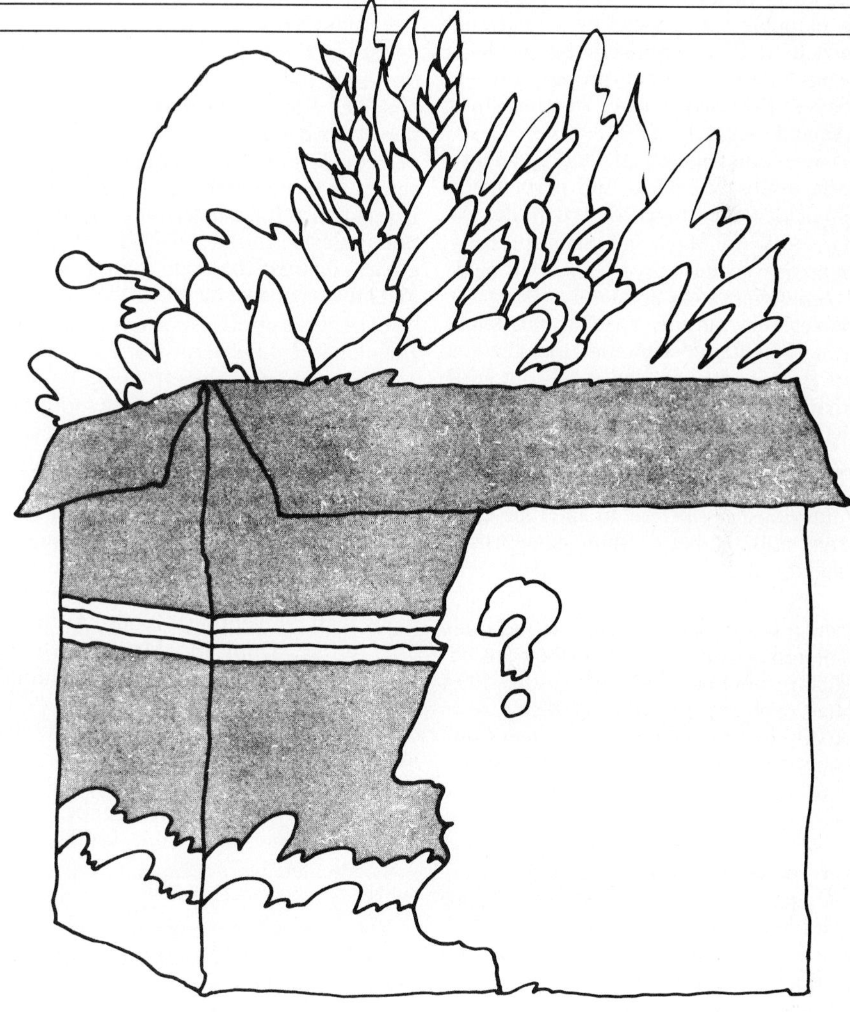

It's probably fair to say that the more people know about food and nutrition the more likely they are to develop eating habits that contribute to good health. Therefore, the growing interest of consumers in the safety and nutritional quality of the American diet is a welcome development. Regrettably, however, much of this interest has been colored by alarmists who state or imply that the American food supply is unsafe or somehow inadequate to meet our nutritional needs.

Advocates of "health," "organic," and "natural" foods—terms for which there is little agreement as to their exact meaning—frequently proclaim that such products are safer and more nutritious than conventionally grown and marketed foods. Although most of these claims are not supported by scientific evidence, it is difficult for the public to evaluate truth from fancy—particularly in regard to use of the term "natural" for everything from whole grain flour or bread to potato chips. Claims or suggestions that certain health foods or diets prevent or cure disease or provide other special health benefits are, for the most part, folklore, and sometimes fabrication.

Almost daily, the public is besieged by claims for new "anti-cancer" foods, "no aging" diets, "no hunger" breads, "new" (nonessential) vitamins, and by endless other quackery. Many consumers do not know that the First Amendment to the Constitution of the United States places some kinds of statements about food and nutrition beyond the reach of Federal regulation through its protection of free speech and free press.

If the label on a food product makes false or misleading claims FDA can take action on the grounds that the product is mislabeled or misbranded. If false claims are made in ads or in other material directly promoting the product, the Federal Trade Commission may be able to take action.

But the labels on or promotions for fad foods or diets often do not make any direct claims that can be shown to be false. Instead, they refer to a book, a pamphlet, a speech, or a magazine article that has praised the product. Thus, these indirect promotions receive the protection of the First Amendment.

Scientific rebuttal of food and nutrition myths published and perpetuated in faddist literature often is futile. As Dr. Edward H. Rynearson, recently retired from the Mayo Clinic, has said, "Americans love hogwash." We have fables that natural vitamins are superior to synthetic vitamins, that the soil in this country is "all worn out," or that use of organic fertilizers results in better crops than manufactured fertilizers. And we have many minor myths: that organic (fertilized) eggs are nutritiously superior to infertile eggs, raw milk is better than pasteurized, and the like.

The terms "organic," "natural," and "health" are so loosely and often interchangeably used that they are difficult to define—so much so that FDA has taken no position on their use in food labeling. The Federal Trade Commission in its proposed Food Advertising Rule would prohibit use of the words "organic" and "natural" in food advertising because of concern about the ability of consumers to understand the terms in the conflicting and confusing ways they are used. FTC also proposes to prohibit the term "health food" in advertising because it is undefined and may fool consumers into thinking one particular food will provide good health.

One thing all health, organic, and natural food products seem to have in common is that they cost the consumer more than conventional foods. A survey by the U.S. Department of Agriculture indicated that the cost at the supermarket can run twice as much for health foods as for regular foods. The price for comparable foods, and sometimes even for the same food, rises steadily from the regular supermarket shelf to the health food section of the supermarket to the health food store. Expanding health food sections in some major foodstores demonstrate the popularity of these items. In 1974 it was projected that organic food retail sales would reach $3 billion in 1980, a rise from $500 million in 1972.

Use of these foods often is tied to the desire for a simpler, pre-technology lifestyle. But the user is misled if he thinks such foods can maintain health or provide better nutritional quality or safety than conventional foods. There is real cause for concern if consumers, particularly those with limited incomes, distrust the regular food supply and buy expensive health foods.

FDA has not tried to arrive at a legal definition of these terms for food labeling because enforcement would be difficult or impossible, and costly. Organically grown foods, once they are removed from the field, cannot be told from commercially fertilized plants. Plant roots absorb nutrients in inorganic form, regardless of the source, and there is no scientific basis for claiming organic foods are more nutritious than conventional foods. According to Dr. Emil M. Mrak, former chancellor of the University of California at Davis and a world authority on agriculture, scientific experiments conducted for 25 years in Michigan, at Cornell University, and in England have established no differences between organic or health foods and foods treated with manufactured fertilizers.

Differences in the nutrient content of food from plants of the same species depend on their genetic nature, the climate, the nutrients available for growth, and the stage of maturity at which they are harvested. For example, wide variation in the vitamin A content has been found in different varieties of carrots and in Valencia oranges grown in different parts of the country.

One of the alleged advantages of organically grown foods is that no pesticides are used on them and thus the so-called organic products consumers buy are supposedly free of traces or residues of pesticides. But the fact is that many of these foods do contain pesticide residues. Even if no pesticides are used on a particular crop, some chemical residues often remain in the soil for years after the last application of a pesticide on a previous crop. In addition, fresh residues may be deposited from drifting sprays and dusts or from rainfall runoff from nearby farms. Traces of pesticides may be found in both organic and conventional foods, but these residues normally are within Federal tolerance levels, which are set low enough to protect consumers.

Since chemically and organically grown foods do not differ in looks, taste, or chemical analysis, the only way to assure that a product labeled as "organically grown" is truthfully labeled would be to keep watch over the product from planting to harvest to sale, and to check soil and water reports. Such a program, of course, would be prohibitively expensive.

The possibility for fraud is apparent when the consumer doesn't know if the storekeeper is honest, when the storekeeper can't tell if the distributor is honest, and when the distributor doesn't know if his suppliers are living up to their promises. Because of this and the premium prices placed on organic foods, it's not surprising that **conventional foods at times have been substituted for organic foods. If FDA can identify fraud in the labeling of a natural or organic or health food, it can take action. The Agency also can act if claims are made suggesting that a certain food or combination of foods can be used to treat a disease condition, if the statements are untrue.**

It would be inaccurate to imply that all elements of the health food industry engage in shady marketing practices. Some distributors and growers supply affidavits or certificates for foods grown and handled according to "or-

ganic and natural" precepts. Many health food operators truly believe in health foods and are sincere in trying to provide consumers the "real" thing.

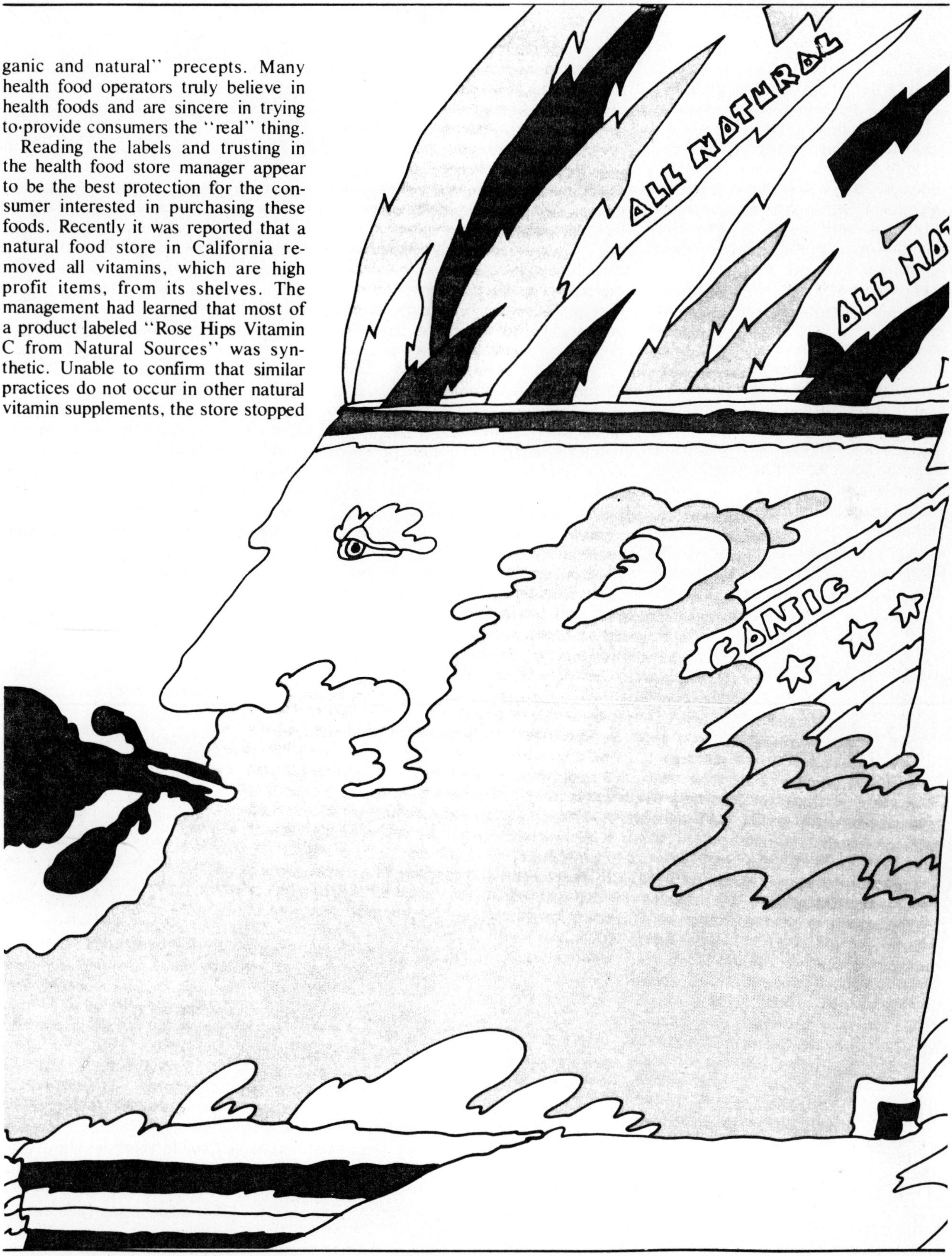

Reading the labels and trusting in the health food store manager appear to be the best protection for the consumer interested in purchasing these foods. Recently it was reported that a natural food store in California removed all vitamins, which are high profit items, from its shelves. The management had learned that most of a product labeled "Rose Hips Vitamin C from Natural Sources" was synthetic. Unable to confirm that similar practices do not occur in other natural vitamin supplements, the store stopped

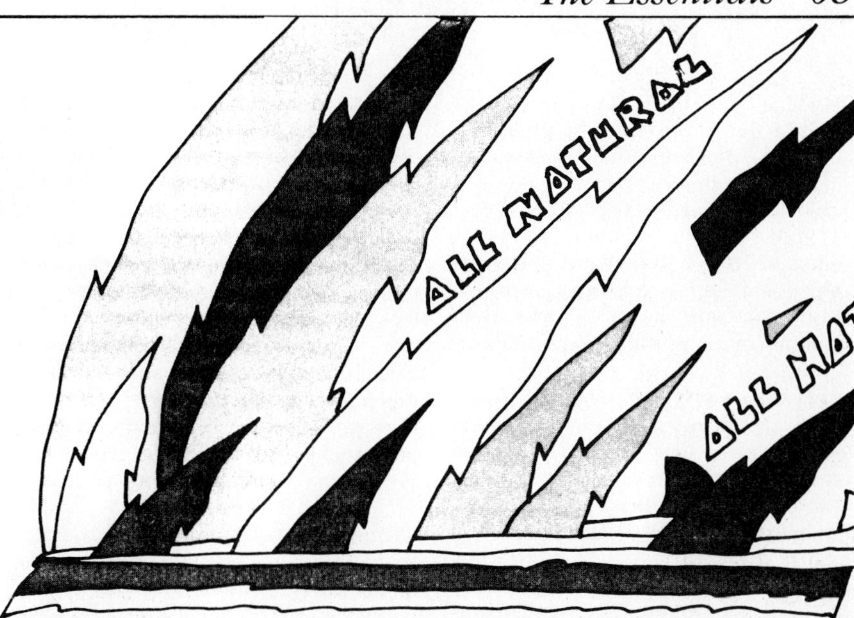

handling vitamins and suggested that people get them from a pharmacy where the pills aren't labeled as natural and they're cheaper.

That's excellent advice from both a scientific and an economic viewpoint. Vitamins from natural sources have no nutritional superiority over synthetic vitamins, and the Food and Drug Administration prohibits such claims in food labeling.

FDA also prohibits claims of nutritional significance in behalf of para-amino-benzoic acid (PABA), rutin and other bioflavonoids, lecithin, and many other such supplements not essential for human nutrition which are sold in health food stores. The continuing market for an ever-increasing variety of these and other food supplements feeds on various myths promoted in the fad literature.

One practice is to falsely promote a substance as a vitamin. A recent example is pangamic acid, which has falsely been called B-15. Vitamins are organic substances required in minute amounts in the diet of animals for normal growth, maintenance of health, and reproduction. Each vitamin has a unique function in the body, and inadequate amounts or the absence of a vitamin in the diet produces a specific deficiency disease condition. For instance, a deficiency or lack of vitamin C causes scurvy.

For a substance to be established as a legitimate vitamin it must be tested under controlled conditions to prove that its absence in the diet causes abnormal body functioning. All animals need some vitamins but not all known vitamins are needed by all animals. Therefore, testing must also establish that a vitamin is essential in the *human* diet before it can be said to be essential in human nutrition. Pangamic acid is not a vitamin because it is not essential in the diet of animals for the normal functioning of the body.

Many people are lured to health foods in the belief that since they're natural they're totally safe, or at least safer than conventional foods. There's not much logic here. Hundreds of toxicants are known to occur naturally in foods. For example, aflatoxin, a mold product which grows naturally under some conditions on corn, peanuts, and other grains, is a powerful carcinogen. FDA monitors foods for aflatoxin and has established safe minimum levels in some foods, such as peanut butter and milk. Peanut butter or milk which contains aflatoxin above these safe levels cannot be marketed. But there's no way FDA or anyone can assure that all foods are entirely free of such naturally occurring toxins.

Herb teas, which are favored by many health food advocates, contain thousands of chemical compounds that have not been tested for safety. Sassafras root was found to contain safrole, which produces liver cancer in rats, and the sale of sassafras tea was banned by FDA in 1976 for that reason.

Lead, arsenic, cadmium, and other heavy metals occur naturally at very low levels in many foods. In extracts and concentrates made from foods, the level of such substances may be much

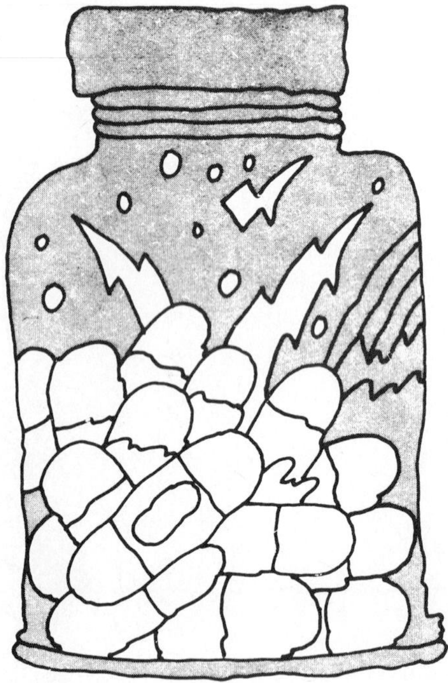

Warning Planned on Potassium Chloride

Potassium chloride, a substance often sold in health food stores as a diet supplement, is potentially dangerous and overuse can be fatal.

Accidental overuse of potassium chloride—sometimes called potassium salt—is known to have caused deaths of otherwise healthy individuals, and potassium chloride supplements and other products labeled as "salt substitutes" which contain potassium should not be used by people with certain medical conditions.

Overuse of potassium chloride supplements by healthy individuals can cause hyperkalemia (excessively high levels of potassium in the blood), a potentially fatal condition. In a recent case that received national publicity, a mother administered large amounts of potassium chloride (3,000 milligrams one day and 1,500 milligrams the next day) to her 2-month old baby as a remedy for "colic." The mother was following the advice of a book by the late Adelle Davis entitled LET'S HAVE HEALTHY CHILDREN. The child died despite medical efforts to reduce body potassium levels.

FDA believes no one should use potassium supplements without medical supervision. The practice is particularly dangerous to children.

At present, potassium chloride supplements and salt substitutes are not required to carry warning labels about potential health hazards. However, FDA soon will propose that all such products be required to carry a warning that they should be used only under medical supervision.

higher. Some bonemeal has been found to contain high levels of lead.

Kelp tablets, a food supplement commonly sold in health food stores, may contain high levels of arsenic, as do many other products from the sea. Studies of industrial workers exposed to arsenic indicate a greater occurrence of cancer among those so exposed. Researchers have found elevated levels of urinary arsenic in individuals who have consumed kelp tablet supplements.

Many commonly used foods, whether sold as health or conventional foods, contain low levels of toxic substances. Oxalic acid is present in several vegetables including spinach. Carrots, lettuce, and celery leaves contain nitrate and nitrite compounds.

Does this mean that we need to be fearful of using these foods? Not at all. The best thing to do is to exercise care and common sense by eating a balanced diet from a wide variety of foods and by practicing moderation in eating any single food.

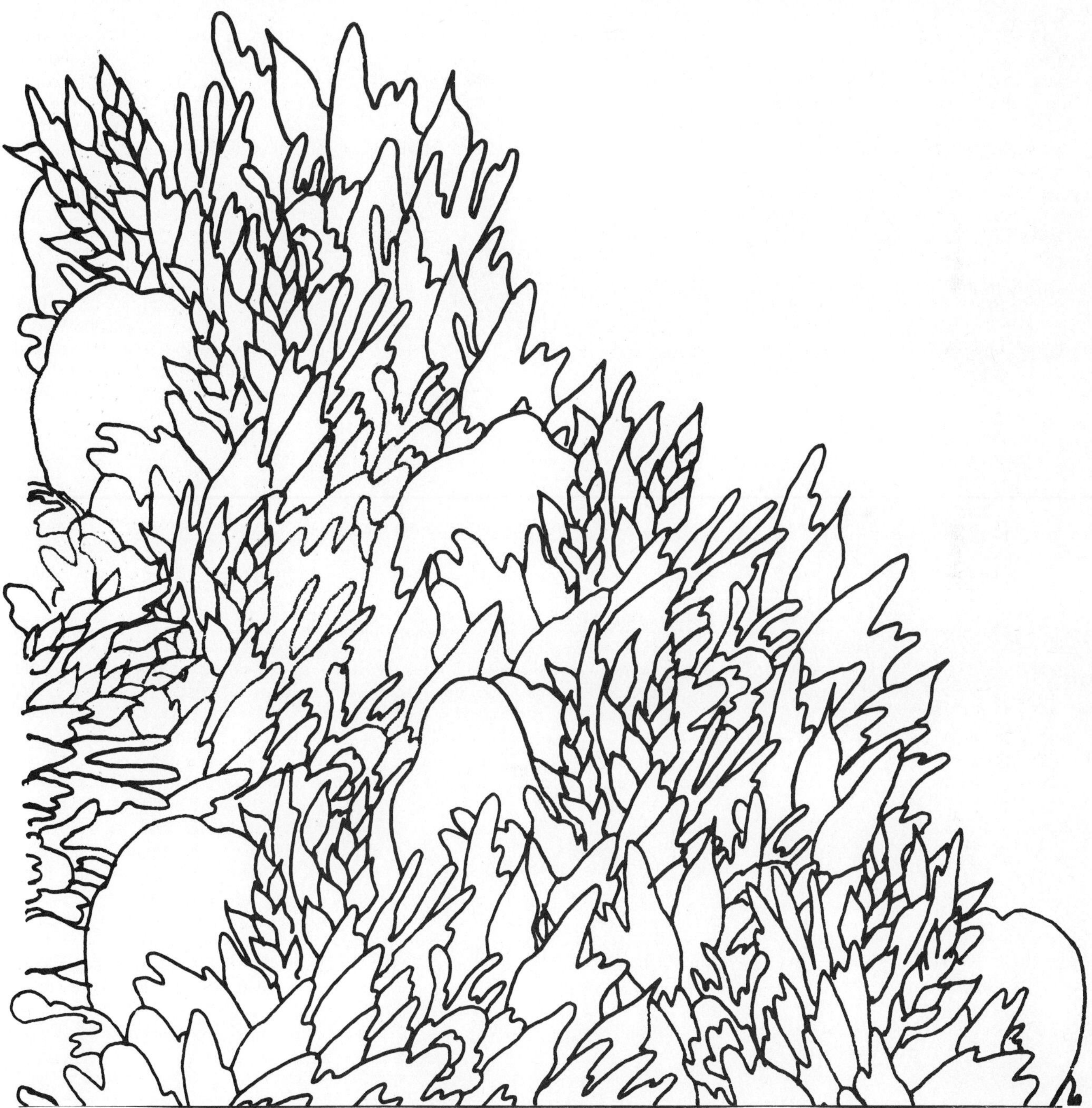

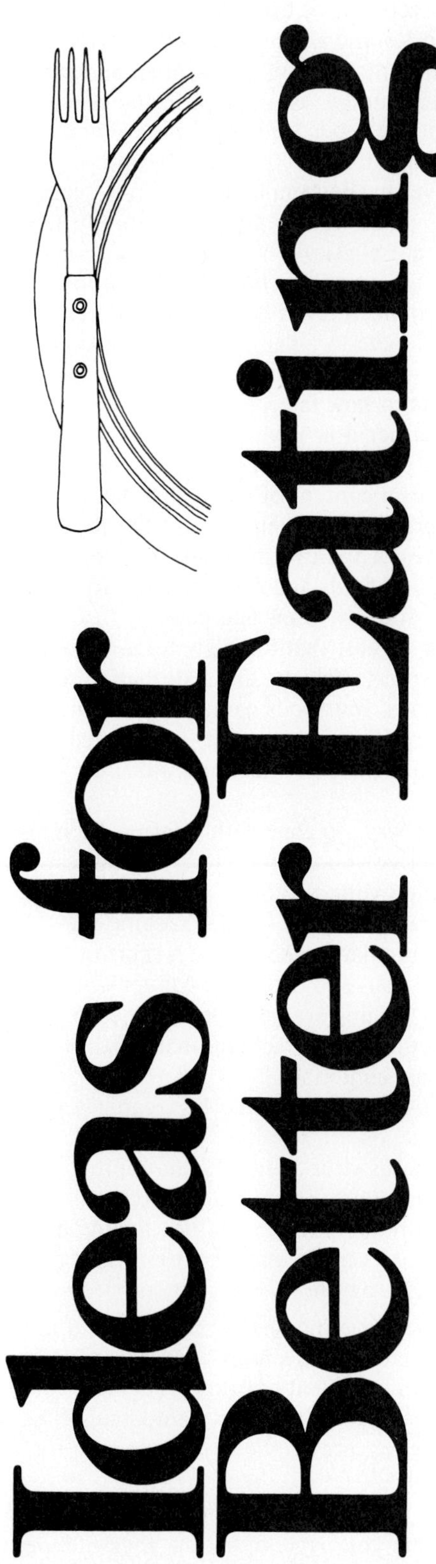

Menus and Recipes That Use U.S. Dietary Guidelines

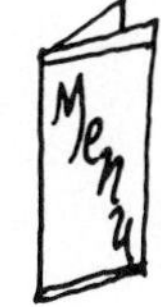

About the Menu Guides

In the past few years, many nutritionists have concluded that we can maintain our health, and even improve it, by modifying our diets. In February 1980, the U.S. Departments of Agriculture and Health and Human Services recommended dietary guidelines in the publication, *Nutrition and Your Health—Dietary Guidelines for Americans.*

There are a lot of good things about the way we eat now. There are also many unanswered questions about the relation of diet and health and of diet and disease—things science has yet to discover. Why should we change the way we eat now?

Many nutritionists recommend we make some prudent changes in our diets based on the best available knowledge. For instance, we know that we need to eat a wide range of nutrients to maintain good health. We know there is a relationship between obesity and eating more calories than we need and between hypertension and eating a lot of salt. Although there is some controversy, many experts believe there is a relationship between heart attacks and eating too much of foods high in fat, saturated fat, and cholesterol.

Nutritionists also recognize that people do not eat for nutritional benefits alone. Food must be appealing and enjoyable or no one will eat it. These menu guides and recipes were developed to help keep our diets appealing and enjoyable as well as healthful.

A final word—moderation is the best guide in eating to maintain health.

I. MAKING A START

By and large, Americans have an adequate diet. With very little effort, they could have a better one. In the process, they would increase their chances of staying healthy.

Nutritionists in the Federal Government have developed a set of guidelines that can help many Americans improve their eating habits. The guidelines are the joint effort of the Departments of Health and Human Services and Agriculture.

Based on what we know today about the relationship of diet to good health, the guidelines recommend that we:

- Eat a variety of foods.
- Maintain ideal weight.
- Avoid too much fat, saturated fat, and cholesterol.
- Eat foods with adequate starch and fiber.
- Avoid too much sugar.
- Avoid too much sodium.
- If you drink alcohol, do so in moderation.

The guidelines help us make informed choices about our food. The object is to get the right balance of vitamins, minerals, and fiber without overdoing the salt or the calories, especially the calories from fat and sugar.

The menus are designed for healthy adults. They can be modified for children and teenagers. The menus are not, however, planned for the use of toddlers, for pregnant or nursing women, for convalescents, or for others with special health or nutrition problems.

There are two versions of each day's menu. One provides 1,600 calories and the other 2,400 calories. They reflect the amounts of food that women and men say they eat, on the average, as reported in the surveys. They also represent the foods we commonly eat and the way we usually eat them.

The calorie level in the sample menu is not necessarily right for you, since we all vary greatly in our need for calories. If you are physically active, you may need more calories than the amounts shown. If you aren't very active, you may need fewer calories to maintain normal weight. You have to judge your own needs depending on your weight and activity.

There are limits to how far you can go. The less food you eat, the harder it is to get all the vitamins and minerals you need. That is particularly true for iron and zinc. The zinc and iron content of a diet that is low in calories can be improved by eating more of the foods that are good sources of the two minerals: lean meat, shellfish, whole grain breads and cereals, some fortified breads and cereals, and dry beans and peas.

Recent studies suggest that the body more readily absorbs the iron in meat, poultry, and fish than it does the iron in plant foods. But foods containing vitamin C—a glass of orange juice, for example—consumed along with plant foods increase the amount of iron absorbed.

There are other ways to cope with calories. Be more active. The more active you are the more you can eat while still maintaining your weight. It's easier to get the vitamins and minerals you need—while keeping the pounds off—if you regularly take part in a sport or some other activity which you enjoy and find convenient. Walking, biking, or jogging are good possibilities. Your doctor can tell you the level of activity that's right for your age and physical condition.

In addition to using up some calories, regular exercise pays other dividends. It develops strength and endurance and increases your agility. It can improve your posture and your appearance in general. Exercise also relieves tension and reduces the risk of developing heart disease. It does more. Exercise may result in better mental performance, less drowsiness, and sounder sleep.

The menus reflect common eating patterns and use ordinary foods. The menus are simply examples of ways to eat for good health and good nutrition. They are consistent with the objectives of the dietary guidelines. The menus are *not*, however, prescriptions that must be followed in every detail.

You could start by looking for those menus that most closely resemble your style of eating. By switching foods from one meal or snack to another, you can create a menu you like better.

Snacks are part of the total nutrition picture in the menus. If you prefer you can tuck them into your meals and forget about snacking.

You aren't going to make all the changes suggested by the guidelines overnight. Start small. Make one change. When you've adjusted to that one, try another.

Don't be too hard on yourself. The important thing is to stay on track—or to get back on it. When you've succeeded in making one change for the better, pat yourself on the back. But don't stop there. Take another step. Keep at it until you've gone the distance.

The menus are based on ordinary foods and standard recipes unless otherwise indicated. The hamburger and french fries in menu 2, for example, are the kind you would eat in a restaurant or in a fast food establishment. Despite their higher sodium and fat content, they fit in with the guidelines. To compensate for the higher fat and sodium content, other foods during the day balance them out.

The recipes provided for items in the menus were developed in test kitchens to moderate the amount of fat, cholesterol, salt, and sugar. If you follow your own recipe, or use different ingredients, you may end up with more calories, fat, cholesterol, salt, or sugar.

The 1,600- and 2,400-calorie menus are most alike at breakfast and dinner, when everyone in the house tends to eat "out of the same pot." Differences are the result of tailoring the menus to the nutritional needs of women and men. On the average, women need fewer calories than men, but have similar requirements for many vitamins and minerals. For women, that leaves less room for calories that don't carry their share of nutrients—calories from fat, sugar, and alcohol.

To adapt the menus to the needs of school-age children and teenagers, add 1 to 2 glasses of fortified milk for 7-to-10-year-olds. Add 2 to 3 glasses for teenagers. For guidance on feeding infants, toddlers, pregnant or nursing women, and convalescents, consult a physician, public health nurse, nutritionist, dietitian, or Extension nutrition specialist.

1 Eat a Variety of Foods.

You can get the vitamins and minerals you need for good health with a variety of foods. Choosing a wide selection of fruits, vegetables, breads and cereals, dairy products, and meat, fish, and poultry products will do the job.

Adding variety to our diets isn't that hard. Most of us vary the way we eat from day to day. It's a good idea nutritionally. If you pick different foods from within each group of foods, you increase the range of nutrients in your diet. Over a period of days, you should come out about right.

To increase the variety of foods, the menus:

- provide more servings of fruits and vegetables than many of us are accustomed to.

- frequently include dark-green vegetables, dry bean dishes, and starchy vegetables.

- use more grain products, especially whole grains.

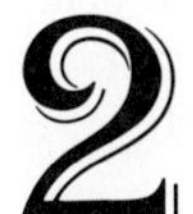

Maintain Ideal Weight.

If you want to lose weight:

- start by cutting back on fats, sugars, and alcohol in your diet.

- cut back on serving sizes.

- increase your physical activity.

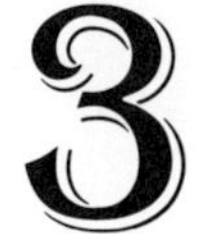

Avoid Too Much Fat, Saturated Fat, and Cholesterol.

Several factors have been linked to heart disease. Among them are high levels of blood cholesterol, high blood pressure, diabetes, a history of heart disease in the family, and obesity. Many scientists believe that certain habits and characteristics raise the risk of heart disease. These traits include smoking, reaction to stress, physical inactivity, and immoderate consumption of fats, saturated fat, cholesterol, and sodium.

Higher levels of blood cholesterol are generally associated with a greater risk of heart disease; lower levels with a lower risk. High levels of blood cholesterol can lead to atherosclerosis (hardening of the arteries), the underlying problem causing most heart and blood vessel diseases. Although levels of blood cholesterol vary among individuals, populations with high consumption rates for saturated fat and cholesterol generally tend to have high levels of blood cholesterol. Differences in heredity explain why some people can follow diets that are high in fat and cholesterol and still maintain relatively low levels of blood cholesterol. Others, consuming less fat and cholesterol, have relatively high levels of blood cholesterol. Your physician can evaluate your blood cholesterol status.

There is debate about whether it is sound to make a general recommendation that people should reduce their dietary fat and cholesterol. Many scientists, including the Surgeon General of the United States, believe it is sensible to consume only moderate amounts of fat and cholesterol. They also believe that this moderation poses no known health risk, and may reduce your risk of heart attack. No diet, however, will insure against heart disease.

Most of the fat and cholesterol in our diets comes from fats and oils, meat, poultry, egg yolks, and dairy products. The menus lower the amount of fat and cholesterol by:

- selecting lean hamburger and lean roasts, chops, and steaks—trimmed of visible fat.
- draining meat drippings.
- limiting the amount of margarine or other fats used on bread and vegetables.
- emphasizing lowfat and skim milk and reducing the amount of fat in other foods when whole milk or cheese is used.
- cutting down the amount of fat used in recipes, added to foods in cooking, or added at the table.
- limiting the number of fried foods, especially breaded or batter-fried foods.
- moderating the amounts of organ meats and egg yolks.
- using fewer creamed foods and rich desserts.
- watching the amount of salad dressing used.

4 Eat Foods with Adequate Amounts of Starch and Fiber.

In order to have enough starch and fiber, the menus:

- provide more vegetables and fruits.
- include potatoes, sweet potatoes, yams, corn, peas, and dried beans more often.
- emphasize whole grain cereal products, such as brown rice, oatmeal, and whole wheat cereals and breads.

When you try the menus, it may seem like more food than you are used to. You are cutting down on the "concentrated calories" from fats and sweets and adding more servings of fruits, vegetables, and whole grains. Your diet is bulkier. There are no more calories, but the volume is larger. Nutritionally, it's an advantage. You are getting more nutrients and fiber for your calories. Since the bulkier diet makes you feel full, it may help curb your appetite. Even so, it may take getting used to.

People who count calories often won't touch starchy foods like potatoes, breads, and grains. They think starches are "fattening." Actually starches are no more fattening than any other food. The question is how much you eat and how much fat or sugar and other sweeteners you add to the starches. Fats have more than two times the calories of starch. Sugar has no more calories than starch, but sugary foods add little more than calories to your diet.

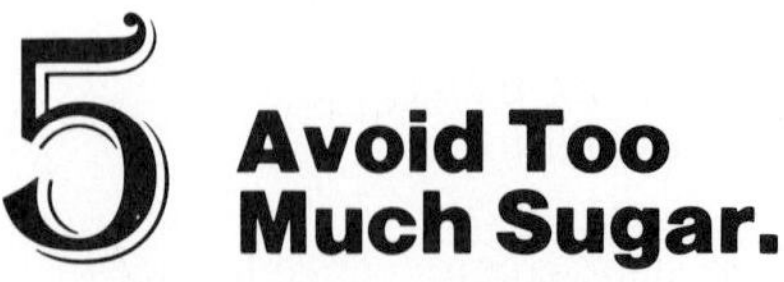

5 Avoid Too Much Sugar.

We get most of our "added sugar" from soft drinks, candy, and desserts, not from the sugar bowl. The menus limit the amount of added sugar by:

- avoiding or cutting down on very sweet foods.

- reducing the amount of sugar in recipes for baked goods and desserts.

- relying more on fresh fruit and canned fruits packed in juice or light sirup.

- limiting the amounts of sugar, jams, jellies, and sirups.

6 Avoid Too Much Sodium and Salt.

Sodium is a component of salt. Aside from the salt we add at the stove and at the table, much of the sodium we consume comes from the salt and other sodium compounds in commercially prepared foods. So choose carefully when you are eating out. When you shop, read the label. Avoid obviously salty foods. Keep the salt shaker off the table. Your appetite for salty foods may be curbed if you make an effort to break the salt habit.

To limit the amount of sodium and salt, the menus:

- use few salty, processed foods.

- use little or no salt and assume that none is added at the table.

- make only sparing use of commercially prepared sauces and condiments; these include such foods as catsup, barbecue sauce, Worcestershire or soy sauce, mustard, relishes and pickles, bouillon cubes, meat tenderizer, monosodium glutamate, gravy mixes, and canned soups.

- use more fresh and frozen vegetables than canned or seasoned frozen vegetables which have salt added.

- limit the use of salty snack foods such as chips, pretzels, and crackers.

For more information, see section titled "The Truth About Salt."

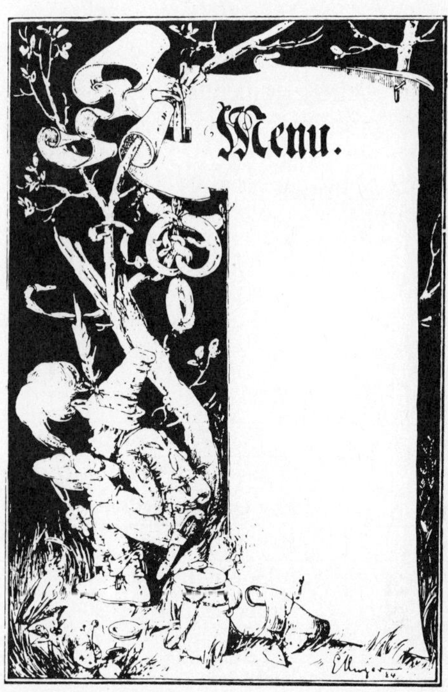

II. MENUS TO GET YOU GOING

Foods alone can't make you healthy. But good eating habits based on moderation and variety, along with regular physical activity, will certainly help.

The menus in the book generally meet or exceed recommended allowances for most nutrients.[1] At the 1,600-calorie level, they fall short of recommended levels for vitamin B_6, folacin (another B vitamin), iron, and zinc. However, the levels of these nutrients in the menus exceed the average amounts consumed at similar levels of calorie intake, according to national surveys. In diets of fewer than 1,800 calories, it is hard to get the recommended levels of all essential nutrients. That is particularly true of vitamins and minerals which are present in many foods but only in low concentrations. To approach the recommended levels of these nutrients at low calorie levels, it is necessary to be more moderate in the use of fat, sugar, and alcohol than many of us are accustomed to, and to eat more nutrient-dense foods.

[1]Nutrient allowances are based on the Recommended Dietary Allowances developed by the Food and Nutrition Board, National Academy of Sciences, Washington, D.C. The Allowances are revised periodically to reflect the latest scientific findings. The most recent RDA's were published in 1980.

Each menu in this book illustrates all the principles suggested in the dietary guidelines, including the principles of moderation and variety. Each menu gives specific examples of modest changes which can be made in your food choices to meet the dietary guidelines. It makes good nutritional sense to choose different foods from meal to meal as well as from day to day.

These menus are not intended to be followed day after day. Choose the menus closest to your style of eating and try the changes suggested to meet the dietary guidelines.

MENU 1

1600 CALORIES		2400 CALORIES
	★ BREAKFAST ★	
¾ cup	Orange juice (fresh or frozen)	¾ cup
None	Egg (soft cooked)	1 large
2 slices	Banana nut bread[2]	2 slices
½ cup	Milk (skim, fortified)	1 cup
	Water, tea, or coffee	
	★ BROWN BAG LUNCH ★	
1 sandwich	Tuna salad sandwich: 2 oz tuna, packed in water; 1 tbsp chopped celery; 1 tsp chopped onion; 2 tsps mayonnaise; 2 slices whole wheat bread	1 sandwich
1 medium	Pear (fresh)	1 medium
1 cup	Milk (skim, fortified)	1 cup
	★ DINNER ★	
4 oz	Pot roast (chuck, lean only)	4 oz
¾ cup	Mashed potatoes	¾ cup
½ cup	Green beans (fresh or frozen)	½ cup
1 cup	Spinach salad	1 cup
1 tbsp	Italian dressing	1 tbsp
1 slice	Italian bread (enriched)	2 slices
1 tsp	Margarine (soft)	1 tbsp
½ cup	Orange-pineapple cup[2]	1 cup
	Water, tea, or coffee	
	★ SNACKS ★	
¼ cup	Chili bean dip[2]	½ cup
1 cup	Raw vegetable sticks: carrot, celery, and green pepper sticks	1 cup
None	Whole wheat crackers	5 to 6 average
None	Juice or alternate[4]	12 oz
	Water, tea, or coffee	

Banana nut bread is a change of pace from plain toast. The two slices have about the same number of calories as a sweet roll, but more vitamins and minerals. The banana nut bread has less fat and sugar and is made with whole wheat flour.

The beef is trimmed of fat. The tuna at lunch was packed in water. Both steps lower the overall fat content of the menu.

NOTE: Foods and quantities highlighted in yellow indicate a difference between the 1,600- and the 2,400-calorie menus. As you can see, the menus are pretty much the same. It is mostly a matter of a little more of this, a little less of that.

[2] Recipe included.

[4] See list of alternates.

Moderation can take the form of a balancing act—balancing more of something at one meal with less at the next. Take the fast food lunch in Menu 2. The somewhat higher fat content at lunch is balanced out by lower fat at breakfast and again at dinner.

1600 CALORIES	MENU 2	2400 CALORIES
	★ BREAKFAST ★	
½ cup	Strawberries (fresh or frozen, unsweetened)	½ cup
2 biscuits ½ medium	Shredded wheat with sliced banana	2 biscuits ½ medium
None	Sugar	**1 tbsp**
  1 cup	Milk 2% lowfat, fortified whole	 **1 cup**
	Water, tea, or coffee	
	★ FAST FOOD LUNCH ★	
 2 oz None 1 bun	Hamburger/cheeseburger ground beef American process cheese enriched bun	 3 oz ¾ oz 1 bun
½ cup	Coleslaw, with mayonnaise-type salad dressing	½ cup
1 small serving	French fries	**1 large serving**
8 oz	Juice or alternate[4]	8 oz
	★ DINNER ★	
1 serving	Chicken cacciatore[2]	1 serving
½ cup	Spaghetti, enriched	**1 cup**
½ cup	Zucchini, cooked fresh	½ cup
1½ cups	Mixed green salad: iceberg lettuce, spinach, green onions, cucumbers	1½ cups
1 tbsp	Italian dressing	1 tbsp
1 slice	Italian bread (enriched)	**2 slices**
1 tsp	Margarine (soft)	**2 tsps**
None	Pear (fresh)	**1 medium**
None	Pineapple juice (unsweetened)	**1 cup**
	★ SNACKS ★	
None	Graham crackers	**2 squares**
  ½ cup	Milk 2% lowfat, fortified whole	 **½ cup**
1 medium	Tangerine	1 medium

[2]Recipe included.

[4]See list of alternates.

The kind of milk is your choice. When you use whole milk in one meal, you might be more moderate in your use of other fats.

Check the recepie. The skin is removed to lower the fat content. No fat or oil used in cooking either.

No fat or salt added to the zucchini. For added zest, try lemon juice, caraway seed, or marjoram.

Sald dressings add calories and sodium. Be moderate in your use of them.

You have cut down on the fats in your diet. Now you have more room for carbohydrates—preferably foods containing starch or fiber or both. Vegetables and grain products are good examples of these foods. Whole grain foods contain all the edible parts of the cereal seed, including the fibrous outer covering and the vitamin and mineral-rich germ. Milling and refining remove some of the vitamins and minerals along with the bran. Some of the vitamins and minerals may be returned as the food is processed. The label will usually tell you which were returned to the food through enrichment or fortification. Vegetables and raw fruits are good sources of fiber and some vegetables, such as potatoes and dry beans or peas, are also good sources of starch.

MENU 3

1600 CALORIES		2400 CALORIES
	★ **BREAKFAST** ★	
¾ cup	**Orange juice (fresh or frozen)**	¾ cup
None	**Scrambled egg**	**1 large**
1 bagel	**Bagel**	1 bagel
1 tbsp	**Cream cheese**	**2 tbsps**
None	**Jam**	**1 tbsp**
1 cup	**Milk (fortified skim)**	1 cup
	Water, tea, or coffee	
	★ **BROWN BAG LUNCH** ★	
1 sandwich	**Sliced chicken sandwich**	**2 sandwiches**
2 oz	sliced chicken	**3 oz**
1 leaf	lettuce	**2 leaves**
2 tsps	mayonnaise-type salad dressing	**3 tsps**
2 slices	whole wheat bread	**4 slices**
1 serving	**Bean salad**[2]	1 serving
None	**Apple (fresh)**	**1 medium**
	Water, tea, or coffee	
	★ **DINNER** ★	
1 serving	**Vegetable chowder**[2]	1 serving
1 serving	**Baked fish with spicy sauce**[2]	**1½ servings**
½ cup	**Broccoli spears (fresh or frozen)**	½ cup
½ cup	**Brown rice**	½ cup
1½ cups	**Mixed green salad: iceberg lettuce, spinach, green onions, cucumbers**	1½ cups
1 tbsp	**French dressing**	1 tbsp
½ cup	**Grapes (seedless)**	**1 cup**
	Water, tea, or coffee	
	★ **SNACKS** ★	
1 serving	**Gingerbread**[2]	1 serving
None	**Pear (fresh)**	**1 medium**

[2]Recipe included.

For safety sake, keep the bag lunch cold until ready to be eaten.

The bean salad adds starch and fiber to the meal. So does the whole wheat bread in the sandwich.

Raw and cooked vegetables are good sources of fiber.

The brown rice and the whole wheat flour in the gingerbread add starch and fiber to the day's menu.

Fruits with edible skins and seeds are good for their fiber.

A lighter hand with sugar and sweeteners leaves extra room for calories that contribute more to your nutrient needs. The fewer total calories you consume, the more important this rule is. The quantity of sweets and sugars in the 1,600-calorie menu is about half the level of the 2,400-calorie menu. Some sweets or foods with added sugar were simply left out. Others appear in smaller portions.

1600 CALORIES	**MENU 4**	**2400** CALORIES
	★ **BREAKFAST** ★	
¼ medium	Cantaloupe	¼ medium
1 large	**Egg (soft cooked)**	**None**
1 average	**Corn muffin**	**2 average**
None	**Margarine (soft)**	**2 tsps**
None	**Jelly**	**2 tsps**
	Milk	
	whole	1 cup
½ cup	1% lowfat, fortified	
	Water, tea, or coffee	
	★ **TWO DIFFERENT LUNCHES OUT** ★	
1 sandwich	**Ham and cheese sandwich: 1 oz lean ham; 1 oz natural swiss cheese; 2 slices rye bread; 2 tsps mayonnaise-type salad dressing; lettuce**	
1¼ cups	**Tossed salad: lettuce, tomato, carrots, green onions**	
1 tbsp	**Italian dressing**	
1 medium	**Orange**	
	Water, tea, or coffee	
	Pork chop (lean only)	**1 large chop**
	Black-eyed peas	**½ cup**
	Rice (enriched)	**½ cup**
	Hard roll (enriched)	**1 large roll**
	Margarine (soft)	**1 tsp**
	Sliced peaches (canned in sirup)	**½ cup**
	Apple cider	**¾ cup**
	★ **DINNER** ★	
1 serving	Flounder Florentine[2]	1 serving
1 medium	Baked potato	1 medium
2 tbsps	Sour cream	2 tbsps
½ cup	Green peas (frozen)	½ cup
1 small roll	Whole wheat roll	1 small roll
1 tsp	Margarine (soft)	1 tsp
4 oz	**Vanilla yogurt (lowfat) mixed with:**	**8 oz**
½ cup	strawberries (fresh or frozen, unsweetened)	½ cup
	Water, tea, or coffee	
	★ **SNACKS** ★	
1 whole muffin	English muffin (enriched)	1 whole muffin
None	**Margarine (soft)**	**2 tsps**
1 tbsp	Marmalade	1 tbsp

Some sugars in the diet are easy to spot-jelly and marmalade, for example. Others are not so obvious, like the sugar in muffins and yogurt.

The higher calorie diet has more room for added sugar, such as the sweetened syrup in canned peaches.

The sugar in flavored yogurt raises the calorie count. Yogurt with fruit preserves has even more sugar in it. We have added our own fruit.

[2]Recipe included.

The salt shaker represents only a part of the sodium in our diets. Sodium is a natural constituent of many foods. It is added to others during processing. Generally, the more calories in a diet, the more sodium. For example, the 1,600-calorie menu here has about two-thirds the sodium of the 2,400-calorie menu. As in all the menus, sodium has been adjusted by modest changes in food choices. Fresh or frozen fruits and vegetables contain little sodium. But salt is generally added to canned vegetables. Meat, fish, poultry, eggs, and dairy products all have a natural supply of sodium. Salt is added in making cheese. Curing meat, fish, or poultry (or other forms of processing) usually adds more sodium. There is salt in margarine, butter, salad dressing, and even peanut butter. Grains start out low in sodium but frequently pick some up as they are turned into breads, cakes, or ready-to-eat cereals. Crackers vary.

MENU 5

1600 CALORIES		2400 CALORIES
	★ **BREAKFAST** ★	
½ medium	**Grapefruit (fresh)**	½ medium
2 slices	**Whole wheat toast**	2 slices
1 tsp	**Margarine (soft)**	1 tsp
None	**Jelly**	**1 tbsp**
1 cup	**Milk (fortified skim)**	1 cup
	Water, tea, or coffee	
	★ **BROWN BAG LUNCH** ★	
6 oz	**Tomato juice (canned)**	6 oz
1 serving	**Luncheon salad**	1 serving
None	turkey	**2 oz**
None	ham	**1 oz**
1½ cups	mixed greens	1½ cups
1½ oz	swiss cheese (natural)	1½ oz
1 tbsp	**French dressing**	**1½ tbsps**
1 serving	**Corn bread**[2]	1 serving
1 small	**Peach (fresh)**	**2 small**
	Water, tea, or coffee	
	★ **DINNER** ★	
4 oz	**Broiled ground beef (lean)**	4 oz
½ cup	**Corn (fresh or frozen)**	**1 cup**
½ cup	**Green beans (fresh or frozen)**	½ cup
None	**Rye rolls**	**2 rolls**
None	**Margarine (soft)**	**1 tsp**
1 serving	**Baked apple with 2 tsps brown sugar**	1 serving
	Water, tea, or coffee	
	★ **SNACKS** ★	
None	**Peanut butter sandwich: 2 slices whole wheat bread; 2 tbsps peanut butter; 2 tsps jelly**	**1 sandwich**
3 squares	**Graham crackers**	**None**
8 oz	**Juice or alternate**[4]	8 oz

There's salt in the tomato juice, as there is in most canned vegetables.

Ham, like most cured or processed meats, adds salt. So, a moderate amount is used.

Check the recipe—less salt than usual.

No condiments added to the ground beef to keep the amount of sodium down. No catsup, mustard, pickles or the like. Try some chopped fresh onions or tomato for a do-it-yourself relish.

Instead of salt, experiment with lemon juice, spices and herbs for flavor.

[2]Recipe included.

[4]See list of alternates.

It can be something of a problem for women to get the recommended amount of iron even though iron is available in a variety of foods. Foods of vegetable origin, for example, can be valuable sources of iron. Enriched and whole grain foods, dry beans and peas, dark leafy greens, and some starchy vegetables are good examples. However, the iron in these foods is in a form that is less available to the body than is the iron in such foods as meat, poultry, and fish. New research shows us how to improve the situation. If you combine a food rich in vitamin C with an iron-containing food, the body can use more of the iron. You can accomplish the same thing by combining some meat, poultry, or fish with some of the vegetable sources of iron.

1600 CALORIES	MENU 6	2400 CALORIES
	★ BREAKFAST ★	
¾ cup	**Orange juice (fresh or frozen)**	**¾ cup**
2 cakes	**Whole wheat pancakes[2]**	**3 cakes**
½ serving	**Blueberry sauce[2]**	**1 serving**
1 cup	**Milk (1% lowfat, fortified)**	**1 cup**
None	**Margarine (soft)**	**2 tsps**
	Water, tea, or coffee	
	★ LUNCH AT HOME ★	
1 taco	**Beef taco[2]**	**2 tacos**
¾ cup	**Fresh fruit cup: oranges, apples, banana**	**¾ cup**
½ cup	**Milk (1% lowfat, fortified)**	**1 cup**
	★ DINNER ★	
4 oz	**Roast loin of pork (lean only)**	**4 oz**
1 small	**Sweet potato (baked)**	**1 medium**
½ cup	**Collard greens (fresh or frozen)**	**½ cup**
1¼ cups	**Tossed salad: lettuce, tomato, green onions, carrots**	**1¼ cups**
1 tbsp	**Italian salad dressing**	**1 tbsp**
1 biscuit	**Biscuits (enriched)**	**2 biscuits**
None	**Honey**	**1 tbsp**
1 tsp	**Margarine (soft)**	**2 tsps**
	Water, tea, or coffee	
	★ SNACKS ★	
4 squares	**Graham crackers**	**4 squares**
8 oz	**Juice or alternate[4]**	**12 oz**
None	**Apple (fresh)**	**1 medium**

[2]Recipe included.
[4]See list of alternates.

Orange juice, a rich source of vitamin C, improves the body's ability to use the iron in whole wheat.

The lean roast pork makes the iron in the sweet potato, collards and biscuit more useful.

When it comes to calories, each individual is different. In addition, women in general need fewer calories than men. Adults need fewer calories as they grow older. The menus show you how you can use essentially the same foods to meet different calorie needs, mostly by varying the size of portions.

1600 CALORIES	MENU 7	2400 CALORIES
	★ BREAKFAST ★	
½ cup	Pineapple chunks (packed in own juice)	¾ cup
½ cup	Oatmeal with cinnamon	1 cup
None	with raisins	3 tbsps
1 tsp	Brown sugar	2 tsps
	Milk	
	whole	1 cup
½ cup	1% lowfat, fortified	
	Water, tea, or coffee	
	★ LUNCH AT HOME ★	
1 serving	Split pea soup[2]	1 serving
1 serving	Chicken salad stuffed tomato: 2 oz cooked, chopped chicken; 1 tbsp chopped celery; 1 tsp chopped onion; 2 tsps mayonnaise; 1 medium tomato	1 serving
3 crackers	Rye crackers	6 crackers
None	Margarine (soft)	2 tsps
None	Lemon sherbet	¾ cup
	Water, tea, or coffee	
	★ DINNER ★	
1 serving	Beef with Chinese-style vegetables[2]	1½ servings
½ cup	Rice (white, enriched)	¾ cup
1 serving	Apple crisp[2]	1 serving
	★ SNACKS ★	
2 slices	Banana nut bread[2]	2 slices
	Milk	
	whole	1 cup
1 cup	1% lowfat, fortified	
1 medium	Orange	1 medium

[2]Recipe included.

The lowfat milk used here reduces calories without reducing essential nutrients.

At 1,600 calories, you can't afford many foods that are high in sugar and low in vitamins and minerals.

The apple crisp fits in because the recipe is lower in fat and sugar than one you may be using.

Snacks are for eating anytime. You could eat the banana nut bread and milk at bedtime, the orange in the afternoon. You could drink the milk at lunch or during your break, instead of coffee.

III. MAKING UP YOUR OWN MENUS

The menus show you how to put together nutritious meals and snacks. They are examples, not commandments. Use them as guides. Pick the ones that suit your own eating habits best, and adapt them to your needs. When you make substitutions, choose foods from the same food group as the ones in the menu. Be varied in your choices.

The menus stress three concepts: moderation, variety, and the avoidance of imbalanced or excessive consumption.

There are two main ideas behind the menus:

- getting enough of the basic foods and nutrients without overdoing the calories.

- cutting back on ingredients or foods which we may eat too much of: fats and oils, salt, and sugar.

To get yourself started, try listing the foods you ate yesterday. Group them according to the same food categories we use. Check your food intake for the number and variety of fruits, vegetables, grains, milk, and meats. Consider the size of servings. Note how frequently you consume fat, sweets, or alcohol.

The menus may not include your favorite foods. Feel free to substitute. While the foods listed below are not exactly equivalent in nutrient content, they are close enough.

Fruits

All fruits contribute fiber and nutrients to your diet, but in different quantities. Citrus fruits and most melons and berries are good sources of vitamin C.

Choices in the menus

Apples
Apple cider
Apple crisp[2]
Baked apple
Bananas
Cantaloupes
Fruit cup
Grapefruit
Grapes
Oranges
Orange juice
Orange-pineapple cup[2]
Peaches, fresh and canned
Pears
Pineapple, canned in juice
Raisins
Strawberries
Tangerines
Tomatoes and tomato juice

Other suggestions

Applesauce
Apricots
Blueberries and other berries
Cherries
Figs
Honeydew melon
Lemons
Mangos
Nectarines
Papayas
Plums
Prunes
Watermelon
Other fruit and fruit juices

[2]Recipe included.

Count as a serving an average size, whole piece of fruit, a melon wedge, 6 ounces of juice, 1/2 cup of berries, or 1/2 cup of sliced or cooked fruit.

Two to three fruits have been included in the menus each day, more in some of the 2,400-calorie menus.

Vegetables

There are three types of vegetables to look for in the menus: dark-green vegetables, starchy vegetables, and other vegetables. Each type makes a somewhat different contribution to your diet.

Dark–green vegetables.

They are low in calories, good sources of fiber, and provide vitamins A and C, along with riboflavin and folacin (B vitamins), and the minerals iron and magnesium.

Choices in the menus

Broccoli
Collard greens
Spinach (cooked or raw)

Other suggestions

Chicory
Endive
Escarole
Greens
  Beet
  Chard
  Dandelion
  Kale
  Mustard
  Turnip
Romaine lettuce
Watercress

Starchy vegetables.

In addition to the starch they contribute, dried beans and peas are generally good sources of fiber, protein, iron, zinc, magnesium, phosphorus, thiamin, vitamin B_6 and folacin. The other vegetables in this group are also sources of these and other nutrients.

Choices in the menus

Black-eyed peas
Chili bean dip[2]
Corn
Green peas
Kidney bean salad[2]
Potatoes
  Baked
  French fried
  Mashed
Split pea soup[2]
Sweet potatoes

Other suggestions

Chickpeas or garbanzos
Lentils
Lima beans
Navy beans
Parsnips
Plantain
Rutabaga
Yams
Other types of dried beans and peas

[2]Recipe included.

Other vegetables.

These vegetables are sources of fiber. Their nutrient content varies. All dark-green or deep-yellow vegetables are reliable sources of vitamin A.

Choices in the menus

Carrots
Celery
Cole slaw (cabbage)
Cucumbers
Green beans
Green peppers
Lettuce (iceberg, bibb)
Onions (mature and green)
Tomatoes and tomato juice
Vegetables in main dish recipes
Vegetables in vegetable chowder[2]
Zucchini

Other suggestions

Artichokes
Asparagus
Bean and alfalfa sprouts
Beets
Brussels sprouts
Cauliflower
Chinese cabbage
Eggplant
Mushrooms
Okra
Pumpkin
Radishes
Turnips
Vegetable juices
Winter squash
Yellow squash
Other vegetables

[2]Recipe included.

You will find a minimum of three servings of vegetables in the daily menus. At least one is a starchy vegetable or a bean dish. Dark-green vegetables show up often.

Vegetables are included in the menus as separate items and as ingredients in main dishes and in soups. The menus and recipes suggest ways to use a variety of vegetables.

Bread, cereals, and grain products

The menus include many different foods made from whole or enriched grain. They are important sources of starch, the B vitamins thiamin, riboflavin, and niacin, and iron. Whole grain products also contribute fiber, vitamin B_6, magnesium, and zinc.

Choices in the menus

Bagel
Banana-nut bread[2]
Biscuits
Brown rice
Corn bread[2]
Corn muffins
English muffins
Gingerbread[2]
Graham crackers
Hamburger bun
Italian bread
Oatmeal
Ready-to-eat cereal (shredded wheat)
Rice
Rye bread
Rye crackers
Rye rolls
Spaghetti
Taco shell
Wheat crackers
Whole wheat bread
Whole wheat pancakes[2]
Whole wheat rolls

Other suggestions

Barley
Buckwheat groats
Bulgur
Cornmeal
Grits
Muffins
Noodles, marcaroni
Popcorn
Pumpernickel bread
Waffles
White bread
Wild rice
Other breads and cereals

[2]Recipe included.

The menus for each day have a minimum of four servings of bread and cereals with more in the 2,400-

calorie menus. Some are always whole grain. Before making your choice, check the ingredient label or the recipe for added salt, sugar, or fat. Quick breads, such as muffins, biscuits, and corn bread, have more fat than most yeast breads. Think about how much fat you add in cooking or at the table.

Meat, poultry, fish, eggs

The menus offer a variety of choices from this group. The important thing is to select and prepare these foods to moderate the amount of fat. To do so, select lean cuts of meat, trim off the visible fat, and remove skin and fat from poultry. It is also important to be moderate in the use of salted meats like ham. Organ meats and egg yolks are sources of many nutrients, but they are also well supplied with cholesterol.

Meat, fish, and poultry products are valued sources of protein, phosphorus, vitamins B_6 and B_{12}, iron, and zinc.

Choices in the menus	Other suggestions
Baked fish with spicy sauce[2]	Beef, marcaroni, and tomato casserole
Beef pot roast	Beef stew
Beef taco[2]	Beef, other lean cuts
Beef with Chinese-style vegetables[2]	Chili
Chicken	Lamb chop or roast (lean)
Chicken cacciatore[2]	Lamb stew
Eggs, scrambled and soft cooked	Meat loaf
Eggs in recipes	Pork, other lean cuts
Flounder Florentine[2]	Shellfish and other fish
Ground beef (lean)	Veal
Ham	
Pork chop	
Pork loin roast	
Tuna fish	
Turkey	

[2]Recipe included.

Two servings of these foods were included almost every day. Dried beans and peas can be used as alternatives for meat, poultry, fish, and eggs. Count the tradeoff as:[7]

1 cup of cooked dried beans or peas + 1 teaspoon fat = 2 ounces lean meat, poultry, or fish + 2 slices of enriched or whole grain bread.

[7]The tradeoff is based on a similar calorie and nutrient content, except for vitamin B_{12}. This vitamin is not found in plant foods.

Milk, milk products, and cheese

Milk and cheese are as popular with most people as they are important to a balanced diet. Adults as well as children need the nutrients found in milk and cheese, particularly calcium and riboflavin. Milk and cheese also contribute protein, vitamins A, B_{12}, and, if fortified, vitamin D.

Choices in the menus	Other suggestions
American cheese	Buttermilk
Lowfat milk (1% and 2%)	Chocolate milk
Milk in vegetable chowder[2]	Cottage cheese[5]
Skim milk	Lowfat yogurt, plain
Swiss cheese	Milk custards
Vanilla lowfat yogurt	Milk puddings
Whole milk	Other cheeses

[2]Recipe included.

[5]Cottage cheese contains considerably less calcium than other cheeses. One-half cup of cottage cheese contains only as much calcium as is found in one-quarter cup of milk, while providing considerably more calories and sodium.

Some tradeoffs you can make:[6]

1 cup whole milk = 1 cup skim milk + 2 teaspoons fat

1 cup 2% milk = 1 cup skim milk + 1 teaspoon fat

1 1/2 ounces natural cheese = 1 cup whole milk + 1 teaspoon fat

8 ounces plain lowfat yogurt = 1 cup 2% milk

1 cup lowfat (2%) chocolate milk = 1 cup 2% milk + 3 teaspoons sugar

8 ounces lowfat vanilla yogurt = 1 cup 2% milk + 4 teaspoons sugar

8 ounces lowfat fruit yogurt = 1 cup 2% milk + 7 teaspoons sugar

1/2 cup ice cream = 1/3 cup skim milk + 2 teaspoons fat + 3 teaspoons sugar

1/2 cup ice milk = 1/3 cup skim milk + 1 teaspoon fat + 3 teaspoons sugar

[6]Tradeoffs are approximations based on calories, calcium, protein, fat, and total carbohydrate content. Individual products vary.

1/2 cup lowfat frozen yogurt = 1/3 cup skim milk + 4 teaspoons sugar

Milk, cheese, or other milk products are included at least twice in each day's menus.

Fats and oils

Animal fats are higher in saturated fat than are most vegetable oils. The exceptions are coconut and palm oil. These vegetable oils are highly saturated. It is not a good idea to use highly saturated fats exclusively. Soft (tub) margarine is a good choice as a spread for bread and vegetables. It is made from liquid vegetable oils that have been only partially hardened (hydrogenated). Remember to use fats and oils with moderation.

Choices in the menus	Some alternates
Cream cheese	Bacon
French and Italian salad dressing	Butter
Margarine (soft)	Cream
Mayonnaise	Half and half
Mayonnaise-type salad dressing	Nondairy creamers
Oil (in recipes)	Margarine (hard)
Sour cream	Other types of salad dressing

Sugars and sweets

Sugars and sweets are listed in the menus. They are also found in prepared foods like salad dressings, peanut butter, vanilla yogurt, lemon sherbet, and quick breads. The amount of sugar we include in the recipes is lower than you will find in many cookbooks.

Calorie levels are somewhat similar for the sugars and sweeteners listed below. They can be substituted, teaspoon for teaspoon. It is hard to tell how much sugar has been added to foods like peanut butter, catsup, or ready-to-eat cereal. Read the label. Ingredients are listed in order of predominance. If sugar or some other caloric sweetener[8] comes first, you know there is more sugar than anything else. It is a great deal easier to control the amount of sugar in your food if you add it yourself. Honey and brown sugar are used for their flavor and color. They have no other special value.

[8]Words used on labels to describe sugar and caloric sweeteners include sugar, sucrose, dextrose, fructose, corn sirups, corn sweeteners, natural sweeteners, honey, and invert sugar.

Choices in the menus	Other suggestions
Blueberry sauce[2]	Corn sirup
Honey	Maple sirup
Jam	Molasses
Jelly	Sugar sirup
Marmalade	
Sugar (white and brown)	
Sirup on peaches	

[2]Recipe included.

Juices and alternates

Several menus list a juice or alternate. An 8-ounce glass of juice contributes about 110 calories. The following alternates contribute about the same number of calories:

8 ounces fruit punch
8 ounces soft drink
1/2 cup sherbet (also contains some fat)
1 popsicle
3/4 cup sweetened gelatin
2 average cookies (also contain some fat)
2 tablespoons sugar, jam, jelly, honey, sirup
1 ounce candy (some contain fat)
8 ounces beer[9]
4 ounces table wine[9]
1 1/2 ounces wiskey[9]

[9]We're not advocating the use of alcoholic beverages. We are only indicating where they fit if you choose to use them.

IV. RECIPES

The recipes in this book have been tested by a taste panel to make sure they will meet with general approval. They are good in their own right. But that doesn't mean they always taste the same as your own favorite version. Try them. Give yourself a chance to enjoy new tastes and flavors.

The recipe for apple crisp, for example, is noticeably different from traditional recipes; it uses much less sugar and combines two whole grain cereals for extra fiber. So, too, the banana nut bread. It uses whole grain flour and cuts back on the sugar. The bean salad recipe calls for less oil than is often used. The chili bean dip and the split pea soup show you other ways to use dried beans and peas.

Beef with Chinese-style vegetables introduces stir-frying, a flavorful way to prepare very lean meat. Our recipe calls for less soy sauce than is traditional, however. Chicken cacciatore cuts calories and fat mostly by removing the skin from the chicken breasts. Herbs and spices are counted on for flavor, rather than salt and fat.

The stone-ground cornmeal in the corn bread is a whole grain cereal. The recipe also uses less salt and fewer eggs than usual. The gingerbread recipe uses whole wheat flour. The honey and molasses in the corn bread and gingerbread are included for their flavor. They offer no caloric or nutrient advantage over other sweeteners. You'll see no salt added to the split pea soup. There's already enough sodium in the ham or ham hock for flavor. The vegetable chowder offers yet another way to increase the number and variety of vegetables in your diet. It is also a good way to use up leftovers. Whole wheat flour is used to thicken the soup. Even the blueberry sauce topping for the whole wheat pancakes has been trimmed of some of its sugar, and thus the number of calories is lower than in most pancake sirups.

So eat and enjoy—new foods and familiar foods, with perhaps a slightly different look or taste.

BANANA-NUT BREAD

1 loaf, 18 slices.
Calories per slice: About 135.

Whole wheat flour	**1¾ cups**
Sugar	**½ cup**
Baking powder	**1 tablespoon**
Salt	**¼ teaspoon**
Walnuts, chopped	**½ cup**
Oil	**⅓ cup**
Eggs	**2**
Bananas, mashed	**2 medium, (about 1 cup)**

1. Preheat oven to 350°F (moderate).
2. Grease 9 × 5 × 3-inch loaf pan.
3. Mix flour, sugar, baking powder, salt, and nuts thoroughly.
4. Mix oil and eggs together. Mix in bananas.
5. Add dry ingredients to banana mixture. Stir until just smooth.
6. Pour into loaf pan.
7. Bake 45 minutes or until firmly set when lightly touched in center top.
8. Cool on rack. Remove from pan after 10 minutes.

APPLE CRISP

4 servings, ½ cup each.
Calories per serving: About 230.

Tart apples, pared, sliced	**4 cups**
Water	**¼ cup**
Lemon juice	**1 tablespoon**
Brown sugar, packed	**¼ cup**
Whole wheat flour	**¼ cup**
Old-fashioned rolled oats	**¼ cup**
Ground cinnamon	**½ teaspoon**
Ground nutmeg	**¼ teaspoon**
Margarine	**3 tablespoons**

1. Place apples in 8 × 8 × 2-inch baking pan.
2. Mix water and lemon juice, pour over apples.
3. Mix sugar, flour, oats, and spices.
4. Add margarine to dry mixture; mix until crumbly.
5. Sprinkle crumbly mixture evenly over apples.
6. Bake at 350°F (moderate oven) until apples are tender and topping is lightly browned, about 40 minutes.

BEAN SALAD

4 servings, ¾ cup each.
Calories per serving: About 280.

Kidney beans, canned, drained	**1 cup**
Garbanzo beans, canned, drained	**1 cup**
Carrots, very thinly sliced	**½ cup**
Onion, chopped	**¼ cup**
Sweet pickle, chopped	**3 tablespoons**
Salt	**¼ teaspoon**
Pepper	**⅛ teaspoon**
Dry mustard	**½ teaspoon**
Vinegar	**3 tablespoons**
Honey	**1 tablespoon**
Oil	**¼ cup**

1. Mix vegetables and pickle in a bowl.
2. Thoroughly mix remaining ingredients.
3. Pour over vegetable mixture. Mix gently.
4. Chill at least 1 hour before serving.

BEEF TACOS

6 servings, 2 tacos each.
Calories per serving: About 340.

Taco shells, fully cooked	**12**
Ground beef, lean	**1 pound**
Onion, chopped	**¼ cup**
Tomato sauce	**8-ounce can**
Chili powder	**2 teaspoons**
Tomato, chopped	**1 cup**
Lettuce, shredded	**1 cup**
Natural sharp Cheddar cheese, shredded	**½ cup (2 ounces)**

1. Brown ground beef and onion in a frying pan. Drain off excess fat.
2. Stir in tomato sauce and chili powder. Bring to a boil.
3. Reduce heat. Cook 10 to 15 minutes uncovered, stirring occasionally, until mixture is dry and crumbly.
4. Fill taco shells with approximately 2 tablespoons of meat mixture.
5. Mix tomato, lettuce, and cheese. Spoon about 2 tablespoons over beef in taco shells.

BEEF WITH CHINESE-STYLE VEGETABLES

4 servings, ½ cup of meat and ½ cup vegetables each.
Calories per serving: About 200.

Beef round steak, lean, boneless	**1 pound**
Green beans, cut in strips	**⅔ cup**
Carrots, thinly sliced	**⅔ cup**
Turnips, thinly sliced	**⅔ cup**
Cauliflower florets, thinly sliced	**⅔ cup**
Chinese cabbage, cut in strips	**⅔ cup**
Boiling water	**⅔ cup**
Oil	**2 teaspoons**
Cornstarch	**4 teaspoons**
Ground ginger	**½ teaspoon**
Garlic powder	**⅛ teaspoon**
Soy sauce	**1 tablespoon**
Sherry*	**3 tablespoons**
Water	**½ cup**

1. Trim fat from beef. Slice beef across the grain into thin strips, about ⅛ inch wide and 3 inches long. (It is easier to slice meat thinly if it is partially frozen.)
2. Add vegetables to boiling water. Simmer, covered, for 5 minutes or until vegetables are tender but still crisp. Drain.
3. While vegetables are cooking, heat oil in nonstick frypan. Add beef and stir-fry over moderately high heat, turning pieces constantly until beef is no longer red, about 2 to 3 minutes.
4. Mix cornstarch, garlic powder, ginger, soy sauce, sherry, and water.
5. Stir cornstarch mixture into beef. Heat until sauce starts to boil.
6. Serve meat sauce over vegetables.

*Sherry may be omitted if desired. Use 3 tablespoons water in place of sherry. About 185 calories per serving when made without sherry.

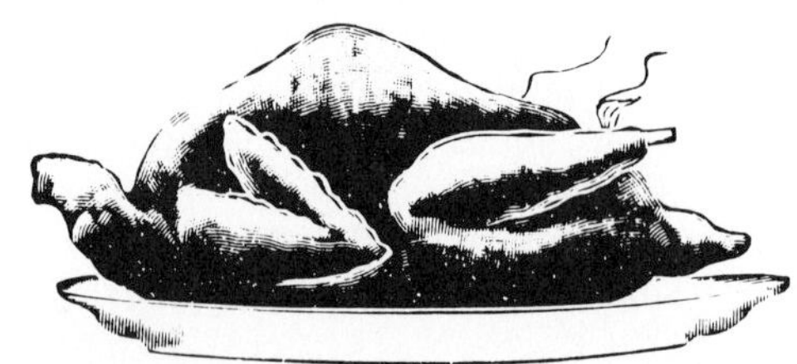

CHICKEN CACCIATORE

4 servings, 1 breast half each.
Calories per serving: About 155.

Onion, chopped	**½ cup**
Boiling water	**¼ cup**
Tomatoes	**8-ounce can**
Tomato puree	**½ cup**
Garlic clove	**1**
Oregano leaves	**1 teaspoon**
Celery seed	**½ teaspoon**
Pepper	**⅛ teaspoon**
Chicken breast halves, without skin	**4**

1. Cook onion in boiling water until tender. Do not drain.
2. Add tomatoes, tomato puree, garlic, oregano, celery seed, and pepper to onions. Simmer 10 minutes to blend flavors.
3. Place breast halves in heavy frying pan. Pour tomato mixture over chicken.
4. Cook, covered, over low heat until chicken is tender, about 60 minutes.
5. Remove garlic clove before serving.

CHILI BEAN DIP

1⅓ cups.
Calories per tablespoon: About 15 without vegetable sticks.

Kidney beans, drained	**16–ounce can**
Vinegar	**1 tablespoon**
Chili powder	**¾ teaspoon**
Ground cumin	**⅛ teaspoon**
Onion, very finely chopped	**2 teaspoons**
Parsley, chopped	**2 teaspoons**
Raw vegetable sticks	**as desired**

1. Place drained beans, vinegar, chili powder, and cumin in blender. Blend until smooth.
2. Remove mixture from blender. Stir in onion and parsley.
3. Serve with raw vegetable sticks.

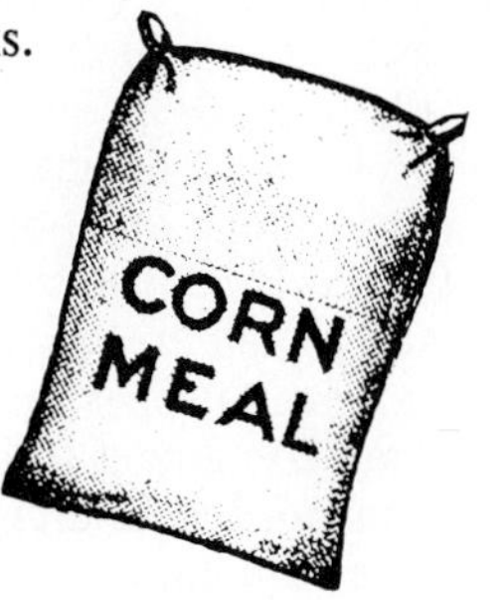

CORN BREAD

8 pieces, 2 by 4 inches each.
Calories per piece: About 220.

Stone-ground cornmeal (see note)	**2 cups**
Baking powder	**1 tablespoon**
Salt	**¼ teaspoon**
Egg, slightly beaten	**1**
Milk	**1 cup**
Honey	**2 tablespoons**
Oil	**¼ cup**

1. Preheat oven to 400°F (hot).
2. Grease an 8 × 8 × 2-inch baking pan.
3. Mix cornmeal, baking powder, and salt thoroughly.
4. Mix egg, milk, honey, and oil. Add to cornmeal mixture.
5. Stir only until dry ingredients are moistened. Batter will be lumpy.
6. Pour into pan.
7. Bake 20 minutes or until lightly browned.

NOTE: Degerminated cornmeal may be used in place of stone-ground cornmeal.

FLOUNDER FLORENTINE

4 servings, about 3 ounces fish and ¼ cup spinach each.
Calories per serving: About 140.

Frozen skinless flounder fillets, thawed	**1 pound**
Boiling water	**1½ cups**
Frozen chopped spinach	**10–ounce package**
Onion, finely chopped	**1 tablespoon**
Marjoram	**½ teaspoon**
Flour	**2 tablespoons**
Skim milk	**1 cup**
Salt	**½ teaspoon**
Pepper	**dash**
Grated Parmesan cheese	**2 tablespoons**

1. Place fish fillets in 1 cup boiling water. Cook, uncovered, 2 minutes. Drain.
2. Place spinach and onion in ½ cup boiling water. Separate spinach with fork.
3. When water returns to boiling, cover and cook spinach 2 minutes. Drain well. Mix with marjoram.
4. Put spinach in 8 × 8 × 2-inch glass baking dish. Arrange cooked fish on top of spinach.
5. Mix flour thoroughly with ¼ cup of milk.
6. Pour remaining milk in saucepan. Heat.
7. Add flour mixture slowly to hot milk, stirring constantly. Cook, stirring constantly, until thickened. Stir in salt and pepper.
8. Pour sauce over fish. Sprinkle with Parmesan cheese.
9. Bake at 400°F (hot oven) until top is lightly browned and mixture is bubbly, about 25 minutes.

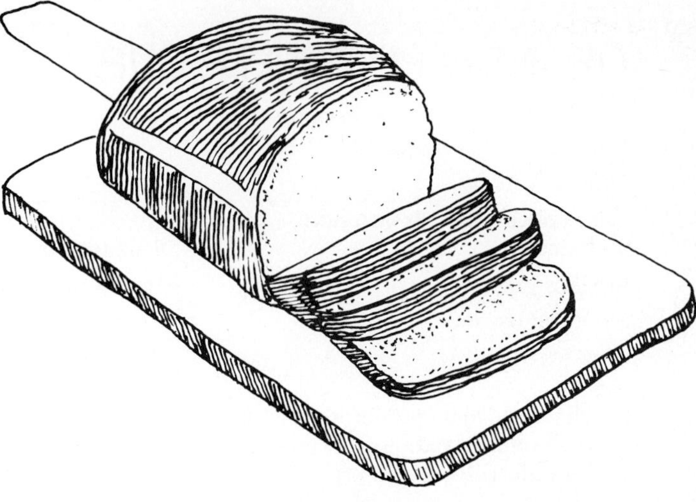

GINGERBREAD

8 servings, about 4 by 2 inches each.
Calories per serving: About 200.

Oil	**⅓ cup**
Water	**⅓ cup**
Molasses, light	**⅓ cup**
Sugar	**⅓ cup**
Egg whites, slightly beaten	**2**
Whole wheat flour, unsifted	**1 cup**
Salt	**¼ teaspoon**
Baking soda	**¼ teaspoon**
Baking powder	**1 teaspoon**
Ginger	**1 teaspoon**
Cinnamon	**½ teaspoon**
Nutmeg	**¼ teaspoon**

1. Preheat oven to 350 °F (moderate).
2. Grease lightly with oil and flour an 8 × 8 × 2-inch baking pan.
3. Mix oil and water. Add molasses, sugar, and egg whites. Stir until sugar is dissolved.
4. Mix flour, salt, baking soda, baking powder, and spices. Add to liquid mixture. Beat until smooth.
5. Pour into pan.
6. Bake 30 minutes or until surface springs back when touched lightly.

SPICY BAKED FISH

4 servings, about 2½ ounces fish each.
Calories per serving: About 110.

Cod fillets, fresh or frozen, without skin	**1 pound**
Onion, chopped	**¼ cup**
Green pepper, chopped	**¼ cup**
Oil	**2 teaspoons**
Tomatoes	**8-ounce can**
Salt	**¼ teaspoon**
Pepper	**⅛ teaspoon**

1. Thaw frozen fish.
2. Grease 9 × 9 × 2-inch baking pan lightly with ½ teaspoon of oil.
3. Cut fish in 4 servings. Place in baking pan.
4. Bake at 350 °F (moderate oven) until fish flakes easily, about 20 minutes. Drain cooking liquid from fish.
5. While fish is baking, cook onion and green pepper in remaining oil until onion is clear.
6. Cut up large pieces of tomatoes.
7. Add tomatoes, salt, and pepper to cooked onion and green pepper.
8. Cook 20 minutes to blend flavors.
9. Pour sauce over drained fish.
10. Bake 10 minutes.

ORANGE-PINEAPPLE CUP

4 servings, about ¾ cup each.
Calories per serving: About 145.

Orange sections	**1 cup**
Pineapple chunks, in own juice, undrained	**8-ounce can**
Seedless grapes	**½ cup**
Shredded coconut	**½ cup**
Mint leaves	**if desired**

1. Mix fruits and coconut together gently.
2. Chill until served.
3. Garnish with mint leaves.

SPLIT PEA SOUP

6 servings, about 1 cup each.
Calories per serving: About 195.

Dry green split peas	**1½ cups**
Smoked ham hock	**1 small**
Onion, chopped	**½ cup**
Pepper	**⅛ teaspoon**
Water	**6 cups**

1. Add peas, ham hock, onion, and pepper to water. Simmer, covered, 1½ hours or until ham hock is tender.
2. Remove ham hock and cut meat from bone. Cut meat into small pieces.
3. Return meat to soup. Heat to serving temperature.

VEGETABLE CHOWDER

4 servings, about 1 cup each.
Calories per serving: About 150.

Onion, chopped	**2 tablespoons**
Celery, chopped	**¼ cup**
Green pepper, chopped	**2 tablespoons**
Margarine	**1 tablespoon**
Potatoes, pared, diced	**½ cup**
Water	**1 cup**
Marjoram, dried	**⅛ teaspoon**
Salt	**¼ teaspoon**
Pepper	**⅛ teaspoon**
Frozen whole kernel corn	**1 cup**
Frozen cut green beans	**½ cup**
Whole wheat flour	**2 tablespoons**
Milk, whole (see note)	**1½ cups**

1. Cook onion, celery, and green pepper in margarine until almost tender.
2. Add potatoes, water, and seasonings.
3. Cover and simmer until potatoes are tender, about 20 minutes.
4. Add corn and beans.
5. Cover and simmer 10 minutes longer or until beans are tender.
6. Mix flour with a small amount of milk; add to remaining milk.
7. Stir milk mixture into cooked vegetable mixture.
8. Cook, stirring constantly, until slightly thickened.

NOTE: Lowfat milk can be used. Calories per serving would be about 125.

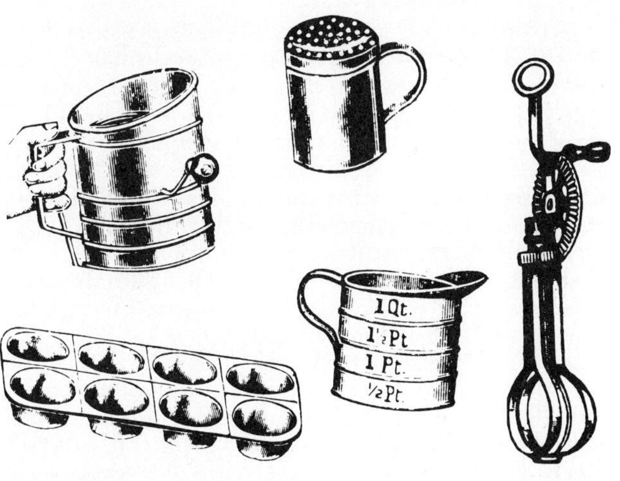

WHOLE WHEAT PANCAKES WITH BLUEBERRY SAUCE

4 servings, 2 pancakes each.
Calories per serving: About 245.

Whole wheat flour	**1⅓ cups**
Baking powder	**2 teaspoons**
Salt	**¼ teaspoon**
Egg, slightly beaten	**1**
Milk	**1⅓ cups**
Brown sugar, packed	**1 tablespoon**
Oil	**1 tablespoon**

1. Grease griddle (see note).
2. Heat griddle while mixing batter. Griddle is hot enough when drops of water sprinkled on it will bounce.
3. Mix flour, baking powder, and salt.
4. Beat egg, milk, sugar, and oil together.
5. Add liquid mixture to flour mixture. Stir only until flour is moistened. Batter will be slightly lumpy.
6. For each pancake, pour about ¼ cup batter onto hot griddle. Cook until covered with bubbles and edges are slightly dry.
7. Turn and brown other side.

NOTE: It is generally unnecessary to grease a well-seasoned griddle or one with a nonstick surface.

BLUEBERRY SAUCE

4 servings, ¼ cup each.
Calories per serving: About 50.

Cornstarch	**2 teaspoons**
Water	**½ cup**
Frozen unsweetened blueberries, thawed, crushed	**¾ cup**
Honey	**2 tablespoons**
Lemon juice	**2 teaspoons**

1. Mix cornstarch with a small amount of water in a saucepan, stir until smooth.
2. Add remaining water, blueberries, and honey.
3. Bring to boil over medium heat, stirring constantly. Cook until thickened.
4. Remove from heat. Stir in lemon juice.
5. Serve warm over whole wheat pancakes.

The Truth About Salt

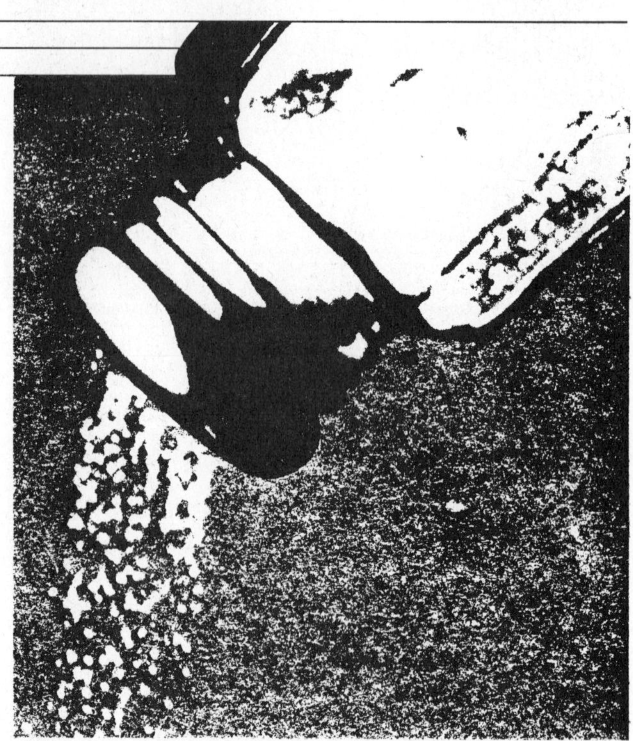

Introduction

Sodium is a mineral element necessary for proper body function. It is involved in maintaining blood volume and cellular osmotic pressure and in transmitting nerve impulses.

Body needs for sodium are not great. Intakes of 1,100 to 3,300 milligrams of sodium per day are considered safe and adequate for the healthy adult by the Food and Nutrition Board of the National Academy of Sciences—National Research Council. Most dietary sodium is found in the form of sodium chloride, the compound we know as table salt, which is 40 percent sodium and 60 percent chloride. One teaspoon of salt contains approximately 2,000 milligrams of sodium. Current estimates of daily sodium intake by individuals are between 2,300 to 6,900 milligrams (about 1 to 3 teaspoons or 6 to 17 grams of salt).

Many Americans consume more sodium than they need. "Nutrition and Your Health—Dietary Guidelines for Americans," published jointly by the Departments of Agriculture and Health, Education, and Welfare in February 1980, suggests that people should "avoid [eating] too much sodium."

Excess sodium in the diet is believed to contribute to high blood pressure or hypertension in some people. Control of body weight and restriction of sodium intake from foods, drinks, and drugs are among treatments prescribed by physicians to control high blood pressure.

In addition to the salt we knowingly sprinkle on our food, many foods contain sodium as a part of their normal chemical composition. Household staples like baking powder and baking soda are sodium compounds. Some popular flavoring agents high in sodium are soy sauce, worcestershire sauce, catsup, pickles, olives, and garlic, onion, and celery salts.

Many processed foods contain added sodium. Salted or brined meats and fish are obviously higher in salt content than the uncured forms. Many canned vegetables are packed in a salt solution or brine.

Frozen vegetables are usually processed without added salt. However, starchy vegetables like lima beans and peas are frequently sorted in brine before freezing. Frozen vegetables with added sauces, mushrooms, or nuts are higher in sodium than the plain varieties.

Canned and frozen fruits are not usually processed with added salt, but some companies add small amounts of salt to prevent darkening of some fruits and to enhance flavor of applesauce. Some canned and frozen fruits, and most canned whole tomatoes, are dipped in sodium hydroxide so that they can be easily peeled. This process causes these foods to have higher sodium levels than are found in the fresh foods. Canned and bottled citrus drinks are sometimes buffered with sodium citrate. Sodium ion exchange is used in processing some wines to reduce sediment and clarify the product.

Chemical ingredients which contain sodium may be added during food processing. Some examples of these ingredients are monosodium glutamate or MSG (a flavor enhancer); sodium saccharin (a sweetener);

sodium phosphates (emulsifiers, stabilizers, buffers); sodium citrate (a buffer); sodium caseinate (a thickener and binder); and sodium benzoate and sodium nitrite (preservatives).

It is especially important for persons on salt-restricted diets to read ingredient labels carefully to see which, if any, sodium compounds have been included in processed foods. Those items listed first on the label are present in the largest amounts. Nutritional information on labels of some foods, such as breakfast cereals, shows sodium values. To allow for variability among packages, cereal manufacturers may show higher values on packages of cereal than those shown in the table.

Some over-the-counter drugs, particularly antacids, contain sodium in significant amounts. Read labels carefully and ask your physician about using such drugs.

Many patients with high blood pressure take diuretics and are advised to increase their potassium intake to replenish that lost in the increased urine volume. Bananas and orange juice are frequently recommended for their potassium content. Most fresh vegetables, fruits, legumes, and uncured meats are also good sources of potassium and add only small amounts of sodium to the diet. If you are thinking of using a potassium substitute for common salt, you should consult your physician before doing so.

Another source of sodium is drinking water. The sodium content of drinking water varies considerably throughout the country. This variation also affects the sodium content of soft drinks and beer produced and bottled at different locations.

Water softeners raise the sodium content of water—the harder the water, the greater amount of sodium needed to soften it. In most States, the State department of public health can supply information on the sodium content of public water supplies and provide help in getting water from individual wells or water supplies analyzed.

Because some products vary considerably in sodium content, table 1 gives representative values. Sodium values shown reflect current processing practices and typical product formulas. If these practices and formulas are changed, sodium values may change also.

Values given in table 1 are for unsalted products, unless specified. Cooked items have been prepared using unsalted water, even though the manufacturers' instructions may call for salt. Canned vegetable values are for total can contents of solids and liquids. The values reported are for common household measures of the foods and include metric equivalents.

Some labels may express sodium content in grams or milligrams. Here's how to convert these measurements and also how to measure the amount of sodium in salt.

Salt and sodium conversions

Grams to milligrams	Multiply weight in grams by 1,000
Sodium into salt (NaCl) equivalent	Milligrams of sodium content ÷ .40 = milligrams of salt
Salt into sodium	Milligrams of salt × .40 = milligrams of sodium
Sodium in milligrams to sodium in milliequivalents[1]	Milligrams of sodium ÷ 23 (atomic weight of sodium) = milliequivalents of sodium
Milliequivalents of sodium to milligrams of sodium	Milliequivalents of sodium × 23 = milligrams of sodium

[1]Medical prescriptions are often given as milliequivalents (mEq).

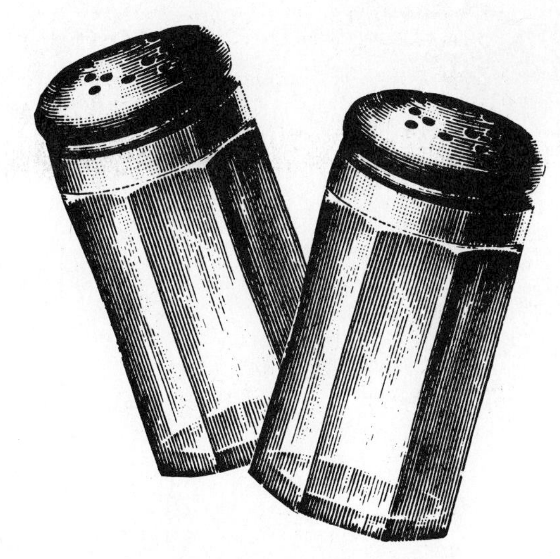

Table 1—Sodium Content of Foods

Beverages and Fruit Juices

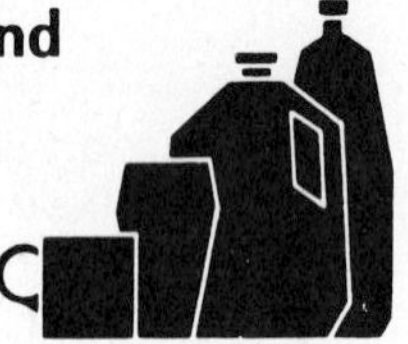

Item	Food	Portion	Weight (grams)	Sodium (milligrams)
	Alcoholic:			
1	Beer	12 fl oz	360	25
2	Gin, rum, whisky	2 fl oz	60	1
	Wine:			
	Red:			
3	Domestic	4 fl oz	120	12
4	Imported	4 fl oz	120	6
5	Sherry	4 fl oz	120	14
	White:			
6	Domestic	4 fl oz	120	19
7	Imported	4 fl oz	120	2
	Breakfast drink, instant:			
8	Grape	8 fl oz	240	0
9	Citrus fruits	8 fl oz	240	14
	Carbonated:			
10	Club soda	8 fl oz	240	39
	Cola:			
11	Regular	8 fl oz	240	16
12	Low calorie	8 fl oz	240	21
	Fruit flavored:			
13	Regular	8 fl oz	240	34
14	Low calorie	8 fl oz	240	46
15	Ginger ale	8 fl oz	240	13
16	Root beer	8 fl oz	240	24
17	Cocoa mix, water added	8 fl oz	240	232
	Coffee:			
18	Brewed	8 fl oz	240	2
	Instant:			
19	Regular	8 fl oz	240	1
20	Decaffeinated	8 fl oz	240	1
21	With chicory	8 fl oz	240	7
22	With flavorings	8 fl oz	240	124
23	Substitute	8 fl oz	240	3
	Fruit drinks, canned:			
24	Apple	8 fl oz	240	16
25	Cranberry juice cocktail	8 fl oz	240	4
26	Grape	8 fl oz	240	1
27	Lemonade	8 fl oz	240	60
28	Orange	8 fl oz	240	77
29	Pineapple-grapefruit	8 fl oz	240	80

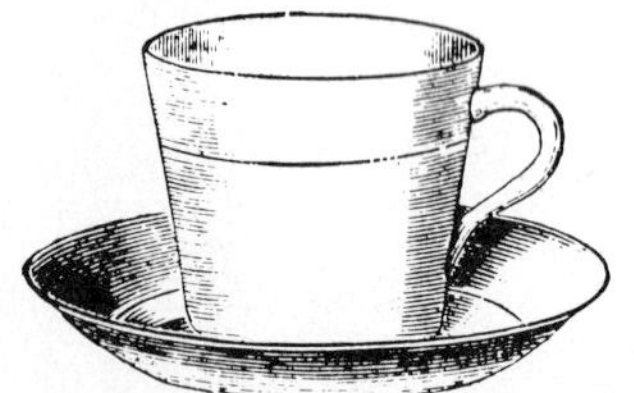

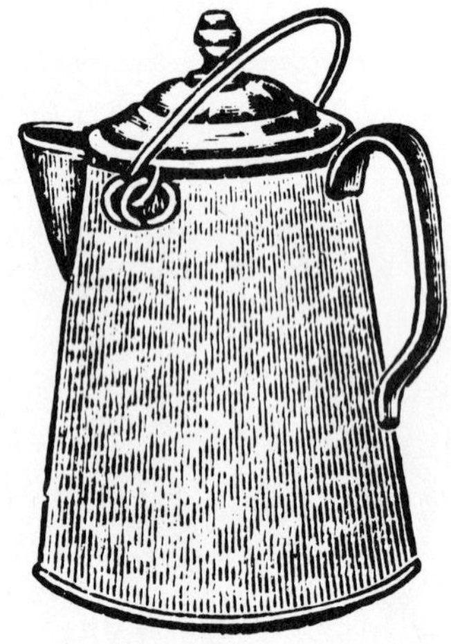

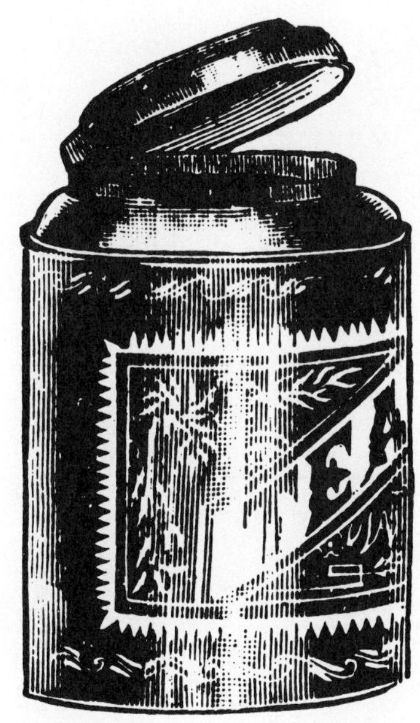

Item	Food	Portion	Weight (grams)	Sodium (milligrams)
	Fruit drinks, dehydrated, reconstituted:			
	Sweetened:			
30	Lemonade-------------	8 fl oz-----	240	50
31	Orange---------------	8 fl oz-----	240	35
32	Other fruit----------	8 fl oz-----	240	0
33	Unsweetened, all flavors	8 fl oz-----	240	0
	Fruit juices:			
34	Apple cider or juice---	1 cup-------	248	5
35	Apricot nectar---------	1 cup-------	251	9
	Citrus:			
	Grapefruit juice:			
36	Canned-------------	1 cup-------	250	4
37	Frozen, diluted----	1 cup-------	247	5
	Lemon or lime juice:			
38	Canned-------------	1 cup-------	244	2
39	Frozen, diluted----	1 cup-------	248	4
	Orange juice:			
40	Canned-------------	1 cup-------	249	5
41	Frozen, diluted----	1 cup-------	249	5
42	Tangerine juice------	1 cup-------	249	2
43	Grape juice, bottled---	1 cup-------	253	8
44	Peach nectar-----------	1 cup-------	249	10
45	Pear nectar------------	1 cup-------	250	8
46	Pineapple juice--------	1 cup-------	250	5
47	Prune juice------------	1 cup-------	256	5
48	Mineral water, imported--	8 fl oz-----	240	42
	Tea:			
	Hot:			
49	Brewed---------------	8 fl oz-----	240	1
50	Instant--------------	8 fl oz-----	240	2
	Iced:			
51	Canned---------------	8 fl oz-----	240	9
	Powdered, lemon flavored:			
52	Sugar sweetened--	8 fl oz-----	240	1
53	Low calorie------	8 fl oz-----	240	15
54	Thirst quencher----------	8 fl oz-----	240	140

Dairy Products

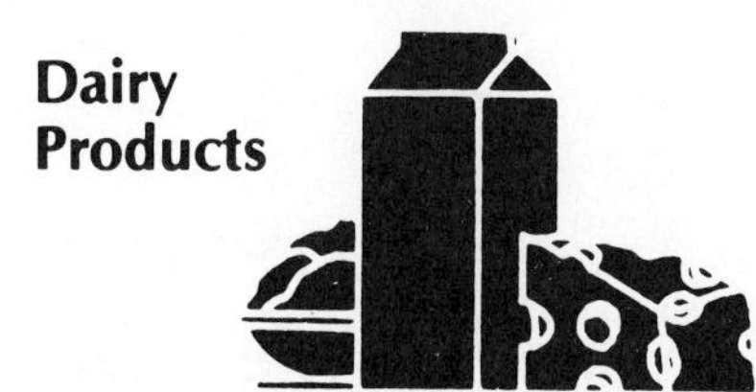

Item	Food	Portion	Weight (grams)	Sodium (milligrams)
	Cheese:			
	Natural:			
55	Blue-----------------	1 oz--------	28	396
56	Brick----------------	1 oz--------	28	159

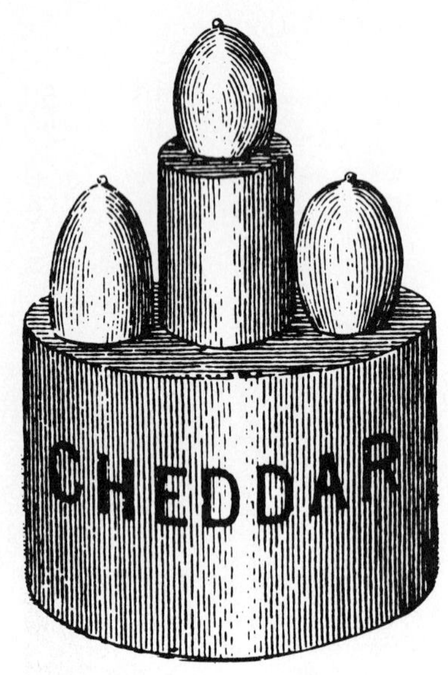

Item	Food	Portion	Weight (grams)	Sodium (milligrams)
57	Brie	1 oz	28	178
58	Camembert	1 oz	28	239
	Cheddar:			
59	Regular	1 oz	28	176
60	Low sodium	1 oz	28	6
61	Colby	1 oz	28	171
	Cottage:			
62	Regular and lowfat	4 oz	113	457
63	Dry curd, unsalted	4 oz	113	14
64	Cream	1 oz	28	84
65	Edam	1 oz	28	274
66	Feta	1 oz	28	316
67	Gouda	1 oz	28	232
68	Gruyere	1 oz	28	95
69	Limburger	1 oz	28	227
70	Monterey	1 oz	28	152
	Mozzarella, from:			
71	Whole milk	1 oz	28	106
72	Part skim milk	1 oz	28	132
73	Muenster	1 oz	28	178
74	Neufchatel	1 oz	28	113
	Parmesan:			
75	Grated	1 oz	28	528
76	Hard	1 oz	28	454
77	Provolone	1 oz	28	248
	Ricotta, made with:			
78	Whole milk	1/2 cup	124	104
79	Part skim milk	1/2 cup	124	155
80	Roquefort	1 oz	28	513
81	Swiss	1 oz	28	74
82	Tilsit	1 oz	28	213
	Pasteurized processed cheese:			
83	American	1 oz	28	406
84	Low sodium	1 oz	28	2
85	Swiss	1 oz	28	388
	Cheese food:			
86	American	1 oz	28	337
87	Swiss	1 oz	28	440
	Cheese spread:			
88	American	1 oz	28	381
	Cream, sweet:			
89	Fluid, all types	1 tbsp	15	6
90	Whipped	1 tbsp	3	4
91	Cream, sour, cultured	1 tbsp	12	6

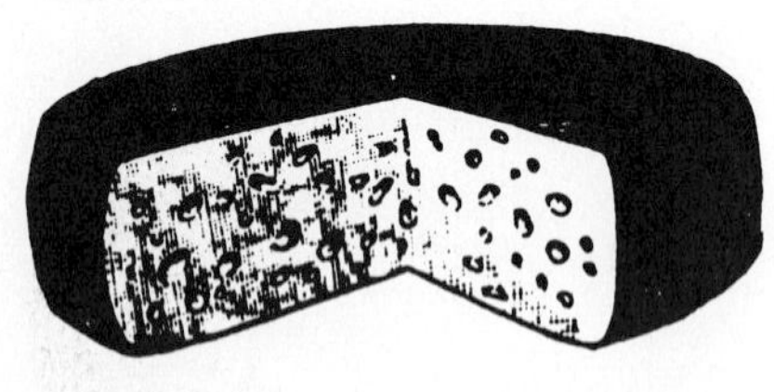

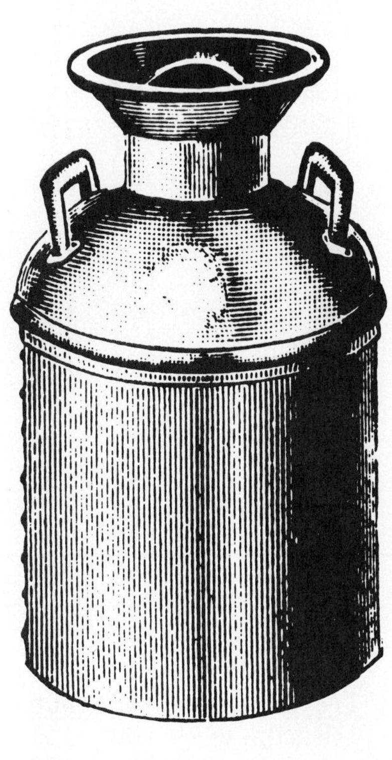

Item	Food	Portion	Weight (grams)	Sodium (milligrams)
	Cream products, imitation:			
	Sweet:			
	Coffee whitener:			
92	Liquid	1 tbsp	15	12
93	Powdered	1 tbsp	6	12
94	Whipped Topping	1 tbsp	4	2
95	Sour, cultured	1 oz	28	29
	Milk:			
	Fluid:			
96	Whole and lowfat	1 cup	244	122
97	Whole, low sodium	1 cup	244	6
	Buttermilk, cultured:			
98	Salted	1 cup	245	257
99	Unsalted	1 cup	245	122
	Canned:			
	Evaporated:			
100	Whole	1 cup	252	266
101	Skim	1 cup	255	294
102	Sweetened, condensed	1 cup	306	389
	Dry:			
	Nonfat:			
103	Regular	1/2 cup	60	322
104	Instantized	1 cup	68	373
105	Buttermilk	1/2 cup	60	310
	Milk beverages:			
106	Chocolate	1 cup	250	149
107	Cocoa, hot	1 cup	250	123
108	Eggnog	1 cup	254	138
	Malted:			
109	Natural flavor	1 cup	265	215
110	Chocolate flavor	1 cup	265	168
	Shakes, thick:			
111	Chocolate or vanilla	1 shake	306	317
	Milk desserts, frozen			
	Ice cream:			
112	Chocolate	1 cup	133	75
113	Custard, French	1 cup	133	84
114	Strawberry	1 cup	133	77
	Vanilla:			
115	French, softserve	1 cup	173	153
116	Hardened	1 cup	140	112
	Ice milk:			
	Vanilla:			
117	Hardened	1 cup	131	105
118	Soft serve	1 cup	175	163

Item	Food	Portion	Weight (grams)	Sodium (milligrams)
	Novelty products:			
	Bars:			
119	Fudge---------------	1 bar-------	73	54
120	Orange cream--------	1 bar-------	66	27
	Vanilla, chocolate coated:			
121	Ice cream---------	1 bar-------	47	24
122	Ice milk----------	1 bar-------	50	31
	Cones, vanilla,			
123	chocolate coated----	1 small-----	71	64
124	Sandwich--------------	1 sandwich--	62	92
125	Sherbet, orange---------	1 cup-------	193	89
	Milk desserts, other:			
126	Custard, baked----------	1 cup-------	265	209
	Puddings:			
	Butterscotch:			
127	Regular, whole milk-	1/2 cup-----	148	245
128	Instant, whole milk-	1/2 cup-----	149	445
129	LoCal, skim milk----	1/2 cup-----	130	130
130	Ready-to-serve------	1 can-------	142	290
	Chocolate:			
131	Home recipe---------	1/2 cup-----	130	73
132	Regular, whole milk-	1/2 cup-----	148	195
133	Instant, whole milk-	1/2 cup-----	149	470
134	LoCal, skim milk----	1/2 cup-----	130	80
135	Ready-to-serve------	1 can-------	142	262
	Vanilla:			
136	Home recipe---------	1/2 cup-----	128	83
137	Regular, whole milk-	1/2 cup-----	148	200
138	Instant, whole milk-	1/2 cup-----	149	400
139	LoCal, skim milk----	1/2 cup-----	130	115
140	Ready-to-serve------	1 can-------	142	279
141	Tapioca, cooked-------	1/2 cup-----	145	130
	Yogurt:			
	Plain:			
142	Regular---------------	8 oz--------	227	105
143	Lowfat----------------	8 oz--------	227	159
144	Skim milk-------------	8 oz--------	227	174
145	With fruit-------------	8 oz--------	227	133

Eggs, Fish, Shellfish, Meat, Poultry, and Related Products

Item	Food	Portion	Weight (grams)	Sodium (milligrams)
	Eggs:			
146	Whole------------------	1 egg-------	50	59
147	White------------------	1 white-----	33	50
148	Yolk-------------------	1 yolk------	17	9

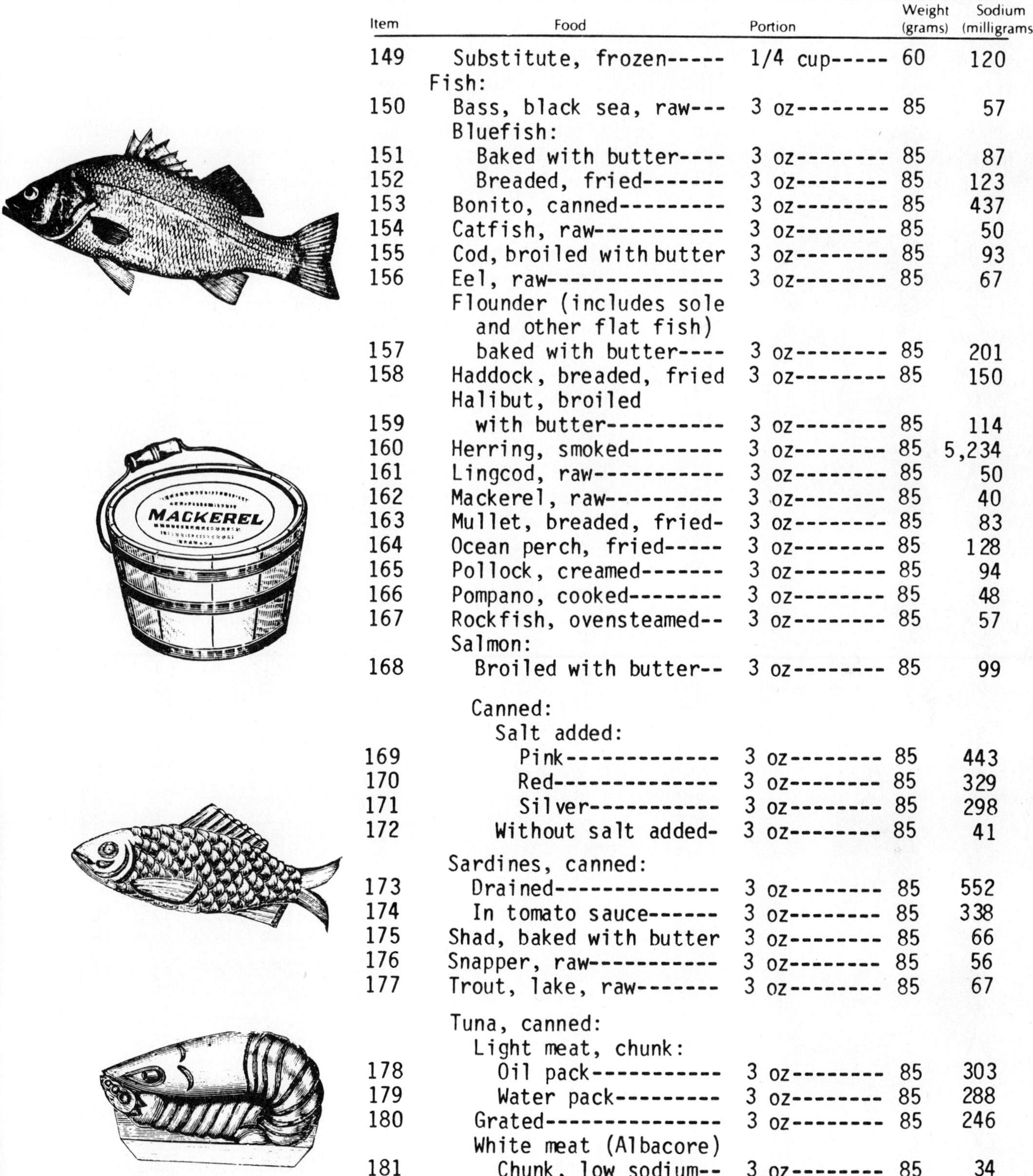

Item	Food	Portion	Weight (grams)	Sodium (milligrams)
149	Substitute, frozen-----	1/4 cup-----	60	120
	Fish:			
150	Bass, black sea, raw---	3 oz--------	85	57
	Bluefish:			
151	Baked with butter----	3 oz--------	85	87
152	Breaded, fried-------	3 oz--------	85	123
153	Bonito, canned---------	3 oz--------	85	437
154	Catfish, raw-----------	3 oz--------	85	50
155	Cod, broiled with butter	3 oz--------	85	93
156	Eel, raw---------------	3 oz--------	85	67
	Flounder (includes sole and other flat fish)			
157	baked with butter----	3 oz--------	85	201
158	Haddock, breaded, fried	3 oz--------	85	150
	Halibut, broiled			
159	with butter----------	3 oz--------	85	114
160	Herring, smoked--------	3 oz--------	85	5,234
161	Lingcod, raw-----------	3 oz--------	85	50
162	Mackerel, raw----------	3 oz--------	85	40
163	Mullet, breaded, fried-	3 oz--------	85	83
164	Ocean perch, fried-----	3 oz--------	85	128
165	Pollock, creamed-------	3 oz--------	85	94
166	Pompano, cooked--------	3 oz--------	85	48
167	Rockfish, ovensteamed--	3 oz--------	85	57
	Salmon:			
168	Broiled with butter--	3 oz--------	85	99
	Canned:			
	Salt added:			
169	Pink-------------	3 oz--------	85	443
170	Red--------------	3 oz--------	85	329
171	Silver-----------	3 oz--------	85	298
172	Without salt added-	3 oz--------	85	41
	Sardines, canned:			
173	Drained--------------	3 oz--------	85	552
174	In tomato sauce------	3 oz--------	85	338
175	Shad, baked with butter	3 oz--------	85	66
176	Snapper, raw-----------	3 oz--------	85	56
177	Trout, lake, raw-------	3 oz--------	85	67
	Tuna, canned:			
	Light meat, chunk:			
178	Oil pack-----------	3 oz--------	85	303
179	Water pack---------	3 oz--------	85	288
180	Grated---------------	3 oz--------	85	246
	White meat (Albacore)			
181	Chunk, low sodium--	3 oz--------	85	34

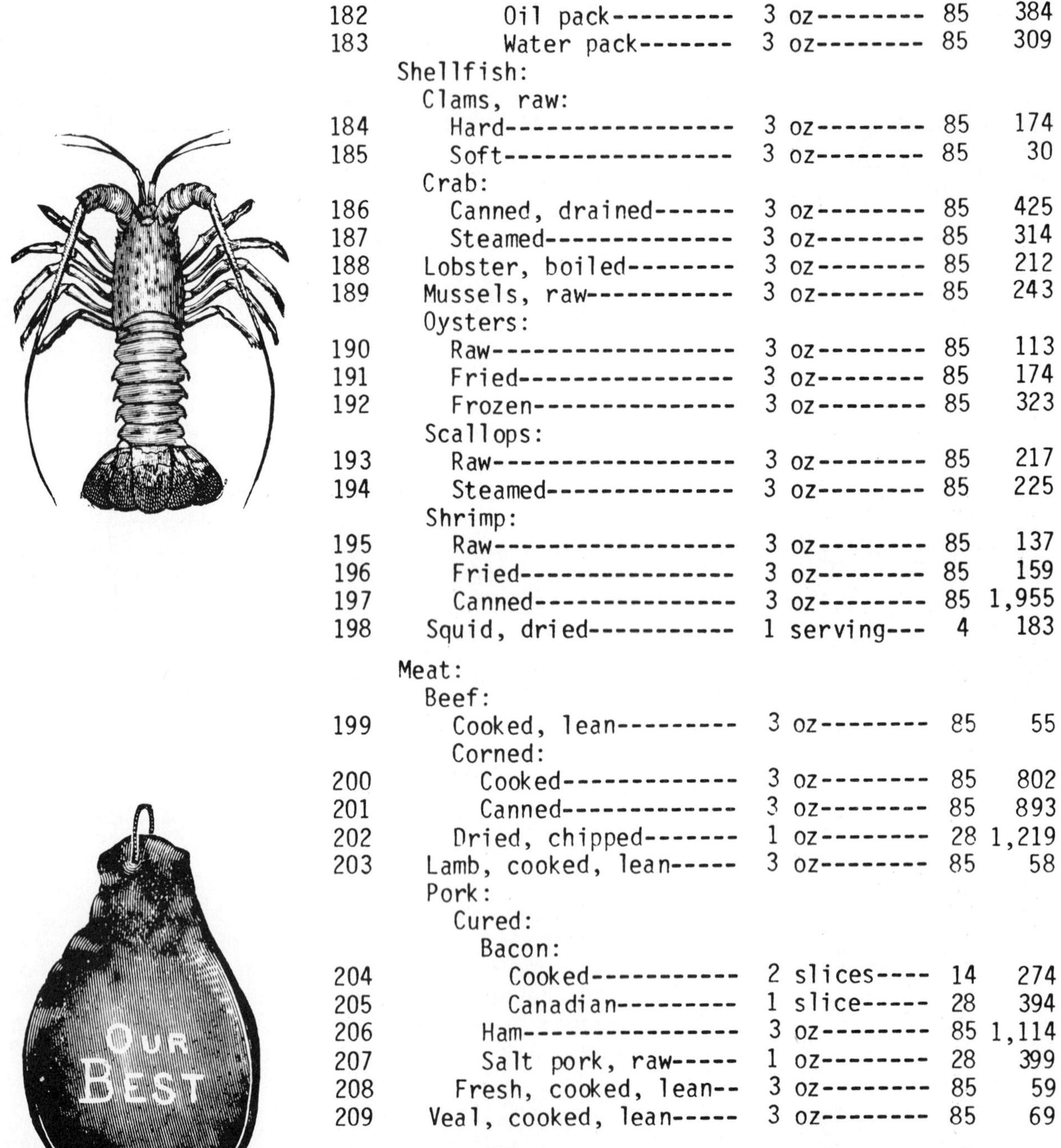

Item	Food	Portion	Weight (grams)	Sodium (milligrams)
	Solid:			
182	Oil pack	3 oz	85	384
183	Water pack	3 oz	85	309
	Shellfish:			
	Clams, raw:			
184	Hard	3 oz	85	174
185	Soft	3 oz	85	30
	Crab:			
186	Canned, drained	3 oz	85	425
187	Steamed	3 oz	85	314
188	Lobster, boiled	3 oz	85	212
189	Mussels, raw	3 oz	85	243
	Oysters:			
190	Raw	3 oz	85	113
191	Fried	3 oz	85	174
192	Frozen	3 oz	85	323
	Scallops:			
193	Raw	3 oz	85	217
194	Steamed	3 oz	85	225
	Shrimp:			
195	Raw	3 oz	85	137
196	Fried	3 oz	85	159
197	Canned	3 oz	85	1,955
198	Squid, dried	1 serving	4	183
	Meat:			
	Beef:			
199	Cooked, lean	3 oz	85	55
	Corned:			
200	Cooked	3 oz	85	802
201	Canned	3 oz	85	893
202	Dried, chipped	1 oz	28	1,219
203	Lamb, cooked, lean	3 oz	85	58
	Pork:			
	Cured:			
	Bacon:			
204	Cooked	2 slices	14	274
205	Canadian	1 slice	28	394
206	Ham	3 oz	85	1,114
207	Salt pork, raw	1 oz	28	399
208	Fresh, cooked, lean	3 oz	85	59
209	Veal, cooked, lean	3 oz	85	69
	Organ meats:			
210	Brain, raw	1 oz	28	35
	Gizzard, poultry,			
211	simmered	1 oz	28	17

Item	Food	Portion	Weight (grams)	Sodium (milligrams)
	Heart:			
212	Beef, braised--------	1 oz--------	28	29
213	Calf, braised--------	1 oz--------	28	32
214	Poultry, simmered----	1 oz--------	28	14
215	Kidney, beef, braised--	1 oz--------	28	71
	Liver:			
216	Calf, fried----------	1 oz--------	28	33
217	Pork, simmered-------	1 oz--------	28	14
218	Poultry, simmered----	1 oz--------	28	16
	Sweetbreads, calf,			
219	cooked---------------	1 oz--------	28	32
220	Tongue, beef, braised	1 oz--------	28	17
	Tripe:			
221	Commercial-----------	1 oz--------	28	13
	Poultry and game:			
	Chicken, roasted:			
222	Breast with skin-----	1/2 breast--	98	69
223	Drumstick with skin--	1 drumstick-	52	47
	Products:			
224	Canned-------------	1 5-oz can--	142	714
225	Frankfurter--------	1 frankfurter	45	617
	Duck, roasted, flesh			
226	and skin-------------	1/2 duck----	382	227
	Goose, roasted, flesh			
227	and skin-------------	1/2 goose---	774	543
	Rabbit:			
228	Leg, raw-------------	4 oz--------	113	40
229	Flesh, cooked--------	4 oz--------	113	70
	Turkey, small, roasted:			
230	Breast with skin-----	1/2 breast--	344	182
231	Leg with skin--------	1 leg-------	245	195
	Sausages, luncheon meats, and spreads:			
232	Beer salami, beef------	1 slice-----	6	56
	Bologna:			
233	Beef-----------------	1 slice-----	22	220
234	Beef and pork--------	1 slice-----	22	224
235	Bratwurst, cooked------	1 oz--------	28	158
236	Braunschweiger---------	1 slice-----	28	324
237	Brotwurst--------------	1 oz--------	28	315
238	Chicken spread---------	1 oz--------	28	115
239	Frankfurter------------	1 frankfurter	57	639
	Ham:			
240	And cheese loaf------	1 oz--------	28	381
241	Chopped--------------	1 slice-----	21	288

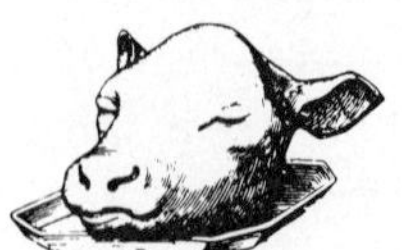

Item	Food	Portion	Weight (grams)	Sodium (milligrams)
242	Deviled	1 oz	28	253
243	Spread	1 oz	28	258
244	Kielbasa	1 slice	26	280
245	Knockwurst	1 link	68	687
246	Lebanon bologna	1 slice	18	228
247	Liver cheese	1 slice	20	245
248	Old fashioned loaf	1 slice	22	275
249	Olive loaf	1 slice	21	312
250	Pepperoni	1 slice	6	122
	Salami:			
	Cooked:			
251	Beef	1 slice	22	255
252	Beef and pork	1 slice	22	234
253	Dry or hard, pork	1 slice	10	226
	Sausage:			
	Cooked:			
254	Pork	1 link	13	168
255	Pork and beef	1 patty	27	217
256	Smoked	1 link	28	264
257	Thuringer	1 slice	22	320
258	Tuna spread	1 oz	28	92
259	Turkey roll	1 oz	28	166
260	Vienna sausage	1 link	16	152

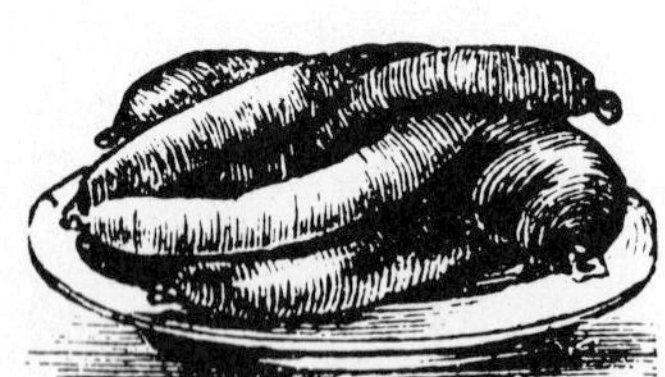

Item	Food	Portion	Weight (grams)	Sodium (milligrams)
	Prepared main dishes:			
	Beef:			
	And macaroni:			
261	Frozen	6 oz	170	673
262	Canned	1 cup	227	1,185
	Cabbage, stuffed,			
263	frozen	8 oz	226	63
	Chili con carne with beans, canned:			
264	Regular	1 cup	255	1,194
265	Low sodium	1 cup	335	100
	Dinners, frozen:			
266	Beef	1 dinner	312	998
267	Meat loaf	1 dinner	312	1,304
268	Sirloin, chopped	1 dinner	284	978
269	Swiss steak	1 dinner	284	682
270	Enchiladas	1 pkg	207	725
271	Goulash, canned	8 oz	227	1,032
	Hash, corned beef,			
272	canned	1 cup	220	1,520
273	Meatballs, Swedish	8 oz	227	1,880

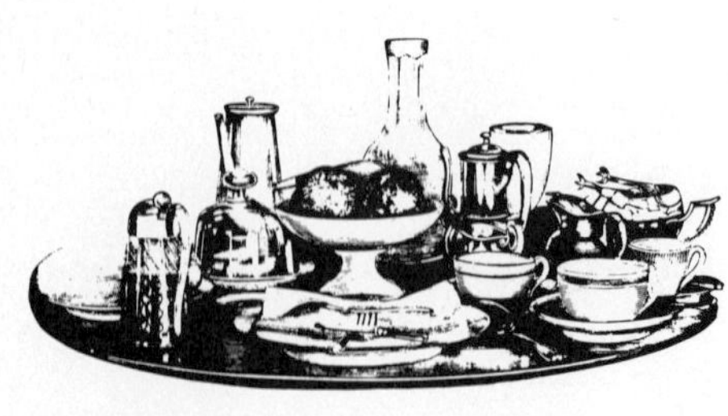

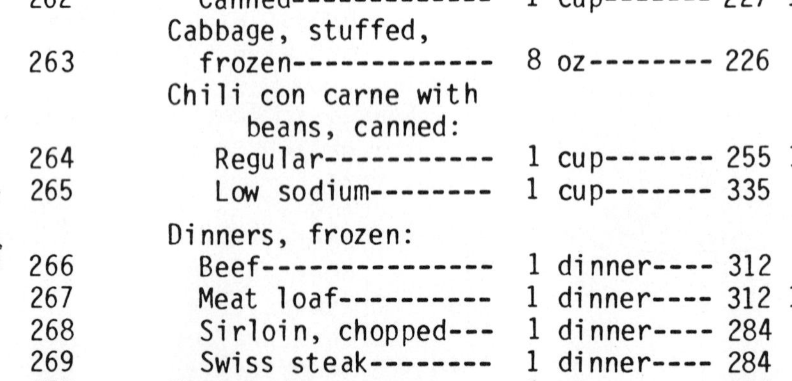

Item	Food	Portion	Weight (grams)	Sodium (milligrams)
	Peppers, stuffed,			
274	frozen------------	8 oz--------	226	1,001
	Pizza, frozen:			
275	With pepperoni-----	1/2 pie-----	195	813
276	With sausage-------	1/2 pie-----	189	967
	Pot pie:			
277	Home baked---------	1 pie-------	227	644
278	Frozen-------------	1 pie-------	227	1,093
279	Ravioli, canned------	7.5 oz------	213	1,065
	Spaghetti, canned:			
280	And ground beef----	7.5 oz------	213	1,054
281	And meatballs------	7.5 oz------	213	942
282	Sauce--------------	4 oz--------	114	856
283	Stew, canned---------	8 oz--------	227	980
	Chicken:			
284	And dumplings, frozen	12 oz-------	340	1,506
285	And noodles, frozen--	3/4 cup-----	180	662
286	Chow mein, home recipe	1 cup-------	250	718
287	Dinner, frozen-------	1 dinner----	312	1,153
	Pot pie:			
288	Home recipe--------	1 pie-------	232	594
289	Frozen-------------	1 pie-------	227	907
	Fish and shellfish:			
290	Fish dinner, frozen--	1 dinner----	248	1,212
	Shrimp:			
291	Dinner, frozen-----	1 dinner----	223	758
292	Egg roll, frozen---	1 roll------	71	648
293	Tuna, pot pie, frozen	1 pie-------	227	715
	Pork, sweet and sour			
294	canned--------------	1 cup-------	275	1,968
	Turkey:			
295	Dinner, frozen-------	1 dinner----	333	1,228
	Pot pie:			
296	Home recipe--------	1 pie-------	227	620
297	Frozen-------------	1 pie-------	233	1,018
298	Veal Parmigiana--------	7.5 oz------	214	1,825
	Without meat:			
	Chow mein, vegetable,			
299	frozen------------	1 cup-------	240	1,273
300	Pizza, cheese--------	1/4 12-in pie	90	447
301	Spanish rice, canned-	1 cup-------	221	1,370

Item	Food	Portion	Weight (grams)	Sodium (milligrams)
	Fast foods:			
302	Cheeseburger	1 each	111	709
303	Chicken dinner	1 portion	410	2,243
304	Fish sandwich	1 sandwich	164	882
305	French fries	2-1/2 oz	69	146
	Hamburger:			
306	Regular	1 each	92	461
307	Jumbo	1 each	236	990
308	Frankfurter	1 frankfurter	93	728
309	Pizza, cheese	1/4 pie	110	599
310	Shake	1 shake	308	266
311	Taco	1 taco	75	401

Fruits

Item	Food	Portion	Weight (grams)	Sodium (milligrams)
	Apples:			
312	Raw or baked	1 apple	138	2
313	Frozen, slices	1 cup	200	28
314	Frozen, scalloped	8 oz	227	45
315	Dried, sulfured	8 oz	227	210
	Applesauce, canned:			
316	Sweetened	1 cup	250	6
317	Unsweetened	1 cup	250	5
318	With added salt	1 cup	250	68
	Apricots:			
319	Raw	3 apricots	114	1
	Canned:			
320	Peeled	1 cup	258	27
321	Unpeeled	1 cup	258	10
322	Dried	1 cup	130	12
323	Avocado, raw	1 avocado	216	22
324	Banana, raw	1 banana	119	2
	Berries:			
	Blackberries (Boysenberries)			
325	Raw	1 cup	144	1
326	Canned	1 cup	244	3
	Blueberries:			
327	Raw	1 cup	145	1
328	Canned	1 cup	250	2
	Raspberries:			
329	Raw	1 cup	123	1
330	Frozen	1 package	284	3

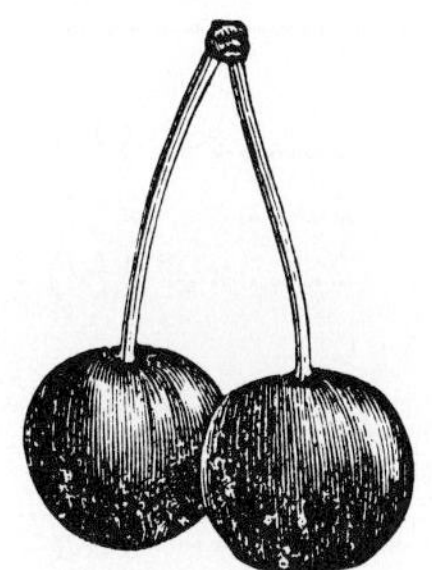

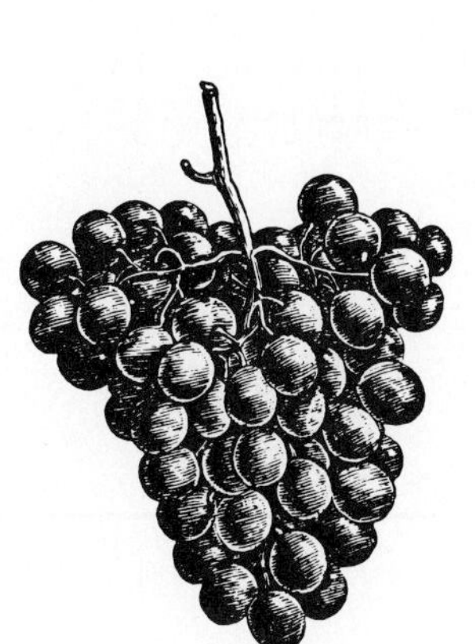

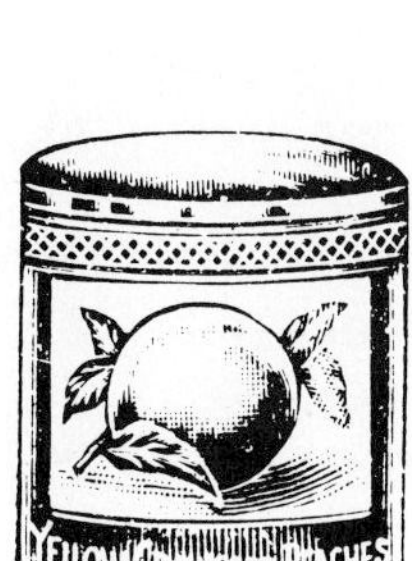

Item	Food	Portion	Weight (grams)	Sodium (milligrams)
	Strawberries:			
331	Raw	1 cup	149	2
332	Frozen, sliced	1 cup	255	6
	Cherries:			
333	Raw	1 cup	150	1
334	Frozen	8 oz	227	3
335	Canned	1 cup	257	10
	Citrus:			
	Grapefruit:			
336	Raw	1/2 grapefruit	120	1
337	Frozen, unsweetened	1 cup	244	6
338	Canned, sweetened	1 cup	254	4
339	Kumquat	1 kumquat	19	1
340	Lemon, raw	1 lemon	74	1
341	Oranges, raw	1 orange	131	1
342	Tangelo	1 tangelo	95	1
343	Tangerine	1 tangerine	86	1
344	Cranberry, raw	1 cup	95	1
345	Cranberry sauce	1 cup	277	75
	Currant:			
346	Raw	1 cup	133	3
347	Dried	1 cup	140	10
348	Dates, dried	10 dates	80	1
	Figs:			
349	Raw	1 fig	50	2
350	Canned	1 cup	248	3
351	Dried	1 fig	20	2
352	Fruit cocktail, canned	1 cup	255	15
353	Grapes, Thompson seedless	10 grapes	50	1
354	Mangos, raw	1 mango	200	1
	Muskmelon:			
355	Cantaloup	1/2 melon	272	24
356	Casaba	1/5 melon	230	34
357	Honeydew	1/5 melon	298	28
358	Nectarines, raw	1 nectarine	138	1
359	Papaya, raw	1 papaya	303	8
	Peaches:			
360	Raw	1 peach	100	1
361	Frozen	1 cup	250	10
362	Canned	1 cup	256	15
363	Dried, uncooked	1 cup	160	10

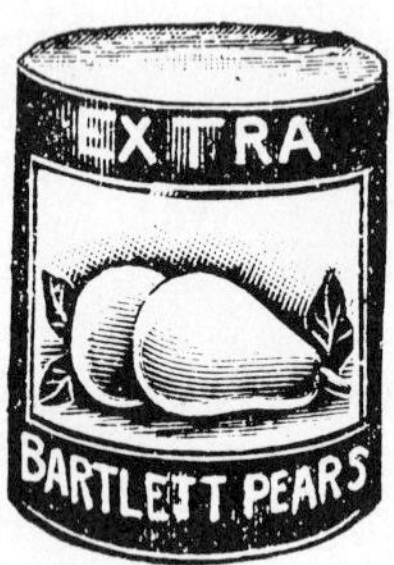

Item	Food	Portion	Weight (grams)	Sodium (milligrams)
	Pears:			
364	Raw	1 pear	168	1
365	Canned	1 cup	255	15
366	Dried	1 cup	180	10
	Pineapple:			
367	Raw	1 cup	135	1
368	Canned	1 cup	255	7
	Plums:			
369	Raw	1 plum	66	1
370	Canned	1 cup	256	10
	Prunes:			
371	Cooked	1 cup	213	8
372	Dried	5 large	43	2
373	Raisins, seedless	1 cup	145	17
	Rhubarb:			
374	Cooked, sugared	1 cup	270	5
375	Frozen	1 cup	270	5
376	Watermelon	1/16 melon	426	8

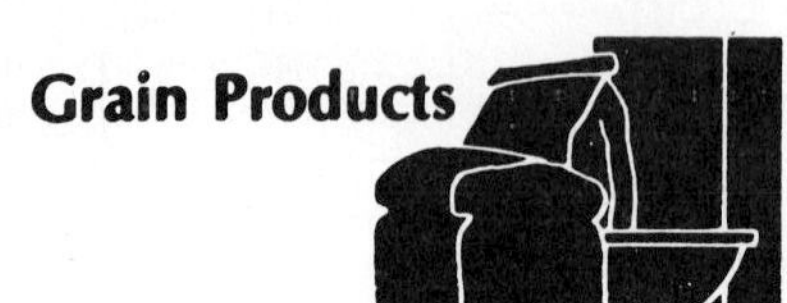

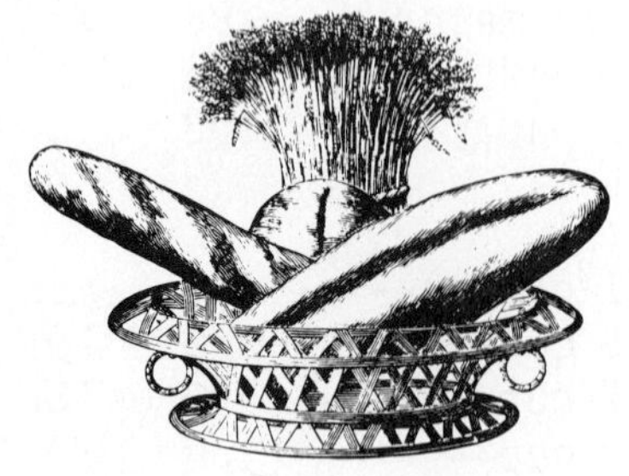

Item	Food	Portion	Weight (grams)	Sodium (milligrams)
377	Barley, pearled, cooked	1 cup	200	6
	Biscuits, baking powder:			
378	Regular flour	1 biscuit	28	175
379	Self rising flour	1 biscuit	28	185
380	With milk from mix	1 biscuit	28	272
381	Low sodium	1 biscuit	28	1
	Bread:			
382	Boston brown	1 slice	45	120
383	Corn, homemade	1 oz	28	176
384	Cracked wheat	1 slice	25	148
385	French	1 slice	23	116
386	Mixed grain	1 slice	23	138
387	Pita	1 loaf	64	132
	Rye:			
388	Regular	1 slice	25	139
389	Pumpernickel	1 slice	32	182
390	Salt rising	1 slice	26	66

Item	Food	Portion	Weight (grams)	Sodium (milligrams)
	White:			
391	Regular	1 slice	25	114
392	Thin	1 slice	16	79
393	Low sodium	1 slice	23	7
394	Whole wheat	1 slice	25	132
	Breakfast cereals:			
	Hot, cooked, in unsalted water:			
	Corn (hominy) grits:			
395	Regular	1 cup	236	1
396	Instant	3/4 cup	177	354
	Cream of Wheat:			
397	Regular	3/4 cup	184	2
398	Instant	3/4 cup	184	5
399	Quick	3/4 cup	184	126
400	Mix 'n eat	3/4 cup	184	350
401	Farina	3/4 cup	184	1
	Oatmeal:			
402	Regular or quick	3/4 cup	180	1
	Instant:			
403	No sodium added	3/4 cup	180	1
404	Sodium added	3/4 cup	180	283
405	With apples and cinnamon	3/4 cup	180	220
406	With maple and brown sugar	3/4 cup	180	277
407	With raisins and spice	3/4 cup	180	223
	Ready-to-eat:			
	Bran cereals:			
408	All-Bran	1/3 cup	28	160
409	Bran Chex	2/3 cup	28	262
410	40% Bran	2/3 cup	28	251
411	100% Bran	1/2 cup	28	221
412	Raisin Bran	1/2 cup	28	209
413	Cheerios	1-1/4 cup	28	304
	Corn cereals:			
414	Corn Chex	1 cup	28	297
	Corn flakes:			
415	Low sodium	1-1/4 cup	28	10
416	Regular	1 cup	28	256
417	Sugar coated	3/4 cup	28	274
418	Sugar Corn Pops	1 cup	28	105
	Granola:			
419	Regular	1/4 cup	34	61

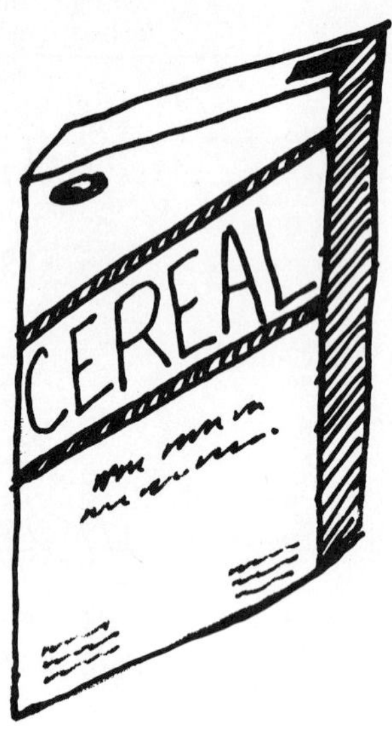

Item	Food	Portion	Weight (grams)	Sodium (milligrams)
420	No sodium added	1/4 cup	34	16
421	Kix	1-1/2 cup	28	261
422	Life	2/3 cup	28	146
423	Product 19	3/4 cup	28	175
	Rice cereals:			
424	Low sodium	1 cup	28	10
425	Puffed rice	2 cups	28	2
426	Rice Chex	1-1/8 cup	28	238
427	Rice Krispies	1 cup	28	340
428	Sugar coated	7/8 cup	28	149
429	Special K	1-1/4 cup	28	265
430	Total	1 cup	28	359
431	Trix	1 cup	28	160
	Wheat cereals:			
432	Puffed wheat	2 cups	28	2
433	Sugar coated	1 cup	28	46
434	Shredded wheat	1 biscuit	24	3
435	Wheat Chex	2/3 cup	28	190
436	Wheaties	1 cup	28	355
437	Wheat germ, toasted	1/4 cup	28	1
	Breakfast sweets:			
	Coffee cake:			
438	Almond	1/8 cake	42	167
439	Blueberry	1/8 cake	35	135
440	Honey nut	1/8 cake	55	110
441	Pecan	1/8 cake	40	172
	Danish:			
442	Apple, frozen	1 roll	72	220
443	Cheese, frozen	1 roll	72	250
444	Cinnamon, frozen	1 roll	72	260
445	Orange, refrigerated dough	1 roll	39	329
	Doughnut:			
446	Cake type	1 doughnut	32	160
447	Yeast leavened	1 doughnut	42	99
	Sweet rolls:			
448	Apple crunch, frozen	1 roll	28	105
449	Caramel, frozen	1 roll	29	118
450	Cinnamon, frozen	1 roll	26	110
451	Honey	1 roll	28	119
	Toaster pastry:			
452	Apple, frosted	1 pastry	52	324

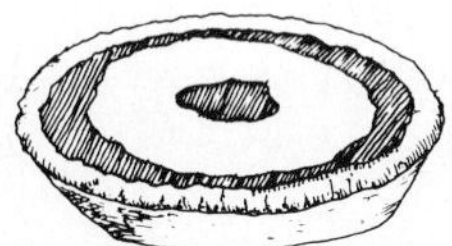

Item	Food	Portion	Weight (grams)	Sodium (milligrams)
453	Blueberry, frosted---	1 pastry----	52	242
454	Cinnamon, frosted----	1 pastry----	52	326
455	Strawberry----------	1 pastry----	52	238
	Cakes, from mix:			
	Angel food:			
456	Regular-------------	1/12 cake---	56	134
457	One step------------	1/12 cake---	57	250
458	Devils food-----------	1/12 cake---	67	402
459	Pound----------------	1/12 cake---	55	171
460	White----------------	1/12 cake---	68	238
461	Yellow---------------	1/12 cake---	69	242
	Cookies:			
462	Brownies, iced--------	1 brownie---	32	69
463	Chocolate chip--------	2 cookies---	21	69
464	Fig bars--------------	2 bars------	28	96
465	Ginger snaps----------	4 cookies---	28	161
466	Macaroons-------------	2 cookies---	38	14
	Oatmeal:			
467	Plain---------------	1 cookie----	18	77
468	With chocolate chips-	2 cookies---	26	54
469	With raisins---------	2 cookies---	26	55
470	Sandwich type---------	2 cookies---	20	96
471	Shortbread------------	4 cookies---	30	116
472	Sugar-----------------	1 cookie----	26	108
473	Sugar wafer-----------	4 cookies---	28	43
474	Vanilla wafer---------	6 cookies---	24	53
	Crackers:			
475	Graham----------------	1 cracker---	7	48
476	Low sodium------------	1 cracker---	4	1
477	Rye-------------------	1 cracker---	6	70
478	Saltine---------------	2 crackers--	6	70
479	Whole wheat-----------	1 cracker---	4	30
480	Macaroni, cooked---------	1 cup-------	140	2
481	Muffin, English---------	1 medium----	57	293
482	Noodles, cooked---------	1 cup-------	140	2
483	Pancakes, from mix-------	1 pancake---	27	152
484	Pancake mix--------------	1 cup-------	141	2,036
	Pies, frozen:			
485	Apple-----------------	1/8 of pie--	71	208
486	Banana cream----------	1/6 of pie--	66	90
	Bavarian cream:			
487	Chocolate-----------	1/8 of pie--	80	78

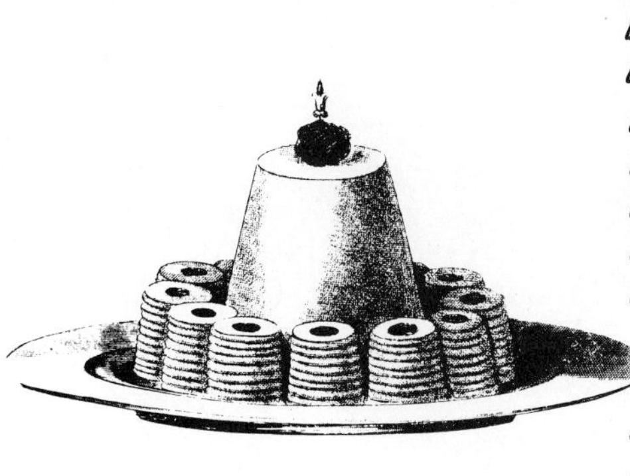

Item	Food	Portion	Weight (grams)	Sodium (milligrams)
488	Lemon----------------	1/8 of pie--	83	71
489	Blueberry--------------	1/8 of pie--	71	163
490	Cherry-----------------	1/8 of pie--	71	169
491	Chocolate cream--------	1/6 of pie--	66	107
	Coconut:			
492	Cream----------------	1/6 of pie--	66	104
493	Custard--------------	1/8 of pie--	71	194
494	Lemon cream------------	1/6 of pie--	66	92
495	Mince------------------	1/8 of pie--	71	258
496	Peach------------------	1/8 of pie--	71	169
497	Pecan------------------	1/8 of pie--	71	241
498	Pumpkin----------------	1/8 of pie--	71	169
499	Strawberry cream-------	1/6 of pie--	66	101
	Rice, cooked:			
500	Brown------------------	1 cup-------	195	10
	White:			
501	Regular--------------	1 cup-------	205	6
502	Parboiled------------	1 cup-------	175	4
503	Quick----------------	1 cup-------	165	13
	Rolls:			
504	Brown and serve--------	1 roll------	28	138
505	Refrigerated dough-----	1 roll------	35	342
	Snacks:			
506	Corn chips-------------	1 oz--------	28	231
	Popcorn:			
507	Caramel coated-------	1 cup-------	35	262
508	Oil, salt------------	1 cup-------	9	175
509	Plain----------------	1 cup-------	6	1
510	Potato chips-----------	10 chips----	20	200
	Pretzels:			
511	Regular twist--------	1 pretzel---	6	101
512	Small stick----------	3 sticks----	1	17
513	Spaghetti, cooked--------	1 cup-------	140	2
514	Stuffing mix, cooked-----	1 cup-------	170	1,131
515	Waffle, frozen-----------	1 waffle----	37	275

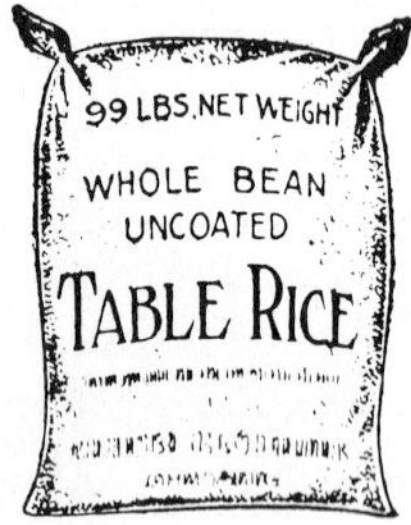

Legumes and Nuts

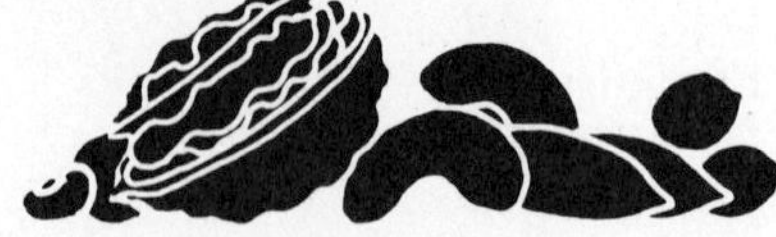

Item	Food	Portion	Weight (grams)	Sodium (milligrams)
	Almonds:			
516	Salted, roasted--------	1 cup-------	157	311

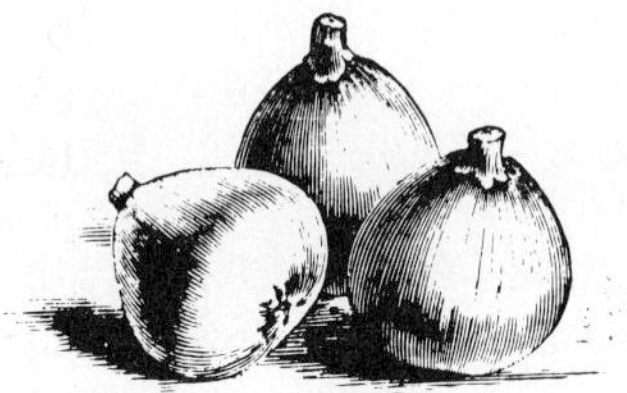

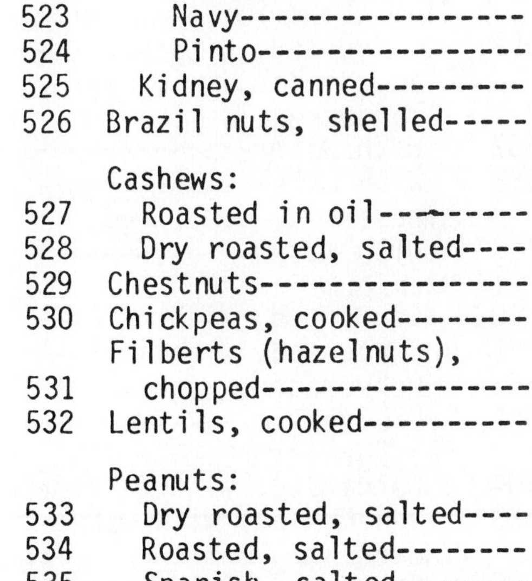

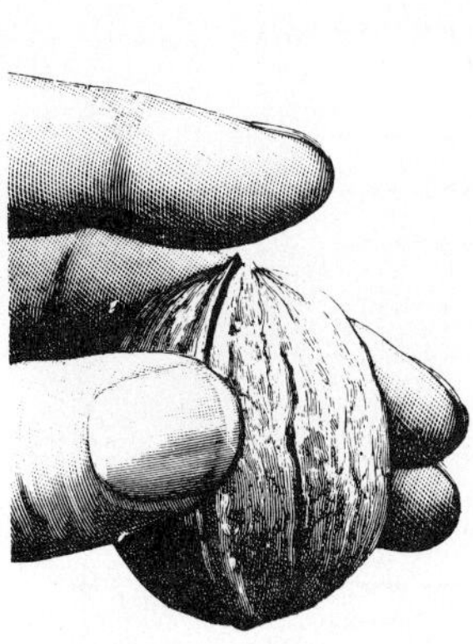

Item	Food	Portion	Weight (grams)	Sodium (milligrams)
517	Unsalted, slivered-----	1 cup-------	115	4
	Beans:			
	Baked, canned:			
518	Boston style---------	1 cup-------	260	606
519	With or without pork-	1 cup-------	260	928
	Dry, cooked:			
520	Great Northern-------	1 cup-------	179	5
521	Lima-----------------	1 cup-------	192	4
522	Kidney---------------	1 cup-------	182	4
523	Navy-----------------	1 cup-------	195	3
524	Pinto----------------	1 cup-------	207	4
525	Kidney, canned---------	1 cup-------	255	844
526	Brazil nuts, shelled-----	1 cup-------	140	1
	Cashews:			
527	Roasted in oil---------	1 cup-------	140	21
528	Dry roasted, salted----	1 cup-------	140	1,200
529	Chestnuts----------------	1 cup-------	160	10
530	Chickpeas, cooked--------	1 cup-------	169	13
	Filberts (hazelnuts),			
531	chopped----------------	1 cup-------	115	2
532	Lentils, cooked----------	1 cup-------	188	4
	Peanuts:			
533	Dry roasted, salted----	1 cup-------	144	986
534	Roasted, salted--------	1 cup-------	144	601
535	Spanish, salted--------	1 cup-------	144	823
536	Unsalted---------------	1 cup-------	144	8
	Peanut butter:			
537	Smooth or crunchy------	1 tbsp------	16	81
538	Low sodium-------------	1 tbsp------	16	1
	Peas:			
539	Blackeye, cooked-------	1 cup-------	204	12
540	Split, cooked----------	1 cup-------	237	5
541	Pecans-------------------	1 cup-------	118	1
542	Pilinuts-----------------	4 oz--------	113	3
543	Pistachios---------------	1 cup-------	125	6
	Soybeans:			
544	Cooked-----------------	1 cup-------	180	4
545	Curd (tofu)------------	1/4 block---	130	9
	Fermented (miso):			
546	Red------------------	1/4 cup-----	72	3,708
547	White----------------	1/4 cup-----	67	2,126
548	Walnuts, English---------	1 cup-------	120	3

Soups

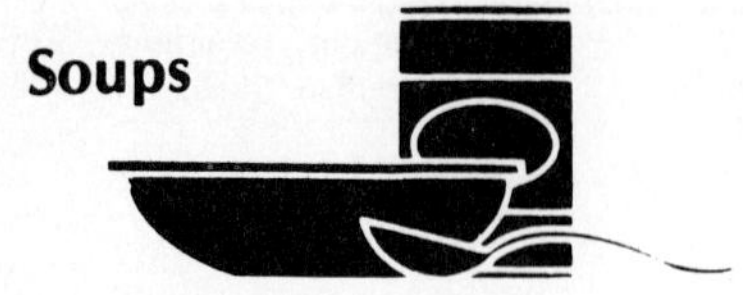

Item	Food	Portion	Weight (grams)	Sodium (milligrams)
549	Beef broth, cubed--------	1 cup-------	241	1,152
	Beef noodle:			
550	Condensed, with water--	1 cup-------	244	952
551	Dehydrated, with water--	1 cup-------	251	1,041
	Chicken noodle:			
552	Condensed, with water--	1 cup-------	241	1,107
553	Dehydrated, with water-	1 cup-------	252	1,284
	Chicken rice:			
554	Condensed, with water--	1 cup-------	241	814
555	Dehydrated, with water-	1 cup-------	253	980
556	Clam chowder, Manhattan, condensed, with water--	1 cup-------	244	1,808
	Clam chowder, New England, condensed:			
557	With water------------	1 cup-------	244	914
558	With milk-------------	1 cup-------	248	992
559	Minestrone, condensed, with water------------	1 cup-------	241	911
	Mushroom:			
560	Condensed, with water--	1 cup-------	244	1,031
561	Condensed, with milk---	1 cup-------	248	1,076
562	Dehydrated, with water-	1 cup-------	253	1,019
563	Low sodium------------	1 cup-------	244	27
	Pea, green:			
564	Condensed, with water--	1 cup-------	250	987
565	Dehydrated, with water-	1 cup-------	271	1,220
	Tomato:			
566	Condensed, with water--	1 cup-------	244	872
567	Condensed, with milk---	1 cup-------	248	932
568	Dehydrated, with water-	1 cup-------	265	943
569	Low sodium------------	1 cup-------	244	29
	Vegetable:			
570	Condensed, with water--	1 cup-------	241	823
571	Dehydrated, with water-	1 cup-------	253	1,146
	Vegetable beef:			
572	Condensed, with water--	1 cup-------	244	957
573	Dehydrated, with water-	1 cup-------	252	1,000
574	Low sodium------------	1 cup-------	244	51

Sugars and Sweets

Item	Food	Portion	Weight (grams)	Sodium (milligrams)
	Candy:			
575	Candy corn------------	1 oz--------	28	60
576	Caramel---------------	1 oz--------	28	74
	Chocolate:			
577	Bitter--------------	1 oz--------	28	4
578	Milk----------------	1 oz--------	28	28

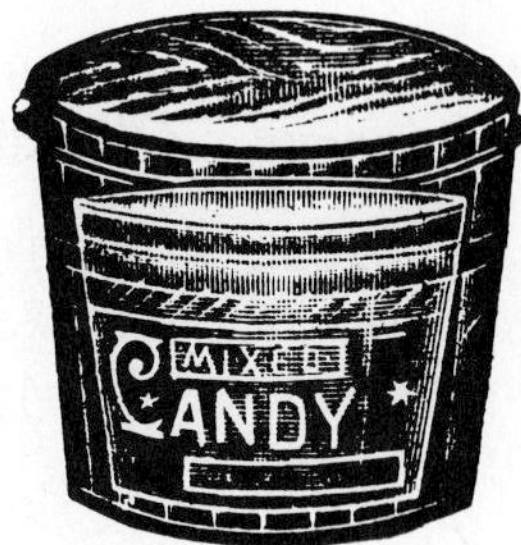

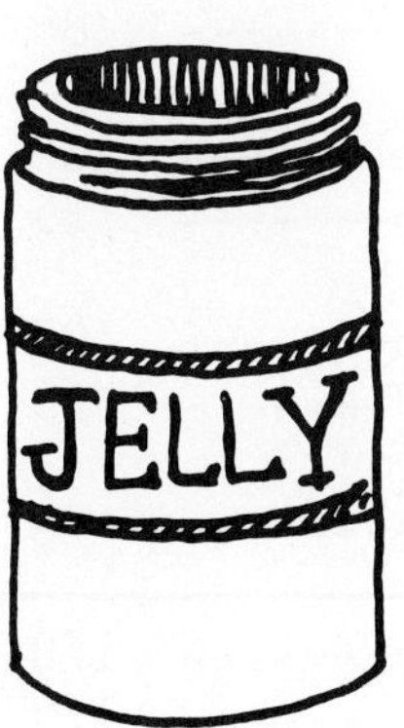

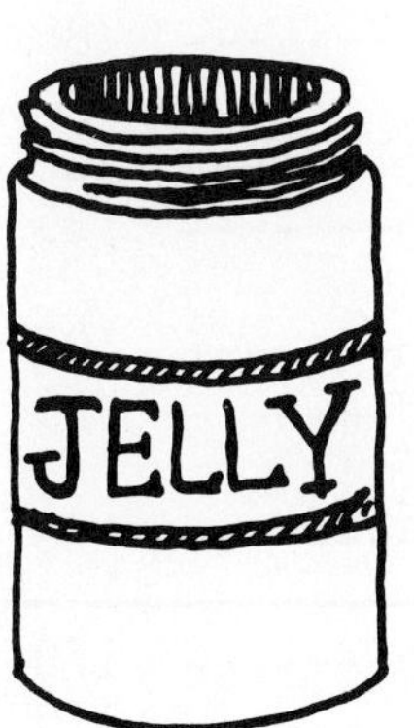

Item	Food	Portion	Weight (grams)	Sodium (milligrams)
579	Fudge, chocolate-------	1 oz--------	28	54
580	Gum drops--------------	1 oz--------	28	10
581	Hard-------------------	1 oz--------	28	9
582	Jelly beans------------	1 oz--------	28	3
583	Licorice---------------	1 oz--------	28	28
584	Marshmallows-----------	1 oz--------	28	11
585	Mints, uncoated--------	1 oz--------	28	56
586	Peanut brittle---------	1 oz--------	28	145
587	Taffy------------------	1 oz--------	28	88
588	Toffee bar, almond-----	1 oz--------	28	65
	Jams and jellies:			
	Jam:			
589	Regular--------------	1 tbsp------	20	2
590	Low calorie----------	1 tbsp------	20	19
	Jelly:			
591	Regular--------------	1 tbsp------	18	3
592	Low calorie----------	1 tbsp------	18	21
	Sirup:			
	Chocolate flavored:			
593	Thin-----------------	1 tbsp------	19	10
594	Fudge----------------	1 tbsp------	19	17
595	Corn------------------	1 tbsp------	20	14
	Maple:			
596	Regular--------------	1 tbsp------	20	1
597	Imitation------------	1 tbsp------	20	20
	Molasses:			
598	Light----------------	1 tbsp------	20	3
599	Medium---------------	1 tbsp------	20	7
600	Blackstrap-----------	1 tbsp------	20	18
	Sugar:			
601	Brown-----------------	1 cup-------	220	66
602	Granulated------------	1 cup-------	200	2
603	Powdered--------------	1 cup-------	120	1

Vegetables, Vegetable Juices, and Salads

Item	Food	Portion	Weight (grams)	Sodium (milligrams)
	Artichokes:			
604	Cooked-----------------	1 medium----	120	36
605	Hearts, frozen---------	3 oz--------	85	40
	Asparagus:			
606	Raw--------------------	1 spear-----	20	1
607	Frozen-----------------	4 spears----	60	4
	Canned:			
608	Regular--------------	4 spears----	80	298
609	Low sodium-----------	1 cup-------	235	7

Item	Food	Portion	Weight (grams)	Sodium (milligrams)
	Beans:			
	Italian:			
610	Frozen	3 oz	85	4
611	Canned	1 cup	220	913
	Lima:			
612	Cooked	1 cup	170	2
613	Frozen	1 cup	170	128
614	Canned	1 cup	170	456
615	Low sodium	1 cup	170	7
	Snap:			
616	Cooked	1 cup	125	5
	Frozen:			
617	Regular	3 oz	85	3
618	With almonds	3 oz	85	335
619	With mushrooms	3 oz	85	145
620	With onions	3 oz	85	360
	Canned:			
621	Regular	1 cup	130	326
622	Low sodium	1 cup	135	3
	Beansprouts, mung:			
623	Raw	1 cup	105	5
624	Canned	1 cup	125	71
	Beets:			
625	Cooked	1 cup	170	73
	Canned:			
626	Sliced	1 cup	170	479
627	Low sodium	1 cup	170	110
628	Harvard	1 cup	170	275
629	Pickled	1 cup	170	330
630	Beet greens, cooked	1 cup	145	110
	Broccoli:			
631	Raw	1 stalk	151	23
	Frozen:			
632	Cooked	1 cup	188	35
633	With cheese sauce	3.3 oz	94	440
634	With hollandaise sauce	3.3 oz	94	115
	Brussels sprouts:			
635	Raw	1 medium	18	1
	Frozen:			
636	Cooked	1 cup	150	15
637	In butter sauce	3.3 oz	94	421
	Cabbage:			
	Green:			
638	Raw	1 cup	70	8
639	Cooked	1 cup	144	16
640	Red, raw	1 cup	70	18

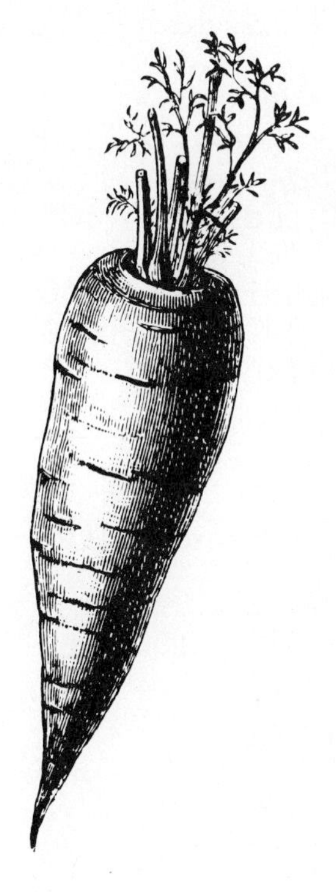

Item	Food	Portion	Weight (grams)	Sodium (milligrams)
	Carrots:			
641	Raw	1 carrot	72	34
	Frozen:			
642	Cut or whole	3.3 oz	94	43
643	In butter sauce	3.3 oz	94	350
644	With brown sugar glaze	3.3 oz	94	500
	Canned:			
645	Regular	1 cup	155	386
646	Low sodium	1 cup	150	58
	Cauliflower:			
647	Raw	1 cup	115	17
648	Cooked	1 cup	125	13
	Frozen:			
649	Cooked	1 cup	180	18
650	With cheese sauce	3 oz	85	325
651	Celery, raw	1 stalk	20	25
652	Chard, cooked	1 cup	166	143
653	Chicory	1 cup	90	6
	Collards:			
654	Cooked	1 cup	190	24
655	Frozen	3 oz	85	41
	Corn:			
656	Cooked	1 ear	140	1
657	Frozen	1 cup	166	7
	Canned:			
	Cream style:			
658	Regular	1 cup	256	671
659	Low sodium	1 cup	256	5
660	Vacuum pack	1 cup	210	577
	Whole kernel:			
661	Regular	1 cup	165	384
662	Low sodium	1 cup	166	2
663	Cucumber	7 slices	28	2
664	Dandelion greens, cooked	1 cup	105	46
665	Eggplant, cooked	1 cup	200	2
666	Endive, raw	1 cup	50	7
	Kale:			
667	Cooked	1 cup	110	47
668	Frozen	3 oz	85	13
669	Kohlrabi, cooked	1 cup	165	9
670	Leek	1 bulb	25	1
671	Lettuce	1 cup	55	4
	Mushrooms:			
672	Raw	1 cup	70	7
673	Canned	2 oz	56	242

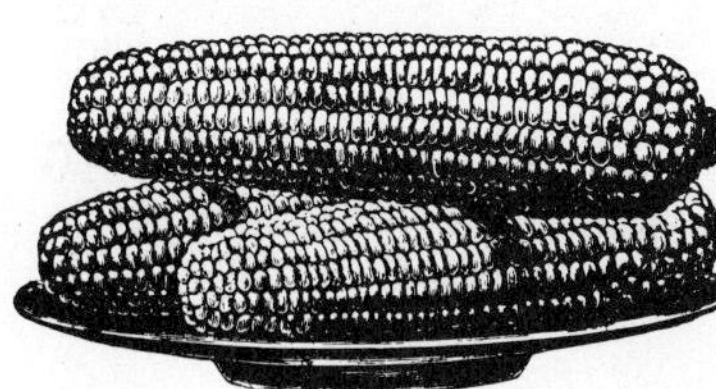

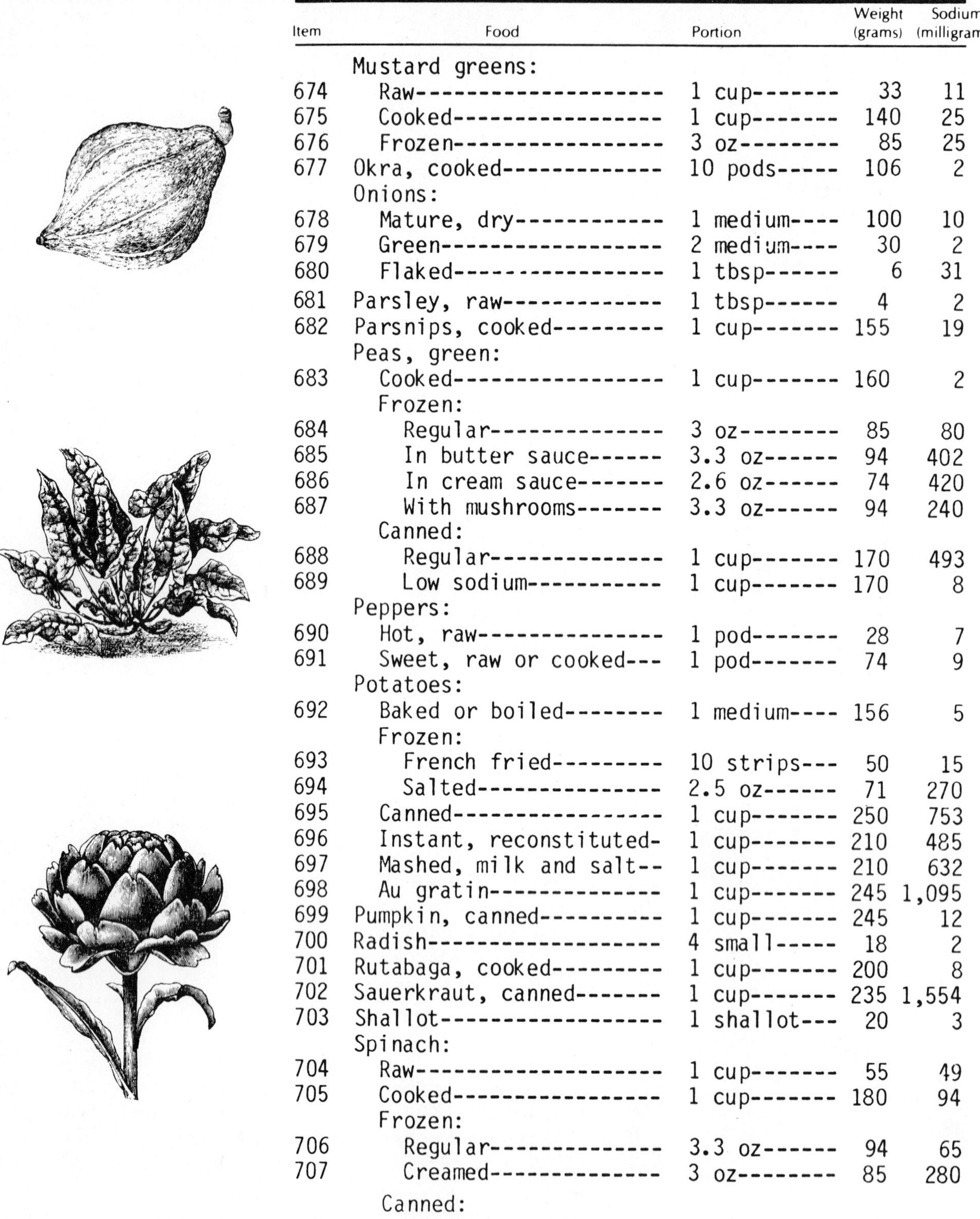

Item	Food	Portion	Weight (grams)	Sodium (milligrams)
	Mustard greens:			
674	Raw	1 cup	33	11
675	Cooked	1 cup	140	25
676	Frozen	3 oz	85	25
677	Okra, cooked	10 pods	106	2
	Onions:			
678	Mature, dry	1 medium	100	10
679	Green	2 medium	30	2
680	Flaked	1 tbsp	6	31
681	Parsley, raw	1 tbsp	4	2
682	Parsnips, cooked	1 cup	155	19
	Peas, green:			
683	Cooked	1 cup	160	2
	Frozen:			
684	Regular	3 oz	85	80
685	In butter sauce	3.3 oz	94	402
686	In cream sauce	2.6 oz	74	420
687	With mushrooms	3.3 oz	94	240
	Canned:			
688	Regular	1 cup	170	493
689	Low sodium	1 cup	170	8
	Peppers:			
690	Hot, raw	1 pod	28	7
691	Sweet, raw or cooked	1 pod	74	9
	Potatoes:			
692	Baked or boiled	1 medium	156	5
	Frozen:			
693	French fried	10 strips	50	15
694	Salted	2.5 oz	71	270
695	Canned	1 cup	250	753
696	Instant, reconstituted	1 cup	210	485
697	Mashed, milk and salt	1 cup	210	632
698	Au gratin	1 cup	245	1,095
699	Pumpkin, canned	1 cup	245	12
700	Radish	4 small	18	2
701	Rutabaga, cooked	1 cup	200	8
702	Sauerkraut, canned	1 cup	235	1,554
703	Shallot	1 shallot	20	3
	Spinach:			
704	Raw	1 cup	55	49
705	Cooked	1 cup	180	94
	Frozen:			
706	Regular	3.3 oz	94	65
707	Creamed	3 oz	85	280
	Canned:			
708	Regular	1 cup	205	910

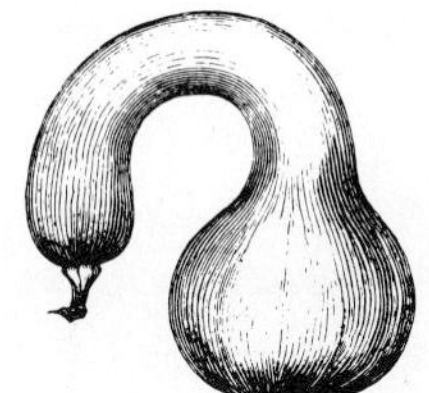

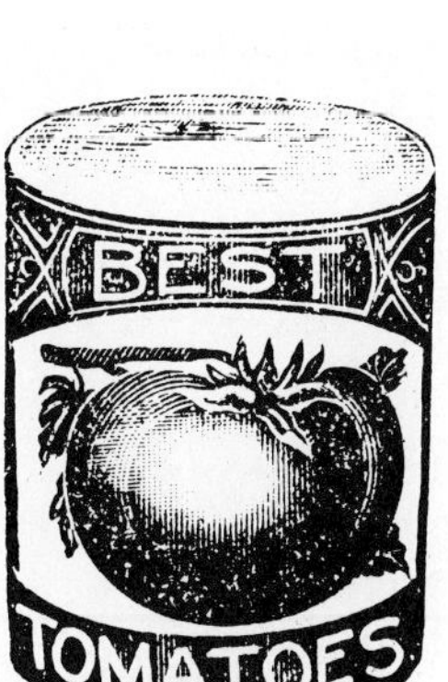

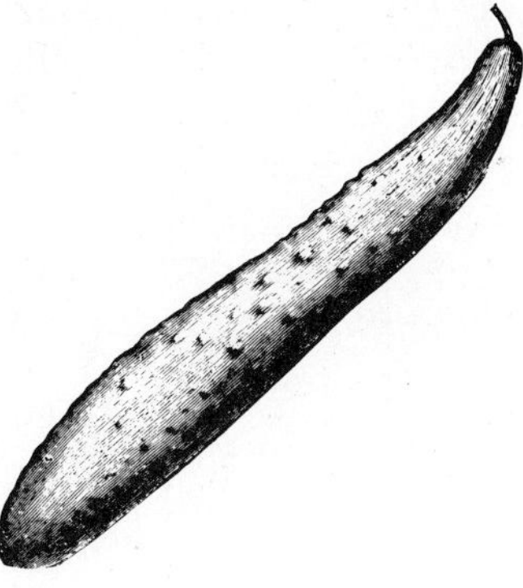

Item	Food	Portion	Weight (grams)	Sodium (milligrams)
709	Low sodium----------	1 cup-------	205	148
	Squash:			
	Summer:			
710	Cooked--------------	1 cup-------	210	5
711	Frozen, with curry---	1/3 cup-----	71	228
712	Canned--------------	1 cup-------	210	785
	Winter:			
713	Baked, mashed--------	1 cup-------	205	2
714	Frozen--------------	1 cup-------	200	4
	Sweetpotatoes:			
715	Baked or boiled in skin--	1 potato----	132	20
	Canned:			
716	Regular-------------	1 potato----	100	48
717	Low sodium----------	1 serving---	113	27
718	Candied---------------	1 potato----	100	42
719	Yam, white, raw--------	1 cup-------	200	28
	Tomatoes:			
720	Raw-------------------	1 tomato----	123	14
721	Cooked----------------	1 cup-------	240	10
	Canned:			
722	Whole---------------	1 cup------	240	390
723	Stewed--------------	1 cup------	240	584
724	Low sodium----------	1 cup-------	240	16
	Tomato juice:			
725	Regular---------------	1 cup------	243	878
726	Low sodium------------	1 cup-------	243	9
727	Tomato paste------------	1 cup-------	258	77
728	Tomato sauce------------	1 cup-------	248	1,498
729	Turnip greens, cooked----	1 cup-------	155	17
	Vegetables, mixed:			
730	Frozen----------------	3.3 oz------	94	45
731	Canned----------------	1 cup-------	170	380
732	Vegetable juice cocktail--	1 cup-------	243	887
	Salads:			
	Bean:			
733	Marinated ----------	1/2 cup-----	130	104
734	Canned--------------	1/2 cup-----	130	537
735	Carrot-raisin---------	1/2 cup-----	63	97
736	Cole slaw-------------	1/2 cup----	60	68
737	Macaroni--------------	2/3 cup-----	127	676
738	Potato----------------	1/2 cup-----	125	625

Condiments, Fats, and Oils

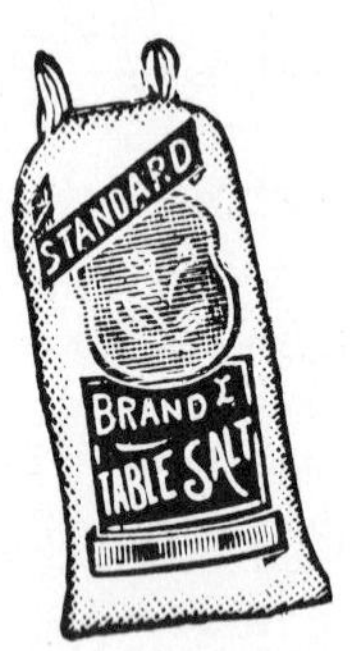

Item	Food	Portion	Weight (grams)	Sodium (milligrams)
739	Baking powder	1 tsp	3	339
740	Baking soda	1 tsp	3	821
	Catsup:			
741	Regular	1 tbsp	15	156
742	Low sodium	1 tbsp	15	3
743	Chili powder	1 tsp	3	26
	Garlic:			
744	Powder	1 tsp	3	1
745	Salt	1 tsp	6	1,850
746	Horse radish, prepared	1 tbsp	18	198
	Meat tenderizer:			
747	Regular	1 tsp	5	1,750
748	Low sodium	1 tsp	5	1
749	MSG (monosodium glutamate)	1 tsp	5	492
750	Mustard, prepared	1 tsp	5	65
	Olives:			
751	Green	4 olives	16	323
752	Ripe, mission	3 olives	15	96
	Onion:			
753	Powder	1 tsp	2	1
754	Salt	1 tsp	5	1,620
755	Parsley, dried	1 tbsp	1	6
756	Pepper, black	1 tsp	2	1
	Pickles:			
757	Bread and butter	2 slices	15	101
758	Dill	1 pickle	65	928
759	Sweet	1 pickle	15	128
760	Relish, sweet	1 tbsp	15	124
761	Salt	1 tsp	5	1,938
	Sauces:			
762	A-1	1 tbsp	17	275
763	Barbecue	1 tbsp	16	130
	Chili:			
764	Regular	1 tbsp	17	227
765	Low sodium	1 tbsp	15	11
766	Soy	1 tbsp	18	1,029
767	Tabasco	1 tsp	5	24
768	Tartar	1 tbsp	14	182
769	Teriyaki	1 tbsp	18	690
770	Worcestershire	1 tbsp	17	206
771	Vinegar	1/2 cup	120	1
772	Yeast, baker's, dry	1 package	7	1

Item	Food	Portion	Weight (grams)	Sodium (milligrams)
	Fats, oils, and related products:			
	Butter:			
773	Regular---------------	1 tbsp------	14	116
774	Unsalted--------------	1 tbsp------	14	2
775	Whipped---------------	1 tbsp------	9	74
	Margarine:			
776	Regular---------------	1 tbsp------	14	140
777	Unsalted--------------	1 tbsp------	14	1
	Oil, vegetable, (includes corn, olive, and			
778	soybean)--------------	1 tbsp------	14	0
	Salad dressing:			
779	Blue cheese-----------	1 tbsp------	15	153
	French:			
780	Home recipe---------	1 tbsp------	14	92
781	Bottled-------------	1 tbsp------	14	214
782	Dry mix, prepared---	1 tbsp------	14	253
783	Low sodium----------	1 tbsp------	15	3
	Italian:			
784	Bottled-------------	1 tbsp------	15	116
785	Dry mix, prepared---	1 tbsp------	14	172
786	Mayonnaise------------	1 tbsp------	15	78
787	Russian---------------	1 tbsp------	15	133
	Thousand Island:			
788	Regular-------------	1 tbsp------	16	109
789	Low cal-------------	1 tbsp------	14	153

A Consumer's Guide to Meat and Meat Substitutes

Beef and Veal

A Guide for Consumers

Meat is a mainstay of the American diet, and beef is the meat that Americans eat in greatest quantity.

Veal, though less popular than beef, is prized for its delicate flavor and fine texture.

Beef and veal abound in flavor and nutritive value. Whether you eat a hearty steak, a quick hamburger, or a savory veal cutlet, you get high-quality protein, B vitamins, and iron. The variety meats (liver, heart, kidney, and other organs of beef and veal) are rich sources of these nutrients. In addition, beef and calf liver are widely acclaimed for vitamin A value.

Lean, well-trimmed beef provides only a moderate number of calories. Calories per serving are included here for some of the beef and veal cuts cooked by various methods, and for all beef and veal recipes.

The average family in this country spends more than one-third of every food dollar for meat, poultry, and fish, so it makes good sense to be informed when you buy and cook it.

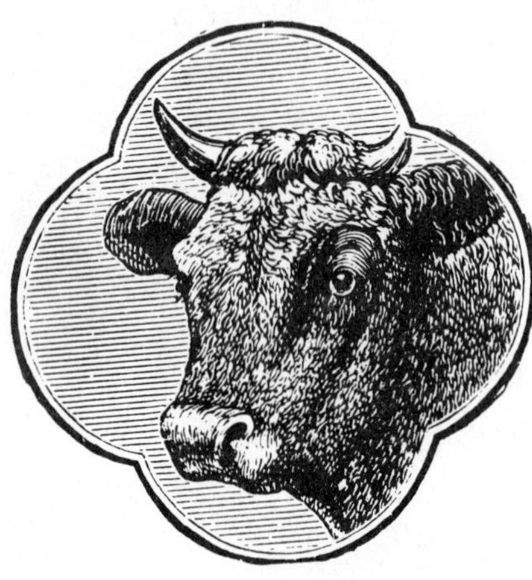

BUYING BEEF AND VEAL

Beef and veal are both produced from cattle—the age of the animal is the difference. Veal usually comes from cattle less than 3 months old. Beef comes from more mature animals—usually 15 to 30 months old. Baby beef comes from animals only 7 to 10 months old.

Veal is grayish pink, smooth textured, and has very little fat. It has a delicate flavor when cooked. Beef is red in color and has a coarser grain.

Identification of Cuts

Learn to identify meat cuts by their appearance. Names given to cuts of meat differ in various parts of the country and sometimes even from store to store in the same town. Names often indicate the section of the carcass from which the meat was cut.

The part of the carcass from which the meat was cut is a good guide to the best cooking methods. Meat from the upper middle sections (rib and loin) is the most tender and can be cooked by dry heat methods. Meat from the shoulder (chuck), round (or rump), shank, and plate is less tender and is usually cooked by moist heat methods.

Other beef and veal cuts (not illustrated) include:

- Filet mignon is the tenderloin of beef.
- Delmonico steak is the rib eye.
- Boneless brisket is a thin flat piece of meat that has been boned; it often is cured and sold as corned beef.
- A crown roast of veal has rib sections "frenched" (meat removed from the end of each rib bone). The ribs are shaped and fastened into a crown. Chops also may be "frenched."
- Kidney chops of veal are loin chops with a slice of kidney.
- Breast of veal may be boned and rolled, or the breast bone may be removed to form a pocket between the ribs and lean for stuffing.
- A cushion shoulder of veal is a square flat piece of meat made by removing the bones from the blade roast. Taking out the bones forms a pocket that can be filled with stuffing.

Ground and Stew Meat

Ground meat is sold in bulk, loaves, or patties. Ground round frequently is leaner than regular ground beef or ground chuck and commands a higher price.

Ground veal is sold as loaves or patties. Mixtures of ground beef, veal, and pork are sometimes sold for meat loaf.

Stew meat—beef or veal—consists of cubes or small pieces of boneless meat.

Variety Meats

Beef variety meats include liver, heart, kidneys, brains, tongue, sweetbreads, and tripe. Variety meats from veal usually are smaller, more tender, finer in texture, milder in flavor, and

TABLE 1.—*Identification of retail cuts of meat.*

Section of carcass	Retail cuts	
	Beef	Veal
Shoulder	Chuck roasts	Shoulder roasts
Rib	Rib roasts and steaks	Rib roasts and chops
Loin	Club, T-bone, and porterhouse steaks	Loin roasts and chops
Sirloin	Sirloin steaks	Sirloin roasts and steak
Round	Round and rump roasts, round steaks	Round and rump roasts, cutlets, and round steak
Foreshank	Shank crosscuts	Shank and shank crosscuts
Short plate	Short ribs	Breast and riblets
Flank	Flank steak	None

lighter in color than those from beef.

Liver is a fine-textured variety meat with a distinctive flavor and high nutritive value. Whole liver should have a moist, smooth surface when bought; sliced liver may appear slightly porous.

Heart is very firm and smooth textured. Long, slow cooking in liquid is needed to make it tender.

Kidneys from beef and veal consist of irregular lobes and deep clefts. Veal kidneys are more tender and delicate than beef kidneys.

Brains are soft, very tender, and delicate in flavor. Veal and beef brains differ little in flavor, texture, and tenderness.

Tongue is one of the less tender variety meats and needs long, slow cooking in liquid. Tongue can be bought fresh, pickled, corned, or smoked.

Sweetbreads, the thymus glands, are made up of two parts—the heart sweetbread and the throat, or neck, sweetbread. They are white and soft and have a very delicate taste. Since the thymus gland disappears as the animal matures, sweetbreads are available only from veal and very young beef.

Tripe consists of the plain or smooth lining from the first beef stomach, the honeycombed lining from the second stomach, and the pocket-shaped part from the end of the second stomach. The pocket-shaped section is smooth on the outside and honeycombed inside. Honeycombed tripe is considered a great delicacy. You can buy tripe partially cooked, pickled, or canned.

Aged Meat

Fresh meat usually reaches the consumer within 6 to 10 days after slaughter. Some high-quality beef, however, is "aged" by holding it at temperatures of 34° to 38° F. for 3 to 6 weeks, or by holding it for 2 days at about 70°. Ultraviolet light is used to reduce bacterial growth in the second method.

Aging develops additional tenderness and characteristic flavor. Since proper aging of meat requires controlled conditions, it is not practical to do it at home.

Cured Meat

In curing, the meat is treated with curing ingredients—primarily salt and sugar. After curing, the meat may be smoked with a nonresinous wood for added flavor. Hickory is a popular wood for smoking cured meats.

Cuts of beef frequently cured are the brisket (called corned beef when cured), the tongue, and some sausages and luncheon meats that contain beef. Dried beef, another cured product, is usually made from the round. Veal tongue may be cured, but other veal cuts usually are not.

Tenderized Meat

Meat sometimes is treated before cooking to increase tenderness. Some tenderizing treatments are applied before the meat is sold; others are applied in the home. The two chief methods of tenderizing meat are—

- *Treatment with liquid or powdered tenderizers.* Meat sometimes is treated with liquid tenderizer before sale. The tenderizer may be injected into the vascular system of the animal before slaughter; this meat usually is sold under a trade name. Or, powdered tenderizers can be bought for home use.
- *Mechanical treatment to cut or break connective tissues and muscle fibers.* Before sale, thin steaks, such as sirloin tip or round steak, may be put through a machine that scores the surface. The meat is then sold as cube steak, "minute" steak, or "sandwich" steak. In the home, round steak and flank steak can be made more tender by pounding them with a mallet.

Signs of Good Quality: Beef, Veal, Pork, and Lamb

Inspection mark and label

This Federal stamp on a meat cut tells consumers that the meat came from a healthy animal, that

38
U.S.
INSP'D & P'S'D
U.S.
INSPECTED
AND PASSED BY
DEPARTMENT OF
AGRICULTURE
EST. 38

it was processed under sanitary conditions, and that it is honestly labeled. It appears on each wholesale cut of an inspected and approved carcass and may or may not appear on the smaller retail cuts. The colored stamping fluid is harmless and need not be trimmed from meat before cooking.

Processed meats—certain cured products, such as corned beef or dried beef, canned meats, and frozen meat products—have a similar circle on the package, can, or label. This stamp indicates that the product carries the same assurance of wholesomeness.

A label for a processed meat product must be accurate and informative, and the product must meet established standards for meat content. Labels may also include information about the nutrient content of the product.

All fresh and processed meat products that are shipped from one State to another must bear a mark of Federal inspection. The Federal Meat Inspection Act of 1967 assures consumers that all meat is inspected by either the Federal Government or an adequate State system. Previously, Federal inspection was required only in plants dealing in interstate or foreign commerce.

Grade stamp or packer's brand

The grade stamp is a colored shield—in contrast to the circular inspection stamp—enclosing the letters "USDA" and the grade designation. These stamps divide the wide range of meat quality into several groups.

Grade stamps appear on most retail beef and veal cuts. Government grading is optional and is paid for by the meat packer.

Not all meat is federally graded. Some meat packers use brand names instead of grades to represent the quality levels of their products. Packers may sell products under several brand names, with each brand representing a different quality level. These may or may not match the standards of Federal grades. Quality-control programs by the packers keep their products within these standards.

Beef grades.—USDA Choice is the beef grade most commonly found in retail markets. USDA Prime, the highest grade, may be found in some retail markets, but most of it goes to hotels and restaurants. Relatively little USDA Good, Standard, and Commercial beef is found in retail markets. Beef of the lowest three grades, USDA Utility, Cutter, and Canner, is used mostly in processed meat products. Samples of grade stamps are shown below.

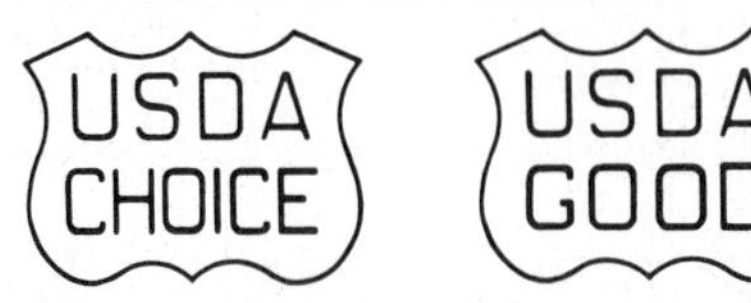

Higher grades of beef generally are more tender and juicy than lower grades of the same cut, but lower grades can be made more tender by slow cooking in water or steam as in pot roasting.

Veal and calf grades.—Veal and calf grades are USDA Prime, Choice, Good, Standard, Utility, and Cull. The lean of USDA Prime veal is light grayish-pink to light pink and is fairly firm and velvety; the bones are small, soft, and quite red. The carcass is given a lower grade as the lean becomes less firm, more moist, coarser in grain, and darker in color, and as the size of bones increases.

Appearance

Appearance of fresh meat is an important guide to quality, especially if the grade or packer's brand does not appear on the meat. Good-quality beef lean is a uniform, bright, light-to-deep red; veal is grayish pink. Fine-textured firm lean is preferable to coarse-textured soft lean.

Color of fat varies with breed, age, and feed of the animal. It is not an indication of quality. Bones become less red and harder as the animal matures. Good-quality beef has red, porous bones; veal bones are soft and very red.

Prices

The economy of a cut of beef or veal depends on the amount of cooked lean meat it provides as well as its price per pound. For example, round steak and beef rib roast may cost the same per pound, but the round steak will provide 2 to 3 ounces more cooked lean meat per pound purchased.

Equal-size servings of cooked lean from different cuts provide similar food value. Generally, cooked lean from pot roast is as nutritious as that from the most expensive steak or chop. Therefore, you can find good buys in food value by comparing the cost of purchased amounts that will provide equal amounts of cooked lean. Or, compare the cost of amounts needed for a family meal.

Retail food stores often feature certain meat cuts as specials. To take advantage of these specials, read newspaper advertisements before you make your shopping list.

Amount To Buy

How much meat is enough? Necessarily the amount you buy at one time depends on available storage space and how you intend to use the meat. Cost is always a factor. So are family size and family preferences.

Some families like to buy favorite cuts in quantity when they are offered at special prices and freeze them for future use. This works well if home freezer space is available. Unless freezer space is available, buy only the amount of meat that can be used within the suggested refrigerator storage periods.

For an estimate of the number of 3-ounce servings of boneless cooked meat to expect from a pound of each retail cut of beef and veal.
Remember that some family members eat large servings; others take small servings.

When buying roasts, it's a good idea to buy enough for two or more meals. Plan to use extra cooked meat in casseroles, salads, and sandwiches. One pound of boneless cooked meat yields about 3 cups of chopped or diced meat. To estimate the yield of chopped or diced cooked meat from a pound of raw meat, see table 2.

Home freezer owners may save money by purchasing wholesale cuts of meat. The price per pound for a side or quarter of beef is likely to be less than the average price per pound of the individual retail cuts from a side or quarter.

A wholesale cut, however, may yield a higher proportion of hamburger and stew meat than you want. Also, the costs of cutting, wrapping, and storing the meat (electricity for home freezer operation or freezer locker rental) may offset the savings made by purchasing a wholesale cut.

TABLE 2.—*Yield of boneless cooked meat from retail cuts of beef and veal*

Kind and cut of meat	Approximate yield of cooked lean and some fat from one pound of raw meat as purchased	
	3-ounce servings	Volume, chopped or diced
	Number	*Cups*
Beef		
Brisket		
Boneless, fresh or corned	3	1½ to 2
Chuck roast		
Bone-in	2½	1½
Boneless	3 to 3½	2
Club or T-bone steak, bone-in	2	....
Flank steak, boneless	3½	....
Ground beef	4	....
Porterhouse steak, bone-in	2¼	....
Rib roast		
Bone-in	2½	1½
Boneless	3	1½ to 2
Round steak		
Bone-in	3¼	....
Boneless	3¾	....
Rump roast		
Bone-in	2½	1½
Boneless	3½	2
Short ribs, bone-in	1½	1
Sirloin steak		
Bone-in	2 to 2½	....
Boneless	2½ to 3	....
Veal		
Breast		
Bone-in	2	1 to 1½
Boneless	3	1½ to 2
Cutlet		
Bone-in	3½	....
Boneless	4	....
Leg roast		
Bone-in	2½	1½
Boneless	3½	2
Loin chops, bone-in	2¾	....
Loin roast		
Bone-in	2½	1½
Boneless	3½	2
Rib chops, bone-in	2½	....
Rib roast		
Bone-in	2¼	1 to 1½
Boneless	3½	2
Shoulder roast		
Bone-in	2½	1½
Boneless	3½	2

STORAGE

Fresh Meat

Fresh meats can be stored at refrigerator temperatures between 35° and 40° F. or at lower temperatures in the special meat compartment of some refrigerators.

Fresh meat generally keeps best if loosely wrapped. However, the transparent wrap on prepackaged meat is designed for refrigerator storage at home for a day or two.

Variety meats, ground meat, and stew meat are highly perishable and cannot be stored as long as other cuts. Suggested home storage times for fresh beef and veal are given in table 3.

Frozen Meat

Fresh meats to be held more than a few days should be frozen. Before freezing the meat, trim off fat and remove bones to save freezer space, if desired. Divide meat into meal-size or serving-size portions.

Wrap meat in moisture-vapor-proof wrappings, such as coated or laminated freezer papers, polyethylene films or bags, or heavy-weight aluminum foil. For easy separation of pieces after freezing, place two pieces of freezer wrap between each steak or chop.

Wrap meat tightly, pressing out as much air as possible. Seal packages well with freezer tape.

Label packages with the cut of meat, the date of freezing, and the date by which the meat should be used for best eating quality.

Meat should be frozen and stored at 0° F. or below. Spread the packages of meat in the freezer so that the meat will freeze quickly. Allow a 1-inch space around packages for air circulation. You can freeze 2 to 3 pounds of meat for each cubic foot of freezer space at one time.

Meats (including cooked meat dishes) purchased frozen should be kept frozen at 0° F. or below until used.

Stored at 0° F., frozen beef and veal will retain high quality for approximately the length of time specified in table 3. The frozen food compartment of a home refrigerator is not designed to maintain 0°. Meats held there usually will retain high quality only for about a week.

In refrigerator-freezer combinations where 0° F. can be maintained in the freezer cabinet, meats may be kept for the same storage periods as in a freezer.

Processed Meats and Meat Products

Cured, smoked, ready-to-serve

Store cured, smoked, and ready-to-serve meats in the refrigerator in their original wrappings, or loosely wrapped. Suggested home refrigerator storage times are given in table 3.

Cured meats do not keep their high quality long in the freezer, because seasonings added in the curing process speed rancidity.

Canned

Canned products containing beef and veal keep well in a cool dry place. Storage in a warm place may change color and flavor. Under proper storage conditions, canned beef and veal will retain their quality for as long as a year. They will be safe to eat as long as the cans are completely airtight.

After opening canned meats, refrigerate and use within a few days.

Cooked Meats and Meat Products

Cooked meats should be covered or wrapped and stored in the refrigerator. Rapid cooling of meats and meat combination dishes helps prevent bacterial growth. Because bacterial growth is favored at temperatures between 40° and 140° F., the food should be taken through this temperature range as quickly as possible.

If you prepare enough of a meat dish for more than one meal,

TABLE 3.—*Suggested home storage periods to maintain high quality in beef and veal*

Product	Storage period	
	Refrigerator (about 40° F.)	Freezer (0° F. or below)
Fresh meat		
Chops and cutlets	3 to 5 days	6 to 9 months
Ground beef or veal	1 to 2 days	3 to 4 months
Roasts		
Beef	3 to 5 days	6 to 12 months
Veal	3 to 5 days	6 to 9 months
Steaks	3 to 5 days	6 to 12 months
Stew meat	1 to 2 days	3 to 4 months
Variety meats	1 to 2 days	3 to 4 months
Cured, smoked, and ready-to-serve meat		
Corned beef	7 days	2 weeks [1]
Frankfurters and wieners	7 days	1 month [1]
Luncheon meat	3 to 5 days	Freezing not recommended
Sausage		
Smoked	7 days	Freezing not recommended
Dry and semi-dry	2 to 3 weeks	Freezing not recommended
Cooked meat		
Cooked meat and meat dishes	3 to 4 days	2 to 3 months
Gravy and meat broth	1 to 2 days	2 to 3 months

[1] Frozen cured meat loses quality rapidly and should be used as soon as possible.

quickly cool and refrigerate or freeze the portion that you intend to serve later. Meat left on the serving platter (part of a roast, for example) should be refrigerated or frozen as soon as the meal is finished.

Cooked meat keeps its quality best if left in large pieces until used. To prevent drying and save storage space, remove cooked meat from the bone if only a small amount of meat remains.

Gravy and meat broth are highly perishable and should be cooled quickly, then refrigerated immediately. Store only 1 or 2 days in refrigerator.

Cooked beef and veal, as well as many combination dishes containing beef or veal, can be stored in the freezer at 0° F. for 2 or 3 months with little or no change in eating quality. Remove cooked meat from the bones, wrap tightly in moisture-vapor-resistant material, and freeze quickly. Cool combination dishes, gravy, or broth quickly, package in meal-size amounts, seal in moisture-vapor-resistant containers, and freeze quickly.

GENERAL PRINCIPLES OF COOKERY

For maximum tenderness and juiciness, cook beef and veal at low to moderate temperatures. The aroma from meat cooked at these temperatures is more pleasant and the color more even than that of meat cooked at high temperatures. Another advantage of low to moderate cooking temperatures is that there is *more meat to serve because of smaller losses through evaporation, shrinkage, and drippings.*

Poorly regulated ovens are sometimes to blame for overcooked meats. Check the oven temperature with an accurate oven thermometer if meat seems to brown too quickly during roasting or if the roast is dry and crusty.

Broiling temperature can be regulated either by changing the distance between the meat and the source of heat or, in some gas ranges, by changing the thermostat setting. Whether the oven door is closed or left open also influences broiling temperature.

Broiling equipment varies greatly in construction and heating capacity. Because of this, it is best to follow the manufacturer's suggestions for the distance to place meat from the source of heat and the position of the door during broiling. Usually the door is left open when broiling in an electric range and closed when broiling in a gas range.

For the same degree of doneness, place thick cuts farther from the source of heat during broiling than thin cuts. This avoids burning the outside of thick steaks before the center is done. If you prefer a steak well done, place it farther from the heat than for a medium or rare steak.

For maximum tenderness in braised and simmered meat, cook at temperatures that maintain the liquid just below the boiling point.

Degree of Doneness

Cook beef as you like it—rare, medium, or well done. Rare beef has a puffy, full appearance, brown exterior, reddish-pink interior, and lots of clear red juice. Beef cooked to a medium degree of doneness has a light pink interior, less juice, and lighter colored juice than rare beef. Well-done beef is light brown throughout with slightly yellow juice.

Veal should be cooked well done to make it tender and palatable. It needs longer cooking because it has more connective tissue than other meats. Veal roasted to the well-done stage has a red-brown exterior and a gray interior color.

The best way to tell when a roast is done is to use a meat thermometer. A meat thermometer is well worth the investment, especially if you like beef on the rare side. Choose a thermometer marked with degrees Fahrenheit, not just stages of doneness for the various meats.

Generally, beef is considered rare when roasted to 140° F., medium at 160°, and well done at 170°. Veal is considered well done at 170°, too. These are internal temperatures taken in the center of the roast. Placement of the meat thermometer is important.

If you don't have a meat thermometer, you can estimate cooking time by a roast-meat timetable. Your roast, however, may not cook to just the stage of doneness you want because several factors affect cooking time besides the size of roast.

The easiest way to tell when a steak is done is to cut into it along the bone and check the interior color.

Cooking Time

Cooking time depends on temperature of meat at start of cooking, cooking temperature, size and shape of cut, composition (proportion of lean, fat, and bone), desired degree of doneness, and whether or not the meat has been aged.

Timetables in this publication are based on meat at refrigerator temperature. More time is needed if the meat is colder than refrigerator temperature—frozen or only partially thawed.

Keep these facts in mind—

- A small roast requires more minutes per pound than a large roast, but its total cooking time is less than for the large roast.
- A longer cooking time is needed for a thick cut than for a thin cut of the same weight.
- Meat with an outside layer of fat takes longer to cook than meat with little or no fat cover.
- Boned and rolled roasts require more cooking time per pound than roasts with bone in.
- Aged meat cooks slightly faster than unaged meat.

Cooking Frozen Meat

If frozen meat is not thawed before cooking, allow extra cooking time. The extra cooking time needed depends on size, shape, and thickness of meat. Large frozen roasts may take up to one and a half times as long to cook as unfrozen cuts of the same weight and shape. Generally, smaller roasts require more extra time per pound than larger roasts.

A meat thermometer may be inserted when the meat has thawed. This will be an aid in determining doneness.

Frozen steaks and chops require up to one and a half times as long to broil. They should be placed at least 4 inches from the source of heat to prevent overbrowning.

If you prefer, thaw frozen meat in the refrigerator, then cook it as fresh meat. Large roasts take 4 to 7 hours per pound to thaw and small roasts take 3 to 5 hours per pound. Cooking time for thawed meat at refrigerator temperature is the same as for meat that has not been frozen.

Frozen meat combination dishes are best when reheated without thawing first. If they are in a watertight container they can be partially thawed by immersing the package in lukewarm water for a few minutes—just long enough to make it easy to remove the food from the container.

Complete thawing of meat combination dishes at room temperature may permit growth of dangerous bacteria, and is not recommended for commercially or home-prepared food of this type.

BASIC COOKING METHODS

Cooking methods commonly used for beef and veal are roasting, rotisserie cooking, broiling, pan broiling, pan frying, braising, pot roasting, and simmering.

Roasting is a method in which meat is surrounded and cooked by heated air, usually in an oven. Meat is not covered and no water is added.

Rotisserie cooking is a method which exposes all sides of the meat to direct and even heat by rotating it on a spit located near a heat source.

Broiling is cooking by direct heat from a flame, electric unit, or glowing coals. Meat is cooked one side at a time.

Pan broiling is cooking in an uncovered pan over direct heat. Fat that cooks out of the meat is drained off as it accumulates.

Pan frying is similar to pan broiling, except that meat is cooked in a small amount of fat.

Braising is cooking in steam trapped and held in a covered container or foil wrap. The source of steam may be water or other liquid added to meat, or it may be meat juices.

Pot roasting is braising large cuts of meat, either on top of range or in oven.

Simmering is cooking meat in liquid just below boiling point.

Consider the tenderness, size, and thickness of any meat cut before you cook it. *Beef* cuts vary greatly in tenderness. Thick, blocky cuts from the rib, loin, and sirloin usually are roasted. Choice grade beef chuck, round, or rump can be oven-roasted. Lower grades of these roasts make excellent pot roasts. Thin steaks usually are best pan broiled or pan fried; thick steaks are best broiled. Braising and simmering are generally recommended for less tender cuts.

Always cook *veal* well done for full flavor. Long, slow cooking does the trick. Braising is good for many veal cuts because the combination of browning and steaming tenderizes the meat and develops its flavor. Large cuts of veal —from the leg and shoulder—can be roasted satisfactorily. Broiling is recommended only for veal patties.

Roasting

Directions

Preheat oven to 325° F. (slow). Place roast with fat side up on a rack in a shallow roasting pan.

If you have a meat thermometer, insert it into roast so that tip is in center but not touching bone or fat.

Roast uncovered, without added liquid, until meat thermometer registers appropriate temperature. The timetable serves as a guide to roasting time at 325°F.

Calories per 3-ounce serving: Beef rib roast—about 375 (lean and fat) or 205 (lean only).

Veal roast—about 230 (lean and fat).

Tips

- A shallow pan is better than a deep one for roasting because it allows heat to circulate around the roast.
- A rack under the roast keeps the meat up from the drippings and increases circulation of heat. The rib bones in standing rib roast can serve as a rack.
- Meat may be seasoned before or after roasting. Either way seasonings penetrate very little below surface of the meat.
- To increase the juiciness of veal roasts that have little outside fat, lay strips of bacon or salt pork across top.
- For easier slicing, allow roast to stand 15 to 20 minutes after removing from oven before carving.
- Boned roasts can be filled with a stuffing for variety.

Timetable for roasting beef and veal

Cut of meat	Approximate ready-to-cook weight	Approximate roasting time at 325° F.[1]	Internal temperature of meat when done
	Pounds	*Hours*	*° F.*
Beef			
Standing ribs[2]			
Rare	4 to 6	2¼ to 2½	140
Medium	4 to 6	2½ to 3⅓	160
Well done	4 to 6	2¾ to 4	170
Rare	6 to 8	2½ to 3	140
Medium	6 to 8	3 to 3½	160
Well done	6 to 8	3½ to 4¼	170
Rolled rib			
Rare	5 to 7	2⅔ to 3¾	140
Medium	5 to 7	3¼ to 4½	160
Well done	5 to 7	4 to 5⅔	170
Rolled rump (choice grade)	4 to 6	2 to 2½	150 to 170
Sirloin tip (choice grade)	3½ to 4	2⅓	140 to 170
	6 to 8	3½ to 4	140 to 170
Veal			
Leg	5 to 8	3 to 3⅓	170
Loin	4 to 6	2⅓ to 3	170
Rib (rack)	3 to 5	2 to 3	170
Shoulder, rolled	3 to 5	2¼ to 3½	170

[1] Meat at refrigerator temperature at start of roasting.

[2] Eight-inch cut. For 10-inch ribs allow about 30 minutes less time.

Rotisserie Cooking

Large, compact roasts—beef rolled rib, rolled rump, and sirloin tip roasts—can be cooked on a rotisserie. The roast should be as regular in shape as possible so that the spit will rotate evenly.

Directions

Mount roast securely on spit so that it does not slip as spit turns. If properly balanced, meat will rotate evenly.

Place a drip pan under roast to catch drippings. If you are cooking meat over coals, arrange pan so that drippings do not fall on coals and cause smoke. For example, if the rotisserie turns so that the meat surface rotates upward at the front the drip pan should be under the front edge of the meat. See where droplets fall and place the pan to catch them.

Insert a meat thermometer at an angle or through end of roast in such a way that tip is in center of roast, but not in fat or touching the spit. Check to see that thermometer clears rotisserie equipment and drip pan as spit turns.

Follow the directions that came with your rotisserie equipment concerning operation of the spit and regulation of temperature. Low to moderate temperatures give best results.

Roast until meat reaches the desired degree of doneness. Cooking time depends on size and shape of roast, cooking temperature, and the degree of doneness you like.

Tips

- Because cooking time varies with intensity of heat produced, a roast cooked on an outdoor rotisserie may require a longer time to cook on a breezy day than on a calm day.
- To maintain an even heat when cooking over charcoal, space coals about an inch apart. Add

Timetable for broiling beef and veal

Cut of meat	Approximate thickness	Degree of doneness	Approximate total cooking time [1]
	Inches		*Minutes*
Beef			
Steaks (club, porterhouse,	1	Rare	15 to 20
rib, sirloin, T-bone,	1	Medium	20 to 25
tenderloin)	1	Well done	25 to 30
	1½	Rare	25 to 30
	1½	Medium	30 to 35
	1½	Well done	35 to 40
	2	Rare	35 to 40
	2	Medium	40 to 45
	2	Well done	45 to 55
Patties	¾	Rare	8
	¾	Medium	12
	¾	Well done	14
Veal			
Patties [2]	¾	Well done	15

[1] Meat is at refrigerator temperature at start of broiling. Regulate broiling temperature as directed on page 10.

[2] Broiling is not recommended for other cuts of veal.

new charcoal around edges and wait until charcoal glows, then push it toward the center.

Broiling

Directions

Adjust broiler rack.

Slash fat around edge of meat to prevent curling.

Place meat on cold broiler grid.

Broil until top side of meat is browned, about half of total cooking time.

Season, turn, and brown other side. Use timetable as a guide for total broiling time.

Calories per 3-ounce serving:

Club steak—about 385 (lean and fat) or 205 (lean only).

Sirloin steak—about 330 (lean and fat) or 205 (lean only).

T-bone or porterhouse steak—about 400 (lean and fat) or 190 (lean only).

Ground beef patties—about 245 if regular ground beef is used; 185 if lean ground beef is used.

Tips

- Put aluminum foil in bottom of broiler pan to simplify cleaning.
- Grease broiler grid to help prevent meat from sticking.
- Turn meat by sticking fork into the fat, not the lean, or use tongs.
- Check doneness by cutting a slit in the meat near the bone and noting interior color. Rare beef is reddish pink, medium is light pink, and well done is light brown.
- Broil frozen meat at a low temperature to prevent surface from charring before interior thaws. Increase cooking time.

Outdoor Broiling

Broiled steaks and hamburgers taste even better when cooked outdoors. Appetites are bigger, too, so be sure to allow for seconds.

Choose thick steaks—at least 1½ inches thick—and plump hamburgers—at least ¾ inch thick—for outdoor broiling. They will be juicier than thinner ones.

Boneless beef cubes cut from sirloin or top round make good shish kebabs.

Directions

Start fire 30 to 45 minutes ahead of time so that coals will be at right temperature. When coals become covered with fine gray ash, spread them about 1 inch apart. No two coals should touch.

Adjust grill so that meat surface is about 6 to 8 inches from coals. This gives even heat without too much intensity. If meat gets too hot, raise grill away from heat.

Tilt grill slightly to let fat run down grids to one side. This prevents fat from dripping on the coals and causing smoke and flame.

Broil meat until it reaches the desired doneness. Turn meat about halfway through the cooking period. The timetable above will help estimate cooking time, but cooking times vary.

Tips

- Meat may be marinated in a marinade of half oil and half vinegar or lemon juice, with your favorite seasonings. Marinate meat for several hours in refrigerator. Drain well before broiling.
- To check doneness, cut a slit in meat near the bone or in center and observe interior color.

• Allow longer cooking time on a breezy day.

Pan Broiling

Thin beef steaks or patties, 1 inch thick or less, can be pan broiled.

Directions

Slash fat around edge of meat to prevent it from curling.

Grease frypan lightly or rub hot frypan with fat edge of meat.

Place meat in hot frypan and cook slowly over moderate heat, turning occasionally as necessary.

Pour off excess fat. Remove meat from pan; drain.

Season and serve.

Total cooking time for patties or 1-inch steaks will be 10 to 20 minutes depending on degree of doneness wanted.

Tips

• If meat is well marbled, it is not necessary to grease pan.

• To test for doneness, cut meat close to the bone near end of cooking period and note interior color of meat.

Pan Frying

Pan frying is suitable for cuts of meat that are 1 inch thick or less.

Directions

Slash fat around the edge of meat to prevent it from curling.

Put a small amount of fat in frypan and preheat over moderate heat.

Cook meat slowly over moderate heat, turning occasionally as necessary to brown both sides.

Remove meat from pan; drain.

Season and serve.

Total cooking time will be about 8 to 10 minutes for rare-to-medium beef steaks 1 inch thick, 25 to 30 minutes for well-done veal cutlets or chops 1 inch thick, and about 15 minutes for well-done veal patties 3/4 inch thick. Thinner cuts take less time.

Tips

• Flouring or breading meat before frying gives it a crisp brown exterior.

• Chilling breaded meats before cooking helps coating stick.

• Frozen meats can be floured and browned without thawing. If egg and crumbs are used, however, the coating will stick better if meat is thawed first.

• To test for doneness, cut meat close to bone near end of cooking period and check interior color of meat.

Braising

Directions

Brown meat slowly on all sides in enough fat to keep the meat from sticking. Use a heavy pan.

Season meat.

Add a small amount of liquid (about ½ cup or less) if necessary to prevent overbrowning.

Cover pan tightly.

Cook slowly over low heat or in a 350° F. oven until tender, adding more liquid if needed. Use timetable above as a guide to braising time.

Calories per 3-ounce serving:

Beef pot roast—about 245 (lean and fat) or 165 (lean only).

Beef flank steak—about 160 (all lean).

Veal shoulder—about 230 (lean and fat).

Tips

• Scoring steaks by cutting slashes across surfaces or pounding steaks with a mallet before braising helps make them more tender.

• Floured cuts brown better than unfloured cuts.

• Chops and steaks can be breaded with fine, dry bread or cracker crumbs.

• Meats that have a considerable amount of fat and that are

Timetable for braising beef and veal

Cut of meat	Approximate ready-to-cook weight or thickness	Approximate total cooking time [1]
		Hours
Beef		
Pot roast, such as chuck or round	3 to 5 pounds	3 to 4
Steak, such as chuck or round	¾ to 1 inch	1 to 1½
Flank steak	½ inch	1½ to 2
Short ribs	2 by 2 by 4 inches	1½ to 2½
Pieces for stew	1½-inch cubes	1½ to 2½
Veal		
Chops	½ to ¾ inch	¾ to 1
Pieces for stew (shoulder)	1-inch cubes	1½ to 2
Shoulder, rolled	3 to 5 pounds	2 to 2½
Steaks (cutlets)	½ to ¾ inch	¾ to 1

[1] Cooking time is for meat braised at simmering temperature. Time needed for braising in a pressure cooker is considerably shorter; follow pressure cooker manufacturer's directions.

not breaded or floured can be browned without added fat.

- Many cuts of beef can be braised without added liquid. Steam from their own juices provides moisture.

Simmering

Directions

Brown meat on all sides, if desired. (Do not brown corned beef.)

Add water to cover meat.

Add desired seasoning. Cover.

Cook slowly over low heat until meat is tender. Do not boil. Use the timetable as a guide to cooking time.

Calories per 3-ounce serving:

Beef shanks—about 245 (lean and fat) or 165 (lean only).

Corned beef—about 315 (lean and fat).

Tips

- To enhance the flavor of beef and veal choose from these seasonings—celery, onion, green pepper, parsley, basil, bay leaves, marjoram, peppercorns, and thyme.
- Simmered meat is more flavorful and juicy if it is chilled quickly in the stock in which it was cooked than if stock is drained from meat before chilling.

Cooking Variety Meats

The choice of a cooking method for variety meats, as for other meats, depends on how tender the particular meat is. Variety meats are usually cooked well done regardless of the cooking method.

Brains, sweetbreads, and veal (calf) liver and kidneys are tender and can be pan fried or broiled. For variety, they can be braised or simmered. Less tender variety meats—heart, tongue, tripe, beef liver and kidneys—require braising or simmering.

Liver

To prepare liver for cooking.—Remove heavy blood vessels and outside membrane if desired.

To broil veal (calf) liver.—Adjust broiler rack so top of liver is exposed to moderate heat.

Dip sliced liver in melted butter or margarine, drippings, or French dressing.

Place on cold broiler grid.

Broil only long enough for liver to lose its red color, about 4 minutes on each side.

For variety, thread cubed liver on skewers alternately with bacon and cooked or canned small whole onions; broil.

To pan fry veal (calf) liver.—Heat a small amount of fat in a frypan over moderate heat.

Dip sliced liver in flour seasoned with salt and pepper. Place in hot fat.

Cook over moderate heat, turning as necessary, until liver is brown and tender, about 5 minutes on each side.

To braise liver.—Heat a small amount of fat in a frypan over moderate heat.

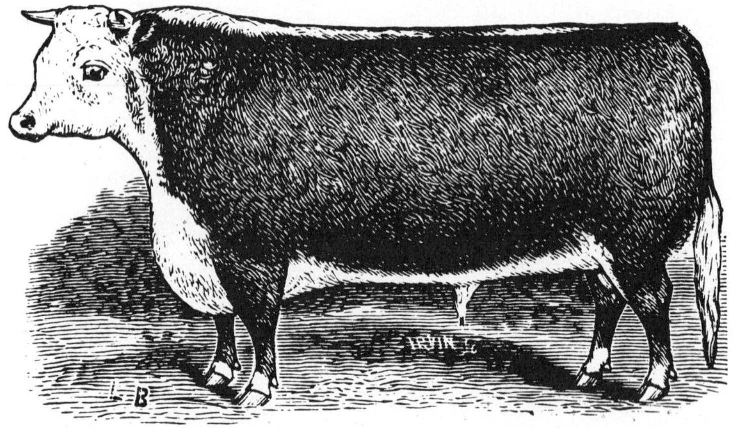

Timetable for simmering beef and veal

Cut of meat	Approximate ready-to-cook weight	Approximate total cooking time
	Pounds	*Hours*
Beef		
Fresh beef brisket or plate	8	4 to 5
Corned beef brisket (whole)	8	4 to 5
Corned beef brisket (piece)	3	3 to 3¾
Beef shanks	4	3 to 4
Pieces for stew (1-inch to 2-inch pieces)		2½ to 3
Veal		
Shanks	¾ to 1 each	2 to 3
Pieces for stew (1-inch to 2-inch pieces)		2 to 3

Dip sliced beef or veal (calf) liver in flour seasoned with salt and pepper.

Brown liver in hot fat over moderate heat.

Cover tightly and reduce heat.

Cook on top of range or in a 350° F. (moderate) oven until liver is tender, about 20 to 25 minutes.

Heart

To prepare heart for cooking.—Wash heart in warm water. Trim away gristle and larger blood vessels.

To braise heart.—Prepare for cooking as directed.

Stuff with a bread stuffing if desired.

Brown on all sides in a small amount of fat. Season.

Add a small amount of water, about ½ cup. Cover tightly.

Cook in a 300° F. (slow) oven or over low heat on top of the range until tender. Beef heart requires 3 to 4 hours; veal heart, 2½ to 3 hours.

To simmer heart.—Prepare for cooking as directed.

Place in a deep pot and add salted water to cover.

Simmer, covered, until tender, 3 to 4 hours for beef heart, 2½ to 3 hours for veal heart.

Kidneys

To prepare kidneys for cooking.—Wash kidneys in cold water.

Remove the outer membrane.

Split kidneys through center, lengthwise; remove inner fat and tubes. Cut up if desired.

To simmer kidneys.—Prepare for cooking as directed.

Place kidneys in a deep pot and add water to cover.

Simmer, covered, until tender, 1 to 1½ hours for beef kidneys, ¾ to 1 hour for veal kidneys.

To eliminate strong odor while cooking beef kidneys, change water once.

For variety, heat cooked kidneys in a spicy sauce, or roll them in seasoned flour and pan fry.

To broil veal kidneys.—Prepare for cooking as directed.

Adjust broiler rack so the top of kidneys is exposed to moderate heat.

Dip kidneys in melted butter or margarine, drippings, or French dressing.

Place on cold broiler grid.

Broil 5 to 10 minutes on each side, or until brown.

For variety, wrap kidneys in bacon slices before broiling.

Brains and Sweetbreads

To prepare brains or sweetbreads for cooking.—Wash in cold water; remove any blood clots.

Soak in cold water 30 minutes.

To simmer brains or sweetbreads.—Prepare for cooking as directed above.

Place in a deep pot and add water to cover.

Add 1 teaspoon salt and 1 tablespoon lemon juice or vinegar for each quart of water.

Simmer, covered, 15 to 20 minutes.

Drain, rinse well in cold water, and remove membrane and blood vessels.

For variety, heat cooked brains or sweetbreads in a cream or tomato sauce. Or, break cooked brains into small pieces and add to scrambled eggs.

To pan fry brains or sweetbreads.—Prepare for cooking as above; remove membrane.

Roll in flour or fine, dry breadcrumbs.

Fry in a small amount of fat in a frypan over moderate heat until tender and lightly browned, about 20 minutes.

Tongue

To simmer tongue. — Wash tongue. Soak corned, pickled, or smoked tongue in water several hours before cooking to make flavor milder, if desired.

Place tongue in a deep pot and add water to cover. Add salt if needed.

Simmer, covered, until tender, 3 to 4 hours for beef tongue, 2 to 3 hours for veal tongue.

Drain tongue; dip in cold water to loosen skin.

Remove skin and cut away bones and gristle at thick end.

Serve tongue hot or cold. If served cold, it will be juicier if it is cooled in the broth.

For variety, use cooked tongue in place of other cooked meats in combination dishes.

Tripe

To simmer tripe.—Place tripe in a deep pot and add water to cover. Add 1 teaspoon salt for each quart of water.

Simmer, covered, until tender, 1 to 1½ hours.

For variety, heat cooked tripe in a spicy tomato sauce.

Making Gravy

The secret of making smooth gravy is to blend the flour thoroughly with fat or with cold liquid before combining it with hot liquid.

Meat drippings often contain both fat and meat juices. Drippings from pan broiled, pan fried, and well-done roasted or broiled meat may consist almost entirely of melted fat and browned crusty bits because most of the meat juices evaporate during cooking. Drippings from braised meat and rare roasted or broiled meat, however, may contain considerable meat juices or broth.

If drippings are scarce or meat broth is weakly flavored, add a bouillon cube or a little meat extract to each cup of liquid.

Method 1

Use with drippings containing only fat and browned crusty bits.

For a thin gravy, use 1 tablespoon each of flour and fat to each cup of meat liquid and water; for a medium gravy, use 2 tablespoons of flour and 1 or 2 tablespoons of fat, as desired.

Measure amount of fat needed and return to pan. Save the rest for other uses.

Stir flour into fat; brown over low heat.

Add liquid slowly, stirring constantly.

Cook until thickened, stirring occasionally.

Season to taste.

Method 2

Use with drippings containing a considerable amount of meat juices or broth.

For a thin gravy, use 1 tablespoon of flour to each cup of liquid; for a medium gravy, use 2 tablespoons of flour per cup of liquid.

Measure drippings or broth; if necessary add water to make desired amount of liquid. Heat.

Mix flour with a small amount of cold water by stirring or shaking until smooth.

Stir flour mixture slowly into hot liquid.

Cook until thickened, stirring occasionally.

Season to taste.

Pork

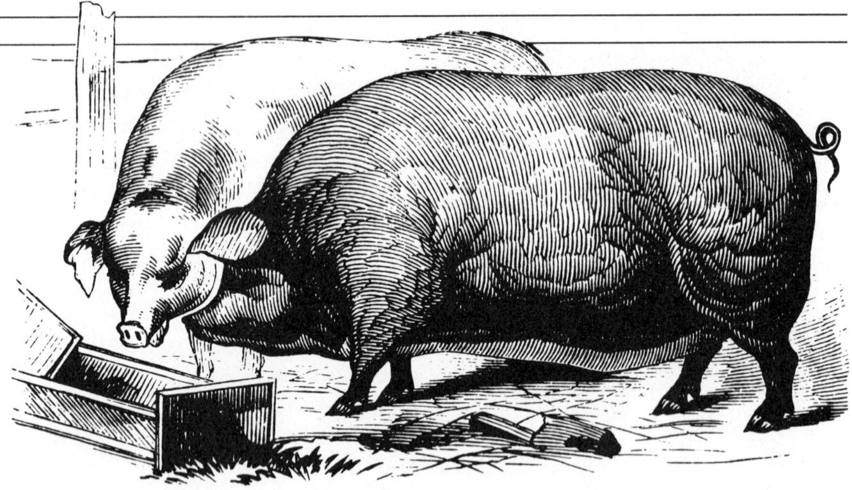

Roast pork, flavorful and juicy . . . crisp bacon, filling the air with tempting aroma . . . and tantalizing baked ham exemplify some of the good eating provided by pork. Many other pork cuts, both fresh and cured, also appear on the table the year around.

Pork is high in nutritive value. An especially rich source of thiamin (vitamin B_1), pork also supplies other B vitamins and iron. It's a good source of protein, too. Variety meats, such as liver and kidneys, are rich in these nutrients. In addition, liver is an especially good source of vitamin A.

Even calorie watchers may include pork in their meals. A 3-ounce serving of roast fresh Boston butt with the fat trimmed off contains approximately 205 calories; a 3-ounce serving of cured ham, fat trimmed off, contains about 160 calories.

BUYING PORK

Pork is meat from hogs, usually under 1 year of age. It is sold fresh, cured, or cured and smoked. Canned and frozen pork products, sausages, and luncheon meats are also available.

Identification of Cuts

Learn to identify pork cuts by their appearance. Names often indicate the section of the carcass from which the meat was cut.

Other pork cuts (not illustrated) are identified as follows:

- **Crown roast** is usually made from the rib sections of two pork loins. The ribs are "frenched" by removing meat from the end of each rib bone. Then the rib sections are shaped into a crown and fastened.
- **Butterfly chops** are boneless double chops, split most of the way through the center and opened to form a butterfly shape.
- **Back ribs, or country ribs,** are made by splitting the loin lengthwise through the rib section near the backbone.
- **Side pork** is trimmed to a rectangular shape. It has alternating layers of lean and fat.
- **Canadian bacon,** cut from boneless pork loin, is cured and smoked. It is usually quite lean.
- **A pork cushion** is a square, flat piece made by removing the bones from the shoulder. This provides a pocket for stuffing.
- **Pigs' feet** are mostly bones and tendons and contain little lean meat. They are sold either pickled or fresh.

Cured Pork

Many pork cuts are cured to add distinctive flavor and variety. Before adequate refrigeration became common, pork was treated with a heavy salt brine to preserve it. Nowadays less salt is used because meats are cured primarily for flavor, not for preservation. "Country style" hams, available in some areas, are heavily salted and may require soaking before cooking.

After treatment with the curing ingredients, the meat may be smoked with a nonresinous wood for added flavor. Hickory is one of the most popular woods used for smoking meats.

Almost all cured and smoked hams are labeled either "fully cooked" or "cook-before-eating."

Other forms of cured pork available include picnic shoulder, shoulder butt, Canadian bacon, bacon, and smoked loin chops.

Sausages and Luncheon Meats

These products can be divided into two categories: fresh and smoked sausages to be cooked before eating; and ready-to-serve sausages and luncheon meats.

Fresh pork sausage is made from ground pork mixed with spices and other seasonings. It is sold in bulk or stuffed into casings or cloth bags. Link sausages may be fresh or smoked, in casings or skinless. Fresh pork sausage must be cooked before eating. Uncooked smoked sausage, such as Polish sausage, must also be cooked before eating.

Ready-to-serve sausages, such as frankfurters and luncheon meats, are fully cooked and can be served cold or heated. Luncheon meat is frequently sold sliced, but bologna and other sausages may be sold in sticks (whole rolls) or in chunks. Included in the ready-to-serve group are specialty loaf-style meats that contain cheese, pickles, olives, macaroni, or pimiento.

Variety Meats

Pork variety meats include liver, heart, kidneys, brains, tongue, and chitterlings.

Liver is fine-textured meat with a distinctive flavor. Whole liver should have a moist, smooth surface when purchased; sliced liver may appear slightly porous.

Heart is firm and smooth textured. It requires long, slow cooking to make it tender.

Kidneys are smooth and bean shaped and have a distinctive flavor.

Brains are soft, tender, and delicate in flavor.

Tongue is firm in texture and is one of the less tender variety meats. Pork tongue usually is sold ready-to-serve.

Chitterlings are the small and large intestines of hogs, emptied and thoroughly cleaned.

See Signs of Good Quality: Inspection mark and label, page 121.

Appearance

Appearance of pork serves as an important guide to quality. Choose meat, either fresh or cured, that has a high proportion of lean to fat and bone. The flesh should be firm and fine textured. Color of the lean in fresh pork may range from grayish pink to red. Lean cured pork has a typical deep pink color.

Visual inspection does not reveal the presence of trichinae, microscopic organisms that can live in pork and be transmitted to man. Severe illnesses can result unless the organism is destroyed by cooking or other procedure. Although a very small percentage of pork is infected with trichinae, raw pork and pork products, including bacon and fresh sausage, should never be tasted before cooking.

In the case of processed pork, packing plants operated under Federal regulations are required to use methods that make certain no live trichinae are present.

To kill trichinae, products such as luncheon meats, processed hams, and frankfurters are heated throughout to at least 137° F.

Cured hams and sausages are freed of trichinae by the combined effects of time, temperature, salt, and drying.

Some pork items are frozen and held for specified periods of time at temperatures between 5° and −20° F to destroy trichinae.

When the United States inspection stamp is on ready-to-eat sausages, frankfurters, and other processed pork products, the consumer can be sure they are safe to eat without cooking.

Packer's brand

Unlike other meats, pork usually is not federally graded. Pork grades have been established but are not widely used. They are based primarily on the proportion of lean to fat.

Some meatpackers use brand names to identify different quality levels of pork products. They maintain standards through their own quality-control programs.

Prices

Price is not a good guide to quality, tenderness, or nutritive value of pork. Popularity of a cut, season of the year, the amount of handling or processing, and the type of retail store—all influence price.

Retail food stores often feature certain meat cuts as specials. Reading the newspaper ads before making a grocery list can help careful shoppers take advantage of these specials.

Amount To Buy

Table 1 shows the number of servings from a pound of pork.

Buy only the amount of pork that you can use within the suggested storage periods given in table 2. Take into consideration family size, ages and food preferences of family members, intended use of the meat, and available storage space.

You may want to buy a large enough roast for two or more meals. Plan to use some of the cooked meat in casseroles, salads, and sandwiches. For the approximate yield of chopped or diced cooked meat from a pound of uncooked fresh or cured pork, see table 1.

TABLE 1.—*Yield of boneless cooked meat from retail pork cuts*

Cut of pork	Approximate yield of cooked lean from 1 pound of pork as purchased	
	3-ounce servings	Volume, chopped or diced
	Number	*Cups*
Fresh:		
Ground pork	3¾ to 4	
Ham:		
Bone-in	2½ to 2¾	1½ to 1¾
Boneless	2¾ to 3	1½ to 1¾
Heart	2¾ to 3	1¾
Liver	3½	
Loin chops, bone-in	2 to 2¼	
Loin roast:		
Bone-in	2 to 2¼	1¼
Boneless	2¾ to 3	1½ to 1¾
Pork cubes (stew meat)	3 to 3¼	
Rib chops, bone-in	1¾ to 2	
Shoulder roast (picnic):		
Bone-in	1¾ to 2	1 to 1¼
Boneless	2½	1½
Shoulder butt roast (Boston butt):		
Bone-in	2½ to 2¾	1½
Boneless	2¾ to 3	1¾
Spareribs	1¼ to 1½	
Cured (mild):		
Ham:		
Canned, boneless:		
Served cold	4¾	2¾
Heated before serving	3½	2
Cook-before-eating:		
Bone-in	2¼	1¼ to 1½
Boneless	2¾ to 3	1½ to 1¾
Fully cooked:		
Bone-in	2¾ to 3	1½ to 1¾
Boneless	3¼	1¾ to 2
Shoulder (picnic):		
Bone-in	2 to 2¼	1¼
Boneless	2¾ to 3	1½ to 1¾
Shoulder butt (Boston butt):		
Bone-in	2¾	1½ to 1¾
Boneless	3	1¾

Home freezer owners may want to buy a whole or half carcass for the convenience of having pork available.

The average price per pound of the meat from the whole or half carcass is likely to be less than the price per pound of the various retail cuts. However, the most desirable cuts, such as loins and hams, make up a relatively small proportion of the carcass. There is some trimming waste too. The costs of cutting, wrapping, and storing (either in home freezer or rented locker) must be added to the cost of the meat. These costs may offset savings made by buying the whole or half carcass.

STORAGE

Fresh Pork

Fresh pork can be stored at refrigerator temperatures between 35° and 40° F or at lower temperatures in the meat compartment of some refrigerators.

Fresh meat generally keeps best if loosely wrapped. However, the transparent wrap on prepackaged meat is designed for refrigerator storage at home for a day or two.

Variety meats and fresh pork sausage cannot be stored as long as other cuts. See table 2.

Frozen Pork

If fresh pork is to be stored for more than a few days, it should be frozen. Before freezing, trim pork carefully to save space, and divide into meal-size portions, if desired.

Wrap the meat in a moisture-vapor-proof wrapping, such as coated or laminated freezer paper, polyethylene film or bags, or heavy-weight aluminum foil. For easy separation of pieces after freezing, place two pieces of freezer wrap between each steak or chop.

Wrap meat tightly, pressing out as much air as possible. Seal packages well with freezer tape.

Label packages with the cut of meat, the date of freezing, and the date by which the meat should be used for best quality.

Meat should be frozen and stored at 0° F or below. Spread the packages of meat in the freezer so that the meat will freeze quickly. Allow a 1-inch space around packages for air circulation. You can freeze 2 to 3 pounds of meat for each cubic foot of freezer space at one time.

Meats (including cooked meat dishes) purchased frozen should be kept frozen at 0° F or below until used. Stored at 0° F, fresh pork will retain high quality for approximately the periods of time specified. The frozen food compartment of a home refrigerator is not designed to maintain 0°. Meats held there will retain high quality only for about a week.

In refrigerator-freezer combinations where 0° can be maintained in the freezer cabinet, meats may be kept for the same time periods as in a freezer.

Fresh pork sausage does not retain quality as long in the freezer as other fresh pork cuts. It soon becomes rancid.

Processed Meats and Meat Products

Cured

Cured and smoked pork requires refrigeration unless stated otherwise on the label. Cured sausages should be wrapped and stored in the refrigerator. Country-style

TABLE 2.—*Suggested home storage periods to maintain high quality in pork*

Product	Storage period	
	Refrigerator, 35° to 40° F	Freezer, 0° F or below
Fresh pork:		
Chops	3 to 5 days	3 to 4 months.
Roasts	3 to 5 days	4 to 8 months.
Sausage	1 to 2 days	1 to 2 months.
Variety meats	1 to 2 days	3 to 4 months.
Cured or processed pork:		
Bacon	7 days	1 month or less. [1]
Frankfurters	7 days	2 weeks
Ham:		
Whole	7 days	1 to 2 months. [1]
Half	3 to 5 days	1 to 2 months. [1]
Slices	3 days	1 to 2 months. [1]
Large canned, unopened	1 year	
Luncheon meat	3 to 5 days	Not recommended.
Sausage:		
Smoked	7 days	Not recommended.
Dry and semidry	2 to 3 weeks	Not recommended.
Cooked pork:		
Cooked pork and pork dishes	3 to 4 days	2 to 3 months.
Gravy and meat broth	1 to 2 days	2 to 3 months.

[1] Frozen cured meat loses quality rapidly and should be used as soon as possible.

cured pork with a high salt content can be kept safely in a cool, dry, dark place. Or it can be refrigerated.

Cured pork stored in the freezer retains high quality for only a short time. Salt added in the curing process hastens rancidity. See table 2.

Canned

Canned hams and picnics should be refrigerated unless directions on label specify that refrigeration is not necessary.

Other canned pork products will retain their quality for as long as a year if stored in a cool, dry place. They will be safe to eat as long as the cans are completely airtight. After opening, canned pork products should be refrigerated and used within a few days. Follow the storage directions given on the label.

Cooked Pork

Cooked meat should be covered or wrapped and stored in the refrigerator. Rapid cooling of meat and meat combination dishes helps prevent bacterial growth. Because bacterial growth is favored at temperatures between 40° and 140° F, the food should be taken through this temperature range as quickly as possible.

Cooked meat keeps best if left in large pieces until used. To save storage space, remove meat from bone. Wrap well to prevent drying.

Gravy and meat broth are highly perishable and should be cooled quickly, then refrigerated immediately. Store only 1 or 2 days.

Cooked pork and many combination dishes containing pork can be stored in the freezer at 0° F for 2 or 3 months with little or no change in quality. Remove meat from the bones, wrap tightly in moisture-vapor-resistant material, and freeze quickly. Cool combination dishes quickly, package in meal-size amounts, seal in moisture-vapor-resistant containers, and freeze quickly.

GENERAL PRINCIPLES OF COOKERY

Cooking Temperatures

Pork cooked at low to moderate temperatures is generally more tender, juicy, and flavorful than pork cooked at high temperatures. Also, there will be more meat to serve because of less shrinkage.

Poorly regulated ovens are sometimes to blame for overcooked meat. Check the oven temperature with an accurate oven thermometer if meat seems to brown too quickly or if roast is dry and crusty.

Broiling temperatures can be regulated either by changing the distance between the meat and heat source, or, in some gas ranges, by changing thermostat setting or flame height. Position of the door also influences broiling temperature. The door is usually closed when broiling in a gas range, and open in an electric range. Follow manufacturer's suggestions.

For maximum tenderness, simmered and braised meats should be cooked at temperatures that maintain the liquid just below the boiling point.

Temperatures in this bulletin are given in degrees Fahrenheit. If you have metric temperature measuring equipment in your home, use the following tabulation to obtain the degrees Celsius.

° F	° C
0	−18
40	4
137	58
140	60
160	70
170	75
300	150
325	165
350	175
375	190

Degree of Doneness

Pork should be cooked long enough to allow heat to penetrate into the center of the meat. Pork heated to 137° F is safe to eat. However, it is more tender and flavorful when cooked to higher temperatures.

A good test for "doneness" of meat is to make small cuts next to the bone and into the thicker part of the meat. If juice is still pink, meat is not done.

For roasts, a meat thermometer helps eliminate guesswork and is well worth the investment. Choose one marked with the degrees Fahrenheit or Celsius not just the stages of doneness for the various meats.

Fresh pork should be cooked to an internal temperature cf 170° F. Cured hams labeled "cook before eating" should be heated to an internal temperature of 160° and cured picnic shoulders to 170°. Fully cooked cured pork can be eaten without further heating but reheating to an internal temperature of 140° enhances the flavor.

If you don't have a meat thermometer, estimate roasting time by the timetable.

Cooking Time

Cooking time depends on—

- Meat temperature at the start of cooking.
- Method of cooking.
- Size and shape of the cut.

- Proportion of lean, fat, and bone.

Timetables in this publication are based on meat at refrigerator or freezer temperature.

A small roast requires more minutes per pound than a large roast, but its total cooking time is less than for the large roast. Longer cooking time is needed for a thick cut than for a thin cut of the same weight. Boned and rolled roasts require more cooking time per pound than roasts with bone in. A roast with an outside layer of fat takes longer to cook than a roast with little or no fat cover.

Cooking Frozen Meat

If frozen meat is not thawed before cooking, allow extra cooking time. The extra cooking time needed depends on size, shape, and thickness of meat. Large frozen roasts may take up to one and a half times as long to cook as unfrozen cuts of the same weight and shape. Generally, smaller roasts require more extra time per pound than larger roasts.

A meat thermometer may be inserted when the meat has thawed. This will be an aid in determining doneness. See timetable for a guide to roasting times for some frozen pork roasts.

Frozen steaks and chops require up to one and a half times as long to broil. They should be placed at least 4 inches from the source of heat to prevent overbrowning.

If you prefer, thaw frozen meat in the refrigerator, then cook it as fresh meat. Large roasts take 4 to 7 hours per pound to thaw, and small roasts take 3 to 5 hours per pound. Cooking time for thawed meat at refrigerator temperature is the same as for meat that has not been frozen.

Frozen meat combination dishes are best when reheated without thawing first. If they are in a watertight container, they can be partially thawed by immersing the package in lukewarm water for a few minutes—just long enough to make it easy to remove the food from the container.

Complete thawing of meat combination dishes at room temperature may permit growth of dangerous bacteria and is not recommended for commercially or home-prepared food of this type.

BASIC COOKING METHODS

Cooking methods commonly used for pork are roasting, broiling, panbroiling, panfrying, braising, and simmering.

Roasting is a method in which the meat is cooked by heated air surrounding it in an oven. The meat is not covered, and no water is added.

In *rotisserie cooking* the meat is rotated on a spit near a heat source. This exposes the meat to direct and even heat.

Broiling is cooking by direct heat from a flame, electric unit, or glowing coals. The meat is cooked one side at a time.

Panbroiling is cooking in an uncovered pan over direct heat. The fat that cooks out of the meat is drained off as it accumulates.

Panfrying is similar to panbroiling, except that the meat is cooked in a small amount of fat.

Braising is cooking in steam trapped in a covered container or foil wrap. The source of steam may be water or other liquid added to the meat, or it may be meat juices.

Simmering is cooking meat in liquid just below the boiling point.

Selection of a cooking method depends on the pork cut. Generally, thick cuts of meat are roasted, braised, or simmered; thin cuts are panbroiled, panfried, or braised. Only thin cuts of fresh or cured pork are recommended for broiling.

Roasting

Directions

Place roast with fat side up on a rack in a shallow roasting pan. If you have a meat thermometer, insert it into roast so that the tip is in the center but not touching bone or fat.

Roast uncovered, without added liquid, until meat thermometer registers appropriate internal temperature.

The timetable serves as a guide to roasting time at 325° F.

Calories per 3-ounce serving: Fresh loin roast—about 310 (lean and fat) or 215 (lean only).

Cured ham—about 245 (lean and fat) or 160 (lean only).

Tips

- Removing rind from ham before roasting is not necessary. It is easier to remove when meat is hot.
- Follow cooking directions on the cured ham wrapper or container when such directions are available.
- A shallow pan is better than a deep one for roasting.
- A rack under the roast holds the meat up from the drippings and allows circulation of heat. The bones in spareribs or pork loin can serve as a rack.
- Cured hams may be glazed about an hour before the end of the cooking period. Remove the rind before glazing.

Timetable for roasting pork

Cut of meat [1]	Approximate ready-to-cook weight	Approximate roasting time at 325° F: Fresh or thawed [2]	Approximate roasting time at 325° F: Frozen	Internal temperature of meat when done
	Pounds	*Hours*	*Hours*	*° F*
Fresh:				
Ham	12 to 16	5½ to 6		170
Ham, half	5 to 7		5 to 5½	170
Ham, boneless, rolled	10 to 14	4⅔ to 5½		170
Loin, center cut	3 to 5	2 to 3⅓	3 to 4	170
Shoulder, picnic	5 to 8	3 to 4	4 to 5	170
Shoulder, picnic, boneless, rolled.	3 to 5	2 to 3		170
Shoulder, Boston butt	4 to 6	3 to 4		170
Shoulder, Boston butt, boneless, rolled.	3 to 5	2¼ to 3¼		170
Spareribs	3 to 4	2		
Cured, cook-before-eating:				
Canadian bacon	2 to 4	1⅓ to 2⅓		160
Ham	5 to 7	2 to 2½		160
Ham	10 to 14	3½ to 4¼		160
Shoulder, picnic, boneless	5 to 8	3 to 4⅔		170
Shoulder, Boston butt, boneless.	2 to 4	1½ to 2⅓		170
Cured, fully cooked:				
Ham	5 to 7	2		140
Ham	12 to 16	3½ to 4		140
Canned ham, boneless	6 to 10	1½ to 2½		140

[1] All cuts of meat listed in the table contain bone unless specified otherwise.
[2] Meat at refrigerator temperature at start of roasting.

● Fully cooked hams may be heated to enhance the flavor.

● For easier slicing, allow the roast to stand 15 to 20 minutes after removing it from the oven before carving.

Rotisserie Cooking

Large, compact fresh or cured pork roasts, such as boneless shoulder butt or boneless ham, can be roasted on a rotisserie. The roast should be as regular in shape as possible so the spit will rotate evenly.

Directions

Mount roast securely on spit so that it will not slip as the spit turns. If properly balanced, the meat will rotate evenly.

Place a drip pan or foil under roast to catch the drippings. If you are roasting meat over coals, place the pan so drippings do not fall on coals and cause smoke.

Insert a meat thermometer at an angle or through the end of the roast so the tip is in center of roast but not in fat or touching the spit. Check to see that the thermometer clears rotisserie equipment and drip pan as the spit turns.

Follow the directions that came with your rotisserie equipment for operation of the spit and regulation of temperature. Low to moderate temperatures give best results.

Roast until the meat thermometer registers the appropriate temperature.

Tips

● Hams may be glazed during the last half hour of cooking. Remove the rind, if any, before glazing.

● Because cooking time varies with intensity of heat produced, a roast cooked on an outdoor rotisserie may require a longer time to cook on a breezy day.

● To maintain even heat when cooking over charcoal, space coals about an inch apart. Add new charcoal around edges and wait until it is glowing before pushing it toward the center.

Broiling

Adjust broiler rack.

Slash fat around edges of meat to prevent curling. Separate bacon slices before broiling.

Place meat on cold broiler grid.

Broil until top side of meat is browned, about half the total cooking time.

Turn and brown other side. Use timetable as a guide for total broiling time.

Calories per slice: Bacon, crisp—about 50.

Canadian bacon—about 45.

Tip

● Line bottom of broiler pan with aluminum foil to simplify cleaning.

Panbroiling

Fresh or cured pork steaks, chops, or slices 1 inch thick or less can be panbroiled.

Directions

Slash fat around edge of meat to prevent curling.

Grease pan lightly with fat or rub hot frypan with fat edge of the meat.

Cook meat slowly over moderate heat, turning occasionally for even cooking.

Remove excess fat as it accumulates.

Remove meat from pan; drain.

Total time for 1-inch ham slices will be about 10 minutes for fully cooked ham and 20 minutes for cook-before-eating ham. Fresh pork chops and steaks will require a little longer.

Be sure that fresh pork is cooked throughout.

To panbroil bacon.—Place bacon slices in a cold frypan.

Cook over moderate heat, turning as necessary to brown evenly.

Remove excess fat as it accumulates.

Drain bacon on absorbent paper.

Total cooking time will be 4 or 5 minutes.

Panfrying

Thin chops and steaks, 1 inch thick or less, are suitable for pan frying.

Directions

Slash fat around edge of meat to prevent curling.

Put a small amount of fat in frypan and preheat over moderate heat.

Cook meat slowly, turning occasionally as necessary to brown both sides.

Remove meat from pan; drain.

Season and serve.

Total time for 1-inch chops or steaks will be about 25 to 30 minutes.

Timetable for broiling pork

Cut of meat	Approximate thickness	Approximate total cooking time [1]
	Inches	*Minutes*
Bacon slices		4 or 5
Canadian bacon	¼	6 to 8
	½	8 to 10
Chops, rib or loin	½ to ¾	30 to 35
Ham slices, cook-before-eating	¾	13 or 14
	1	18 to 20
Ham slices, fully cooked	1	10

[1] Meat at refrigerator temperature at start of broiling.

Braising

Directions

Brown meat slowly on all sides in a small amount of fat. Use a heavy pan.

Remove the excess fat; season meat.

Add a small amount of liquid, if necessary, to prevent overbrowning.

Cover pan tightly.

Cook slowly over low heat or in a 350° F oven until tender. Use timetable on page 16 as a guide to braising time.

Calories per 3-ounce serving: Spareribs—about 375 (lean and fat).

Tips

- Floured meat browns better than unfloured meat.
- Chops and steaks can be breaded with fine, dry bread or cracker crumbs.
- Meats that have considerable fat and that are not breaded or floured can be browned without added fat.
- Many cuts of pork can be braised without added liquid. Steam from meat juices provides enough moisture.
- If you add a liquid, such as water or tomato juice, use just enough to keep meat from scorching.

Timetable for braising pork

Cut of meat	Approximate weight or thickness	Approximate braising time [1]
		Hours
Chops, rib or loin	¾ to 1½ inches	¾ to 1
Spareribs	2 to 3 pounds	1½
Steaks, shoulder	¾ inch	¾ to 1
Cubes	1 to 1¼ inches	¾ to 1

[1] Meat at refrigerator temperature at start of braising.

• Spareribs may be braised in a barbecue sauce.

Simmering

Simmering is recommended for less tender cuts and "country-style" cured ham. "Country-style" cured ham needs to be soaked overnight in water to cover, in order to remove the salt before simmering. Drain and use fresh water for simmering.

Directions

Place meat in a large pot.
Add water to cover meat.
Add desired seasonings. Cover.

Cook slowly over low heat until meat is tender. Do not boil. Use the timetable on page 16 as a guide to cooking time.

Calories per 3-ounce serving: Fresh picnic—about 320 (lean and fat) or 180 (lean only).

Tips

• Cured and smoked pork is especially tasty when cooked with potatoes, carrots, green beans, or cabbage. Add vegetables just long enough before the meat is tender to cook them.

• If the meat is to be served cold, it will be more flavorful and juicy if it is chilled quickly in the liquid in which it was cooked.

• "Country-style" cured hams may be roasted after simmering. Use directions for fully cooked hams.

Timetable for simmering pork

Cut of meat	Approximate ready-to-cook weight	Approximate total cooking time
	Pounds	*Hours*
Cured "country-style" ham, whole	12 to 16	4 to 5
Cured ham, shank or butt	5 to 8	2 to 3
Cured picnic shoulder	5 to 8	3 to 4
Cured shoulder butt, boneless	2 to 3	1½ to 2
Pork hocks	¾ to 1, each	2½ to 3

Cooking Variety Meats

Pork liver, kidneys, heart, and chitterlings generally require braising or simmering to make them tender; brains are tender and can be pan fried or broiled. Pork tongue usually is sold ready to serve.

Liver

To prepare for cooking.—Remove heavy blood vessels and outside membrane if desired.

To braise.—Heat a small amount of fat in a frypan over moderate heat.

Dip sliced liver in flour seasoned with salt and pepper.

Brown liver on both sides. Add a few tablespoons of water, then cover tightly.

Turn heat to very low or place pan in a 350° F (moderate) oven.

Cook about 20 minutes longer or until meat is tender and juice is no longer pink.

Heart

To prepare for cooking.—Wash in warm water. Trim away gristle and the larger blood vessels.

To braise.—Prepare for cooking as directed.

Stuff with a bread stuffing if desired.

Brown on all sides in a small amount of fat. Season.

Add a small amount of water, about ½ cup. Cover tightly.

Cook in a 300° F (slow) oven or over low heat on top of the range until tender, 2½ to 3 hours.

To simmer.—Prepare for cooking as directed.

Place in a deep pot and add salted water to cover.

Simmer, covered, until tender, 2½ to 3 hours.

Kidneys

To prepare for cooking.—Wash in cold water.

Remove the outer membrane.

Split through the center, lengthwise; remove inner fat and tubes. Cut into pieces if desired.

To simmer.—Prepare for cooking as directed.

Place in a deep pot and add water to cover.

Simmer, covered, until tender, ¾ to 1 hour.

Change water once during cooking to eliminate any strong odor.

For variety, dip cooked kidneys in egg and dry breadcrumbs; fry in deep fat. Or roll cooked kidneys in seasoned flour and fry. Cooked kidneys may also be added to a well-seasoned sauce with or without added vegetables.

Brains

To prepare for cooking.—Wash in cold water; remove any blood clots.

Soak in cold water 30 minutes.

To simmer.—Prepare for cooking as directed.

Place in a deep pot and add water to cover.

Add 1 teaspoon salt and 1 tablespoon lemon juice or vinegar for each quart of water.

Simmer, covered, 20 minutes.

Drain, rinse well in cold water, and remove membrane and blood vessels.

For variety, heat cooked brains in a cream or tomato sauce. Or, break cooked brains into small pieces and add to scrambled eggs.

Cooked brains may be dipped in melted butter or margarine and broiled until lightly browned on both sides, using moderate heat.

Chitterlings

To simmer.—Place chitterlings in a deep pot.

Add enough salted water to cover.

Simmer, covered, until tender, about 1 to 1½ hours.

For variety, dip cooked chitterlings in batter and fry in deep fat, or fry in a little hot fat until brown. Serve with vinegar.

Making Gravy

The secret of making smooth gravy is to mix the flour thoroughly with the fat or with the cold liquid before mixing with the hot liquid.

Meat drippings often contain both fat and meat juices. Drippings from panbroiled, panfried, and well-done roasted or broiled meat may consist almost entirely of melted fat and browned crusty bits because most of the meat juices evaporate during cooking. Drippings from braised, roasted, or broiled meat, however, may contain considerable meat juice or broth.

The proportions of flour, fat, and meat juices or other liquid for gravy depend on how thick you like it. For moderately thick gravy, use 2 tablespoons of flour and 1 to 2 tablespoons of fat to each cup of meat juices or other liquid. For thin gravy, use only 1 tablespoon each of flour and fat.

Method 1.—*Use with drippings containing only fat and browned crusty bits.*

Measure amount of fat needed and return to pan. Save the rest for other uses.

Stir flour into fat; brown over low heat.

Add liquid slowly, stirring constantly.

Cook until thickened, stirring occasionally.

Season to taste.

Method 2.—*Use with drippings containing a considerable amount of meat juices or broth.*

Measure drippings or broth; if necessary add water to make desired amount of liquid. Heat.

Mix flour with a small amount of cold water by stirring or shaking until smooth.

Stir flour mixture slowly into hot liquid.

Cook until thickened, stirring occasionally.

Season to taste.

Lamb

Let lamb lend variety and appeal to your weekly menus.

Once a seasonal meat served chiefly in the spring, juicy and flavorful lamb is now available throughout the year. You can serve tasty lamb shish kebabs in summer, hearty lamb stew in winter, and, of course, the traditional spring roast leg of lamb.

Lamb, like other meats, is rich in essential body-building protein, in iron, and in the B vitamins—niacin, thiamin, and riboflavin. Lamb liver and kidneys are especially good sources of these nutrients.

Improved breeding, feeding, and marketing practices are steadily improving the quality of lamb cuts. As a result, today's lamb has more protein, less fat, and fewer calories than it used to have, and you can usually buy it well trimmed and ready to cook.

Best of all—because all cuts of lamb are tender—even the least expensive cuts can become appetizing and satisfying main dishes when you prepare them with imagination.

BUYING LAMB

Lamb is meat from young sheep usually less than 1 year old. Most of the sheep annually sold for meat are marketed as lamb.

Lamb is pinkish red in color with white, brittle fat. The bones are porous and reddish.

While most lamb is marketed fresh, some is sold as frozen products and some as canned products.

Identification of Cuts

Learn to identify meat cuts by their appearance. Names often indicate the section of the carcass from which the meat was cut.

Other lamb cuts

Boneless stew lamb, small pieces or cubes of meat, usually are cut from the neck and shoulders, but they may come from any part of a lamb carcass.

Ground lamb generally is made from neck, breast, shanks, and flank, although boneless lamb from any cut can be used. Sometimes ground lamb is shaped into patties.

A *lamb cushion shoulder* is a square, flat piece of meat formed by removing bones from a shoulder and leaving a pocket which can be stuffed.

A *leg steak* is a slice usually cut from the middle of the leg, containing a round bone.

Saratoga chops are boneless lamb chops made from the inside shoulder muscle.

Variety meats

Brains are soft, very tender, and delicate in flavor.

Heart is very firm and smooth textured. It is one of the less tender variety meats and requires long, slow cooking.

Kidneys are smooth and bean shaped, and comparatively mild in flavor.

Liver is fine textured, and distinctive and mild in flavor. Whole liver should have a moist, smooth surface when purchased; sliced liver may appear slightly porous.

Sweetbreads, the thymus glands, are white and soft and have a very delicate flavor.

Tongue is firm in texture and is one of the less tender variety meats. Lamb tongue is usually sold cooked and ready to serve.

See Signs of Good Quality: Inspection mark and label, page 121.

Grade stamp or packer's brand

The grade stamp is a guide to the quality of federally graded retail cuts of lamb. It tells whether a lamb cut is USDA Prime, Choice, Good, Utility, or Cull.

Grade depends on the proportion of meat to bone, the color and texture of the lean, the firmness of lean and fat, and the degree of marbling (flecks of fat throughout muscle). Most of the federally graded lamb on the retail market is USDA Prime or USDA Choice.

Because meat grading is optional and is paid for by the meatpacker, not all lamb is federally graded. Some meatpackers use brands, instead of grades, to represent the quality levels of their products. Each packer may sell products under several brand names, with each brand representing a different quality level. These may or may not match the standards of Federal grades.

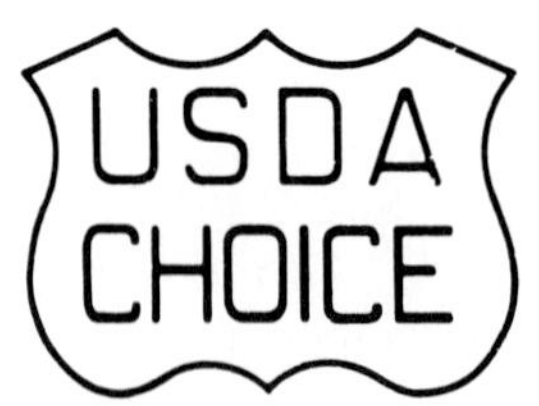

Appearance

Appearance of fresh lamb is an important guide to quality—especially if the grade or packer's brand does not appear on the meat.

Meat from high-quality, young lambs has pink, firm, fine-textured lean. Cross sections of bones appear red, moist, and porous. The lean meat from older, high-quality lambs is light red; the bones appear drier, harder, and less red than bones of younger lambs.

External fat should be firm. However, its color should not be taken as an indication of the quality of the lamb. The color of fat varies with the breed and age of the animal, and with the type of feed it has been fattened on.

Prices

Many factors influence the retail price of lamb: The store where it is sold, the popularity of the cut or brand, the amount of handling or processing necessary to get the meat to market, and the season of the year.

Price is not indicative of the quality, tenderness, or nutritive value of a cut of lamb. Lean meat from all parts of the lamb furnishes high-quality protein.

Amount To Buy

The amount of lamb to buy depends on the number in your family, their ages and preferences, how you plan to use the meat, and available storage space. Unless you have adequate freezer storage space, buy only the amount of lamb that you can use within the refrigerator storage periods suggested in the table.

To estimate the number of servings of boneless, cooked meat from a pound of various retail lamb cuts, see table below.

Yield of boneless, cooked meat from retail lamb cuts

Cut of lamb	Approximate yield of cooked lean and some fat from 1 pound of fresh lamb as purchased [1]	
	3-ounce servings	Volume, chopped or diced
	Number	*Cups*
Ground lamb	3½	---------
Leg roast:		
Bone-in	2½ to 3	1½
Boneless	3½	2
Shoulder roast:		
Bone-in	3	1½
Boneless	3 to 3½	2
Stew lamb	3	2

[1] Assumes that most fat is trimmed from meat before it is eaten. These figures allow no more than 10 percent fat on a cooked, bone-in cut and no more than 15 percent fat on a cooked, boneless cut.

STORING LAMB

Fresh Lamb

Refrigerator storage

Fresh lamb can be stored at refrigerator temperatures between 35° and 40° F. or at lower temperatures in the meat compartment of some refrigerators. It generally keeps best if loosely wrapped. However, prepackaged fresh lamb may be refrigerated in the original wrapper if it is to be used within 1 or 2 days.

Lamb variety meats, ground lamb, and stew lamb are highly perishable and cannot be stored as long as other lamb cuts. Suggested home storage times for fresh lamb are included in the table .

Freezer storage

Fresh lamb should be frozen if it is to be stored for more than a few days. Trim it carefully to save freezer space, and divide it into meal-size portions. Wrap portions tightly in a packaging material that is both moisture and vapor resistant.

Suggested storage periods to maintain high-quality in lamb

Product	Storage period	
	Refrigerator, (about 40° F.)	Freezer, 0° F.
Fresh lamb:	*Days*	*Months*
Chops and steaks	3 to 5	6 to 9
Ground lamb	1 to 2	3 to 4
Roasts	3 to 5	6 to 9
Stew lamb	1 to 2	3 to 4
Variety meats	1 to 2	3 to 4
Cooked lamb:		
Cooked lamb and lamb dishes	3 to 4	2 to 3
Gravy and meat broth	1 to 2	2 to 3

Meats (including cooked meat dishes) purchased frozen should be kept frozen at 0° F. until used.

Stored at 0° F. (in a freezer or freezer-cabinet of a refrigerator-freezer combination), fresh lamb retains its high quality for the approximate lengths of time specified in table on this page. In frozen food compartments of home refrigerators, which do not maintain 0° F., lamb retains high quality only a few days. If you have a refrigerator-freezer combination that maintains 0° F. in the freezer cabinet, your meats will keep as well in it as they do in a freezer.

Cooked Lamb

Cover or wrap cooked lamb and lamb combination dishes, and refrigerate promptly. Rapid cooling will help prevent bacterial growth. Refrigerate or freeze lamb left on a serving platter (part of a roast, for example) as soon as you finish your meal.

Cooked lamb keeps best if you leave it in large pieces until you are ready to use it. However, to prevent drying and to save storage space, you may want to remove cooked lamb from the bone—especially if only a small amount of meat is left.

Lamb gravy and broth are highly perishable and should be cooled quickly, refrigerated, and used within 1 or 2 days.

Cooked lamb, as well as many combination dishes containing lamb, can be stored in the freezer at 0° F. for 2 or 3 months. Remove cooked meat from bones, wrap tightly in moisture-vapor-resistant material, and freeze. Cool combination dishes quickly, package in meal-size portions, seal in moisture-vapor-resistant containers, and freeze.

Canned Lamb and Lamb Products

Canned products containing lamb keep well in a cool, dry place. Under proper storage conditions, canned lamb products retain their quality up to a year and will be safe to eat as long as the cans remain airtight.

Once opened, canned lamb products should be refrigerated and used within a few days.

GENERAL COOKING PRINCIPLES

Cooking Temperature

Generally, lamb should be cooked at low to moderate temperatures. Slow cooking usually makes it more tender, juicy, and flavorful than it would be if cooked faster. Also, color is more even, aroma more pleasant, and yield higher.

- When braising or simmering lamb, keep the temperature of the cooking liquid just below boiling for maximum tenderness.
- When broiling lamb, follow manufacturer's suggestions for the distance from heat source to place meat being broiled, and for the position of broiler door (open or closed).

To prevent the outside of a thick cut of lamb from charring before the inside cooks, place the meat farther from the heat source than you would a thinner cut. Cook it longer.

- When roasting lamb, check a timetable for approximate roasting time. If there is any reason to doubt your oven's accuracy, check its temperature with a good oven thermometer. A faulty oven may either brown your roast too quickly, or undercook it.

Cooking Time

Cooking time depends on several factors: The temperature of your lamb at the start of cooking, the cooking temperature, the size and shape of the lamb cut, the composition of the cut (proportion of lean, fat, and bone), and the doneness desired.

A small lamb roast requires more minutes of cooking per pound than a large roast, but less total cooking time. A thick cut of lamb needs more cooking time than a thin cut of the same weight. Lamb with an outside layer of fat takes longer to cook than lamb with little or no fat covering. Boned and rolled roasts require more cooking time per pound than roasts with bone in.

Degree of Doneness

Lamb is usually preferred medium or well done. Medium lamb has a grayish-tan interior with a tinge of pink. Well-done lamb is grayish tan with no trace of pink.

To check the doneness of a lamb steak or chop, cut along the bone and observe interior color of the meat.

The best way to tell when a lamb roast is done the way you want it is to use a meat thermometer (illustration above). Generally, lamb is considered well done when the internal temperature, taken in the center of the roast, is 180° F.; medium lamb has an internal temperature of 170° F.

If you don't have a meat thermometer, you can estimate cooking time from a roast meat timetable. However, following such a table does not assure that your roast will be cooked to just the doneness you want.

Cooking Frozen Lamb

Frozen lamb need not be thawed before cooking, but it requires extra cooking time. The extra cooking time needed depends on size, shape, and thickness of meat. Large roasts may take one and a half times as long to cook as fresh roasts of the same weight and shape. Small roasts require less additional time. A meat thermometer may be inserted when meat is thawed. Frozen steaks and chops require up to one and a half times as long to broil. They should be placed at least 4 inches from the source of heat to prevent overbrowning.

Thawed lamb can be cooked the same as fresh lamb. But you should thaw your frozen meats in the refrigerator, since *thawing meat or meat combination dishes at room temperature may permit dangerous bacterial growth.*

Frozen lamb combination dishes are best if reheated without thawing. However, if you wish to transfer them from their containers to heatproof utensils for reheating, immerse the containers for a few minutes in lukewarm water. The food then can be easily removed, and its quality will be unchanged.

HOW TO COOK LAMB

Selecting a Cooking Method

Nearly all lamb cuts are tender enough to be cooked without added liquid. They can be roasted, broiled, pan broiled, or pan fried; but for variety, they are delicious simmered or braised. *Lamb cooked by any method tastes best if served piping hot or chilled, rather than warm.*

To help you select the right cooking method for various lamb cuts, see timetables listing cuts usually cooked by each of the procedures.

Broiling is cooking meat one side at a time by direct heat from a flame, electric unit, or glowing coals.

Pan broiling is cooking in an uncovered pan over direct heat. Fat that cooks out of the meat is drained off as it accumulates.

Pan frying is similar to pan broiling, except that meat is cooked in a small amount of fat.

Roasting is a method in which meat is surrounded and cooked by heated air, usually in an oven. Meat is not covered and no water is added.

Rotisserie cooking is a method which exposes all sides of meat to direct and even heat, by rotating it on a spit located near a heat source.

Braising is cooking by steam trapped and held in a covered container or foil wrap. The source of steam may be water or other liquid added to the meat, or it may be meat juices alone.

Pot roasting is braising large cuts of meat, either on top of a range or in an oven.

Simmering is cooking meat in liquid kept just below boiling.

To add to lamb's natural good flavor, choose any of these seasonings: Basil, bay leaves, celery, dill, garlic, marjoram, mint, onion, parsley, oregano, rosemary, savory, tarragon, and thyme. The kinds and amounts of seasonings you use will, of course, depend on your family's preferences.

When braising, broiling, or frying lamb, brown the meat and then sprinkle seasonings on. When roasting lamb, rub seasonings into the meat before cooking (garlic pieces can be inserted beneath the fat).

Special sauces, either homemade or commercially prepared, also enhance the flavor of lamb. Of these, mint sauce and jelly are probably the most commonly used.

Broiling

Directions

Adjust broiler rack according to broiler manufacturer's directions.

Slash fat around edge of meat to prevent curling.

Place meat on cold broiler grid.

Broil until top of meat is brown, about half total cooking time.

Season and turn. Brown on other side. Use timetable as a guide for total broiling time.

Calories per serving: Lamb loin chop (5-ounce), about 315 (fat and lean); lamb rib chop (4-ounce), about 260 (fat and lean).

Tips

- Turn meat by sticking a fork into fat, not lean; or use tongs.
- Check doneness by cutting a slit in the meat near the bone (or in center of patties) and noting interior color.
- Broil frozen lamb at a low temperature to prevent surface from charring before interior thaws. Increase cooking time.

Outdoor Broiling

Broiled lamb tastes especially good when cooked outdoors. Appetites are bigger, too, so be sure to allow for seconds.

Choose thick chops and patties for outdoor broiling. Chops at least 1½ inches thick and patties at least ¾ inch thick will be juicier than thinner ones.

Cubes cut from lamb shoulder or leg make delicious shish kebabs.

Directions

Light fire 30 to 45 minutes ahead of time, so coals will be the right temperature. When coals are covered with fine gray ash, spread them about 1 inch apart. No two coals should touch.

Adjust grill so that meat surface is about 6 to 8 inches from the coals. This gives even heat without too much intensity. If meat cooks too fast, raise grill away from heat.

Turn meat when about half cooked. Broil until meat reaches desired doneness. The timetable above will help estimate cooking time, but cooking times vary.

Tips

- Marinate lamb in a seasoned mixture of half oil and half vinegar or other acid ingredient for several hours in the refrigerator before broiling.
- Check doneness by cutting a slit in the meat near the bone (or in the center of patties) and observing interior color.
- Allow meat more time to cook on a windy day than on a calm one.

Timetable for broiling lamb

Cut of meat	Approximate thickness	Approximate total cooking time[1]
	Inches	*Minutes*
Chops, loin, rib, or shoulder	1	12 (medium)
		14 (well done)
	1½	18 (medium)
		22 (well done)
Patties	1	15 to 18 (medium)
		20 (well done)
Steaks, leg	1	12 to 14 (medium)
		16 to 18 (well done)

[1] Meat is at refrigerator temperature at start of broiling.

Pan Broiling

Directions

Choose thin (1-inch thick or less) lamb chops, steaks, or patties for pan broiling.

Slash fat around edge of meat to prevent it from curling.

Grease frypan lightly or rub hot frypan with fat edge of meat.

Place meat in hot frypan and cook slowly over moderate heat, turning occasionally as necessary.

Pour off excess fat as it accumulates.

Remove meat from pan; drain.

Season and serve.

Total cooking time for ¾- to 1-inch chops or steaks, 10 to 15 minutes.

Pan Frying

Directions

Thin (¾- to 1-inch thick) cuts of lamb are best for pan frying.

Slash fat around edge of meat to prevent it from curling.

Add a small amount of fat to frypan.

Preheat pan over moderate heat.

Cook meat slowly over moderate heat; turn occasionally, to brown both sides.

Remove meat from pan; drain. Season and serve.

Total cooking time, 10 to 15 minutes.

Roasting

Directions

Preheat oven to 325° F. (slow).

Place roast with fat side up on rack in shallow roasting pan. Season as desired.

If you have a meat thermometer, insert it into roast so that its tip is in center of roast, not touching bone or fat.

Timetable for roasting lamb

Cut of meat	Approximate ready-to-cook weight	Approximate roasting time at 325° F.[1]
	Pounds	*Hours*
Leg	5 to 8	3 to 4.
Leg, boneless, rolled	3 to 5	2 to 3.
Rib (rack)	4 to 5	3 to 3⅓.
Shoulder	4 to 6	2⅓ to 3.
Shoulder, cushion-style	3 to 5	1¾ to 2½.
Shoulder, boneless, rolled	3 to 5	2¼ to 3⅓.

[1] Meat at refrigerator temperature at start of roasting.

Roast uncovered, without added liquid, until meat thermometer registers appropriate temperature (180° F. for well-done lamb; 170° F. for medium-done lamb).

The timetable below serves as a guide to roasting time for well-done lamb. Medium-done lamb will require slightly less roasting time.

Calories per 3-ounce serving: Lamb leg roast (Choice grade), about 235; lamb shoulder roast (Choice grade), about 285.

Tips

- For a "frenched" leg of lamb, ask your butcher to remove enough meat from the shank end of a leg roast to expose an inch or more of bone. For special occasions, decorate this bone with a paper frill.
- Removing the "fell" (the thin, paperlike covering on lamb roasts) before roasting is not necessary.
- For easier slicing, remove roast from the oven and let stand 15 to 20 minutes before carving.
- Lamb roast is especially good served with mint sauce or jelly.

Rotisserie Cooking

Use only large, compact lamb roasts, such as boneless rolled shoulder and boneless rolled leg, for rotisserie cooking. To make even rotation possible, choose a roast that is regular in shape.

Directions

Mount roast securely on spit so that it does not slip as the spit turns. If properly balanced, meat will rotate evenly.

Place a drip pan under roast to catch drippings. If you are cooking meat over coals, observe where drippings fall and arrange pan so that drippings do not fall on coals and cause smoke. Arrange coals in front of and in back of drip pan, to provide even heat.

If you have a meat thermometer, insert it at an angle, or through the end of the roast, so the tip is in the center of roast. Be sure it is not in a fat pocket or touching the spit. And check to be certain that the thermometer does not hit the rotisserie equipment or drip pan as the spit turns.

To operate spit and regulate temperature, follow the directions that came with your rotisserie equipment. Low to moderate temperatures give best results.

Cook until meat reaches desired doneness. Cooking time depends on size and shape of roast, cooking temperature, and doneness desired.

Tips

● Lamb roasts may be basted with a mint sauce or other sauce during roasting. If sauce contains sugar or other ingredients that burn easily, baste only during the last half hour of roasting.

● If you are cooking a roast on an outdoor rotisserie, it may take longer on a windy day than on a calm one.

● To maintain an even heat when cooking over charcoal, space coals about an inch apart. Add new charcoal around edges and wait until the coals glow; then push them toward the center.

Braising

Directions

Brown lamb slowly on all sides in a heavy pan, with enough added fat to prevent sticking; season.

Add a small amount of liquid (about ½ cup for a roast) if necessary.

Cover pan tightly.

Cook slowly over low heat or in a 350° F. oven until tender, adding more liquid if needed. Use timetable as a guide to braising time.

Tips

● Lamb cuts that have a considerable amount of fat and that are not breaded or floured can be browned without added fat.

● Many cuts of lamb can be braised without added liquid, because their own juices provide enough moisture. If you do add water or tomato juice, use just enough to keep meat from scorching.

Simmering

Directions

Brown meat on all sides, if desired.

Add enough water to cover meat.

Add seasonings; cover.

Cook slowly over low heat until meat is tender. (1- to 2-inch lamb cubes require 1½ to 2 hours.)

Cooking Variety Meats

Since most lamb variety meats are tender, they can be prepared in any of several ways. They are usually cooked well done.

Here are a few of the cooking methods most commonly used with each of the lamb variety meats.

Liver

To prepare for cooking.—Remove heavy blood vessels and outside membrane.

To braise.—Heat small amount of fat in frypan over moderate heat.

Dip sliced liver in flour seasoned with salt and pepper.

Brown in hot fat over moderate heat.

Cover pan tightly and reduce heat.

Cook on top of range or in 350° F. (moderate) oven until tender, about 20 to 25 minutes.

To broil.—Adjust broiler rack for moderate heat. Dip sliced liver in melted butter, drippings, or french dressing.

Place on cold broiler grid.

Broil until liver loses its red color, about 4 minutes on each side.

As a variation, thread cubed liver on skewers alternately with bacon and small, whole onions; broil.

To pan fry.—Heat a small amount of fat in a frypan over moderate heat.

Dip sliced liver in flour seasoned with salt and pepper. Place in hot fat.

Cook over moderate heat, turning as necessary, until liver is brown and tender, about 5 minutes on each side.

Heart

To prepare for cooking.—Wash in warm water. Trim away gristle and larger blood vessels.

To braise.—Fill cavity with bread stuffing, if desired.

Brown on all sides in small amount of fat; season.

Add small amount of liquid, about ½ cup. Cover tightly. Cook in 300° F. (slow) oven or over low heat on top of range until tender, about 2½ to 3 hours.

To simmer.—Place in a deep pot and add salted water to cover.

Timetable for braising lamb

Cut of meat	Approximate ready-to-cook weight or thickness	Approximate total cooking time [1]
		Hours
Breast, boneless, rolled	1½ to 2 pounds	1½ to 2
Breast, stuffed	2 to 3 pounds	1½ to 2
Neck slices	¾ inch	1
Riblets		1½ to 2
Shanks	¾ to 1 pound each	1½ to 2
Shoulder chops	¾ to 1 inch	¾ to 1
Pieces for stew	1½ inches	1½ to 2

[1] Cooking time is for meat braised at simmering temperature.

Simmer, covered, until tender, 2½ to 3 hours.

Kidneys

To prepare for cooking.—Wash in cold water and remove outer membrane. Split through center, lengthwise, and remove inner fat and tubes. Cut up if desired.

To broil.—Adjust broiler rack for moderate heat.

Dip kidneys in melted butter, drippings, or french dressing.

Place on cold broiler grid. Broil 5 to 10 minutes on each side, until brown.

As a variation, wrap kidneys in bacon slices before broiling.

To simmer.—Place in a deep pot, with water to cover.

Simmer, covered, until tender, 45 to 60 minutes.

As a variation, heat cooked kidneys in a spicy sauce, or roll them in seasoned flour and fry.

Brains and sweetbreads

To prepare for cooking.—Wash in cold water and remove any blood clots.

Soak in cold water 30 minutes.

To simmer.—Place in a deep pot with water to cover.

For each quart of water, add 1 teaspoon salt and 1 tablespoon lemon juice or vinegar.

Simmer, covered, 15 to 20 minutes.

Drain, rinse well in cold water, and remove membrane and blood vessels.

As a variation, heat cooked brains or sweetbreads in a cream or tomato sauce. Or, break cooked brains into small pieces and add to scrambled eggs.

To broil.—Simmer, following method above.

Dip in melted butter or margarine and place on cold broiler grid. Broil until lightly browned, turning once. Total broiling time, 10 to 15 minutes.

Lamb Gravy

The secret of making smooth gravy is to blend flour thoroughly with fat or with cold liquid before combining it with hot liquid.

Meat drippings often contain both fat and meat juices. Drippings from pan broiled, pan fried, and well-done roasted or broiled meat may consist almost entirely of melted fat and browned crusty bits because most of the meat juices evaporate during cooking. Drippings from braised meat and medium roasted or broiled meat, however, may contain considerable meat juice or broth.

The proportions of flour, fat, and meat juices or liquid for gravy depend on how thick you like it. For moderately thick gravy, use 2 tablespoons of flour and 1 to 2 tablespoons of fat to each cup of meat juices or other liquid. For thin gravy, use only 1 tablespoon each of flour and fat.

Method 1

Use with drippings containing only fat and browned crusty bits.

Measure amount of fat needed and return to pan. Save the remainder for other uses.

Stir flour into fat; brown over low heat.

Add liquid slowly, stirring constantly.

Cook until thickened, stirring occasionally.

Season to taste.

Method 2

Use with drippings containing a considerable amount of meat juices or broth.

Measure drippings or broth. If necessary, add water to make desired amount of liquid. Heat.

Mix flour with an equal amount of cold water by stirring or shaking until smooth.

Stir flour mixture slowly into hot liquid.

Cook until thickened, stirring occasionally.

Season to taste.

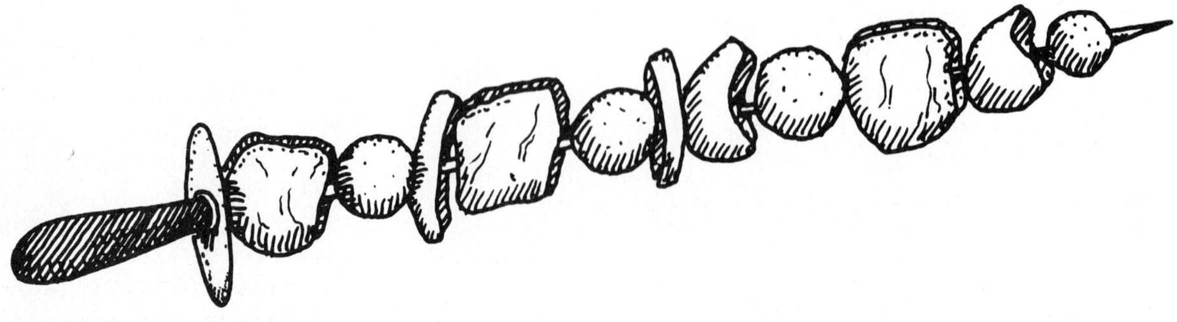

Please Don't Pass the Meat: The Case for Soybeans

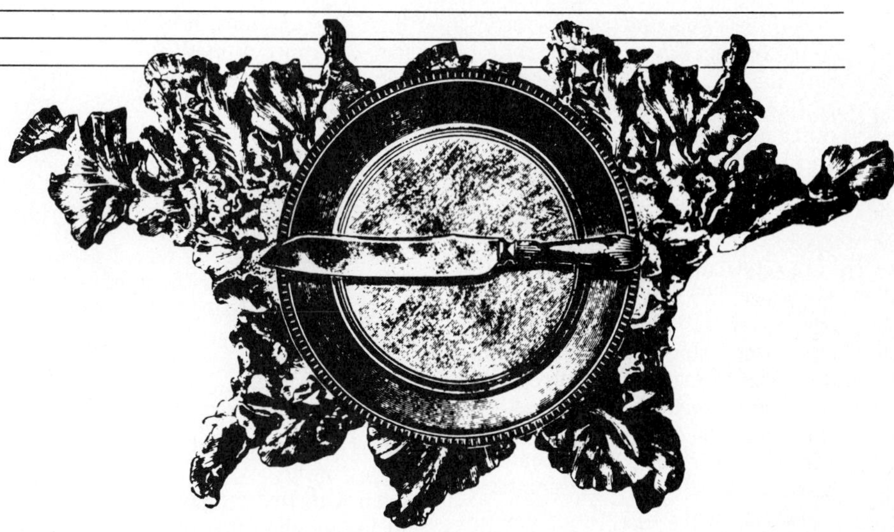

Inflation and the trend toward more "natural" lifestyles have heightened the interest in vegetarianism. The experts say that extreme vegetarian diets can be dangerous, but there are also indications that other meatless diets may be quite beneficial.

Let's hear it now for vegetarians! No, they're not a band of religious fanatics who wear their hair shirts by denying themselves some of the finer moments of dining, and in the process jeopardize their health with deficiencies of vitamins and nutrients.

The fact is that vegetarians as a group may be a whole lot healthier than the rest of us. They can also be credited with adopting a very efficient means of getting their body essentials—a consideration of no small merit on this planet of finite resources.

True, vegetarians have to go through life tortured by the smell—and only the smell—of barbecued ribs, frying bacon, Big Macs, and other such animal delicacies. And it also may be true that because they don't eat hot dogs they don't get much out of baseball. But that doesn't make them un-American.

Economists, ecologists, philosophers, and nutritionists who look at vegetarians often have to come up with plus marks for these flesh teetotalers. With hamburger about to break the $2 a pound barrier, it's not hard to understand why economists can applaud vegetarians. And with cattle having to eat 16 pounds of grain to produce 1 pound of meat, it's easy to see why vegetarians get approving nods from ecologists.

Philosophers can admire the discipline that vegetarians impose to maintain their proper diets. And nutritionists have to agree that vegetarians, because they eat less fat and are more careful about their diets, are less likely to suffer from obesity.

The idea that vegetarians can't get what their bodies need without meat was pretty well put into the myth category in 1974 when the Food Nutrition Board of the National Academy of Sciences issued a statement on vegetarian diets. Concluded the board: "A vegetarian can be well nourished *if* he eats a variety of plant foods and gives attention to the critical nutrients (needed by all people)."

The underscoring of the "if" in that statement was provided by the Food and Nutrition Board. The underscoring is necessary because the more restricted the diet, the more difficult it is to get all of the nutrients needed.

The people who—in the words of one of civilization's better known vegetarians, George Bernard Shaw—"refuse to dine off the carcasses of dead animals" generally fall into categories based on the animal foods left in their diets. The categories are:

- Vegans, or pure vegetarians—consume only plant food, and the purists among them only raw plant food.
- Lacto vegetarians—eat dairy products as well as plant foods. Many Seventh-Day Adventists practice this type of vegetarianism.
- Lacto-ovo vegetarians—tolerate eggs as well as dairy products along with their plant foods.

Other vegetarians may consume poultry and fish, leaving only red meat to the gastronomic heathens. The more restrictive the vegetarian's diet the more likely nutrition will be limited. Of concern in recent years have been the extremist diets of groups such as the very restrictive levels of the Zen macrobiotics regimen. Indeed, the Food and Nutrition Board warned in its 1974 statement that such extremely restrictive diets endanger health.

Families who practice stricter forms of vegetarianism should be sure that their growing children are getting enough calories and some other nutrients, such as vitamins D and B_{12}. Studies to date indicate that children may not be able to thrive as well as adults on the more limited diets.

In addition to George Bernard Shaw and the Seventh-Day Adventists, other well-known vegetarians include the Trappist Monks and Hindus. The Monk group shuns meat because it considers it a luxury and thus in conflict with its quest for the simple life. Hindus avoid meat because they believe in transmigration of souls; thus, butchering an animal would be tantamount to butchering a person.

Studies on the health of vegetarians aren't too definitive. It is known that Seventh-Day Adventists generally have fewer deaths due to heart disease, but this may also be traced to the fact that they usually don't smoke or drink. The saturated fats in animal products contribute to high blood cholesterol levels, which is one of the risk factors for heart disease.

Some 40 to 45 percent of the calories in the average American's diet comes from fat. Much of that fat, of course, comes from animal sources. The high fat content in our diets may be related to several diseases including colon and some other forms of cancer.

Needless to say, the high content of fat in the U.S. diet also contributes to obesity. Overweight people are more prone to heart disease, high blood pressure, and diabetes.

Still another advantage to never saying "please pass the meat" is that vegetarians, because of the high fiber content in their diets, usually don't contribute to America's several hundred million dollar a year laxative habit.

The high fiber intake may also discourage overeating, and therein deny those extra pounds a chance to attach themselves. One fills up fast on grains and such. Consequently, fat vegetarians are a rare species. The high fiber content, however, may make it more difficult for some people, such as growing children and pregnant women, to obtain enough calories. Also, high fiber may interfere with the absorption of zinc, iron, and other minerals.

A leading proponent for the vegetarian way of life in recent years has been Frances Moore Lappe, author of DIET FOR A SMALL PLANET. Lappe pointed out that eating meat to get protein is about as efficient as paddling a canoe with a tennis racket. It takes 16 pounds of grain to add 1 pound to beef in the feedlot, Lappe notes. With a ratio like that or even with the average livestock ratio, including chickens, of 7 or 8 pounds of grain or soybeans for 1 pound of flesh, it's easy to see how the world's food shortages might be greatly lessened if vegetarianism swept the world.

However, if meat is hard to produce, it does a good job of providing protein as well as iron and B vitamins once it is inside a person's stomach. Meat provides high quality protein, and protein is required throughout life. Indeed, protein provides building blocks for muscle and tissue. Protein is made from amino acids. Meat contains more of the indispensable or essential amino acids that the body cannot make by itself in the quantities and proportions needed.

Plant foods do not contain the amount or balance of essential amino acids needed by humans. However, if certain combinations of plant foods are eaten or if plant foods are taken with some animal protein, the missing amino acids are filled in. A number of these combinations have been around a long time, indicating that some of those old wives who told tales possibly knew what they were talking about. For example, baked beans and brown bread complement each other, with one providing the amino acid the other is low in. The same is true for macaroni and cheese and the beans and cheese combination that is served as tamale pie. Lentil-rice soup makes a good protein combination, as does breakfast cereal and milk.

Dairy products, including eggs, provide high-quality protein, and are thus good meat substitutes. Legumes (soybeans, chickpeas), nuts including peanuts, and meat substitutes made from plant protein (usually with a soybean base) are also protein sources for vegetarian diets. In addition to providing protein, these meat alternatives supply varying amounts of other essential nutrients.

In its statement on vegetarianism, the Food and Nutrition Board cited a 1954 study of vegetarians, which found that nutrient intake for all vegetarian groups equaled or exceeded necessary amounts, with the exception of vitamin B_{12}. That vitamin was low in the total vegetarian diet. B_{12} is found in all animal products including eggs and milk products. Additional sources are fortified foods including soy milk, cereals, and meat substitutes. B_{12} substitutes are also available.

The Food and Nutrition Board said that vegetarians will get along nutritionally well by using a good variety in the diet. "The greatest risk comes from undue reliance on a single plant food source, usually a cereal grain or starchy root crop," the board said.

Here are the board's recommendations for filling the tummy with the right stuff while sparing the lives of animals:

• Legumes (particularly soybeans)—rich in protein, B-vitamins, and iron. (It's difficult for women to get enough iron in their usual diets, and even more difficult when red meats are left out.)

• Grains—for carbohydrates, proteins, thiamin, iron, and trace minerals.

• Nuts and other seeds—provide fat (which supplies energy), and B-vitamins in addition to protein and iron.

• Dark green, leafy vegetables—sources of calcium, riboflavin, and carotene (used to make vitamin A). These vegetables should be used liberally by vegetarians.

Vegetarians are advised to provide themselves with two servings daily of the high-protein meat alternatives of legumes, nuts, peanuts, eggs, meat analogs, and dairy products.

So, let's hear it again for vegetarians. Many of them have earned and deserve their wholesomer-than-thou attitude.

in family meals

Soybeans can make a valuable addition to the foods we eat for a balanced diet.

Soybeans are available in many forms. Fresh green soybeans are in the market in late summer or fall and make a succulent vegetable.

Canned green soybeans are usually available in all seasons.

Dry soybeans may be purchased the year around and are prepared for eating in the same ways as other dry beans.

Soybean sprouts may be purchased or grown at home. They make a tasty addition to salads and can also be served as a vegetable.

Soybean milk, prepared from dry soybeans, may replace cow's milk in most recipes and can be used as a beverage.

Soybean mash or pulp is the solid material left after soybean milk is prepared.

Soybean curd is prepared from soy milk and may be purchased fresh, canned, or as an instant powder.

Soy sauce, a fermented product made from soybeans, is used as a seasoning, especially in Oriental foods.

Soybeans are also a valuable source of oil, flour, and grits.

The soybean is processed into several forms that are used as ingredients in commercial foods. Soy protein concentrate, protein isolate, and textured protein are an important part of the developing food picture.

Because soybeans contribute good-quality protein, they are used in products designed as substitutes for meat, or combined with meat as an extender. They may also be used with other foods.

NUTRITIVE VALUE

Soybeans are a valuable and economical source of several essential nutrients.

Green soybeans are a dependable source of a number of minerals and vitamins including calcium, phosphorus, iron, vitamin A, thiamin, and riboflavin. However, a considerable portion of the vitamin A is lost during drying.

Dry soybeans contain 1-1/2 times as much protein as other dry beans and 11 times as much fat.

The protein in soybeans contains all the essential amino acids in varying amounts and is of good quality. Amino acids are the units of which protein is made. Those amino acids that the body requires but cannot make are called essential and must come from foods.

The fat or oil of soybeans is high in polyunsaturated fatty acids.

Soy grits and full-fat flours are made from whole dry soybeans and are similar to dry soybeans in nutritive value.

Defatted soy flours, which are prepared after the oil is extracted, are much lower in fat content and higher in protein and carbohydrate than full-fat flours.

Soy milk is lower in food value than cow's milk. The protein content is similar, but soy protein is not utilized by the body quite as well as milk protein.

Soy milk contains less calcium, phosphorous, vitamin A, and some other nutrients, but more iron than cow's milk. The fat content is about one-half to two-thirds that of whole milk.

Commercially, soy milk is often fortified with vitamins and minerals to make it an acceptable substitute for cow's milk.

USING SOYBEANS

Fresh Soybeans

Fresh green soybeans are available in some areas in the late summer or fall. Vegetable-type soybeans are the kind used for cooking. They are somewhat larger and milder in flavor than field-type soybeans, which are used for oil and commercial flour production.

Vegetable-type soybeans are ready to use when the pods are bright green and plump. Each pod usually contains two beans. The pods have a fuzzy surface and are not edible.

To shell fresh soybeans, cover with boiling water and let stand 5 minutes. Drain and cool. Break the pods crosswise and squeeze out the beans. One pound in the pod yields about 1-2/3 cups ready-to-cook soybeans.

To cook, add 2 cups shelled soybeans to 1 cup boiling water. Add 1/2 teaspoon salt. Return to a boil, cover, and cook gently 10 to 20 minutes until tender.

Cooked soybeans are similar to green peas or lima beans in color and flavor but have a firmer texture. They are not soft or mealy.

Season cooked soybeans with butter or margarine and serve as a vegetable or use them in favorite recipes in place of lima beans.

Fresh soybeans must be used as soon as possible to maintain optimum quality. If they must be stored, refrigerate them in covered containers. Shelled soybeans may be frozen to extend their use over a longer period of time. Blanch and freeze in meal-size portions as for lima beans.

Green soybeans may also be purchased in the canned form. A 15-ounce can, drained, contains about 2 cups of soybeans. To serve, heat thoroughly and season as desired or use in recipes that call for cooked lima beans.

Dry Soybeans

Sort dry soybeans before cooking to remove any discolored, cracked, or shriveled beans. After sorting, measure beans and wash thoroughly. To soak and cook, follow the directions below. One cup of dry soybeans will yield about 2-1/2 cups cooked beans.

To soak, use 4 cups water for each cup of dry beans. To soak them quickly, boil beans 2 minutes, remove from heat, and let stand 1 hour. Or if you prefer, boil beans 2 minutes and let them stand overnight in the refrigerator.

To boil, soak beans as directed above. Add 1 teaspoon salt for each cup of dry beans. Simmer, covered, in soaking water 2 to 3 hours until beans are tender. Add water, if necessary, during cooking. When done, the beans will be firm but tender, and not mealy. To reduce foaming, add 1 to 2 teaspoons oil or meat drippings to the cooking water.

To cook in pressure cooker, soak beans as directed above. Place beans and soaking water in pressure cooker. Add 1 teaspoon salt for each cup of dry beans. *Fill pressure cooker no more than one-third full of beans and water.* If cooker is too full, food may clog the vent tube and cause an explosion. Follow manufacturer's instructions for use of your pressure cooker.

Cook about 30 minutes at 15 pounds pressure. Cool immediately under cold running water. Soybeans cooked under pressure are softer than boiled beans.

Store dry soybeans in a cool, dry place. After cooking, store covered in the refrigerator. Cooked soybeans may be stored about 1 week.

Soybean Sprouts

Soybeans can be sprouted at home. They increase in volume about six times as they sprout. In other words, 1/3 cup of dry beans will yield 2 cups of sprouts. Any dry soybeans may be used. There are also special varieties developed for sprouting.

Select a container with good drainage for sprouting beans. A clean clay flowerpot or a milk carton is suitable. Cover the hole in the pot with cheesecloth to hold beans in while allowing water to drain out freely. Punch small holes in the sides and bottom of the milk carton.

Soak the beans overnight in water. Use three times as much water as beans.

Rinse soaked beans well and place in prepared container. Set the container in a cool place (about 65° F.). Rinse beans with cool water four or five times a day. It is important that all the water drains out to prevent growth of mold. If any beans become molded, discard them. The sprouts will be 2 to 3 inches long in 3 to 5 days.

Soybean sprouts grown at home or purchased should be thoroughly rinsed and drained before they are used. Discard any discolored beans and, if desired, remove root ends from sprouts. The sprouts are more attractive with the root ends removed.

One pound fresh sprouts as purchased or prepared at home yields 4 cups ready-to-use sprouts.

Soybean sprouts may be stored for 3 to 5 days in the refrigerator. Store in a tightly sealed plastic bag in the vegetable crisper of the refrigerator. To maintain crispness, rinse with water and shake off excess moisture or place a dampened paper towel in the bag.

Because of the firm texture of the bean, bean sprouts used in recipes in this bulletin were parboiled.

To parboil, drop sprouts into boiling water, using 1/2 cup water and 1/4 teaspoon salt for each cup of sprouts. Boil gently 10 to 15 minutes until beans and sprouts are of desired tenderness.

Since vitamin C content is decreased by cooking, cook sprouts as little as possible. Serve tender-crisp. Two cups raw sprouts yield 1 cup cooked sprouts.

Soy Flour

There are three types of flour made from soybeans.

Full-fat flour contains over 35 percent protein and about 20 percent fat, which is all of the fat present in whole soybeans.

Lowfat flour contains about 6 percent fat and nearly 45 percent protein.

In defatted flour, the fat has been removed by hexane extraction. This flour contains less than 1 percent fat and about 50 percent protein.

Full-fat flour is the type generally available in stores and was used in recipes in this bulletin.

Although full-fat flour can be prepared in the home, special steps are needed to obtain flour with acceptable flavor and keeping quality. Simply grinding any kind of soybeans is not satisfactory.

Soy flour has many uses in baking. It helps keep baked products from becoming stale. When used in doughnuts, it reduces fat absorption. Soy products have a richer color, finer texture, and are more tender and moist than products made with other flour.

Soy flour cannot completely replace all-purpose flour because it does not contain gluten. Gluten, a protein present in all-purpose flour, provides the structure for baked products.

The recipes in this bulletin were developed using as much soy flour as possible without altering the quality of the final product.

Stir soy flour before measuring, because it tends to pack in the container. After stirring, spoon the flour lightly into a measuring cup and level with a spatula.

To increase nutritive value in products made with all-purpose flour, place 1 or 2 tablespoons of soy flour in a measuring cup before filling with all-purpose flour. Products containing soy flour brown more quickly than other products, so baking time or temperature may need to be adjusted slightly.

Store soy flour in a cool, dry place. Because of its high fat content, it may become rancid if stored at too high a temperature.

Soy Grits

Soy grits are available only in defatted form. They are similar to soy flour but are more coarsely ground.

When preparing soy grits, follow cooking instructions on the package. After opening, cover tightly and store in a cool, dry place.

Soy Milk

Soy milk is available commercially in dry, concentrated, and ready-to-use forms. Instructions for preparing, serving, and storing are on the package. Soy milk may also be prepared at home.

Commercial soy milk is often fortified with vitamins and minerals to approximate the composition of cow's milk.

Soy milk may be used in place of cow's milk in most recipes. Due to the flavor difference between soy and cow's milk, you may prefer to use half soy milk and half cow's milk.

To prepare about 2 quarts of soy milk, use 1 pound (2-1/2 cups) dry soybeans. Sort and wash beans thoroughly.

Using 2 quarts of water, soak beans overnight or use the 2-minute-boil method. Drain soaked beans and discard the soaking water. Remove the skins from the beans if you wish to use the bean mash or pulp after the milk is made.

Using 3 quarts of water, grind the soaked beans in a blender. Place part of the beans and enough water to cover in blender container; grind until very fine (about 2 minutes). Repeat until all beans have been ground and the 3 quarts of water have been used.

Strain ground beans through two layers of cheesecloth into a large kettle. Wring as much liquid from the mash as possible. (To use mash, see below.)

Boil the soy milk for 30 minutes, stirring occasionally to prevent scorching. It is necessary to cook the milk thoroughly to destroy a substance which interferes with trypsin, one of the digestive enzymes.

While the milk is still warm, add 2 tablespoons sugar and 1 teaspoon salt. Stir until dissolved. Cover milk tightly and store in the refrigerator.

Strain milk before use because a skin often forms on the surface.

Soybean Mash

The mash or pulp is the solid material left after soybean milk has been prepared. Some protein is retained in the mash.

Mash has a bland flavor and a rather coarse texture. Use it in combination with other foods for its nutritive value or as an extender in ground meat dishes. Several recipes are included in this bulletin as suggestions for using mash.

Mash must be heated thoroughly to eliminate the beany flavor and to prevent spoilage. Place mash in the top of a double boiler. Cook slowly over boiling water for about 1 hour. If mash becomes too dry, moisten it with a little soy milk or water. Stir occasionally during cooking. Add 1 teaspoon salt. Cool and store in refrigerator.

One pound of beans, prepared for milk, will yield 1 quart of mash.

Soybean Curd

Soybean curd may be purchased fresh in many grocery stores and specialty markets. Fresh curd is purchased in squares called cakes.

Select cakes that are slightly firm and unbroken; they retain their shape better when cut. One-and-one-half cakes (2-1/2 by 2-1/2 by 1 inch) yield 1 cup of 1/2-inch cubes.

To use fresh curd in recipes, cut the curd and let stand a few minutes. Drain off liquid before adding to recipe.

To store fresh bean curd, cover with water and store, tightly covered, in the refrigerator. Change the water daily. The curd will remain fresh several days.

Canned soybean curd is also available. It is cut into 1-inch cubes. A 10-ounce can (drained weight) yields 2 cups of 1-inch cubes. Canned curd is darker in color and has a slightly different flavor and texture than fresh curd. Drain canned curd thoroughly before using.

Packaged instant bean curd powder is another form available. Prepare according to package directions. Cut and use it in the same way as fresh or canned bean curd.

Soybean Oil

Soybeans are rich in polyunsaturated oil, which is extracted for commercial use. Many commercial vegetable oils contain soybean oil.

Processed soybean oil is light in color, has a mild flavor, and can be used as oil in any recipe.

Unrefined soybean oil is dark brown and has a strong flavor and aroma. When used in recipes, it may alter the color and flavor of the final product.

Soybean oil keeps best at refrigerator temperature after opening.

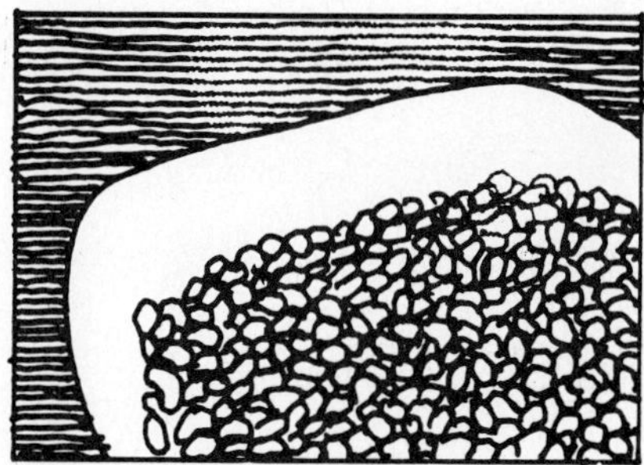

Seafoods for Health

Why Fish?

Nutrition is a key to good health, and fish and shellfish can play more than a nominal role in this aspect of our living. Also, fishery products when properly prepared can be delicious and satisfying to appetite and taste. **Historically,** fish and shellfish have been an important component in the diet of man. Food from the sea and fresh water has been sought by man since primitive times because it is nutritious and delicious. An old Chinese proverb recognized the nutritional value of fish: "Give a man a fish and he will live for a day, teach him to fish and he will have food for life."

Fish were often used as a medium of exchange or as payment for services rendered. In the 29th year of Ramses III, the Union of Grave Diggers in Egypt filed a petition with the royal authorities for higher wages. As part of their wages, these workers received large amounts of fish four times each month. The petition requested a pay increase, pointing out that the petitioners came to the authorities without clothes and ointments—and even without fish—the indispensible food.

As early as the 5th century B.C., it was recognized that fish could be farmed, just as hunters had previously come to realize that certain land animals could be domesticated. Ponds were constructed and stocked with fish by both the rich and the poor. Legal documents of the time indicate the importance of these food reservoirs.

Throughout recorded history the significant role of aquatic products in the diet is well documented. Until recently, however, only tacit recognition has been given to their nutritional and dietary attributes. We have come to recognize that fish and shellfish are not only satisfying to appetite and taste, but they are also highly nutritious.

The nutritional characteristics of fish and shellfish should be of vital interest to the consumer. The reasons are many. Dieticians must provide balanced and appealing meals, at economical prices, for large numbers of people. Certainly, fishery products are highly nutritious and an excellent means of obtaining dietary essentials, like protein, minerals, and vitamins. Moreover, the cost per pound of edible flesh from most fish is no more —and is often less—than that of many cuts of meat from domestic animals.

Individual consumers may be concerned about the caloric content of foods. The fat content of fish varies greatly between different species, and those with low amounts of fat are particularly suited for weight-control diets. Moreover, the fat in fish contains a high proportion of polyunsaturated fatty acids. Because a high proportion of polyunsaturates in the diet may help to decrease the incidence of atherosclerosis, heart specialists are particularly interested in the nutritional quality and composition of fishery products. Many doctors are now recommending generous portions of fish in the diet to increase the intake of polyunsaturated fatty acids, while insuring an adequate intake of protein.

Fishery products are also easily digested. They thus can play a major role in the diets of young children and elderly people, where ease of digestibility is of critical importance.

Custom-tailored diets can be prepared by the proper selection and inclusion in the diet of either fat or lean species of fish. Like people, fish come in many sizes and shapes, and may be classified as lean, medium, and fat. Of course, fat is only one of the major components of fish. The others are protein, minerals, and water. In general, an inverse relationship exists between the fat and water content of fish. These two components account for approximately 80 percent of the weight of fish, and when one of these is high the other tends to be low.

There are variations in the composition of fish and shellfish within a single species, and variations also occur between different species. Based on their gross composition, we can divide fish and shellfish into four main groups. In these groups are species with:

- Low-fat and high-protein content;
- Medium-fat and high-protein content;
- High-fat and low-protein content;
- Low-fat and low-protein content.

The terms "fat" and "oil" can be used interchangeably, since they refer to the same class of compounds. At room temperature, "fat" usually is in the solid form, while "oil" is in the liquid form.

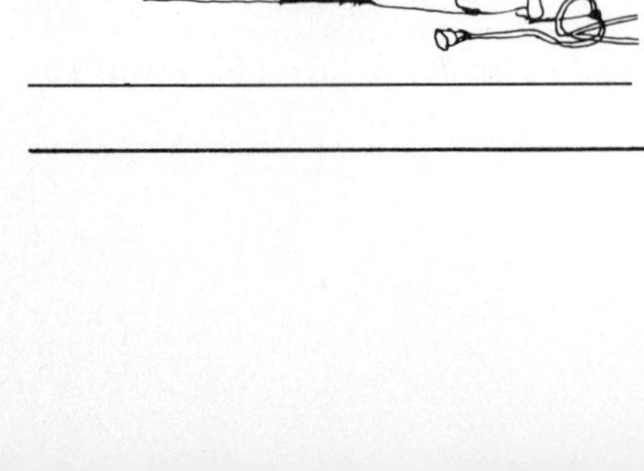

Most fish and shellfish fall into the low fat-high protein group. These fishery products have less than 5 percent fat and more than 15 percent protein. Included in this group are tunas, halibut, cod, flounders, haddock, pollock, mullet, ocean perch and other rockfishes, carp, whiting, crabs, scallops, shrimp, and lobsters. Tunas and halibut are particularly good sources of protein and may contain up to 25 percent. The fat content of many species in this class is closer to zero than to 5 percent.

Medium fat-high protein fish are those with 5 to 15 percent fat and more than 15 percent protein. Included in this group are anchovies, herring, mackerel, salmon, and sardines. The composition of fish in this group—as in other groups—varies during certain seasons of the year. For this reason, these species occasionally may be classified in other groups. Variation in composition is related to the feeding habits and sexual development of fish, as well as to other related factors. Both fat and protein content of fish can vary, depending on the amount and kinds of food eaten. Also, prior to spawning, the fat content of most fish is at its highest level, and it tends to be at its lowest level after spawning.

Only a few species of fish are in the high fat-low protein group—those that contain more than 15 percent fat and less than 15 percent protein. The fish in this category include certain subspecies of lake trout, and during particular seasons, herring, mackerel, and sardines. A particularly interesting representative of this group is the Siscowet lake trout. Individuals weighing more than 50 pounds have been caught in Lake Superior. The peculiar feature of these fish is that they contain a phenomenal amount of fat. Studies have revealed that fillets may contain from 20 to 70 percent fat; whereas protein content ranges from 6 to 16 percent. The fat, however, has been shown to contain the high levels of polyunsaturated fatty acids normally found in fish.

Oysters and clams are in the low fat-low protein group. These shellfish have a fat content of less than 5 percent and a protein content of less than 15 percent. The other major component, water, is present in amounts of about 80 percent.

Fish and shellfish can furnish many of the nutrients that are required by the body—and in generous amounts. No natural food by itself, however, including fish, can supply all essential nutrients required by people of all ages. Some foods may furnish adequate amounts of certain vitamins, while others may be a good source of protein. To insure adequate intake of all essential nutrients, it is important that a variety of foods be eaten.

About 45 nutrients must be included in our diet in sufficient quantities for normal body function and growth. These can be divided into six groups: water, proteins, carbohydrates, fats, vitamins, and minerals.

An adequate supply of water is often taken for granted, because it is on tap in almost every household. Water in one sense can be considered the most essential nutrient. A person can survive without food for 5 weeks or more; but without water, the fire of life flickers out in a few days.

Protein is a particularly critical dietary essential, and it is required in relatively large amounts. Unfortunately, protein is a costly dietary ingredient, and worldwide it is in short supply. The main function of protein is to supply the building blocks—amino acids—that are needed to make and repair body tissues, such as hair, skin, and muscles.

Carbohydrates and fats simply provide the fuel, or calories, required to keep the human engine running. Fats also contain compounds called fatty acids, which play a significant role in human health. As with most foods of animal origin, the carbohydrate content of fish and shellfish is low, and we will no longer consider it in our discussion.

The next group of nutrients are the vitamins. There are 13 vitamins that are essential for human health and that must be supplied by the diet. Included

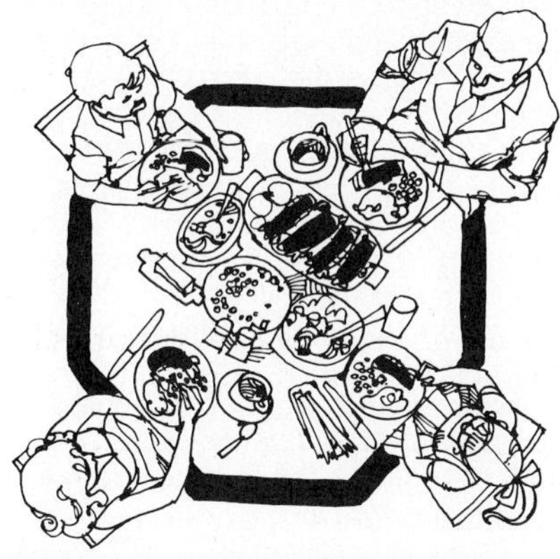

are vitamins A, C, D, E, K, and eight members of the vitamin B family. Vitamins are required in extremely minute amounts. They function as the sparks that ignite numerous chemical reactions throughout the body.

The remaining 17 essential nutrients are minerals. Based on the amounts required by the body, the minerals may be classified as either macroelements or microelements.

An ounce of each of the macroelements will meet the body's requirements for 1 month to 100 years, depending on the element. Minerals in the macro group include calcium, chlorine, iron, magnesium, phosphorus, potassium, sodium, and sulfur.

The microelements—or trace minerals—include chromium, cobalt, copper, fluorine, iodine, manganese, molybdenum, selenium, and zinc. As little as 0.1 ounce of some microelements is sufficient to meet the body's requirements for 100 years.

Fish and shellfish are excellent sources of high-quality protein. For centuries, it has been observed that those who obtain their food from the ocean and inland waters are well nourished. A scientific study in 1952 showed that the physical and nutritional condition of people in Northeast Brazil depended on the type of protein available. Tall, healthy individuals were found along the coast where most of the protein in the diet came from fish. In the jungle, where foods of vegetable origin formed the principal dietary staple, people were shorter in stature and malnutrition was, and still is, more prevalent.

Such studies have shown that fish and shellfish contain protein of excellent quality that clearly place them in a unique and enviable class. There is no mystery surrounding the attributes of protein from fish. Simply stated, protein in fish and shellfish contains generous amounts of the amino acids that are needed to construct body protein. Moreover, fish protein is easily and almost completely digested.

Protein contain four basic elements: carbon, oxygen, hydrogen, and nitrogen. By combining these four elements in various ways, molecules called amino acids are formed. In turn, amino acids combine to form protein molecules, which are further linked together to form muscle fibers or other tissues.

Unlike the building blocks used to construct buildings, amino acids are not of uniform shape, size, or composition. Rather, there are some 22 different amino acids that are required by the body in order to synthesize protein. Of these, 13 are called "nonessential" amino acids because they can be manufactured by the body if sufficient nitrogen is supplied by the diet. The remaining 9 amino acids are termed "essential," since they cannot be synthesizd by the body but must be supplied by the food that we eat.

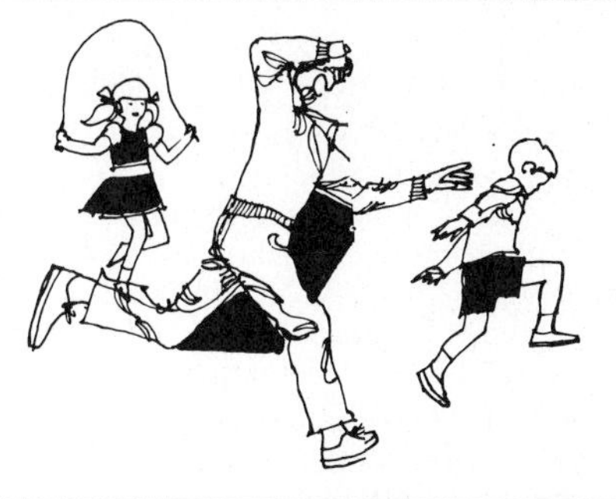

Essential amino acids are as vital to human health as are the more publicized vitamins. But amino acids are needed in much larger quantities than vitamins. As we have seen, protein is an essential part of the diet for two basic reasons. First, protein furnishes nitrogen, which the body uses to synthesize nonessential amino acids. Second, it supplies the essential acids, which the body uses—together with the nonessential amino acids—to manufacture muscle and tissue protein

Food protein varies considerably in its ability to furnish amino acids that the body requires. Some foods contain small amounts of protein and thus supply small amounts of amino acids.

Often proteins in some foods severely lack one or more essential amino acids. Such is the case with proteins from many, but not all, grains and vegetables. Sometimes, these foods have relatively small amounts of protein, and generally this protein does not contain a well-balanced mixture of essential amino acids.

Unfortunately, many people especially in developing countries, have no choice but to obtain most of their dietary protein from cereal grains and vegetables. These people often suffer from protein malnutrition, which may seriously retard mental as well as physical development. Research shows that children who experience protein malnutrition in early life may suffer permanent mental damage. Thus the success of improved feeding programs may ultimately depend on whether or not the nutritional needs of the child are met during prenatal development.

Fish, meat, and dairy products are examples of foods that have proteins of excellent quality, and in abundant amounts. Also, the essential amino acids in proteins from animal foods are well balanced in relation to our body's requirements. Scientists have found that the amino acid composition of proteins from most animal sources is similar to that of human tissue. Because of this similarity, proteins in fish, meat, and dairy products usually have high nutritive values.

A serving as small as 4 ounces of lean fish will supply about half the total amount of protein required each day by the body. The other half can easily be supplied by a normal intake of protein of nonanimal origin. Although total protein content varies between lean and fatty fish, amino acid composition and quality of the protein is remarkably constant. Thus, the quality of the protein is high, regardless of whether it comes from lean or fatty fish.

Fish and a few other foods are often referred to by food faddists as brain food. There is no basis for this claim. In fact, no such thing as brain food exists, anymore than there is a big-toe food or a little-finger food. As we have pointed out, fish is a particularly good source of high-quality protein. When it is included in a balanced diet, it provides nourishment to all body tissues and shows no special preference for any particular part of the body.

Certain shellfish contain protein that is especially high in quality. Oysters, for example, are extremely well suited for man and are frequently used in therapeutic diets. The protein content of oysters is low, compared to that of most other fish and shellfish. The quality of oyster protein, however, is superior to that of most fish and to that of beef. Although oysters are excellent food, we have no scientific basis for the commonly held view that sexual potency is increased when generous amounts are consumed.

Ease of digestibility is another factor that is related to the quality of food proteins. Digestion may be defined as the breakdown of large food particles into smaller units so that they are available for absorption and utilization by the body. Absorption of amino acids from proteins by humans is directly related to the ease to which the digestive tract is able to split proteins into their individual amino acids. Proteins in some food are difficult to split; therefore, these proteins are poorly utilized. Poor digestibility may be related to the inherent natural characteristics of the protein, or it may be caused by the methods used to process the food.

Normal processing—like boiling, steaming, canning, or freezing—has little or no effect on the digestibility or nutritive quality of protein. But, when foods are exposed to high temperatures or pressures for an extended period of time, the digestibility and nutritive quality of protein may be markedly decreased. For example, improper drying, salting, or cooking of fishery products may decrease the nutritive quality of protein. Or severe heat treatments used to manufacture toasted or puffed breakfast cereals can be especially damaging to the quality of protein.

For many centuries, fish and shellfish have been considered to be easily digestible. Recent research has shown that 90 to 100 percent of fish protein is digestible. The digestibility of protein in fish and shellfish is considered to be slightly higher than that of beef and chicken.

We do not fully understand the reasons for the relative ease of digestion of fish and shellfish, but two partial explanations can be advanced. Compared with mammals, fishery products have a much greater ratio of muscle protein (e.g., tropomyosin and actomyosin) to connective tissue protein (e.g., collagen and elastin). Muscle protein is believed to be more readily digestible than connective tissue protein. Also, the relatively shorter length of fish muscle fiber (compared with mammalian muscle fiber) may play a role by allowing enzymes in the stomach to react more quickly with the protein. Once this initial stage of digestion is completed, fish protein quickly moves through succeeding stages of digestion and then assimilation by body tissues. This protein, so vitally needed for body building and tissue repair, is made available for utilization sooner.

Because fishery products are easily digested and well utilized, they are included in many special diets for people with digestive disorders. Fish and shellfish are used liberally in diets often recommended for convalescent ulcer patients.

Since fishery products contain low amounts of connective tissue and fibrous components, they are especially suited for low-bulk, bland diets. Here, the goal is to minimize the amount of undigested food in the digestive tract and still provide a diet that is nutritionally adequate. Often, fishery products can be included in diets for people with digestive disorders to provide a wider variety of main dishes that are flavorful and appealing, but still suited to special dietary needs.

Oil in fish and shellfish can play a significant roll in human health. A great deal of attention has recently been given to the relationship between the amount and type of fat in the diet and the incidence of heart disease. This relationship has not been conclusively established—though evidence does suggest that a high intake of meat fat may be one of the predisposing factors contributing to heart disease. Because fat in fish and shellfish has a unique chemical nature, fishery products are often recommended in diets designed to minimize the risk of heart disease. The reason for this can be better understood by a brief examination of the chemistry of fats.

In almost all foods, fat (or oil) is composed primarily of "triglycerides." A triglyceride molecule can be pictured as being shaped like the letter "E." The vertical side contains three carbon atoms that are connected like the links of a chain. This is the "glycerol" portion of the triglyceride. The three arms of the triglyceride molecule are termed "fatty acids." The skeleton of each fatty acid may contain from 4 to 32 carbon atoms that are connected in chainlike fashion. The key that determines the type of fat or oil in a given food is locked in the kinds of fatty acids in the triglyceride.

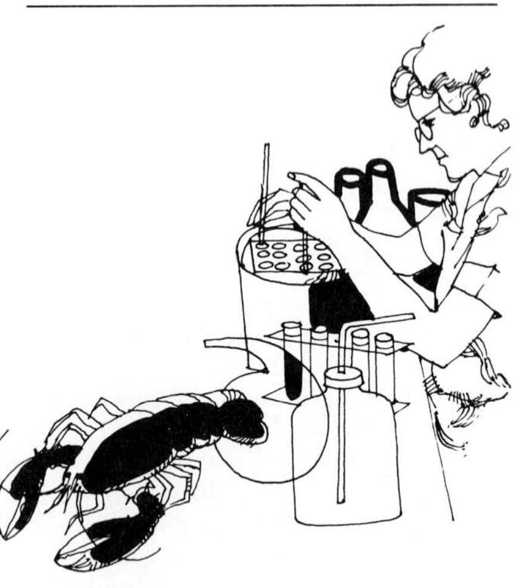

Fatty acids may differ in two ways. The first is in the size or length of the fatty acid chains. As indicated, they may contain as few as 4 and as many as 32 carbon atoms. The second way in which fatty acids differ is in the number of hydrogen atoms attached to each carbon atom in the chain.

- If two hydrogen atoms are attached to each carbon atom, we say that the fatty acid is "saturated."
- If two adjacent carbon atoms each contain only one hydrogen atom, the fatty acid is "unsaturated."
- If more than one pair of unsaturated carbon atoms is present, the fatty acid is referred to as "polyunsaturated."

This is the basic explanation of terms that have become common household words.

The content of polyunsaturated fatty acids in the oil of fish and shellfish is uniformly high, even though the total amount of oil may vary widely between different species. As noted previously, the oil content of fish may range from zero to well over 15 percent. Most fish, however, contain less than 5 percent oil. Meat from land animals also varies widely in fat content. Lean cuts of beef contain about 5 percent fat, whereas prime porterhouse steak may contain over 40 percent fat. The two main features that distinguish fish oil from other animal fat are: the unusually long fatty acid chains in fish oil and an exceedingly high degree of unsaturation in the fatty acid chains.

Meat fat and vegetable oil contain only small amounts of fatty acids with more than 18 carbon atoms. In fish oil, one-third or more of the fatty acids have more than 18 carbon atoms. Most fatty acids in fish oil contain either 16, 18, 20, or 22 carbon atoms. As much as 60 to 85 percent of these fatty acids are unsaturated, and many are polyunsaturated. Many of the fatty acids with 20 carbon atoms contain 5 pairs that are unsaturated. Many with 22 carbon atoms contain 6 pairs that are unsaturated.

Thus, compared with meat fat, fish oil contains more unsaturated fatty acids; also, fish fatty acids possess a greater number of unsaturated pairs of carbon atoms. Vegetable oil may contain more unsaturated fatty acids than fish oil. But, since fatty acids in vegetable oil rarely contain more than two pairs of unsaturated carbon atoms, the total number of unsaturated sites is less than that in fish oil. The total effectiveness of the polyunsaturates in fish oil is therefore much greater than that of vegetable oil.

The relationship of diet and heart disease has been the subject of much research in recent years. Evidence from some studies has indicated that diets—containing large amounts of fat composed mostly of saturated fatty acids—tend to produce high amounts of cholesterol in the blood. People with high blood cholesterol levels tend to run a higher risk of developing atherosclerosis. We should point out that diet is only one of many factors that is apparently related to the incidence of heart disease. This is a particularly complex medical problem, for which there is, as yet, no simple answer.

Two dietary modifications are often recommended to reduce the incidence of heart disease among vulnerable groups. The first is to reduce the fat content and the total caloric content of the diet. The second is to partially substitute polyunsaturated fatty acids for saturated fatty acids.

The American Heart Association has recommended that vulnerable persons should reduce fat consumption under medical supervision. Drastic reduction in dietary fat is seldom recommended, however, since this forces a high consumption of carbohydrates and proteins to maintain caloric levels for active men. Some evidence indicates that large amounts of carbohydrates increase the amount of blood cholesterol, which would offset any benefits from using a low-fat diet.

The Association has also advised that, in some instances, a diet higher in unsaturated and lower in saturated fats would lead to a reduction in blood cholesterol levels. This might reduce the chances of developing various undesirable heart conditions. In this respect, it is interesting to note the results of a study reported in the *Journal of the American Medical Association* in 1966.

In this study, over 800 male members—aged 40 to 59—of an Anticoronary Club were compared with 475 volunteers picked at random. The purpose was to test the efficacy of a special anticoronary diet. In this diet, total calories and calories from saturated fat were reduced, while the amount of polyunsaturated fat was increased. Meat was de-emphasized and a minimum of four seafood meals per week was prescribed. At the end of four years, significant reductions in obesity, hypertension, high blood pressure, and blood cholesterol were noted. The incidence of coronary diseases among the members of the Anticoronary Club was only one-third as great as that for the volunteers, who were not on the special diet.

A relationship between serum cholesterol and heart disease was demonstrated in a study conducted in Framingham, Mass. Men, aged 40 to 49, were studied for 10 years. A progressive increase in susceptibility to coronary disease was found with increasing concentrations of blood cholesterol. The death rate of individuals with high cholesterol levels was three times greater than in the group with low cholesterol levels.

Much controversy and confusion still surrounds the problem of what does and does not cause heart disease, but a few clear points have emerged. First, we have no proof that high blood cholesterol levels cause heart disease, nor do we have any assurance that low blood cholesterol levels will prevent heart disease. Second, the risk that coronary disease will develop is related to a number of factors, including body weight and blood cholesterol levels. This last point was recognized by the Council on Foods and Nutrition of the American Medical Association. It recommended that the physician consider regulating dietary fat to prevent the increase of serum cholesterol and other lipids, which may occur with increasing age in men, thus putting them in a high-risk category. The Council also emphasized the desirability of regulating dietary fat to reduce the amount of cholesterol in the serum of individuals who are especially susceptible to heart disease.

Fishery products can play a major role in helping to regulate the fat in diets, thereby reducing the incidence of heart disease. Many studies have shown that ingestion of oil containing large amounts of polyunsaturated fatty acids will tend to suppress the blood cholesterol level and lower the incidence of atherosclerosis. Few people, however, will want to consume oil directly for its polyunsaturated properties. A much more palatable method is simply to include generous portions of fishery products in the diet. To illustrate, some salmon average nearly 15 percent oil. A 6-ounce serving would furnish nearly an ounce of oil rich in polyunsaturated fatty acids.

Not only do fish contain high proportions of polyunsaturated fatty acids, but they also contain relatively small amounts of cholesterol. Fishery products generally contain about as much cholesterol, or cholesterol-like compounds, as meat and milk products. Certain cuts of beef and some egg products, however, contain up to 10 times as much cholesterol as is found in fish and shellfish.

Reducing the total intake of calories, however, is often as important as including liberal quantities of polyunsaturated fatty acids in the diet. In this case, fish that are low in oil can form the main entree of a meal. Total caloric intake will be reduced, while still providing adequate protein to meet the body's requirements. Low-fat fish and shellfish normally contain less than 100 calories in a 4-ounce serving. On the other hand, a 4-ounce serving of many cuts of good-quality beef may supply well over 300 calories. For those who are calorie conscious, substituting seafoods offers a distinct advantage over meats that are high in fat.

Vitamins in fishery products have been given little consideration thus far. We can divide the 13 common vitamins into two major groups: fat-soluble vitamins and water-soluble vitamins. In fishery products, fat-soluble vitamins are found in oil. Vitamins in the water-soluble group are in the water that is dispersed throughout.

In the history of vitamins, it was early recognized that fish liver oil was a rich

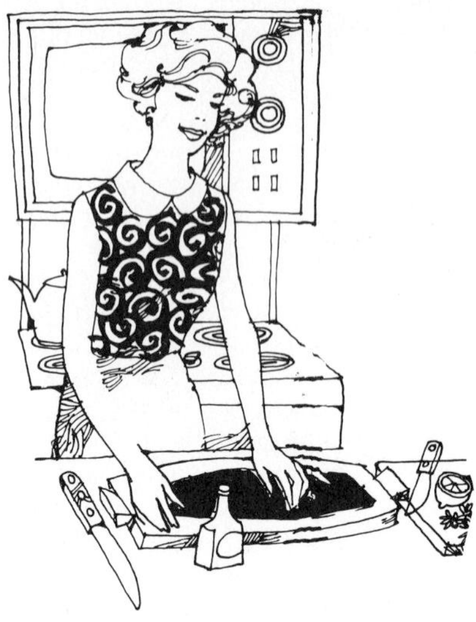

natural source of fat-soluble vitamins, especially vitamins A and D. Many people, who were raised during the first half of the 20th century, can recall the ritual of taking a daily dose of cod liver oil. Although fish liver oil was long considered the primary source of fat-soluble vitamins, its use has dwindled since the introduction of synthetically produced vitamins. Vitamin pills have been promoted and sold so successfully that people give little consideration to the amounts of vitamins that are supplied in the diet. Most nutritionists agree that a well-balanced diet will supply sufficient amounts of all vitamins.

Although fish liver oil in an extremely rich source of fat-soluble vitamins, the flesh of fish contains relatively little of these vitamins. Food consumed by fish contains large amounts of most fat-soluble vitamins, and fish simply store these in their liver. Vitamin A in fish liver oil results from the large amount of carotene that is present in the food of fish.

Fish oil generally has a higher content of fat-soluble vitamins than the fat of land animals. In turn, it should not come as a great surprise to learn that fatty fish contain more of these vitamins than do lean fish. Some fatty fish are an excellent source of vitamin D; lean fish contain very small amounts. The vitamin A content of the flesh of most fish is relatively low. It has been reported, however, that swordfish and whitefish contain high amounts of vitamin A.

As for water-soluble vitamins, four of the eight members of the vitamin B family can be supplied in adequate amounts by fish and shellfish. These four vitamins are B_6, B_{12}, biotin, and niacin. The remaining four B vitamins are found in fishery products, but generally are not present in appreciable quantities. Larger amounts of B vitamins are usually found in high-fat fish than in low-fat fish. It has also been found that the B vitamin content of the dark meat of fish is many times higher than that of the white meat. The B vitamin content of fish is about the same as that of meat from land animals.

Fishery products are also a valuable source of many essential minerals. The mineral content of fish and shellfish has been the subject of much investigation. Most of the research, however, has dealt with the macroelements. It is well established, for example, that fish contain relatively large amounts of phosphorus, potassium, and iron. Conversely, the sodium and chlorine content of fish is relatively low, despite the relative richness of sea water in sodium chloride.

Since the advent of the low-sodium diet, much attention has been focused on the sodium content of fish and shellfish. Occasionally, doubt is expressed about the advisability of using fish in low-sodium diets that are prescribed for people suffering from hypertension. This doubt is not well founded, even in the case of salt-water fish.

The maximum sodium content of the low-sodium diet is 100 milligrams per 100 grams of food. With the exception of most shellfish, no species of fish contains as much sodium in an average serving as this maximum permitted level. Fresh oysters and soft clams are low in sodium. Other shellfish often contain about 200 to 400 milligrams of sodium per 100 grams. If salt has been added during processing, fish will contain sodium levels in excess of the maximum permissible level. Normally, however, fish may be used quite freely in low-sodium diets. Since fish vary considerably in flavor and texture, they offer the possibility of variety and diversification in low-sodium diets.

Fish and shellfish contain at least as much of the macroelements as is found in meat from domestic animals. Fish contain greater amounts of calcium magnesium, and chlorine than meat does. The potassium, phosphorus, and sulfur levels are about equal to those of meat. In general, the iron and sodium content of fish is less than that of beef. Certain shellfish contain more.

Fishery products are noted for a high content of microminerals, or "trace minerals." Because trace minerals perform vital functions, fish and shellfish are viewed with special interest. Most essential trace minerals are present in fishery products in amounts at least equivalent to those in meat, and usually in much higher amounts than in vegetables and dairy products.

Marine foods are by far the richest source of iodine in the ordinary diet. The importance of iodine in preventing goiter has been recognized since the turn of the 20th century. As might be expected, salt-water fish and shellfish contain considerably more iodine than do fresh-water varieties. Of the salt-water varieties, shellfish generally contain the highest amount of iodine.

Fishery products are an excellent source of fluoride, and for this reason their inclusion in the diet should be encouraged. Several years ago, medical research established that the intake of small amounts of fluoride by children helps prevent tooth decay. The low incidence of tooth decay in some people has been attributed to high consumption of fish. This is true of people in the Orient who eat large quantities of fresh and processed fish and who generally have excellent teeth. More recent medical evidence strongly indicates that a high dietary intake of fluoride by older people may be desirable to help prevent arteriosclerosis and certain bone diseases, like osteoporosis.

Several other essential trace minerals are abundant in fishery products. These include copper, zinc, manganese, cobalt, molybdenum, and

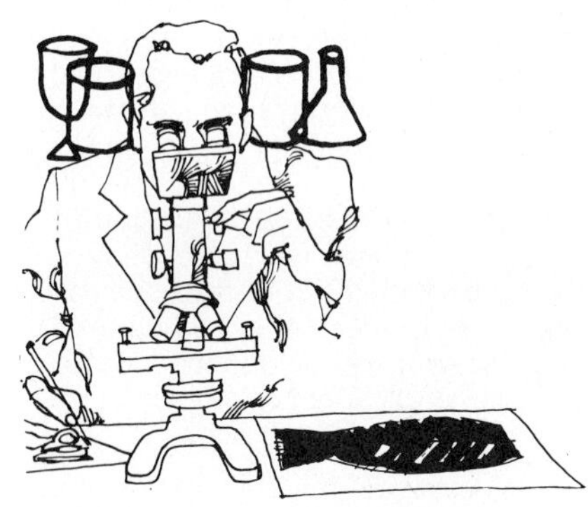

selenium. Especially interesting is that large quantities of these trace elements are found in fish eggs (cod roe) and in shellfish. Oysters are a particularly good source of micronutrients. An average serving of these seafoods will supply sufficient amounts of the trace minerals to meet daily requirements. Microminerals in the flesh of fish and shellfish are completely absorbed and fully utilized by the human body.

Nutritionally, fish and shellfish can make major contributions to our diet. Adequate nutrition is critical for each of the more than 3 billion people in the world. Unfortunately, not everyone is equally concerned about good nutrition. For some, the basic concern is simply to have a sufficient quantity of food to relieve pains of hunger. These are the people who represent nearly two-thirds of the world population, and to whom undernutrition and malnutrition are facts of life.

Fishery products can be a major weapon against hunger and malnutrition. For this reason, scientists are striving to develop the resources of the sea so that fishery products can be a more effective and available source of food for those in need.

What about adequate nutrition for people in affluent societies where food is abundant and the choices are many? Again, the nutritional quality of the diet is not the primary concern of these people. Their lack of concern, however, is much different from that of the people who are undernourished. Where food is plentiful, convenience and good taste are overriding factors which determine the foods that people select. Nutrition often takes a back seat in today's modern world, and many people who can most afford an adequate diet are the ones who have an inadequate nutrient intake. This is particularly true of teenagers who consume large quantities of foods that are high in carbohydrates. Yet, good nutrition, good taste, and convenience can be compatible.

Fish and shellfish can also contribute to the enjoyment of eating. Over 150 varieties—either fresh or processed—are available to the consumer. With this multiplicity of choice, it is possible to find fishery products to please even the most discriminating palate. Seafood, however, is a most delicate food and must be handled with care from the time it is caught until it is placed on the table. Natural goodness and taste is easily lost if improper preservation and processing techniques are used. Whereas meats tend to improve with "aging," fish and shellfish are at their best when freshly caught.

In the past, fresh fishery products were available only to those who lived near the sea or inland waters. Today, modern rapid transportation has made it possible for seafood to be available to many people, regardless of distance from the sea. Also, science has greatly improved methods of preserving seafoods. With the advent of frozen foods it is now possible to purchase all kinds of seafoods anywhere in the United States any time of the year. We may look to the future and expect to have fresh seafood available that has been preserved by irradiation from atomic energy. Fortunately, most modern methods that are used to preserve fish or shellfish have little effect on their nutritional value.

Many new and appetizing fishery products have become available in recent years. Fish sticks and portions have proven popular. They are nutritious and appetizing, especially to children and teenagers. Moreover, these products are exceptionally good buys, in terms of price per pound of edible food.

The methods used in preparing fish and shellfish for the table are just as important as the methods used in preservation and processing. Good fish can be easily spoiled if improperly cooked. The flesh of fish may be likened to egg white. Fish should be cooked only until the flesh "sets" and can be easily flaked from the bones. Fish may be baked, broiled, boiled, or fried. Certain types of fish are more suitable for particular methods of cooking. For example, fatty fish are considered better for broiling and baking and lean fish are more appropriately broiled, boiled, or steamed. The important point to remember is that overcooking should be avoided to preserve the natural texture and flavor.

Fish and shellfish can be delicious in taste and prepared with ease. They should be thought of as more than a substitute for meat. They can be used as a first course or an appetizer or as the main attraction. Even the most discriminating connoisseur can find the right seafood to suit his particular purpose and taste. When cooked and flavored with appropriate herbs and spices—and consumed with a special vintage wine—seafoods can be a truly enjoyable experience in eating.

"Fish must swim thrice—once in the water, a second time in the sauce, and a third time in wine of stomach."
John Ray: *English Proverbs* (1670).

How to Buy Red Snapper and Others

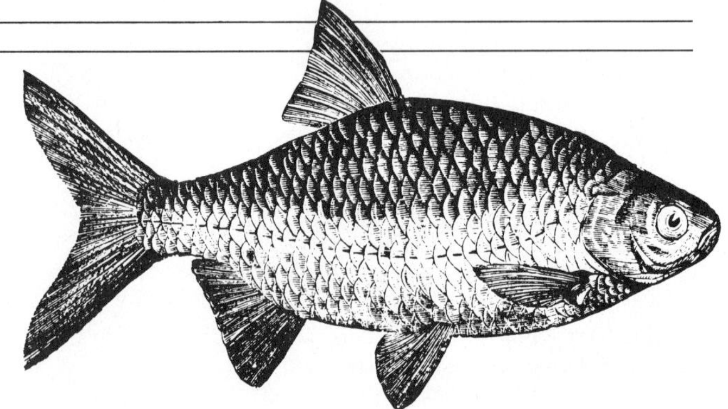

Each year, about three billion pounds of fish and shellfish are caught commercially for food in the United States. The consumer may buy these fresh and frozen in a variety of forms.

* Whole or round fish are marketed just as they come from the water. Before cooking, they must be scaled and eviscerated. Usually, head, tail, and fins are removed.

* Drawn fish are marketed with only the entrails removed. They need to be scaled and head, tail, and fins are removed before cooking.

* Dressed or pan-dressed fish are both scaled and eviscerated; usually, head, tail, and fins are removed and they are ready for cooking. Smaller fish, called pan-dressed, usually have head and tail left on, and are ready for cooking. Larger, dressed fish are frequently cut into steaks or fillets.

* Steaks are cross-section slices of the larger types of dressed fish. They are ready to cook as purchased.

* Fillets are the sides of dressed fish, cut lengthwise away from the backbone. They are practically boneless, may be skinned, and require no preparation before cooking.

* Butterfly fillets are two sides or fillets of the fish held together by the uncut belly skin and are usually boneless.

* Fish sticks are pieces of fish cut from frozen fish blocks into uniform portions usually about 1 inch wide and 3 inches long. They weigh up to 1 1/2 ounces.

* Fish portions, so very popular today, are cut from frozen fish blocks into uniform portions weighing not less than 1 1/2 ounces and up to 6 ounces.

* Shellfish (such as clams, lobsters, oysters, and some varieties of crabs) should be alive if purchased in the shell.

* Shucked shellfish have shells removed.

* Shrimp are usually sold headless. "Green" shrimp applies to raw, headless shrimp in the shell in most areas. Peeled shrimp are headless shrimp with the shells removed. Deveined shrimp are shrimp with the intestinal track or black vein down the back removed. Cooked shrimp, available fresh, frozen, and canned, is usually sold peeled and deveined, ready to use.

PURCHASING FRESH FISH

Check your fish dealer for information on when to purchase fish. Different varieties of fish are abundant at different times of the year. Check with your dealer.

When buying fish whole or round, watch for bright, clear eyes; reddish-pink gills free from odor or slime; and bright-colored scales adhering tightly to skin. Flesh is firm and elastic (springs back when pressed gently) and free from objectionable odors.

Fish is perishable and must be handled with utmost care. Fresh fish should be packed in ice and kept in the coolest part of the refrigerator.

PURCHASING FROZEN FISH

Excellent variety of products with built-in labor bonus makes these items a good buy.

Frozen fish should be stored at -10 degrees F. or lower until ready to use. Dressed frozen fish, fillets, and steaks may be cooked in frozen form but require extra cooking time.

Thawing is necessary for cleaning and dressing of frozen whole and drawn fish. Thawing at refrigerator temperatures (40 degrees to 45 degrees F.) is accepted practice. But fish should be held this temperature only long enough to permit ease of preparation. Never refreeze thawed or partially thawed fish.

PURCHASING CANNED FISH

Wide variety is offered in canned fish, shellfish, and speciality products. These include canned clams, salmon, sardines, shrimp, and tuna in addition to fish balls, chowders, cakes, and roe.

Five species of salmon are canned on the West Coast and Alaska. The higher priced varieties are deeper red in color and have a higher oil content. Salmon may be purchased in 3 3/4-, 7 1/2-, 15 1/2-, and 64-ounce cans.

There are two broad classifications of canned tuna--white meat, which in the United States, may be canned only from albacore, and light meat, which is canned primarily from yellowfin, bluefin, and skipjack species. Tuna may be purchased in 3 1/2-, 7-, 13-, and 60- to 66 1/2-ounce cans.

Store canned fish in a cool, dry place; avoid high temperatures and humidity.

FISH FAVORITES

Some of the more popular fresh or frozen fish varieties regularly used by food service operators are:

Catfish: Available whole, dressed, fresh, and frozen. Deep-fat fry or use in catfish stew.

Cod: Available breaded, raw and precooked in sticks or portions; fillets, fresh, frozen, or dry-salted. Deep fat-fry, broil, poach, or bake fresh or frozen portions; use salt cod in creamed dishes and in fish cakes.

Halibut: Available drawn, dressed in steak form, fresh, and frozen. Broil or bake; stuff and broil or bake. Cooked flakes may be used in casseroles.

Perch: Available fresh or frozen dressed whole and filleted. Pan-fry, deep-fry, or baked in sauce.

Pollock: Available dressed as fillets; fresh or frozen. Deep fat-fry, broil,or bake; cook in sauce.

Red Snapper: Available dressed, steaks, and fillets, fresh and frozen. Deep fat-fry, broil, or bake.

Salmon: Available dressed, fresh or frozen in steaks or fillets; also smoked and canned. Poach, bake, broil, pan-fry; flakes of fresh or canned salmon are used for fried patties or cakes and in salads.

Sole: Available whole or in fillets; fresh or frozen. Deep-fry, stuff and bake, broil, pan-fry.

Trout: Brook trout and rainbow trout, raised on trout farms, are usually purchased whole, frozen, and dressed. The 6- to 12-ounce fish are most popular. Broil, bake, stuff and bake, saute, or pan-fry.

Whitefish: Available whole, drawn, dressed, in fillets, fresh or frozen. Bake, broil, or poach.

SHELLFISH FAVORITES

Shellfish are divided into two classifications: crustaceans, which include crabs, crayfish, lobster, and shrimp; and mollusks, which include clams, oysters, and scallops.

Shellfish are among the most delicate and perishable of foods. Bargains should never be considered unless top quality is assured. Purchase only the best at all times, but not necessarily the most expensive. Once purchased, shellfish must be kept refrigerated until preparation time.

CRUSTACEANS

Shrimp: Raw or "green" shrimp varies from a greenish-grey to reddish-brown depending on the species and where it is caught. The common varieties are: white or common; brown or grooved; pink or coral; red or royal. When cooked, all are similar in appearance, flavor, texture, and yield.

The term "shrimp" refers to the fresh, frozen, or cooked tail section of the shrimp.

These tails are graded according to number per pound--a unit known as the "count". The shrimp are usually designated by such terms, corresponding to number per pound, as jumbo, large, medium, small, etc. Regular, non-peeled shrimp are divided into the following catagories: 15 and under; 16 to 20; 21 to 25; 26 to 30; 31 to 42; 42 and over.

Shrimp are marketed headless, peeled and deveined, cooked in the shell, cooked, peeled, and deveined, and breaded.

Shrimp are also marketed as broken, imperfect pieces for use in salads or mixed dishes where shape is unimportant. Shrimp in the shell are usually marketed frozen in 5-pound boxes. Shelf-ready, freezer-dried shrimp are also available in hermetically sealed cans. The water is removed from the shrimp in a special freezing and drying process.

Shrimp may be boiled for use as hors d'oeuvres, in cocktails, salads, sandwiches; cooked in Newburg, creole, and other sauces; sauteed or dipped in breading or batter and then deep fried. Large shrimp may be stuffed and baked.

Breaded uncooked shrimp ready for deep-frying, and precooked, breaded shrimp, ready to heat-and-serve are also available.

Prawns are large shrimp, and the term usually refers to jumbo Gulf shrimp.

Lobster: Live northern or Maine lobsters may be purchased for shipment to all parts of the country. They are also available alive, through the use of holding tanks, in many areas of the country. Lobsters may also be obtained in three other forms: cooked in the shell, fresh or frozen lobster meat, and canned lobster meat. Except in the producing areas, fresh lobsters cooked in the shell and lobster meat are not found on the market in large quantities.

A live lobster may weigh from 3/4-pound to 3 pounds or heavier. The meat comes from both the tail and claws. Northern or Maine lobsters must not be confused with crayfish or rock lobster, which have marketable tails only.

The frozen tails of the rock lobsters are imported to the United States largely from South Africa, Australia, and New Zealand. Rock lobster tails usually run from 4 ounces to 1 pound each.

Whole lobsters may be broiled, or baked stuffed and served in the shell. Lobster meat is used for salads, cocktails, sandwiches; in Newburg; in chowders and bisques.

Lobster tails may be treated in the same manner as other lobsters, but are used most successfully broiled, baked, and baked stuffed.

Crabs: Varieties available are the hard-shell or blue crab from Atlantic waters, the Dungeness crab from Pacific waters, and King and tanner or queen crab from Pacific waters off Alaska. Soft-shell crabs are molting blue crabs that have shed their hard shells.

Crabs may be purchased in the following forms: live; cooked in the shell; fresh, frozen, or pasteurized meat, and canned meat. Near the fishing grounds, crabs are generally sold alive or freshly cooked.

Hard-shell crabs are frequently cooked by steaming or boiling almost as soon as taken from the water. As the meat is very perishable, the crabs must be refrigerated or packed in ice till used.

The meat is picked from cooked crabs and shipped in iced containers.

Cooked blue crab meat is available in the following forms:

* Lump meat--comes from the larger muscles. It is known as "special" or back-fin. The meat is white.

* Flake meat--also white in color is the remaining portion of the body meat.

* Flake and lump meat--in some sections both kinds of white meat are packed together.

* Claw meat--as the name implies, comes from the claws. The outer surface of the meat is brownish in color. There is only one grade.

Crab meat may be sauteed, creamed, served in New burg, salads, cocktails, sandwiches, and hors d'oeuvres. Whole crabs may be steamed and served with drawn butter.

King crabs weigh from 6 to 20 pounds each. The leg meat is available cooked and frozen in 5 pound blocks; cooked and frozen leg sections in the shell are available whole and split. Whole legs may be broiled, baked in the shell, or served cold with mayonnaise.

Soft-shell crabs are available fresh or frozen. They are marketed by size or number to the pound. They are usually cleaned prior to freezing and may be eaten shell and all. Soft-shell crabs may be sauteed or deep fried.

Canned and pasteurized crab meat are available in all parts of the country and can be used interchangeably in recipes calling for cooked crab meat.

Deviled crab in aluminum foil "shells" are now marketed frozen ready to heat-and serve.

MOLLUSKS

Bay and Sea Scallops: Bay scallops, taken from inshore waters, are small and considered a delicacy. The supply is very limited. The large sea scallop, an inhabitant of offshore banks and deep waters, is the one used extensively in quantity food operations. Both species have sweet, firm, white meat.

Scallops can be served broiled, en brochette (on a skewer), sauteed, breaded and deep fried, au gratin, in Newburg sauce, and in soups and chowders.

Clams: Clams in the shell should be alive when purchased. Gaping shells that will not close when handled mean that the hard-shell clam is dead and no longer usable. With other varieties, the siphon or neck of a live clam will twitch when touched. Shell clams will remain alive for several days if refrigerated at about 40 degrees F. They are sold by the peck, bushel, and barrel.

Shucked clams should be plump, with clear liquor, and free from any pieces of shell. They should be kept refrigerated or packed in ice. When properly handled, they will remain fresh and in good condition for a week to 10 days. Shucked clams are usually purchased by the gallon for chowders, for frying, or sauced entrees.

Frozen shucked clams should not be thawed until ready to use; once thawed, they should never be refrozen.

Cherrystone and Little Neck clams can be served raw on the half shell.

Soft-shell clams can be steamed and served with broth in which they were cooked and with drawn butter.

Frozen fresh clam strips are available for deep frying.

Shucked clams are canned whole, minced, or as clam chowder and are widely used in many quantity food establishments.

Oysters: Oysters vary in size, texture, and flavor according to where they are harvested. They inhabit the Atlantic and Pacific Coasts and the Gulf of Mexico. Those taken from the waters of the Atlantic, from the Canadian Maritime Provinces to Texas, are known as Eastern oysters. The Olympia, a small delicately-flavored oyster, is found in Puget Sound. The giant Japanese oyster is taken from the Pacific.

Oysters may be purchased in three forms; live in the shell, fresh and frozen shucked, and canned.

Shell oysters are sold by the bushel, sack, and barrel. They should be alive when purchased, as indicated by a tightly-closed shell. Oysters with gaping shells that do not close when handled are dead and unfit to eat. Shell oysters refrigerated at 40 degrees F. or lower will keep alive for several days.

Shucked oysters should be plump and have a natural cream color, with clear liquor free from shell particles. Fresh shucked oysters are packed in metal containers or waxed cartons and should be kept refrigerated. They are sold by the pint, quart, and gallon. When properly refrigerated, they will remain fresh from a week to 10 days.

Oysters may be served raw on the half shell as appetizers or baked on the half shell with various toppings. Shucked oysters may be escalloped, breaded and fried, or used for chowders, stews, bisques, and in stuffing mixtures.

Eastern oysters are designated by terms corresponding to number of meats to the gallon: small,301 to 500; select, 211 to 300, preferred for frying; extra selects, 160 to 210, and counts, under 160 to the gallon.

PREPARING FISH AND SEAFOOD

Frying: Most fish cooked in quantity food operations is deep fried. When properly fried, fish and seafoods are appetizing and inviting. They have an attractive brown color, a crisp, non-greasy crust, a thoroughly cooked interior without being overcooked, and the characteristic flavor of the specific fish.

Frying Fats: The quality of the frying fat is of prime importance because it affects the flavor of the fish. For this reason, the fat must be frequently checked.

The following fats are the ones commonly used for deep frying: hydrogenated shortening; salad oils of good quality produced from cotton seed, peanut, or corn oil; and modern lards that have an anti-oxidant added.

Do not overload frying kettle. The ratio to use is 1:8, that is 1 pound of fish to 8 pounds of fat.

Frying Temperatures: The temperature of frying fat also affects the quality of the fish. Fish fried at too low a temperature absorbs a great deal of fat, while that cooked at the correct temperature absorbs little fat. Temperature should not be lower than 325 degrees F. or higher than 385 degrees F.; 360 degrees F. is optimum.

CAUTION: DO NOT OVERCOOK FISH

Broiling: Frozen fish is usually thawed before broiling. Fresh or thawed fillets and steaks are placed in a pre-heated broiler 3 to 4 inches from the broiling unit. The distance from the source of heat for split fish varies from 2 to 6 inches. Frozen fish or fish of a very delicate texture is placed about 4 inches from the direct heat.

The fish is brushed several times with oil, melted butter, or margarine. Some chefs prefer to dust the fish lightly with seasoned flour when preparing it for broiling.

Steaks are turned once; fillets are never turned.

When fish is charcoal grilled, the grill should be sufficiently hot to mark the fish.

Steaming: Steaming, simmering, and poaching are closely related, the difference being in the amount of cooking liquid used. In steaming, the product is placed on a rack over the liquid, covered tightly, and cooked. Steaming may be done in top-of-the-stove, shallow pans; in the oven in covered pans or wrapped tightly in foil; or in steam cooking equipment.

In simmering, the liquid must cover the fish. The fish is steamed, boiled, or simmered in water or a prepared stock called court bouillon. It may be necessary to wrap the fish tightly in cheesecloth to prevent flaking or breaking apart during steaming and later handling. This is particularly true when cooking whole fish such as fresh salmon.

Fish cooked in moist heat requires very little cooking time and is usually accompanied by a sauce.

Cod, halibut, haddock, salmon, and similar fish, as well as shellfish, may be steamed. Cod, flounder, haddock, halibut, ocean perch, pompano, salmon, sea bass, and sole are the varieties that lend themselves to poaching in liquid to which a little white wine has been added.

Baking: Unlike meat, fish and seafoods even in the raw state are already tender. They are flavorful and moist when baked at a moderately high temperature (400 degrees to 425 degrees F.) for the shortest period of time.

Sauteing and Pan-Frying: The fish is floured and sauteed in the usual manner with a small amount of hot butter or other fat. Ordinary butter may be used if the fish are quite small but clarified butter is preferable to prevent burning for both small and larger fish. When fish are browned on one side, they are then carefully turned for completion of cooking and browning.

Flounder, perch, salmon, sole, crab pieces, lobster chunks, whole soft-shell crabs, and shucked oysters are some of the fish and shellfish which lend themselves to sauteing and pan-frying.

Boiling "Green" Shrimp: Shrimp may be peeled, deveined, and cooked; or cooked, peeled, and deveined. Some chefs believe that shrimp cooked in the shell are more flavorful.

The amount of salt varies according to the method. For every 15 pounds of peeled shrimp, allow 3 gallons of water and 1 1/2 cups of salt. Bring salted water to a boil. Add shrimp. Cover, return to boil and simmer 3 to 5 minutes.

If the recipe calls for further cooking in a sauce or casserole, reduce initial cooking time for shrimp.

Breaded Frozen Shrimp: No kitchen preparation is necessary; no thawing is needed. The shrimp are cooked from their hard-frozen state in 2 to 3 minutes in 350 degrees F. deep fat. This convenient product can be cooked to order, with no delay even during busy rush periods.

While large-size shrimp will cook from a hard-frozen state in about 2 to 3 minutes in 350 degree F. deep fat, jumbo shrimp require 3 to 4 minutes.

Boiled Live Lobsters: Live lobsters are usually plunged headfirst into a large pot of boiling, salted water and simmered for 12 to 15 minutes. Large lobsters (over a pound) may take up to 20 minutes.

For cold boiled lobster or to prepare lobsters for meat,

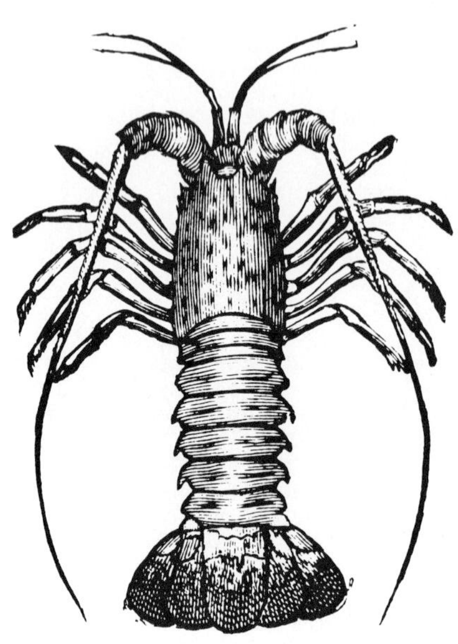

cool cooked lobster in cold running water. For hot boiled lobster, serve directly from range with drawn butter. Claws should be disjointed and cracked, or portion of the shell removed for ease of eating. Body may be split from head to tail down to the back shell, the stomach and intestinal vein removed, and the cavity filled with parsley, stuffing, or mayonnaise.

Some operators split live lobsters before dropping in boiling water.

Broiled Lobster: Rinse live lobsters thoroughly in cold water. Chop off claws and legs. Place lobster on chopping board with back down. Starting at the head, insert a sharp knife between body and tail segments and split lobster lengthwise, but do not cut through back shell. Remove the stomach, which lies just back of the head, and the intestinal vein. Fill cavity with stuffing of bread crumbs and butter or other stuffing. Place under broiler, about 4 inches from the heat, 12 to 15 minutes or on bake sheets or roast pans in 400 degrees F. oven 15 to 20 minutes, depending upon size of the lobster. Large claws may be baked in oven with a little water to retain moisture.

Crack claws after cooking for convenience of patrons and arrange near body in a natural way.

Broiled Lobster Tails: Frozen rock lobster tails should be thawed only in time to be used, not far in advance of actual preparation. Split lengthwise down to, but not through, the back shell. Brush with butter and broil 15 to 17 minutes, depending upon size.

HANDLING AND PREPARATION TIPS

Do not over-cook fish or shellfish. Fish is tender as it comes from the waters. It is cooked to heat or brown, to develop the flavor, and to soften the small amount of connective tissue present.

Do not over-season. Fish and seafoods have a delicate flavor that should not be overwhelmed by too much seasoning.

Cook fresh fish within 1 day. To store fresh fish, place dry, dressed fish in dish and loosely wrap with foil or plastic wrap or in pan surrounded with fresh crushed ice. Keep fresh shellfish in cracked ice in the refrigerator or in meat compartment.

Do not refreeze thawed seafoods. to store frozen fish or seafoods, keep solidly frozen in original wrapper, with best storage temperature -10 degrees F. Use immediately after defrosting.

Do not thaw frozen seafood at room temperature. Partially thaw fillets and steaks in the refrigerator, or under cold water in water-tight wrappings if in a hurry. Defrost only until portions separate easily. Do not thaw breaded fish portions, sticks, or shellfish. They go directly from the freezer to oven, broiler, frypan, or deep fryer. If you do your own breading, thaw seafoods before deep frying.

Cheese: An Essential Source of Protein

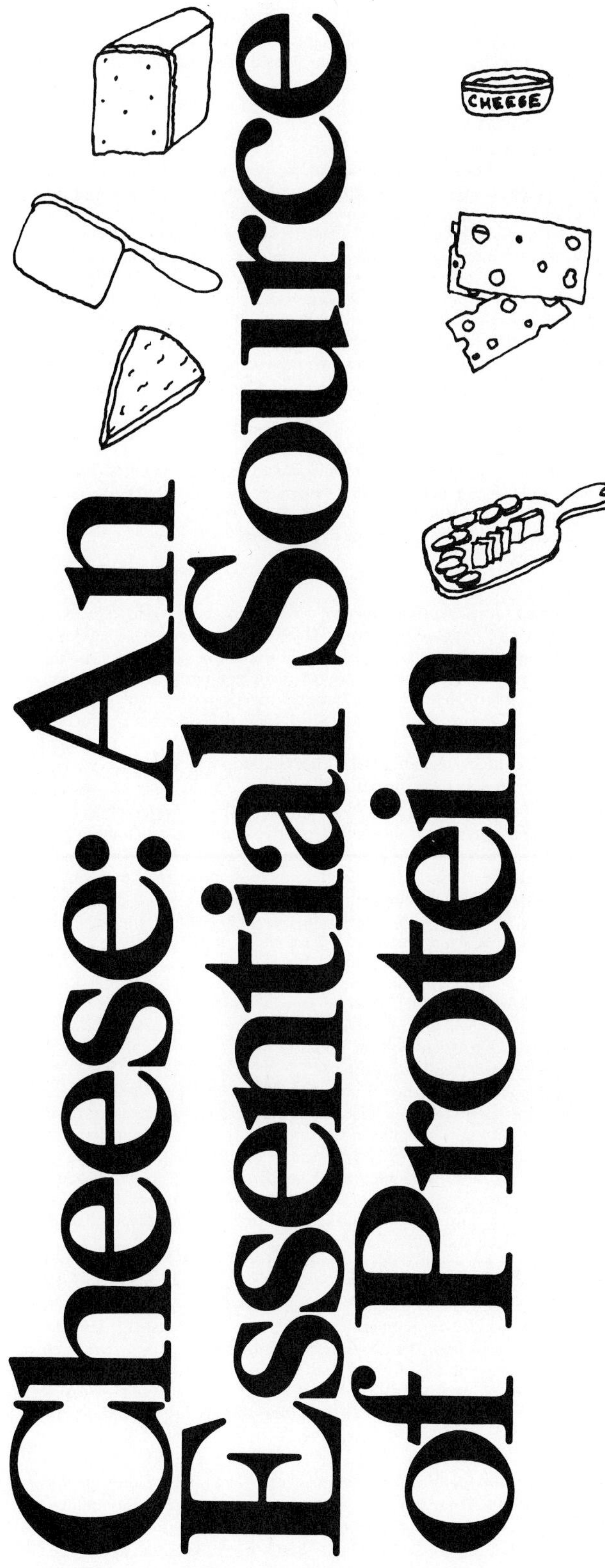

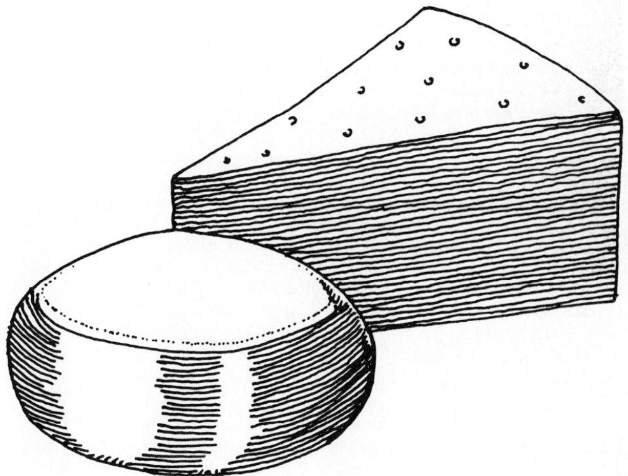

Cheese is a highly nutritious and palatable food. It is of value in the diet because it contains in concentrated form almost all the protein and usually most of the fat, as well as essential minerals, vitamins, and other nutrients, of milk.

Cheese is made wherever animals are milked and produce more milk than the people use in fluid form. Most cheese is made from cow's milk, simply because cows are milked more generally throughout the world than other animals. Smaller quantities are made from the milk of goats and ewes. Cheese is also made in some countries from the milk of other animals, such as camels, asses, mares, buffaloes, and reindeer.

People all over the world like and eat cheese. People in the United States are no exception. Although we do not eat nearly so much cheese per capita in the United States as do people in some countries, we eat nearly twice as much now as 20 years ago, or about 14 pounds (all kinds) per capita per year. This increased consumption is the result, at least in part, of improvements made in recent years in the quality and uniformity of many kinds of cheese.

No one knows who made the first cheese, but according to an ancient legend it was made accidentally by an Arabian merchant. The merchant put his supply of milk into a pouch made of a sheep's stomach when he set out on a long day's journey across the desert. The rennet in the lining of the pouch combined with the heat of the sun caused the milk to separate into curd and whey. He found at nightfall that the whey satisfied his thirst and the cheese (curd) satisfied his hunger and had a delightful flavor. Thus, according to the legend, the making of one of our most useful foods was begun.

According to ancient records, cheese was used as a food more than 4,000 years ago. It was made and eaten in Biblical times. Travelers from Asia are believed to have brought the art of cheesemaking to Europe. Cheese was made in many parts of the Roman Empire when it was at its height. Then cheesemaking was introduced to England by the Romans. During the Middle Ages—from the decline of the Roman Empire until the discovery of America—as well as later, cheese was made and improved by the monks in the monasteries of Europe. Gorgonzola was made in the Po Valley in Italy in 879 A. D. and Italy became the cheesemaking center of Europe in the 10th century. Roquefort was mentioned in the ancient records of the monastery at Conques, France, in 1070. The Pilgrims included cheese in the ship's supplies when they made their famous voyage to America in the Mayflower in 1620.

Until the middle of the 19th century, however, cheesemaking was a local farm industry. Housewives made cheese from the surplus milk produced on the farm. In 1851 the first cheese factory in the United States was built by Jesse Williams near Rome, Oneida County, N. Y. Herkimer County, which adjoins Oneida County, was the center of the cheese industry in the United States for the next 50 years. For many years during this period the largest cheese market in the world was at Little Falls, N. Y.; there cheese from about 200 factories was sold, in addition to farmmade cheese. As the population increased in the East, and there was a corresponding increase in the demand for market milk, the industry gradually moved westward, centering in the rich farm lands of Wisconsin. Cheesemaking in the United States and in the other leading cheese-producing countries of the world is now largely a factory industry, only small amounts being made on farms for home use.

Almost 2 billion pounds of cheese is now made in the United States each year. About 15 percent of the annual milk production is used in making this cheese.

"Natural" cheese is made directly from milk (or whey, in some instances). It is made by coagulating or curdling milk, stirring and heating the curd, draining off the whey, and collecting or pressing the curd. Desirable flavor and texture are obtained in many cheeses by curing the cheese, that is, holding it for a specified time at a specific temperature and humidity. Process cheese is made from a combination of one or more batches or kinds of natural cheese heated to pasteurization temperatures and packaged.

It is difficult, if not impossible, to classify the different cheeses satisfactorily in groups. There probably are only about 18 distinct types or kinds of natural cheese. No two of these are made by the same method; that is, the details of setting the milk, cutting, stirring, heating, draining, pressing, and salting the curd, and curing the cheese are varied to produce characteristics and qualities peculiar to each kind of cheese. The following cheeses are typical of the 18 kinds: Brick, Camembert, Cheddar, Cottage, Cream, Edam, Gouda, Hand, Limburger, Neufchâtel, Parmesan, Provolone, Romano, Roquefort, Sapsago, Swiss, Trappist, and whey cheeses (Mysost and Ricotta).

Accidental modifications or changes in one or more steps of the cheesemaking process throughout the centuries were largely responsible for the development of the different kinds of cheese. These changes were little understood and difficult to duplicate because scientific knowledge of bacteriology and chemistry was lacking. As a result, cheesemaking was considered an art, and the making process was a closely guarded secret passed down from father to son.

With increased scientific knowledge, especially since 1900, has come an understanding of the bacteriology and chemistry involved in the making of many cheeses. Thus it has become possible to control more precisely each step in the making process and to manufacture a uniform product. Now, cheesemaking is becoming a science rather than an art.

Brick

Brick cheese, one of the few cheeses of American origin, is made in considerable quantities in numerous factories, particularly in Wisconsin. It is a sweet-curd, semisoft, cow's-milk cheese, with a mild but rather pungent and sweet flavor, midway between Cheddar and Limburger but not so sharp as Cheddar and not so strong as Limburger. The body is softer than Cheddar but firmer than Limburger, is elastic, and slices well without crumbling. Brick has an open texture with numerous round and irregular shaped eyes (holes). Although the exact derivation of the name is unknown, it may refer to its brick-like shape or to the bricks used in pressing.

High-quality whole milk, preferably pasteurized, is warmed to a temperature of 88° to 92° F. Lactic starter is added, and enough rennet so the curd will be firm enough to cut in about 30 minutes. After the curd is cut into cubes and stirred gently for 15 to 25 minutes, it is warmed in about 45 minutes to a temperature of 106° to 110°, or even as low as 96° and as high as 115° in some cases (depending on the size of the cubes and the rate of acid development). The final cooking temperature is maintained until the curd is transferred to the forms. Part of the whey is removed, and the curd either is stirred in the remainder of the whey or warm water (at the cooking temperature) is added and stirring is continued. When the curd reaches the desired degree of firmness, the curd-whey mixture is dipped into the forms.

The forms, which are made of wood or perforated metal and have no top or bottom, are rectangular (10 inches long, 5 inches wide, and 5½ inches deep). They are placed on a mat or metal screen on a drain table.

A flat-sided pail or scoop is used to transfer the curd to the forms. As soon as the curd settles, a cover (10 by 5 inches) is placed on each form, if necessary, to reduce loss of heat. The forms are turned about five times at 30-minute intervals, and about the second or third time a 5-pound weight (usually a brick) is placed on each. Draining continues under this pressure overnight; the forms are kept covered if the room is cold.

The next morning the forms are removed, and either dry or brine salting is begun. For dry salting, the cheeses are rubbed with salt and laid on one of their broad sides on a salting table. Salting is repeated daily for 3 days. Then the cheeses are scraped smooth and placed on shelves in the curing room. For brine salting, the cheeses are floated in a saturated salt solution at a temperature of 55° to 60° F. for a day, and salt is sprinkled on the upper surface. After 24 hours, they are turned and left in the brine for another day, or 48 hours in all.

The cheese is cured at a temperature of 60° F. and a relative humidity of 90 percent. The bricks are placed close together for 10 to 12 days to prevent drying and cracking of the rind. Micro-organisms grow on the surface and produce a reddish-brown color. This is desirable in normal curing. The cheeses are washed frequently with salty water. After about 12 days, they are separated so the air can circulate around them and dry them, or they are removed to a cooler, drier room to dry; then they are dipped in paraffin or cheese wax, wrapped in parchment and an overwrapper of heavy paper, and packed in boxes. The cheese usually is stored for further curing for 2 to 3 months at 40° to 50° F. If the cheese is made from raw milk, it is cured for at least 60 days at not less than 35° F. unless it is to be used for manufacturing and is designated "Brick cheese for manufacturing."

Brick cheese that measures about 10 inches long, 5 inches wide, and 3 inches thick, will weigh aproximately 5 pounds. The yield is about 9.5 pounds of cheese per 100 pounds of milk containing 3.5 percent of fat.

Analysis: Moisture, not more than 44 percent (usually 39 to 42 percent); fat, 31 percent (not less than 50 percent of the solids); protein, 20 to 23 percent; and salt, 1.8 to 2 percent, or slightly more.

Camembert

Camembert, a soft, surface-ripened, cow's-milk cheese, was first made in 1791 by Marie Fontaine (Madame Harel) at Camembert, a hamlet in the Department of Orne, France. It is said that Napoleon was served this cheese, which was as yet unnamed, and he thereupon named it Camembert. The industry soon extended from Orne to the Department of Calvados, and these two Departments are still the principal centers of production. However, Camembert-type cheese is made also in other parts of France and in other countries, including the United States.

Each cheese is about 4½ inches in diameter, 1 to 1½ inches thick, and weighs about 10 ounces. The interior is yellow and waxy, creamy, or almost fluid in consistency, depending on the degree of ripening. The rind is a thin, felt-like layer of gray mold and dry cheese interspersed with patches of reddish yellow. Camembert is made in much the same way as Brie, but it is smaller and the characteristic flavor differs.

The method of making Camembert is in general as follows: Good-quality whole milk or milk standardized to a fat content of 3.5 percent is put in small vats or in flat-bottomed, conical metal cans that hold about 200 pounds. Lactic starter is added, and the milk is warmed to a temperature of approximately 85° F. A little color may be added, and enough rennet is added so the curd will be firm enough to dip in 1 to 1½ hours. The curd may be cut before it is put into the hoops to hasten drainage of the whey, but usually it is hooped without cutting.

The curd is ladled carefully—a slice at a time and with as little breaking as possible—into perforated, circular hoops that rest on rush mats on drain boards on a draining table. The hoops are about 4½ inches in diameter and 5 inches deep and are open at both ends. In some factories half hoops just large enough to slip over the deeper hoops easily (4⅝ inches in diameter and 2½ inches deep) are used, and in some factories heavy metal disks are placed on the curd to aid in settling it evenly. The temperature of the room should be about 70° F.

The hoops are turned and the mats are changed after a few hours, and this procedure is repeated frequently for about 2 days. At the end of the first day, the cheeses will have settled to a thickness of 1½ to 1¾ inches, and the deeper hoops may be removed. At the end of the second day, the cheeses are removed from the hoops, salted with fine dry salt, and may be inoculated with a culture of mold and bacteria. The culture either is mixed with the salt and rubbed on the surface of the cheeses, or it is dissolved in water and sprayed on. Then the cheeses are moved to the curing room.

Curing the cheese is the most difficult part of the manufacturing process for there must be a uniform and progressive development of the ripening agents and at the same time the curd must dry gradually but not too rapidly. The cheeses are cured on open board frames or shelves at a temperature of about 55° F. and a relative humidity of 85 to 90 percent for about 3 weeks; then at a temperature of 48° to 50°. In the United States, if the cheese is made from raw milk it is cured for at least 60 days. Cheeses are turned frequently. A primary surface growth of a grayish-white felt-like layer of mold is followed by a secondary fermentation that produces a trace of sliminess and changes the surface to show spots of yellow and finally a reddish or russet color; at the same time the interior of the curd becomes creamy and somewhat yellow.

The cheeses are wrapped in paper, parchment, or cellophane and may be covered with metal foil; they usually are packed in round, flat, wooden or plastic boxes. Sometimes they are cut in pie-shaped segments for marketing, but they are said to cure more normally if they are not cut. From 13 to 15 pounds of Camembert cheese is obtained per 100 pounds of whole milk.

Analysis: Moisture, 52.3 percent in domestic Camembert, and 43 to 54.4 percent in imported; fat, 24 to 28 percent (at least 50 percent in the solids); protein, 17 to 21 percent; and salt, 2.6 percent.

Cheddar

Cheddar cheese is named for the village of Cheddar in Somersetshire, England, where it was first made. The exact date of origin is not known, but it has been made since the latter part of the 16th century.

Colonial housewives made the first Cheddar cheese in America; and the first cheese factory in the United States was a Cheddar-cheese factory, established in 1851 by Jesse Williams, near Rome, Oneida County, N. Y.

Production increased rapidly with the establishment of the factory system. At present, nearly 1.3 billion pounds of Cheddar (and Cheddar-type) cheese is made in the United States each year, which is about 67 percent of all the cheese made. In fact, it is made and used so widely that it often is called American cheese, or American Cheddar cheese, and cheeses similar to Cheddar but made by a slightly modified process are called American-type cheeses.

In addition to being the name of the cheese, Cheddar is the name of a step in the manufacturing process and also the name of the most common style, which is about 14½ inches in diameter, 12 inches thick, and weighs between 70 and 78 pounds. Other styles are: Daisy, which is about 13¼ inches in diameter, slightly more than 4 inches thick, and weighs 21 to 23 pounds; Flat or Twin, which is 14½ inches in diameter, slightly more than 5 inches thick, and weighs 32 to 37 pounds; Longhorn, which is 6 inches in diameter, 13 inches long, and weighs 12 to 13 pounds; Young American, which is 7 inches in diameter, 7 inches thick, and weighs 11 to 12 pounds; Picnic or Junior Twin, which is 9¾ inches in diameter, 5 inches thick, and weighs 11 to 12 pounds; and rectangular blocks or prints, which usually are 14 inches long, 11 inches wide, 3¼ inches thick, and weigh 20 pounds. However, they are made in barrel sizes that weigh up to 600 pounds. The blocks are often cut into prints and packaged (see Natural Rindless Loaf). In many stores, the 1-pound print is most popular.

Cheddar is a hard cheese, ranging in color from nearly white to yellow. It is made from sweet, whole cow's milk, either raw or pasteurized. (If it is made from partly skimmed or skim milk, it must be so labeled.)

Research has shown that pasteurizing the milk improves the quality of the cheese; and that cheese of uniformly good quality can be made from pasteurized milk by the so-called time-schedule method. Use of the time schedule systematizes the cheese-making operations and makes it possible to control the amount of acid that develops and the rate of its development during the making process. More than 90 percent of the Cheddar cheese made in the United States is now made from either heat-treated or pasteurized milk.

The pasteurized milk is cooled to the setting temperature (86° to 88° F.) and run into the cheese vat. Starter is added and the milk is agitated (stirred) usually for about an hour as the milk ripens (develops acidity). The amount of starter and the length of the ripening period are adjusted so that acid will develop at the desired rate during the making process. Then rennet and color are mixed in thoroughly and stirring is stopped. When the curd is sufficiently firm, usually about 30 minutes after setting, it is cut with curd knives into ¼-inch or ⅜-inch cubes. It is stirred continuously from cutting to dipping (draining the whey). About 15 minutes after cutting is completed, the curd is heated gradually (in about 30 minutes) to a temperature of about 100°.

About 2¼ hours after the rennet was added, the curd is pushed back from the gate end of the vat, and the whey is drained. Draining should be completed in 15 minutes; then a ditch is made down the middle of the vat and the curd is packed about 7 or 8 inches deep on each side. When it is firm enough to be turned without breaking it is cheddared or matted, that is, it is cut into slabs 5 or 6 inches wide which are turned frequently and, finally, when firm enough, piled in layers. Then the curd is run through a curd mill and spread evenly over the bottom of the vat and stirred. About 2½ to 3½ pounds of salt for each 1,000 pounds of milk is mixed in; and the curd is piled on either side of the vat while the whey drains.

When the salt has dissolved completely, the curd is transferred to cloth-lined metal hoops and pressed for about 30 minutes. Then the hoops are removed from the press, the cheeses are dressed, pressed again for 12 to 24 hours, and then removed from the hoops and dried for 3 or 4 days at a temperature of 50° to 60° F. before dipping in paraffin or wax.

When rindless cheese is made the press cloths are removed after pressing and the cheese wrapped in a heat-sealing plastic film.

Cheeses are cured usually at a temperature between 40° and 50° F., but it may be as low as 35° or as high as 60°. They are cured for at least 60 days, usually for 3 to 6 months, and in some instances for as long as a year. Between 9½ and 11 pounds of cheese is obtained per 100 pounds of milk.

Analysis: Moisture, 37 to 38 percent (not more than 39 percent); fat, 32 percent (fat in the solids, not less than 50 percent); protein, 25 percent; and salt, 1.4 to 1.8 percent.

Cottage

Cottage cheese, sometimes called Pot cheese and also Dutch cheese or Schmierkäse, is a soft, uncured cheese made from skim milk or from reconstituted concentrated skim milk or nonfat dry milk solids.

Large-grained, low-acid cheese is made by adding rennet to the milk, cutting the curd into large cubes, and washing the curd thoroughly to reduce the acid flavor. It is known as sweet-curd Cottage cheese, flake-type Cottage cheese, and low-acid rennet-type Cottage cheese. The large particles of curd resemble kernels of popped corn, and in some localities this kind of cheese is called Popcorn cheese. Small-grained Cottage cheese sometimes is called country-style or farm-style cheese.

Usually some cream is mixed with the cheese curd before it is marketed or consumed. If the cheese contains 4 percent or more of fat, it is called Creamed Cottage cheese. Flavoring materials, such as peppers, olives, and pimientos, may be added also.

Large quantities of Cottage cheese are made and consumed in the United States; it is highly nutritious and palatable and is used as a table cheese and in salads. It is easy to make both in the home and in the factory. In the home, about 1 pound of cheese is obtained from 1 gallon of skim milk; in the factory, from 12 to 15 pounds of curd is obtained from 100 pounds of skim milk and this makes from 14 to 18 pounds of Creamed Cottage cheese.

Cottage cheese may be made by either the short-setting method or the long-setting method. In the short-setting method, more lactic starter is added to the milk than in the long-setting method; the milk is set at a higher temperature; and the coagulation period is shorter. In both methods, the milk is pasteurized and cooled to the setting temperature. Lactic starter is added; rennet may be added; and the milk is held at the setting temperature until it curdles.

The curd is ready to cut when it is firm but not hard and brittle. It is cut into cubes, the size determining to some extent the size of the curd particles in the finished cheese. Then the curd is heated, with careful stirring. The temperature to which the curd is heated and the length of the heating period depend on the characteristics of the curd and the acidity of the whey. When the curd has attained the proper firmness, the whey is drained off and the curd washed first with cool tap water, then with ice water. Then the water is drained off. When the curd is firm and dry, it is salted. It may be creamed and packed in consumer-size cartons. However, it is customary for the manufacturer to pack the curd in tubs or tins that hold as much as 50 pounds for shipping to the distributor, who creams and packs it in consumer-size cartons to supply his daily needs. The curd may be held for several days at a temperature of 32° to 35° F.

Analysis: Moisture, not more than 80 percent (usually 70 to 72 percent).

Cream

Cream cheese is a soft, mild, rich, uncured cheese made of cream or a mixture of cream and milk, and used as a spread for bread, in sandwiches, and with salads. It is similar to unripened Neufchâtel but has a higher fat content. It is one of the most popular soft cheeses in the United States and is made in many factories throughout the country, especially in New York and Wisconsin. In addition, there are several French Cream cheeses.

The method of making Cream cheese varies in the different factories in the United States; following is a general description:

The cream, or milk-and-cream mixture, which usually is homogenized, is pasteurized, cooled to a temperature of 75° to 85° F., and lactic-acid culture, with or without rennet, is added. After the curd forms, it is stirred until it is smooth and then is heated by one of two methods. In one method, the curd is heated in the vat, with stirring, to a temperature of 115° to 125° and held at that temperature until the whey begins to separate from the curd. Then the curd is ready to drain. It may be placed in draining bags immediately or it may be cooled before it is placed in the bags. In the other method, the curd is stirred until it is smooth, and stirring is continued as hot water (equal to the volume of curd) is added. The temperature of the water should be about 170° to 180°. When the curd-water mixture reaches a temperature of 120° to 130°, it is poured into the draining bags.

When whey has practically stopped draining from the curd, the cheese is packaged by either the cold-pack method or the hot-pack method. In the cold-pack method, the curd is pressed and chilled, and salt is added; it is then mixed until it is smooth, and flavoring materials—such as pimientos, olives, pineapple, or relish—may be added. Usually cream cheese is packed in metal foil or in glasses sealed with metal tops.

In the hot-pack method, the curd is stirred and salted, and any one of several dairy ingredients may be added. Then the mixture is pasteurized, it may be homogenized, flavoring material may be added, and it is packed immediately (while it is in a semifluid condition) in the final package.

Analysis: Moisture, not more than 55 percent (usually 48 to 52 percent); fat, not less than 33 percent (usually 35 to 38 percent); protein, 10 percent; and salt, 0.8 to 1.2 percent.

Edam

Edam cheese was first made in the vicinity of Edam in the Province of North Holland, Netherlands. It is known in the Netherlands by various local names, such as Manbollen, Katzenkopf, and Tete de Maure. Like Gouda, it is a semisoft to hard, sweet-curd cheese made from cow's milk. Originally it was made from whole milk but now the fat content of the milk is usually reduced to about 2.5 percent. When the cheese is made for export, the fat content is indicated on the label, according to Government specifications. Edam is made also in the United States.

Edam has a pleasingly mild, clean, sometimes salty, flavor and a rather firm and crumbly body, free of holes and openings. It usually is shaped like a flattened ball, but in the United States it is made also in a loaf shape. The cheeses usually weigh from 3½ to 4½ pounds but sometimes weigh as much as 14 pounds. In the United States, they sometimes weigh only about ¾ to 1 pound.

High-quality milk should be used in making Edam; if the milk is pasteurized, as is common in the United States, lactic starter is added. Color may be added and the milk is set with rennet extract. About 15 minutes later the curd is cut into ⅜-inch cubes, then stirred and heated to a temperature of 90° to 95° F. When the curd is sufficiently firm, part of the whey is drained off. When enough whey has drained so that the curd is exposed, the curd is pushed to the side of the vat and more whey pressed out. The curd is stirred and may be salted. The temperature of the curd should be at least 88° when it is put into the molds for pressing.

Special pressing molds, preferably metal but sometimes hardwood and lined with cheesecloth, are used. Each has a round lower section about 6 inches deep and 6 inches in diameter, with holes in the bottom for drainage, and a round cover. In the United States the cheese sometimes is pressed in rectangular loaf-shaped molds.

The molds are filled with curd, covered, and then pressed for about 30 minutes with a pressure of 20 to 30 pounds. Then the cheeses are removed from the molds and dipped in warm whey (at a temperature of 125° to 130° F.). The rough edges of curd are trimmed off, and the cheeses are bandaged and again pressed for 6 to 12 hours with a pressure of 60 to 120 pounds.

The cheeses then are rubbed with fine salt and placed in salt in special salting molds that are the same shape as the pressing molds but have no covers. Salting is continued for 5 or 6 days, and the cheeses are turned daily. In the United States, and less commonly in the Netherlands, the cheeses are salted by immersion in a salting bath for about a week; however, dry salting is preferable as it aids in producing a smooth rind.

The cheeses are scrubbed with a brush in warm water or whey, wiped dry, and then cured on shelves at a temperature of 50° to 60° F. and a relative humidity of 80 to 90 percent. They are piled in layers on the shelves to aid in flattening the top and bottom surfaces. They are washed, dried, and turned daily for a week or two, then less frequently. In some factories they are washed in a churn-like machine, and the surfaces may be smoothed by rotating the cheeses in a machine that resembles a lathe.

In the Netherlands, cheese for export is colored red, rubbed with oil, and wrapped in some transparent material; the red coating is an identifying characteristic of Edam cheese. However, cheese made for consumption within that country is rubbed with oil but not colored.

In the United States, Edam cheese is covered with red paraffin or some other tightly adhering red coating.

The cheeses are packed usually 8 to 12 in a box; for export to warm climates they may be sealed in tins. Between 8 and 9 pounds of cured cheese is obtained per 100 pounds of milk.

Analysis: Moisture, not more than 45 percent (usually 35 to 38 percent); fat, 26.5 to 29.5 percent (not less than 40 percent in the solids); protein, 27 to 29 percent; and salt, 1.6 to 2 percent.

Gouda

Gouda, first made in the vicinity of Gouda in the Province of South Holland, Netherlands, is a semisoft to hard, sweet-curd cheese similar to Edam except that it contains more fat. It is made from whole or partly skimmed cow's milk, but skimmed less than milk used in making Edam. Gouda usually is shaped like a flattened sphere and pressed in molds with rounded ends. The molds vary in size but usually are nearly 14 inches in diameter and 4½ to 5 inches deep. The cheeses usually weigh between 10 and 25 pounds but may weigh as little as 6 or as much as 50 pounds. Gouda is made also in a loaf weighing about 8 pounds. A so-called "baby Gouda" is oval, weighs a pound or slightly less, may be coated with red wax, and wrapped in a cellophane-type wrapper. The red surface is not necessarily an identifying characteristic, however, as it is of domestic and imported Edam.

Gouda is made in much the same way as Edam. (See Edam.) Some slight modifications in the details of manufacture are mentioned here. Although the milk may be set at any temperature between 84° and 90° F., it usually is set at 90°. After the curd is cut, the whey is drained off, heated, and poured back into the vat. This procedure is repeated once or twice, in order to increase the temperature of the curd to between 100° and 106°. Other factors being equal, cheese made from curd heated to the higher temperatures (within this range) will have a firmer body, will cure more slowly, and will have better keeping quality. Some salt is added to the curd before it is put into the hoops (molds) for pressing. Salting is usually completed by immersing the cheese in a salt solution; however, it may be completed in the curing room by rubbing dry salt on the cheese daily for 7 to 10 days. The cheese cures in 2 to 3 months, but it improves in flavor if it is cured for 5 to 6 months.

About 12½ pounds of uncured cheese can be made from 100 pounds of whole milk, and about 8 pounds of cured cheese from 100 pounds of milk containing from 3 to 3.5 percent of fat.

Analysis: Moisture, not more than 45 percent (usually 36 to 43.5 percent); fat, 29 to 30.5 percent (not less than 46 percent in the solids); protein, 25 to 26 percent; and salt, 1.5 to 2 percent.

Hand

Hand cheese, a small, sour-milk, surface-ripened cheese, is so named because originally is was molded in final shape by hand, and still is in some parts of Europe. It is very popular among Germanic peoples and is made in several countries. There are many local names for Hand cheese, among which are the following: In Germany—Mainzer Handkäse or Harzkäse, Alte Kuhkäse, or Berliner Kuhkäse, Ihlefeld, Satz, and Thuringia Caraway cheese; in Austria—Olmützer Quargeln and Olmützer Bierkäse; and in Russia—Livlander. Some of these are described under their particular names.

The method of making Hand cheese differs in different localities. Following is a general description: Buttermilk or lactic starter is added to skim milk, which is then coagulated at room temperature. The curd is broken up or cut, stirred, and heated slowly to a temperature of about 120° F. It is held at this temperature for about 3 hours, and stirred for the first hour. At the end of the heating period, the curd is put in cloths or in forms, while the whey drains either with or without pressure. Then the curd is either mixed thoroughly or ground in a curd mill, and salted. Sometimes caraway seed is added. The cheeses then are molded by hand, or pressed in small forms, into the desired shape. They are dried in a warm room and then placed on shelves in a cool, moist cellar to cure. The cheeses are kept clean while curing. When surface ripening has begun, they are wrapped and packed in boxes. They are cured for 6 to 8 weeks at a temperature no higher than 50°. At higher temperatures they cure too rapidly. Well-ripened Hand cheese has a very sharp, pungent flavor and aroma; the consumer sometimes must become accustomed to it before he finds it agreeable.

In the United States, cheese of this type is made by farm families of German descent in Pennsylvania and in a few factories in New York, Wisconsin, and northern Illinois. The curd is prepared in much the same way as Cottage-cheese curd, either with or without rennet. The drained curd is salted and either molded by hand or pressed in forms into cakes 2 to 3 inches in diameter and less than an inch thick. The cheeses then are cured in a cool, moist room. Action of bacteria, yeasts, and molds causes surface ripening, and a smear usually appears. Regulation of the temperature and humidity in the curing room is essential to control surface ripening; it is controlled also by frequent rubbing or washing of the cheese.

Queso de mano (Hand cheese) is a sour-milk, cooked-curd, small, round cheese made in small quantities in Venezuela and some other Latin-American countries for local consumption. Usually it is made from cow's milk, but it is said to be made also from goat's milk. The cheeses are 6 or 7 inches in diameter.

Limburger

Limburger is a semisoft, surface-ripened cheese with a characteristic strong flavor and aroma. Usually it contains small irregular openings. The cheeses vary in size from a 3-inch cube that weighs less than a pound to a cheese 6 inches square and 3 inches thick that weighs about 2½ pounds.

Limburger was first made in the Province of Lüttich, Belgium, and is named for the town of Limburg, where originally much of it was marketed. It is made also in other parts of Europe, especially in Germany and Austria, and in the United States, especially in Wisconsin and New York. Other similar European cheeses are: Allgäuer Limburger and Stangen, made in Bavaria; Romadur and Hervé, made in Belgium; Schloss, made in Germany and Austria; Marienhofer and Tanzenberger, made in Carinthia, Austria; Backsteiner, made in Germany; and Void, made in France.

The method of making Limburger differs in different factories, but in general is as follows: Fresh milk, preferably whole milk, may be pasteurized, and it is warmed in a vat or kettle to a temperature usually between 86° and 92° F., but in some factories to as high as 96°. Lactic starter and rennet are added. Usually about 30 minutes after setting, but in some factories an hour later, the curd is cut into cubes about ½ inch in diameter. If the milk was set at the lower temperatures, the curd is stirred slowly as it is warmed to about 96°, and it is stirred gently at intervals as it acquires firmness. When the curd is sufficiently firm, most of the whey is drained off. In some factories, the curd is washed with weak salt brine to lower its acidity.

The curd is dipped into large rectangular metal or wooden forms that rest on a drain table. Sometimes the forms are divided into sections the size of the individual cheeses; sometimes the forms are not divided, and after the block of curd is removed from the forms, it is divided to make the individual cheeses. In some factories, a light-weight board is placed on the curd to furnish light pressure. The forms of curd are turned frequently.

When the cheeses are firm enough to retain their shape, they are removed from the forms and salted. In some factories, they are packed close together in dry salt on a salting table for at least a day, and they are turned frequently until they have absorbed salt on all surfaces; in other factories, they are rubbed with salt daily for about 3 days; and in still other factories, they are immersed in salt brine for a day at a temperature of 55° to 60° F.

After the cheeses are salted, they are cured on shelves at a temperature of 50° to 60° F. and a relative humidity of about 90 percent. According to some authorities, surface-ripening micro-organisms are responsible for the characteristic flavor and aroma. Yeasts, which reduce the acidity, predominate at first, and these are followed by *Bacterium linens*, which produces a characteristic reddish-yellow pigment.

The cheeses are placed close together on the shelves at first, and separated later. As the cheese cures, slime forms on the surface and the rind acquires a reddish-yellow color. In some factories, the cheeses are rubbed and turned every 2 or 3 days; in other factories, they are washed with salty water. The older cheeses are rubbed or washed before the younger ones; in this way, the younger ones are inoculated with the surface-ripening micro-organisms. After they have cured for 2 or 3 weeks, they are wrapped in parchment or waxed paper and an outer layer of metal foil, and curing is continued at a lower temperature. If the cheese was made from raw milk, it is cured for at least 60 days. From 11 to 13 pounds of cured cheese is obtained per 100 pounds of whole milk.

Analysis: Moisture, not more than 50 percent (usually 43 to 48 percent); fat, 26.5 to 29.5 percent (not less than 50 percent of the solids); protein, 20 to 24 percent; ash, 4.8 percent; and salt, 1.6 to 3.2 percent.

Mysost

Mysost cheese is made in the Scandinavian countries (Norway, Sweden, and Denmark) and in a few factories in the United States, principally in northern Illinois, Michigan, New York, and Wisconsin, from the whey obtained in the manufacture of other cheeses. There is considerable variation in the composition of the whey used in different factories and in different localities, and in the manufacturing procedure and the composition of the cheese; and it is known by different local names. Mysost is made from cow's-milk whey. Similar cheese made from goat's-milk whey is called Gjetost. In some instances a small proportion, usually not more than 10 percent, of buttermilk or whole milk, or even cream is added to the whey. Cheese made from such whey contains more fat and is softer and sometimes is called Primost or Fløtost. Cheese made by the same method from whole milk rather than whey is called Gomost.

The cheese consists principally of caramelized lactose (milk sugar) but contains also the fat, protein, and minerals present in the whey. It is light brown in color, has a buttery consistency and a mild, sweetish flavor. It does not undergo appreciable ripening but keeps well when packaged properly.

Sometimes, if the whey contains considerable acid, neutralizer is added to prevent a sour or bitter flavor in the cheese. If sweet whey is used, lactic starter usually is added. The whey is strained into a kettle and boiled (condensed) until it is a viscous mass, which may take 5 hours or longer. It is stirred while boiling. The albuminous material that rises to the surface is skimmed off. When the whey is reduced to about one-fourth its original volume and has the consistency of heavy cream, the albumin skimmed off earlier is stirred in thoroughly. Some manufacturers also stir in as much as 10 percent of brown sugar and some add spices, such as cloves or cumin seed. Then, while hot, it is poured or dipped into a round tank or vat equipped with a stirrer, and, while cooling, it is stirred constantly to prevent the formation of lactose crystals. When cool, it is poured into greased round or rectangular forms. When hard (firm), the cheeses usually but not always are cut into pie-shaped or small rectangular segments. Then, the whole cheese or, if cut, the individual segments may be dipped in wax or paraffin, and they are wrapped tightly, preferably in metal foil, to prevent contamination, and packed in cartons. The flat, cylindrical cheeses frequently weigh about 18 pounds.

Analysis: Moisture, frequently about 13 percent and preferably not more than 18 percent; fat in the solids, frequently 10 to 20 percent but preferably not less than 33 percent.

Neufchâtel

Neufchâtel cheese (Fromage de Neufchâtel), as made originally in France—especially in the Department of Seine Inférieure—is a soft, mild cheese made from whole or skim milk or a mixture of milk and cream. It may be eaten fresh or it may be cured. Bondon, Malakoff, Petit Carré, and Petit Suisse are other French cheeses that differ from Neufchâtel mainly in fat content and in size and shape.

Lactic starter is added to fresh milk at a temperature of 82° to 86° F., and enough rennet is added to coagulate the curd in 16 to 18 hours, or overnight. The coagulated curd is poured into a cloth, and it is either hung up to drain or placed in a drainer for 2 to 4 hours or longer. When the whey has practically stopped dripping, the curd is gathered up in the cloth, as in a bag, and chilled with ice. Then it is pressed between boards with a weight on top for 6 to 8 hours. The pressed curd is removed from the cloth bag, salted, either run through a curd mill or kneaded by hand, and then pressed in molds about 2½ inches in diameter and 2 or 3 inches deep. Salt may be rubbed on the surface of the cheeses when they are removed from the molds. Next, they are dried on a draining board for about 24 hours. Then they are transferred to a cool, damp curing room or cellar where they are kept clean and are inverted frequently. While curing, microorganisms—including *Mycoderma casei, Penicillium candidum,* and *P. camemberti,* as well as the so-called red cheese bacteria—grow on the surface of the cheese; a thin coating of white mold develops, followed by a yellow or reddish growth. The cheese, which is ready to market in 3 to 4 weeks, is wrapped in parchment or tinfoil. About 15 pounds of cured Neufchâtel cheese can be made from 100 pounds of rich, whole milk.

Neufchâtel frais (fresh) refers to Neufchâtel cheese made in France that is eaten without curing. It is cylindrical and flat, about 2 inches in diameter and 2½ inches thick, and weighs less than 8 ounces. It is made usually from whole milk and contains at least 45 percent of fat in the solids.

In the United States, Neufchâtel is made from pasteurized milk or a pasteurized milk-and-cream mixture in much the same way as Cream cheese, but it contains less fat and more moisture. (See Cream cheese.)

Analysis (fresh, domestic Neufchâtel): Moisture, 55 to 60 percent (not more than 65 percent); fat, not less than 20 percent but less than 33 percent; protein, 18 percent; and salt, 0.8 to 1.2 percent.

Parmigiano

Parmigiano, which is about the same as Reggiano, is one of the subvarieties of Grana (commonly called Parmesan), the hard Italian cheeses used for grating. It is made in Parma (hence the name Parmigiano), Reggio Emilia, Modena, Mantua, and Bologna, usually between April and November. The cheeses usually are from 12½ to 18 inches in diameter, from 7 to 9 inches thick, and they weigh between 48 and 80 pounds. The surface of the cheese is colored dark and coated with oil; the interior is the color of straw. The cheese may have no eyes or it may contain a few small eyes. It is cured for 1 to 2 years or longer. (See Grana, Parmesan, and Reggiano.)

Analysis: Moisture, 27 to 32 percent at 2 years; 18 to 27 percent at 3 years; fat in the solids, 32 to 38 percent; salt, 2.4 to 3 percent.

Provolone

Provolone, an Italian plastic-curd (pasta filata) cheese, was first made in southern Italy but is now also made in other parts of Italy and in the United States, principally in Wisconsin and Michigan. It is light in color, mellow, smooth, cuts without crumbling, and has an agreeable flavor.

Provolone is made in various shapes and sizes, each of which is identified by a more or less distinguishing name. Typically, the style called Provolone is pear-shaped and in the United States weighs about 14 pounds; in Italy, it weighs between 6 and 9 pounds and is called Provolone affetale if it weighs between 9 and 14 pounds. Larger styles, weighing as much as 50, 100, or 200 pounds, are called Provolone giganti. Smaller styles, weighing from 1 to 5 pounds, usually are spherical and are called by various names such as Provoletti, Provolotini, and Provoloncini. Another style is sausage-shaped and is called Salame (Italian, sausage) if it weighs about 10 to 12 pounds, Salamini if it is smaller, and Salame giganti if it is larger (up to 200 pounds or more).

The Italian method for making Provolone and Caciocavallo are almost identical. However, Provolone contains more fat and the cheeses usually are smoked after they are salted and dried. After the cheeses are smoked, they may be dipped in paraffin; if they are not paraffined, they are oiled. Although Caciocavallo may be used as a table cheese after it has cured for 2 to 4 months, usually it is cured for longer periods and is especially suitable for grating. On the other hand, Provolone is an excellent table cheese after it has cured for 6 to 9 months, and the larger styles are still suitable for use as table cheese after curing as long as 14 months. Sometimes the surface of the cheese is grooved, because it was hung in strings or ropes or because it was molded in a grooved form. The cheeses are kept clean while curing. The yield is 9½ to 10½ pounds of uncured cheese, or 7½ to 8¾ pounds of cured cheese per 100 pounds of milk.

The method for making Provolone in the United States differs in some respects from the Italian method. The milk, which may be either raw or pasteurized, is put in a Cheddar-type vat and starter is added. The milk is set with rennet paste or rennet extract plus an enzyme preparation. After the curd is cut and the whey is removed, as in the Italian method, the curd is matted, like Cheddar curd, and then cut into slabs about 2 by 8 by 24 inches which are worked and stretched in hot water. In some factories, the curd is worked in a mixing machine. The machine, which holds about 500 pounds of curd, is a metal container equipped with an irregular-shaped metal-rod stirrer, with paddle-like elbows, that revolves on a horizontal axis. The water is added at a temperature of about 180° F. and usually is changed at least once during the mixing process. The curd is worked for about 15 minutes and reaches a temperature of about 135°. Then the mass of curd—now shiny, elastic, and stringy—is removed from the machine and cut into pieces for the individual cheeses. These are treated further as described under Caciocavallo. The yield of uncured cheese is from 9 to 9½ pounds per 100 pounds of cow's milk from which very little of the fat has been removed. If the cheese is made from raw milk, it must be cured at least 60 days.

Analysis (domestic Provolone): Moisture, not more than 45 percent (usually 37 to 43.5 percent); fat, 25 to 33 percent (fat in the solids, at least 45 percent and usually 47 percent); and salt, 2 to 4 percent.

Ricotta

Ricotta cheese is made from the coagulable material (principally albumin) in the whey obtained in the manufacture of other cheeses, such as Cheddar, Swiss, and Provolone. It was first made in Italy and, therefore, is classed as an Italian cheese. However, it is now made in all the countries of central Europe and in some parts of southern Europe. It is made also in the United States, principally in Wisconsin and New York. It is sometimes called whey cheese or albumin cheese; other names for it are Ziger or Schottenziger, Recuit, Broccio, Brocotte, Sérac, Ceracee, and Mejette.

Cheddar-cheese whey usually contains between 0.2 and 0.35 percent of fat, and Swiss-cheese whey contains at least twice as much. In making Ricotta, usually all of the fat is left in the whey, and in the United States from 5 to 10 percent of either whole milk or skim milk is added. Usually whole milk is added if fresh Ricotta is being made, and skim milk if dry Ricotta is being made. The fat is incorporated in the cheese with the coagulated albumin, and it improves the body, flavor, and food value of the cheese.

The manufacturing process should begin soon after the whey is removed from the original cheese, before it has developed excessive acidity; the acidity should not be more than 0.20 percent. The sweet whey is heated in a kettle with a steam jacket to a temperature of 200° F. (near the boiling point). Sometimes live steam is injected into the whey. Sour whey or other coagulant is stirred in. Much of the coagulated albumin rises to the surface, and is dipped out with a perforated ladle or removed with a dipping cloth. The curd may be hung in the dipping cloth to cool and drain, or it may be dipped into perforated forms or spread on a screen platform in a vat. To improve the flavor and promote ripening, lactic starter may be mixed in after the curd has cooled to about 100°. From 1 to 1.5 percent or more of salt may be added at this time.

At this stage the curd is moist, grainy, and lacks cohesiveness; it resembles cottage-cheese curd in consistency. If it is to be marketed as fresh or moist Ricotta, draining is continued or the curd may be pressed for several hours in cheesecloth-lined hoops; then it is packed in paper cartons that usually hold 5 pounds. If it is to be marketed as dry Ricotta, the curd is placed in perforated forms about 6 inches in diameter and 9 inches deep, and it is pressed heavily for a longer period. Then it is salted on the surface, if it was not salted earlier, and it is dried in a curing room at a temperature of 100° F., or slightly higher. Dry Ricotta is suitable for grating.

Approximately 5 pounds of fresh, moist curd is obtained from 100 pounds of unskimmed cheese whey with 5 pounds of added whole milk.

Analysis: Fresh, moist Ricotta—Moisture, 68 to 73 percent; fat, 4 to 10 percent; protein, 16 percent; carbohydrate, 3 percent; and salt, 1.2 percent. Cured, dry Ricotta—Moisture, 60 percent; fat, 5.2 percent; protein, 18.7 percent; carbohydrate, 4 percent; ash, 3.6 percent; and salt (in the ash), 1.5 percent.

Romano

Romano, which is sometimes called Incanestrato, is one of the most popular of the very hard Italian cheeses. It was first made from ewe's milk in the grazing area of Latium, near Rome, but it is now made also from cow's and goat's milk and in other regions in southern Italy and in Sardinia. When made from ewe's milk, it is called Pecorino Romano; from cow's milk, Vacchino Romano; and from goat's milk, Caprino Romano. Romano-type cheese made in Sardinia is called Sardo. Some Romano cheese is made in the United States from cow's milk, and considerable quantities are imported from Italy and Sardinia.

The cheeses are round, with flat ends; they vary in size but frequently are about 10 inches in diameter and 6 inches thick. A single cheese usually weighs between 15 and 20 pounds but may weigh as much as 25 pounds. The interior is somewhat granular and has practically no holes or eyes.

The milk usually is partly skimmed, and it may be pasteurized. It is put into a vat, warmed to a temperature of about 90° F., and rennet is added. If the milk is pasteurized, starter must be added. After a coagulation period of 15 to 20 minutes, the curd is cut, and then heated with stirring to about 118°. In some factories, the curd is dipped from the whey into the hoops, which are circular and lined with cloth; in other factories, the whey is drained off, then the curd is stirred and part of the salt is mixed in before the curd is hooped. The hoops of curd are pressed, and they are turned frequently. Sometimes in Italy the cheeses are punched with holes to aid drainage; this practice, however, may result in growth of mold within the cheese.

When the cheeses are removed from the press, they are immersed in salt brine and later salt is rubbed on the surface. They are cured on shelves at a temperature of 50° to 65° F. They are kept clean (they may be scraped to clean them), and they are turned frequently. They may be colored black on the surface, and may be rubbed with olive oil toward the end of the curing period.

Romano is cured for not less than 5 months. It is used as a table cheese after curing for 5 to 8 months, and after longer curing—usually at least a year—it is hard, very sharply piquant, and suitable for grating. About 8 pounds of Romano is obtained per 100 pounds of milk.

Analysis: Moisture, not more than 34 percent (usually 32 percent); fat in the solids, not less than 38 percent; and salt, 5 to 6 percent.

Roquefort

Roquefort, a blue-veined, semisoft to hard cheese, is named for the village of Roquefort in the Department of Aveyron in southeastern France, where its manufacture has been an important industry for more than two centuries. At one time shepherds prepared the curd, but now the milk is collected and the curd is prepared in centralized dairies.

A French regulation limits use of the word Roquefort to cheese made in the Roquefort area from ewe's milk. Other French cheese of the blue-veined type is called Bleu cheese, and blue-veined type cheese made in the United States and other countries is known as Blue cheese. In addition, these are the distinctive blue-veined cheeses of England (Stilton) and Italy (Gorgonzola).

Roquefort cheese is characterized by its sharp, peppery, piquant flavor, and by the mottled, blue-green veins throughout the curd and the whiteness of the curd between the veins. Powder containing spores of *Penicillium roqueforti* mold is added to the curd as it is being put into the hoops, and the veins result from growth of the mold during the curing period. The powder is prepared by inocculating loaves of fresh bread with a pure culture of mold; when the mold has permeated the bread—in 4 to 6 weeks—the interior is crumbled, dried, ground, sifted, and stored for use in the cheese.

Following is a brief description of the making process: Ewe's whole milk is set with rennet at a temperature between 76° and 82° F. It is customary to heat fresh milk to between 122° and 140° and then to add enough cold milk to adjust the mixture to the setting temperature. After a coagulation period of 1½ to 2 hours, the curd is cut, the free whey is removed, and the curd either is transferred onto a cloth to drain or is mixed and drained in the vat. Then it is transferred to perforated metal hoops, about 7½ inches in diameter and 6 inches deep, which rest on drain mats on drain boards. The curd is put into the hoops in 3 or 4 layers, and blue-mold powder is sprinkled between each layer.

The curd is not pressed, but the hoops are turned several times the first day, and two or three times daily for the next 4 or 5 days. Then the cheeses are removed from the hoops, and they are taken to the caves for salting and curing. There are many natural caves in the Roquefort area and additional excavations have been made. The caves are a network of caverns and grottoes connected with one another and with the outside surface by numerous channels through which a brisk movement of cool, moist air keeps the temperature at not more than 50° F. (often as low as 40°) and the relative humidity at about 95 percent throughout the year, thus providing natural conditions that are favorable to mold growth and ripening of Roquefort cheese.

The cheeses are dry salted, piled in two or three layers for 3 days, then salted again and piled in layers for another 3 or 4 days—making a total salting period of a week. Besides improving the flavor, the rather heavy salting retards growth of slime-forming micro-organisms and foreign molds and is one of the factors that control normal ripening. When salting is completed, each cheese is punched with 60 or more holes, which permit air to reach the interior of the cheese so that the blue mold can grow. The cheeses are then placed on edge on racks, and they are cleaned every 2 or 3 weeks by scraping and brushing. The curing period is 2 to 5 months, depending on the extent of ripening desired. When ripened sufficiently, the cheeses are cleaned, wrapped in tinfoil, and boxed. They may be stored at a temperature of 40° F. The yield of cured cheese is said to be nearly 20 percent of the weight of milk used.

Analysis: Moisture, 38.5 to 41 percent (not more than 45 percent); fat, 32.2 percent; fat in the solids, not less than 50 percent; protein, 21.1 percent; ash, 6 1 percent; and salt (in the ash), 4.1 percent.

Sapsago

Sapsago cheese has been made in the Canton of Glarus, Switzerland, for at least 500 years and perhaps more; it is made also in Germany. It is known by various other names, including Schabziger, Glarnerkäse, Grünerkäse, Krauterkäse, and Grünerkrauterkäse. It is a small, very hard cheese that frequently is dried. A powder prepared from clover leaves is added to the curd, which gives it a sharp, pungent flavor, a pleasing aroma, and a light-green or sage-green color. The cured cheeses are cone-shaped, 3 inches thick at the base, 2 inches at the top, and 4 inches tall, and weigh 1 to 2¼ pounds. The fully cured, dry cheese can be used for grating.

Sapsago is made from slightly sour, skim milk. The milk is put into a round kettle and stirred while it is heated to boiling temperature. Cold buttermilk is added slowly as heating and stirring are continued. The coagulum that appears on the surface is removed, set aside, and added to the curd when it is put into the forms. Then enough sour whey is added to precipitate the casein, as in making Ricotta, and stirring is stopped. If too little whey is added, the curd will be too soft and moist; if too much or too sour whey is added, the curd will be too firm and dry. The curd is collected in a cloth or strainer and spread out to cool as the whey is drained off. Then the coagulum that was set aside is mixed with the curd, salt may be added, and it is placed in perforated wooden forms, covered with a press lid, and pressed under heavy pressure at a temperature of 60° F. The curd is ripened (cured) under light pressure at this temperature for at least 5 weeks. At this stage, it is ready for use in making the cheese. In many cases it is sold and transported in large sacks or casks to a distant factory where the cheese is made.

The ripe, dry curd is ground, and about 5 pounds of salt and 2½ pounds of dried, powdered leaves of the aromatic clover, *Melilotus coerulea,* are added to each 100 pounds of curd. The mixture is stirred into a homogeneous paste, then packed in the small cloth-lined, cone-shaped forms.

About 10 or 11 pounds of fresh curd is obtained per 100 pounds of skim milk and about 65 pounds of Sapsago is obtained per 100 pounds of fresh curd.

Analysis: Moisture, as much as 40 to 43 percent but usually much less (cheese imported into the United States, not more than 38 percent); fat, 5 to 9.4 percent; protein, 40 to 42.5 percent; and salt, 4 to 5 percent.

Swiss

Swiss (Emmentaler) cheese, which is a large, hard, pressed-curd cheese with an elastic body and a mild, nut-like, sweetish flavor, is best known because of the holes or eyes that develop in the curd as the cheese ripens. The eyes often are ½ to 1 inch in diameter and from 1 to 3 inches apart. The cheeses are about 6 inches thick, frequently more than 36 inches in diameter, and usually weigh between 160 and 230 pounds.

Switzerland is famous for this so-called King of Cheeses, and a large part of the milk produced in Switzerland is used in its production. It was first made, probably about the middle of the 15th century, in the Canton of Bern in the Emmental Valley (which accounts for its native name Emmentaler). The industry was well developed and cheese was being exported by the middle of the 17th century. Only the best cheese is exported, and it is commonly called "Switzerland Swiss."

Swiss cheese is made in many other countries besides Switzerland, including France, Denmark, Germany, Bavaria, Italy, Austria, Finland, Russia, Argentina, and the United States. Allgäuer Emmentaler, Bellunese, Formaggio Dolce, Fontina, Fontine d'Aosta, and Traanen are local names for similar cheeses made in Switzerland and nearby countries. Gruyère, made mostly in France, is similar to Swiss but is smaller and cures somewhat differently. Danish Swiss is called Samso.

The first Swiss cheese in the United States was made about 1850 by Swiss immigrants, and much of it is still being made by their descendants. Among the hard cheeses, Swiss ranks third in the quantity produced each year. About two-thirds of the annual production of 130 million pounds is made in Illinois and Wisconsin. Idaho, Minnesota, Ohio, Utah, and Wyoming also are producers. In the United States, Swiss cheese is often called Schweizer or Sweitzer.

Swiss cheese is one of the most difficult kinds of cheese to make. Control of the quality and composition of the milk, propagation and use of the essential bacterial starters, and the details of manufacture are complicated procedures that require the services of a skilled cheesemaker, and its successful manufacture is a factory operation that requires special equipment.

Three species of bacteria are used as starters: *Streptococcus thermophilus*, called the coccus culture; a lactobacillus—*Lactobacillus bulgaricus* or *L. lactis*—called the rod culture; and *Propionibacterium shermanii* (a propionic-acid-forming micro-organism), called the eye former. The lactobacillus and streptococcus produce lactic acid, which aids in expelling the whey, and they probably contribute to the breakdown of the curd during ripening. The propionic-acid bacteria are largely responsible for the characteristic flavor and eye formation.

Although there are slight differences between the methods used for making Swiss cheese in Switzerland and in the United States, following is a brief description of the general method:

Swiss cheese is made in round copper kettles that hold at least 2,000 pounds of milk, and frequently 3,000 or 3,200 pounds. The kettles are double-jacketed or have a steam chamber in the bottom. Good-quality, fresh milk is essential. It is advisable to clarify and standardize the milk. Clarification increases the elasticity of the curd in the cheese and improves eye formation. Standardizing the fat content of the milk assures cheese of uniform composition; usually slightly more than 10 percent of the fat is removed.

As the milk flows from the clarifier into the kettle, steam is turned on in the jacket or steam chamber under the kettle, and the milk is warmed to setting temperature (88° to 94° F.). Stirring is begun, the starter is added, and shortly thereafter enough rennet extract is added so the curd will be firm enough to cut in 30 minutes (the first indication of thickening appears in from 20 to 22 minutes).

As soon as the curd is firm enough to cut, the surface is "turned under"—that is, the creamy top layer is skimmed off with a wide, flat scoop and pushed to the back of the kettle, in order to mix this creamy layer with the rest of the curd. The curd is cut with a Swiss-cheese harp—from back to front and from side to side—into long rectangular strips about 1 inch square. Then the curd is turned under from top to bottom with a scoop, so that which was underneath will be on the surface, and the pieces are cut into 1-inch cubes. About 5 minutes after cutting is completed, the curd is harped (cut and mixed) until the particles are about ⅛ inch in diameter. This usually requires about 15 minutes.

Then the curd is "foreworked"—that is, stirred slowly, either continuously or at intervals—for 30 minutes to an hour or more as it acquires firmness. When it is sufficiently firm, steam is turned on and the curd is heated, usually in 30 minutes, to a temperature between 120° and 127.5° F. It is stirred continuously while it is being heated, and stirring is continued for at least 25 minutes and sometimes for an hour or longer after the final cooking temperature is reached. This is called "stirring out." As soon as the particles of curd can be broken apart easily without sticking when compressed in the hand, the curd is ready to be dipped. Some cheesemakers add several gallons of cold water at this point. Stirring is discontinued, so the curd will settle, and some of the whey is drawn off.

The curd is enclosed in a large, coarsely woven dipping cloth, and it is hoisted slowly over the kettle with a block and tackle, and the excess whey drains into the kettle. The bag of curd is then lowered into a circular wooden or stainless-steel hoop, which rests on a circular pressboard on a drain table. The curd is pressed gently down into the hoop, the edges of the cloth are smoothed over the curd, a circular pressboard is laid on top of the curd, and the curd is pressed from above with a screw- or lever-press.

About 5 minutes later, the hoop is removed; a clean, light cloth and a clean, heavy burlap cloth are substituted for the dipping cloth; the hoop is replaced; the cheese is turned over and another pressboard is placed on it; and it is pressed again. This process is repeated at definite intervals for 24 hours.

Then the cheese is removed from the press and, still in the hoop, it is taken to the so-called cold room (temperature about 55° F. and relative humidity 80 to 85 percent), where it is salted in brine. The cheese may be removed from the hoop and placed in the salt tank at once; or, still in the hoop, it may be placed on a shelf to cool for a day or so before it is salted. It is left in the salt brine for 2 or 3 days, the time depending on the size of the cheese, the amount of salt absorbed, and the rind formation desired. It is turned over and sprinkled with salt daily. Then it is placed on a circular board on a shelf in the cold room for a week or 10 days; it is washed, turned, and sprinkled with dry salt daily.

Then it is transferred to a clean board on a shelf in the warm room (temperature 65° to 72° F. and relative humidity 80 to 85 percent), where the principal ripening process takes place. The cheese is washed with salty water, it is turned and placed on a clean board, and salt is rubbed on the surface every few days. The eyes begin to form when the cheese is about 3 weeks old; eye formation is controlled to some extent by regulating the temperature of the room. The cheese usually remains in the warm room for 4 to 6 weeks; then it is returned to the cold room for further but slower curing, or to a storage room where it is held at about 40°.

Much of the cheese made in the United States is marketed after curing for 3 or 4 months (the minimum curing period is 2 months). Most of the cheese exported from Switzerland is cured for 6 to 10 months and has a more pronounced flavor.

A cheese weighing between 185 and 210 pounds can be made from a 2,500-pound kettle of milk. Several cheeses are packed in a round, wooden box for shipment; the box may contain more than 1,000 pounds of cheese. Swiss cheese is also made in rectangular blocks, about 28 inches long and 8 inches square, that weigh 25 to 28 pounds.

So-called rindless Swiss cheese is made by a somewhat modified method. The milk (in some instances as much as 20,000 pounds) is set in a rectangular vat, and the curd is prepared in the usual way. The curd and whey are transferred to a so-called press vat. Then, in a procedure similar to that used in making Herrgårdsost, the curd is pressed under the whey into a flat, rectangular block. The block of curd is subdivided into sections, each of which makes a cheese. Each cheese is placed in a cloth-lined box and pressed, then removed from the box, salted in brine, and dried. Then it is wrapped in film and placed in a box to cure.

Analysis (Domestic Swiss): Moisture, 39.4 percent (not more than 41 percent); fat, 27.5 percent (not less than 43 percent in the solids); protein, 27.4 percent; and salt, 1 to 1.6 percent.

Trappist

Trappist cheese was first made in 1885 in a monastery near Banjaluka in Bosnia, Yugoslavia. It is made also in monasteries in Hungary, Czechoslovakia, southern Germany, and other parts of Europe. It is much the same as the Port du Salut cheese made in France and the Oka cheese made in Canada, but there are variations in the manufacturing process.

The cheese is pale yellow and has a mild flavor. Although it is a semisoft cheese, it is cured more like the hard cheeses. It is washed frequently during the curing period, which largely prevents the growth of mold on the surface, and it ripens throughout rather than only from the surface. The size varies, the smallest being about 7 inches in diameter and weighing 2½ to 3 pounds. A larger size is about 10 inches in diameter and weighs about 5 pounds—the usual size of Port du Salut. There are still larger sizes, weighing about 10 pounds or more.

Trappist cheese is made from fresh, whole milk, usually cow's milk but some ewe's or goat's milk may be added. The milk is set with rennet at a temperature of about 82° to 90° F. After a coagulation period of 30 to 40 minutes (or as long as 90 when the setting temperature is low) the curd is cut, stirred, and heated, in some instances to a temperature of 95° to 108°. The whey is removed and the curd is transferred to forms. In Bosnia, the curd is pressed lightly, and the cheese is rather soft and tender. In Hungary and Czechoslovakia, the curd is pressed more heavily, and the cheese is somewhat firmer. The ripening period is from 5 to 6 weeks. The salted cheese is cured initially in a humid room at a temperature of 62° to 68° and later in a cooler cellar. The yield is 9 to 11 pounds of cheese per 100 pounds of cow's milk.

Analysis: Moisture, 45.9 percent; fat, 26.1 percent; protein, 23.3 percent; and salt, 1.3 to 2.5 percent.

Cereals and Pasta: A Surprising Source of Food Energy

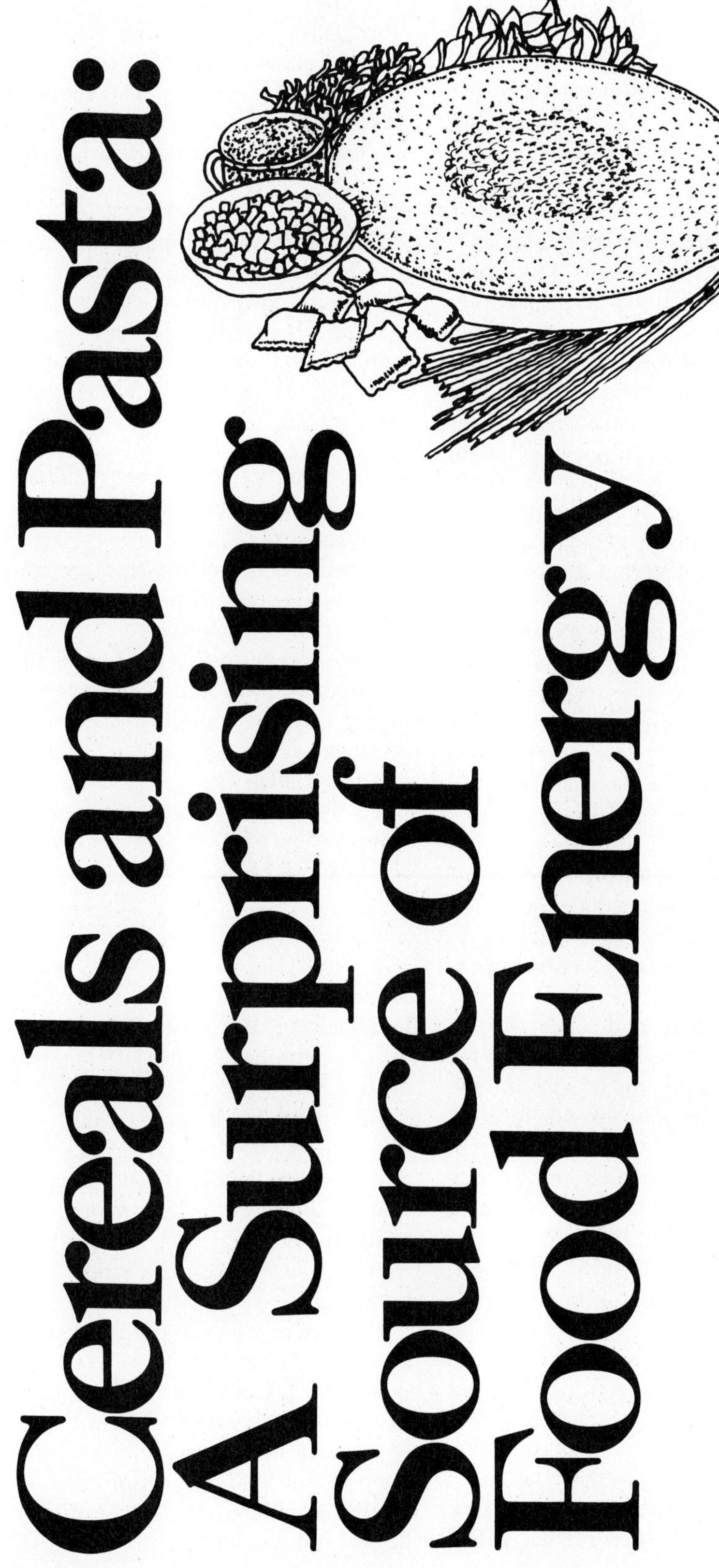

For hearty eating at mealtime, count on cereals and pasta. These grain products are good sources of food energy at relatively low cost.

Besides the diverse forms of corn, wheat, oats, and rice that appear at the family table, cereals and cereal products are used widely in combination dishes and in baked products, including breads, cookies, and pastries.

Whole grain cereals furnish a number of nutrients such as carbohydrate, protein, important trace minerals, iron, B vitamins including thiamin, riboflavin, and niacin, and certain other vitamins. Since whole grain cereals contain much of the bran portion of the grain that is largely indigestible, they contribute fiber to the diet. Other cereals are made wholly or in part from the inner portion of the cereal grain that contains smaller amounts of nutrients than are found in the whole grain. Most of these products have one or more nutrients, or wheat germ, added during processing to improve their nutrient content.

The protein in cereals is supplemented by the milk, meat, or other high-protein foods often served with cereals.

Then there's pasta, which includes all members of the spaghetti, macaroni, and noodle family. The bland flavor of pasta teams well with a variety of foods, from mild cheese to highly seasoned tomato sauce. Pasta helps stretch the food dollar by making meat and other protein foods go farther.

Enriched pasta provides useful amounts of thiamin, niacin, riboflavin, and iron. Pasta also supplies some protein; this protein is supplemented by the protein in meat, poultry, fish, cheese, eggs, and milk—foods that are often combined with pasta.

BUYING CEREALS

Breakfast Cereals

Ready-to-eat cereals come in a variety of textures, flavors, and shapes. You can select breakfast cereals made from corn, wheat, oats, rice, or a mixture of grains—in flaked, puffed, granular, and shredded forms.

Some ready-to-eat cereals are flavored with cocoa, molasses, fruit, or spices; some are combined with raisins or nuts. Cereals with fruit or nuts usually cost more per ounce than plain cereals.

Labels give clues to the economy of ready-to-eat cereals. Ingredients are listed in order from the item weighing the most to the item weighing the least. Sugar and other sweeteners add to the cost of the cereal. Cereals that have some form of sweetener, such as sugar, molasses, corn sirup, and honey listed first or several sweeteners listed as ingredients usually cost more per ounce than other cereals.

Most ready-to-eat cereals contain sugar or other sweeteners. Some contain much more than others. Those that contain the most list sugar as the first or second ingredient or list several sweeteners as ingredients. Some manufacturers show on the label the grams of sugar and other sweeteners per ounce of cereal. Sugar and other sweeteners furnish calories in the form of carbohydrate but supply little or no other nutritive value.

Most cereals are available in large and small size packages. If you can store and use it, the large package may be more convenient, reduce trips to the store, and save money, too. To find out if the large package saves money, compare the cost per unit—per ounce or per pound—of cereal from different size packages. Most stores now show the price per unit on the shelf where the cereal is displayed. Individual serving boxes of one kind of cereal or an assortment of cereals may be packaged together. These individual packs cost more but help preserve freshness and give family members a choice.

Labels on ready-to-eat cereals also give information about their nutritive value. The food energy (calories), the amount of protein, carbohydrate, and fat and the percent of the U.S. Recommended Daily Allowance (U.S. RDA) of certain vitamins and minerals in a serving are shown.

Whole grain and bran cereals provide fiber which is needed for normal functioning of the intestinal tract. They also provide more of certain nutrients than other cereals.

Ready-to-eat cereals may have nutrients added that are short in many diets—iron, thiamin, and vitamin B_6, for example. However, you do not need to choose cereals with 100 percent of the U.S. RDA for all nutrients listed in order to have a well-balanced diet. These cereals are usually expensive.

Hot cooked cereals—so appealing on cold mornings—may be made from wheat, oats, corn, or rice. Popular choices are farina, rolled oats (called oatmeal when cooked), whole-wheat cereal, and hominy (corn) grits. Some of these cereals are flavored with malt, cocoa, fruits, spices, or maple by the manufacturers.

You can also buy quick-cooking cereals that are specially processed and require only minutes to cook.

Instant hot cereals need only to be heated a few seconds after mixing with hot water or milk. Other instant cereals can be prepared right in the cereal bowl—all you do is add boiling water, stir, and serve. This type of cereal comes in individual-serving packages.

Cereals to be cooked and served hot usually cost less per serving than ready-to-eat cereals.

Both ready-to-eat and cooked cereals may have added food value in the form of vitamins, minerals, or wheat germ (the embryo of the wheat kernel).

To learn the food value and composition of a cereal food, read the label carefully.

Rice

Rice is economical and versatile. It is easy to prepare and its bland flavor combines well with many ingredients.

Rice may be long, medium, or short grain. Buy long-grain rice for use in main dishes, salads, curries, soups, and stews. Use short- or medium-grain rice in croquettes, meat and fish loaves, rice rings, and puddings.

You can buy rice in the following forms:

Regular white rice has been milled to remove the hull, germ, and practically all of the bran. Milling removes some of the vitamins and minerals. White rice has a bland flavor and tender texture. Cooked long-grain rice is light and fluffy, with grains that are separate and distinct. Cooked short- or medium-grain rice has moist grains that tend to cling together.

Enriched rice is white rice plus added vitamins and iron.

Parboiled rice is treated by a special steam-pressure process before milling. This forces the vitamins and minerals from the hull, bran, and germ into the starchy part of the grain, so that much of the natural vitamin and mineral content is retained after milling. Parboiled rice is also enriched. Parboiled rice takes longer to cook than regular white rice. The cooked grains are fluffy, separate, and plump. They are slightly firmer and more chewy than regular milled rice.

Precooked rice is long-grain white rice that has been cooked and dried. It takes less preparation time than regular white rice but costs more.

Brown rice is whole-grain rice from which only the hull and a small amount of the bran has been removed. It retains more of the natural vitamins and minerals than white rice. It has a nutlike flavor and a slightly chewy texture. Brown rice needs to cook a little longer than regular white rice.

Wild rice is not a true rice, but the seed of a grass that grows wild in shallow lakes and marshes. It is dark brown, distinctive in flavor, and costs considerably more than other types of rice.

Convenience foods containing rice are also available. You can get canned or frozen rice that is cooked and ready to heat and serve. Rice is a major ingredient in many canned and frozen combination foods. Mixes containing precooked rice, regular long-grain rice, or wild rice combined with spices, herbs, or other ingredients are also on the market.

Cornmeal and Hominy (Corn) Grits

Degerminated cornmeal is made from ground, mature, white or yellow corn from which the bran and germ have been removed. Also available is stone-ground (whole-ground) cornmeal. This is slightly coarser than degerminated cornmeal.

Hominy (corn) grits are also made from hulled, degerminated corn, but are much coarser than degerminated cornmeal.

White cornmeal and grits are traditional in the South; yellow cornmeal and grits are more likely to be found in the North. Besides color, there are also differences in flavor in these products.

Most cornmeal and hominy (corn) grits on the market are enriched with thiamin, niacin, riboflavin, and iron according to U.S. Government standards. Calcium and vitamin D also may be added to these corn products.

Bulgur

Bulgur—a wheat food eaten for centuries in certain countries of the Near East—is considered a gourmet food in the United States.

In the making of bulgur, wheat is parboiled and dried, and some of the bran is removed. Bulgur may be sold whole or cracked.

Cooked bulgur has a nutlike flavor and a slightly chewy texture. You can use bulgur in many of the same ways you use rice.

BUYING PASTA

Pasta includes macaroni, spaghetti, and noodles—in a great variety of shapes and sizes. Pasta dough is made from one or more of the following—semolina (made from durum wheat), farina, and wheat flour—and water. Pasta products made with semolina hold their shape well during cooking. Farina products are quick cooking and may be somewhat more tender than semolina products. Noodles are made with the same ingredients as macaroni and spaghetti but also contain eggs.

Machines form the dough into more than 150 shapes, ranging from long, thin spaghetti to broad, flat lasagna noodles—from elbow macaroni to jumbo macaroni shells—and from alphabet noodles to noodle bows and ribbons.

Some common forms of pasta are listed below.

Macaroni is usually shaped like a hollow tube; elbow macaroni is short and curved. Shell macaroni, as the name indicates, is shaped like a seashell.

Spaghetti is formed into long, thin, solid rods. Spaghettini is thinner than regular spaghetti, and vermicelli is thinnest of all. Short, curved spaghetti is also available.

Noodles are flat, ribbon-like strips cut in varying widths—fine, medium, and broad.

Among the more unusual forms of pasta are the Italian specialties—manicotti, rigatoni, green noodles (which contain spinach), and cresta di gallo (shaped like a rooster's crest).

A number of convenience foods combining pasta with sauce mixes or canned sauces are available, too.

Most pasta products are enriched with thiamin, riboflavin, niacin, and iron. Check the label.

STORING CEREALS AND PASTA

Store cereals and pasta at room temperature in tightly closed containers to keep out dust, moisture, and insects. Choose a relatively cool, dry place in your kitchen—not above the range or refrigerator, or below the sink. Do not store cereals and pasta near soap or other products with strong odors.

Open cereal packages carefully—follow instructions on the packages—and close them tightly after use. Refold the inner wrap on ready-to-eat cereals to help protect flavor and crispness.

When humidity is high, ready-to-eat cereals may soon lose crispness. To restore crispness, heat the cereal in a shallow baking pan in a preheated oven at 350° F. for about 5 minutes.

The following home storage guide gives the approximate length of time cereals and pasta will maintain flavor and crispness in a cool, dry place. When these products are held longer than the time indicated, off-flavors may develop.

	Maximum storage time for best quality
Breakfast cereals	2 to 3 months
Bulgur	6 months
Degerminated cornmeal and hominy (corn) grits	4 to 6 months
Pasta (except egg noodles)	1 year
Egg noodles	6 months
Rice:	
White	1 year
Parboiled	1 year
Precooked	1 year
Brown	6 months
Wild	6 months
Seasoned mixes	4 to 6 months

USING CEREALS AND PASTA

Preparing and Serving Breakfast Cereals

Ready-to-eat cereals

These cereals—ready to serve directly from the package—save time on hurried mornings. They are especially convenient when family members eat breakfast at different times. Children enjoy helping themselves to ready-to-eat cereals.

Keep an assortment on hand so everyone can choose his or her favorite cereal or combine two or more in a cereal medley.

To spark new interest in breakfast, provide one or more of the following toppings for cereal.

- Fresh, frozen, or canned fruit.
- Cooked or uncooked dried fruit.
- Softened ice milk (good on hot days).
- Honey or molasses.

Cooked cereals

When cooking breakfast cereals, use the proportions of ingredients and the cooking times recommended on the package.

Here are some general directions that apply to all breakfast cereals that require cooking.

- Have water boiling rapidly before adding cereal.
- Sprinkle cereal slowly over boiling water while stirring constantly to prevent lumping. Boiling should not stop.
- Stir cereal as it thickens to prevent sticking. Excessive stirring may break up the cereal and make it pasty.

Reduce heat, cover, and continue cooking for length of time given on package. During this step, regular-cooking cereals can be cooked either over direct heat or over boiling water in a double boiler. Quick-cooking cereals are usually cooked over direct heat. Although a certain amount of cooking is necessary to develop the flavor, overcooking makes cereal gummy.

To vary the flavor of cooked cereals, cook them in milk or with raisins or cut-up dried fruits or add fresh, frozen, or canned fruit to the cereal after cooking.

To cook cereal in milk, use a little more milk than the amount of water called for. Heat the milk to just below the boiling point before stirring in and cooking the cereal.

To add variety to cooked cereals, try these suggestions.

- Add cinnamon, nutmeg, or mace (1 teaspoon for 6 servings) to water just before adding cereal.
- Stir wheat germ, coconut, or nuts into cooked cereal before serving.
- Serve with honey or molasses.

Serve cooked cereal immediately. When cooked cereal is allowed to stand exposed to the air, a rubbery film quickly forms on the surface. If cooked cereal must wait for latecomers, cover it and keep it hot in the top of a double boiler over hot water.

To reheat leftover cooked cereal, place it in a saucepan and add just enough water or milk for the desired consistency. Cook over low heat, stirring to prevent sticking, until the cereal is hot.

Or if you prefer, add the liquid and reheat cereal in the top of a double boiler over boiling water. Cover and heat without stirring.

Cereals as ingredients

Breakfast cereals can add flavor and texture to many foods. They are familiar ingredients in cookies, quick breads, and desserts. When added to meatballs and meat loaves, they help keep the meat moist.

Many recipes call for crushed cereals. You can buy packaged cereal crumbs or you can crush most crisp ready-to-eat cereals by hand. Place cereal in a plastic bag or between two sheets of waxed paper and crush it with a rolling pin. Or crush cereal in an electric blender.

One cup of ready-to-eat cereal makes 1/4 to 1/3 cup of crumbs; the yield of crumbs depends on the kind of cereal and how fine you crush it.

Add a crunchy texture to foods by using breakfast cereals in the following ways:

As a crisp coating for meat, poultry, or fish—

Use crushed, unsweetened ready-to-eat cereal flakes, packaged cereal crumbs, or degerminated or stone-ground cornmeal in place of breadcrumbs or flour as a coating. Season crumbs or cornmeal with salt, pepper, and your favorite herbs, if desired.

As a topping for casseroles—

Combine crushed, unsweetened, ready-to-eat cereal with melted butter or margarine. If desired, add shredded Cheddar or grated Parmesan cheese, an herb such as basil or oregano, or poultry seasoning. Top your favorite casserole with this cereal mixture instead of buttered breadcrumbs, and bake as directed in casserole recipe.

As croutons—

Use unsweetened puffed corn, puffed wheat, or bite-size shredded wheat, corn, or rice. Combine the cereal with melted butter or margarine and grated Parmesan cheese or your favorite herb seasoning. Use on tossed salads or hot soups.

As a crunchy coating for cookies or biscuits—

Drop cooky dough from a teaspoon into crushed ready-to-eat cereal. Roll dough into balls and bake on a greased baking sheet as directed in cooky recipe.

Dip rounds of refrigerated or homemade biscuit dough in undiluted evaporated milk; then roll in fine cereal crumbs and bake in a foil-lined pan. To make cinnamon biscuits, mix sugar and cinnamon with the cereal crumbs.

As a dessert topping—

Serve on ice cream, fruits, or a chilled pudding.

Cooking Rice

Rice is easy to cook—you can boil, steam, oven-cook, or fry it.

Keep in mind that most kinds and brands of rice swell during cooking. One cup of uncooked white, parboiled, or brown rice yields 3 to 4 cups cooked rice; 1 cup of precooked rice yields from 1 cup to slightly more than 2 cups.

To keep as many nutrients as possible in cooked rice, follow these rules:

- Do not wash rice before cooking. Packaged rice is clean.
- Use only the amount of water that the rice will absorb during cooking.
- Do not rinse rice after cooking.

Rice is done when a grain of rice pressed with a spoon or between two fingers is soft throughout.

Leftover cooked rice can be used in most combination dishes that call for cooked rice.

Cooked rice may be kept up to 1 week in the refrigerator. Cooked rice may also be frozen and kept in the freezer at 0° F. or below for 6 to 8 months.

To reheat cooked rice, steam it in a colander or sieve over boiling water. Or add 2 tablespoons water for each cup of cooked rice, and reheat in a covered pan over low heat or in the oven. While rice is heating, occasionally stir it gently with a fork. If rice has been frozen, thaw and reheat as for refrigerated rice.

Regular or enriched white rice

Some persons like rice fluffy and dry, firm yet tender, with the grains well separated. Others prefer rice soft and moist with the grains clinging together. Here are cooking directions for fluffy rice and a variation for softer rice.

Boiled white rice (fluffy)

6 servings, about 1/2 cup each

Salt	1 teaspoon
Water	2 cups
White rice, uncooked	1 cup
Butter or margarine	1/2 teaspoon

Add salt to water and bring to a boil.

Stir rice into rapidly boiling water.

Add fat to reduce foaming.

Bring back to boiling point and lower heat until water is just bubbling.

Cover tightly and boil *gently* 20 minutes. Don't stir during cooking; stirring may mash the grains and make the rice gummy. Do not uncover rice during cooking.

Rapid boiling may break the grains and make the rice boil over.

After cooking, remove pan from direct heat, but *do not remove cover.*

Let rice stand 10 to 15 minutes, covered tightly, to finish cooking in its own steam.

Fluff rice with a fork.

For softer rice.—Increase water to 2¼ cups and boil gently 25 minutes. Let stand 10 minutes, covered.

Calories per serving: About 120.

Oven-cooked white rice (fluffy)

6 servings, about ½ cup each

White rice, uncooked	1 cup
Salt	1 teaspoon
Butter or margarine	½ teaspoon
Boiling water	2 cups

Preheat oven to 350° F. (moderate).

Place rice, salt, and fat in a 1-quart casserole or pan. Pour boiling water over rice; stir and cover.

Bake 35 minutes or until rice is tender.

Calories per serving: About 120.

Other kinds of rice

Parboiled rice.—Follow either of the methods—boiling or oven cooking—as for white rice, but increase water to 2½ cups for each cup of uncooked rice. Boil parboiled rice 25 minutes. For oven-cooked parboiled rice, increase baking time to 40 minutes. One cup uncooked rice makes six servings cooked rice. Calories per serving are about the same as for white rice.

Brown rice.—Use either method—boiling or oven cooking—as for white rice. Boil brown rice 45 minutes or until tender and water is absorbed. Or cook in oven about 55 minutes. One cup uncooked rice makes six servings cooked rice. Calories per serving are about the same as for white rice.

Precooked rice.—Follow directions on package.

Cooking Bulgur

For variety in your meals, serve cooked bulgur as a breakfast cereal or as a vegetable. Or add bulgur to soups or stews at the start of cooking. You can also use cooked bulgur in meat loaves, meatballs, stuffed peppers, or casserole dishes.

Cooking methods for bulgur are similar to those for rice. Like rice, bulgur is not washed before cooking or rinsed after cooking. Cook in just the amount of water that will be absorbed during cooking.

One cup of dry, cracked bulgur yields 3 to 3½ cups cooked bulgur.

Boiled bulgur

6 servings, ½ cup each

Water	2 cups
Salt	½ teaspoon
Bulgur, dry, cracked, unseasoned	1 cup

Heat water to boiling; add salt.

Stir bulgur into boiling water.

Cover tightly and cook over very low heat 25 minutes. Do not remove cover while cooking.

Calories per serving: About 100.

Oven-cooked bulgur

6 servings, ½ cup each

Bulgur, dry, cracked, unseasoned	1 cup
Salt	½ teaspoon
Boiling water	2 cups

Preheat oven to 350° F. (moderate).

Place bulgur and salt in a 1-quart casserole.

Pour boiling water over bulgur; stir and cover.

Bake 25 minutes or until tender.

Calories per serving: About 100.

Try These Variations

Cook rice or bulgur in a flavorful liquid instead of water. Try chicken or beef broth or equal parts of tomato or fruit juice and water.

Add flavor with spices, herbs, or other seasonings.

- Add curry powder, cumin, thyme, turmeric, mace, saffron, or dried parsley flakes to the water with the rice or bulgur. For most spices or herbs, use ½ to 1 teaspoon for 1 cup uncooked rice or bulgur. For dried parsley flakes, use 1 tablespoon. For saffron, use ⅛ teaspoon.
- Cook chopped onions, celery, or mushrooms in a little fat or oil until tender; add to rice or bulgur at start of cooking.
- Add raisins to rice or bulgur before cooking. Or add nuts, chopped olives, or toasted sesame seeds after cooking.
- Add chopped fresh or frozen parsley or chives to cooked rice or bulgur.

Cooking Cornmeal and Hominy (Corn) Grits

Cornmeal can be served as a breakfast cereal, but it is used most often as an ingredient in breads. Cornbread, johnnycake, and spoonbread are popular versions.

When a recipe calls for "yellow cornmeal" or "white cornmeal," you will get the best results if you use the kind specified. But if the recipe simply calls for "cornmeal," you can use either yellow or white.

If you use self-rising cornmeal, you will need to omit or decrease the amount of salt and baking powder. Self-rising cornmeal contains ½ teaspoon salt and the equivalent of 1½ teaspoons baking powder for each cup of cornmeal.

Cornmeal mush

8 servings, ½ cup each

Cornmeal	1 cup
Cold water	1 cup
Salt	1 teaspoon
Boiling water	3 cups

Mix cornmeal, cold water, and salt.

Stir cornmeal mixture slowly into boiling water.

Stir until thickened.

Cover and cook over low heat 15 minutes, stirring occasionally to keep from sticking.

Serve cornmeal mush hot.

Calories per serving: About 70.

VARIATION

Fried cornmeal mush.—Chill mush thoroughly in loaf pan. Cut mush into ½-inch slices and fry in 2 tablespoons fat until brown. About 100 calories per serving.

Hominy (corn) grits

8 servings, ½ cup each

Salt	1 teaspoon
Water	5 cups
Hominy (corn) grits, regular, uncooked	1 cup

Add salt to water; bring to boil.

Stir in hominy grits slowly. Lower heat and stir until thickened.

Cook for 15 minutes longer, stirring occasionally to keep from sticking.

Hominy grits are usually served with meat or eggs—for breakfast, lunch, or supper.

Calories per serving: About 70.

Cooking Pasta

Well-cooked pasta is tender yet firm—not sticky. For best results, pasta should be added to rapidly boiling, salted water, and cooked only until tender.

Thick pasta products, such as lasagna noodles, need more water for cooking than other pastas. To cook thick pasta products, follow directions on the package.

General directions for cooking other pasta products are given here.

Boiled pasta

3 to 4 cups cooked pasta

Salt	1 tablespoon
Water	3 quarts
Pasta, uncooked (macaroni, spaghetti, or noodles)	8-ounce package

Add salt to water. Bring water to a full rolling boil.

Add pasta gradually to rapidly boiling water so that boiling does not stop. To fit long spaghetti into pan, break long spaghetti strands in half. Or place one end of spaghetti strands in the boiling water, then, as the spaghetti softens, gradually coil the strands around the pan until they are completely underwater.

Leave pan uncovered.

Stir occasionally to keep pasta from sticking to pan.

Cook pasta just until tender; consult directions on package for cooking time. To test for doneness, press a piece of the pasta with a fork or spoon against the side of the pan. Pasta should break easily and cleanly when done.

Drain pasta at once in a colander or strainer. Do not rinse pasta after cooking. If pasta tends to stick together, add a sauce or a little fat or oil.

Calories per cup: About 260 for macaroni, 345 for spaghetti, 235 for egg noodles.

Tips

Be careful not to overcook pasta; overcooking makes it soft and unappetizing.

Shorten the cooking time slightly if pasta is to be used in a combination dish that needs further cooking.

Pasta is best, of course, when cooked just before it is to be served or mixed with other ingredients. But if it must be cooked ahead of time, keep it hot in a strainer over hot water. The steam will reduce sticking. Cooking oil, butter, or margarine stirred into cooked pasta also helps reduce sticking.

If cooked pasta is to be used cold in salads, add the salad dressing while the pasta is still hot. This helps prevent sticking. Flavors blend more thoroughly, too.

Different kinds of pasta can be used interchangeably in most recipes that call for a given weight of **uncooked pasta**—an 8-ounce package, for example. But in recipes that call for a given measure—such as 1 cup—you may not be able to substitute so successfully, because a cupful of one kind of uncooked pasta may weigh more or less than a cupful of another kind.

Different kinds of **cooked pasta,** however, can be used interchangeably, measure for measure, in recipes.

Vegetables: High in Vitamins, Low in Calories

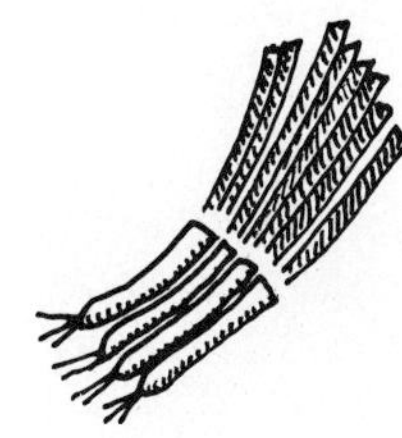

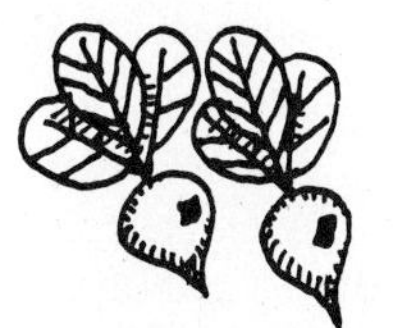

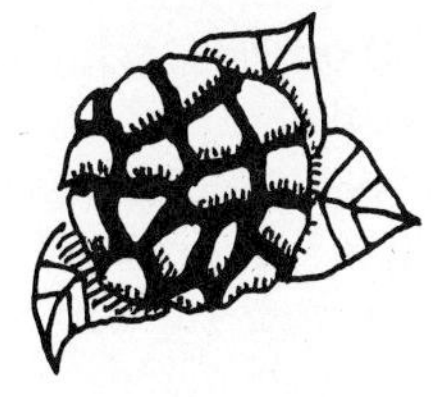

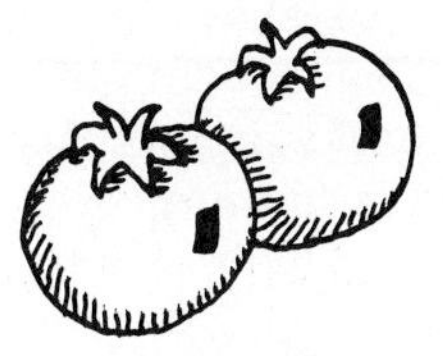

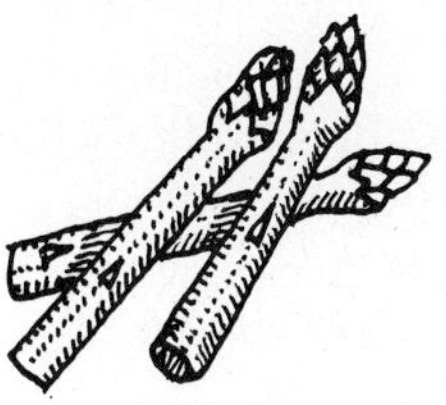

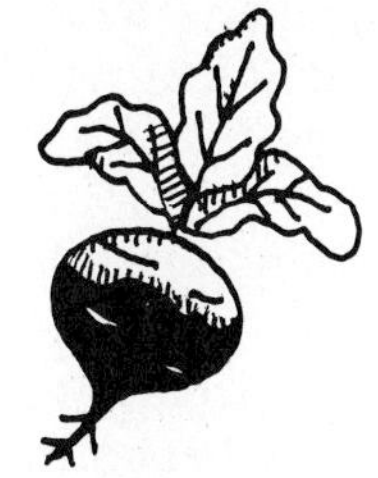

Vegetables grow in great variety—from A (asparagus) to Z (zucchini). Often they are low in cost and calories and a number of them rank high in vitamins and minerals. One-half cup of most boiled vegetables contains less than 50 calories. Starchy vegetables like lima beans, peas, corn, and plain, boiled potatoes supply from 50 to 100 calories in a half-cup serving.

Most dark-green and deep-yellow vegetables excel as dependable and inexpensive sources of vitamin A. In fact, unless your meals include several servings of carrots, spinach, sweetpotatoes, winter squash, broccoli, kale or other greens each week, your family may not get enough vitamin A. As a bonus, many dark-green vegetables supply valuable amounts of vitamin C, iron, and other vitamins and minerals.

The mature dry legumes—dry peas and members of the bean family including navy, pinto, and soybeans—are outstanding among the vegetables for the protein they contain. They also contribute B vitamins, iron, and other nutrients.

And how drab our diets would be without the color and crispness of fresh-tossed salads, the tang and texture of relishes, and the distinctive flavors of our vegetable dishes.

Raw vegetables are becoming increasingly popular as a low-calorie between-meal snack. Weight watchers do well to keep a supply of celery sticks, carrot sticks, radishes, or green pepper slices ready in the refrigerator to eat when hunger strikes.

BUYING VEGETABLES

Besides a variety of fresh vegetables now available the year round, you usually have the choice of buying other forms—canned, frozen, or dehydrated.

Here are points you may want to consider in making your choice:

- Fresh vegetables are generally highest in quality and lowest in price *when in season.* In selecting, look first for freshness. Vegetables should be comparatively dry; excessive moisture hastens decay.
- Canned vegetables are probably the most convenient because they need only brief reheating and do not require refrigerated storage until the can is opened.
- Frozen vegetables closely resemble fresh vegetables in color, flavor, and texture, and usually cost more than canned vegetables.
- Dehydrated vegetables usually take up less storage room than fresh, canned, or frozen vegetables. Some dehydrated vegetables cost slightly more than comparable fresh products, but can be prepared much more quickly.
- Dry legumes—including dry beans, peas, and lentils—are inexpensive but take a relatively long time to prepare.

Purchase Units

Canned vegetables come in a variety of can sizes. The most popular family size is one that holds 16 ounces. If you have a one- or two-person family, the 8-or 8½-ounce can is a good choice. Can sizes most commonly available and the approximate amount of vegetable in each follow.

Can size	*Approximate amount of contents*
8 or 8½ ounces	1 cup
12 ounces	1½ cups
16 ounces	2 cups
27 to 29 ounces	3½ cups
104 to 117 ounces (6½ pounds to 7 pounds 5 ounces)	12 to 13 cups

Most frozen vegetables come in the familiar "family-size" 10-ounce package. A few come in 8-, 9-, and 12-ounce packages. Many retail markets also offer 16- and 32-ounce packages of some vegetables.

Some frozen vegetables are sold in heavy polyethylene bags. You can get 16, 24, and 32 ounces of cut green beans, corn, peas, peas and carrots, potatoes, and mixed vegetables packaged this way. The advantage of this type of packaging is that the vegetables are usually separate enough to pour from the bag, making it possible to use part of the package and return the rest to the freezer.

For good-quality frozen vegetables, follow these suggestions:

- Select clean, firm packages. If packages are soft, you can be sure the food has already lost quality. However, a hard-frozen package does not assure high quality. Frozen food is safe to eat as long as the package remains frozen, but a storage temperature of 0° F. or lower is necessary to maintain high quality.
- Buy only frozen foods that are displayed in a properly refrigerated cabinet made for that purpose. Do not buy frozen vegetables stacked outside the frozen food cabinet even if they are packed in dry ice.
- Select packages only from clean cabinets in which foods are stacked no higher than the proper fill line. This line, which is marked on the inner side of many cabinets, indicates the level above which frozen foods should not be stacked.
- Look for a thermometer in the cabinet; if there is one, it should register 0° F. or below.
- Plan to pick up frozen foods last when shopping. For the trip home, it's a good idea to protect frozen foods in an insulated bag or a double paper bag, particularly in warm weather. At home, get packages into home freezer or freezing compartment as quickly as possible.

Number of Servings

The number of servings you get from a common-size purchase unit of a vegetable varies widely with the kind of vegetable and whether it is fresh, frozen, canned, or dried.

Necessarily, the inedible parts of fresh vegetables—pods, husks, parings, and trimmings—lower the yield of edible food per pound. Some fresh vegetables shrink because they lose water during cooking; others absorb water and swell as they cook.

Yield from a pound of fresh vegetables may vary from two to six servings (½ cup each) of cooked food.

Frozen vegetables usually do not lose much weight or volume during preparation. For the approximate amount of each vegetable to buy for six servings, see the Boiling Guide for Home Frozen Vegetables.

Some loss of volume occurs during preparation of canned vegetables for serving if the liquid is drained from the vegetables or if the liquid is concentrated during cooking. From a 16-ounce can of most vegetables you can expect three or four servings (½ cup each) of drained vegetables and two or three servings of canned greens, such as kale or spinach.

Dried vegetables increase considerably in weight and volume during cooking because they absorb water. See the Boiling Guide for Dry Beans, Peas, and Lentils, for the approximate yield of cooked food from a cup of dry beans, peas, or lentils.

STORING VEGETABLES

Fresh

Even under ideal storage conditions—the right temperature and humidity—most fresh vegetables retain top quality only for a few days.

Green, leafy vegetables quickly wilt and change flavor as water evaporates from tissues. Other vegetables—corn, beans, and peas—lose sweetness within a short time as sugar converts to starch.

Most fresh green vegetables keep well and stay crisp if put in covered containers or plastic bags and stored in the refrigerator. If you wash lettuce, celery, and other leafy vegetables before storing, drain thoroughly because too much moisture can hasten decay. Tops should be removed from beets, carrots, and radishes.

Always sort vegetables before storing. Discard or use at once any bruised or soft vegetables; do not store them with sound, firm vegetables.

To maintain high quality in the following fresh vegetables, store them in the refrigerator in the crisper or in plastic bags, and use within the time specified.

Asparagus—2 or 3 days.

Beans, snap (green or wax)—1 week.

Beets—2 weeks.

Broccoli, brussels sprouts—3 to 5 days.

Cabbage—1 or 2 weeks.

Carrots—2 weeks.

Cauliflower—1 week.

Celery—1 week.

Cucumbers—1 week.

Greens—spinach, kale, collards, chard, beet, turnip, and mustard greens—3 to 5 days.

Lettuce and other salad greens—1 week.

Mushrooms—1 or 2 days.

Okra—3 to 5 days.

Onions, green—3 to 5 days.

Parsnips—2 weeks.

Peppers—1 week.

Radishes—2 weeks.

Squash, summer—3 to 5 days.

Here are specific directions for storing other vegetables and the length of time they can usually be held:

Beans, lima. Store uncovered in pods in refrigerator—3 to 5 days.

Corn. Store unhusked and uncovered in refrigerator—1 or 2 days.

Eggplant. Store at cool room temperature (approximately 60° F.). If air is dry, keep eggplant in plastic bag to retain moisture—1 or 2 days.

Onions, mature. Store at room temperature or slightly cooler (60° F. is best). Put in loosely woven or open-meshed containers with good circulation of air. Onions sprout or decay if temperature or humidity is high, but will keep several months in a cool, dry place.

Peas, green. Store uncovered in pods in refrigerator—3 to 5 days.

Potatoes. Store in a dark, dry place with good ventilation and a temperature of 45° to 50° F. May be held several months under these conditions.

Squash. Store hard-rind winter varieties in cool, dry place (about 60° F.). Keeps several months.

Sweetpotatoes, rutabagas. Store at cool room temperature (about 60° F.). Temperatures below 50° may cause chilling injury. Stored this way, these vegetables keep several months.

NOTE: Mature onions, potatoes, winter squash, sweetpotatoes, and rutabagas can be kept at room temperature for a short time if it is not possible to store them at the temperatures recommended. Buy only enough for a week.

Tomatoes. Store ripe tomatoes uncovered in the refrigerator. Keep unripe tomatoes at room temperature away from direct sunlight until ripe, then refrigerate. Too much sunlight prevents development of even color.

Frozen

Frozen vegetables should be stored at 0° F. or lower. Stored at 0°, they retain quality and nutritive value several months.

Most home freezers and freezer sections of refrigerator-freezer combinations can maintain a temperature near 0° F., but freezing compartments of most conventional home refrigerators cannot. Before buying large quantities of frozen vegetables, check the temperature of your frozen food storage area. If the temperature is above 0°, plan to use frozen vegetables within a few days.

Exactly how long commercially frozen vegetables will retain high quality when stored at 0° F. depends on the kind of vegetable and condition at time of purchase. Maximum storage suggested for commercially frozen asparagus, beans, cauliflower, corn, peas, and spinach is 8 months. Home-frozen vegetables should maintain high quality 8 to 12 months.

Canned and Dried

Store unopened canned vegetables in a cool, dry place. For best quality, use canned vegetables within a year of purchase. Vegetables lose quality if stored too long, but remain indefinitely safe to eat if the seal is not broken.

Freezing does not make canned vegetables unsafe to eat unless it breaks the seal and lets in bacteria that cause spoilage. Rust on the can caused by dampness is not harmful to the food unless it penetrates the can.

Food may be left in tin cans after opening. Put a cover on the can and store in refrigerator. Some vegetables, particularly acid vegetables like tomatoes, develop an unpleasant, but harmless, metallic taste from a chemical reaction of the food to the can lining after opening. Use canned vegetables within 2 or 3 days after opening.

Store dried vegetables in tightly closed containers in a cool, dry place. Most dried vegetables will keep several months.

COOKING FRESH VEGETABLES

Preparing

Remove bruised, wilted, yellowed, or tough portions from fresh vegetables. Trim sparingly to avoid excessive loss of food and nutrients. If root vegetables and potatoes are pared before cooking, make parings thin.

Dark-green outer leaves of cabbage, lettuce, and other leafy green vegetables contain valuable nutrients, so don't discard them unless they are wilted or tough. Remove woody midribs from kale leaves—there is little loss of nutritive value and the kale tastes better.

Wash vegetables thoroughly before cooking. Use plenty of water for leafy greens; lift them from water to let sand and grit settle.

Soak fresh brussels sprouts and broccoli in cold salt water for a short time to remove insects if any are present. Cover potatoes with water to prevent darkening if held after paring. Long soaking of most vegetables, however, is not desirable because some nutrients dissolve in the water.

Boiling

To insure the best flavor, color, texture, and food value in vegetables, cook them only until they are tender. Vegetables cooked whole in skins retain most of their nutritive value. To shorten cooking time—cut, slice, dice, or coarsely shred vegetables.

The amount of water used in cooking is important—the less water, the more nutrients retained in the cooked vegetables.

For young, tender vegetables, ½ to 1 cup of water is usually enough for six servings. Use water to cover for root vegetables when cooked whole, because they require longer cooking. Corn-on-the-cob also requires water to cover. Spinach and other greens need only the water clinging to their leaves from washing if cooked over low heat in a pan with tight-fitting lid. Tomatoes can be cooked in their own juice.

Here are directions for boiling fresh vegetables:

- Bring salted water to a boil (use ½ to 1 teaspoon salt for six servings of vegetable).
- Add vegetable. Cover and quickly bring water back to a boil.
- Reduce heat and cook gently until vegetable is just tender. (See boiling guide).
- Serve immediately; flavor and nutritive value may be lost if vegetables are allowed to stand.

Pressure Cooking

In cooking vegetables, follow the directions that came with your cooker, but learn to adjust cooking time to suit the quality of vegetable being cooked. Very young, tender vegetables may require a shorter cooking time than is recommended. Even 1 or 2 minutes extra cooking can cause undesirable color, changes in texture, and loss of nutrients.

Here are directions for pressure cooking:

- Bring pressure up quickly.
- Time the cooking period exactly.
- Reduce pressure as quickly as possible when time is up.

Boiling Guide for Fresh Vegetables

Vegetable	Cooking time after water returns to boil	Approximate amount as purchased for six servings) (about ½ cup each)
	Minutes	*Pounds*
Asparagus	10 to 13 (whole)	2½
Beans, lima	25 to 27	2¾ in pods
Beans, snap (green or wax)	13 to 15 (1-inch pieces)	1
Beets	38 to 41 (whole)	2½ with tops or 1½ without tops
Broccoli	9 to 12 (heavy stalk, split)	2
Brussels sprouts	15 to 17	1½
Cabbage	6 to 8 (shredded)	1¼
	10 to 13 (wedges)	1½
Carrots	20 to 22 (whole)	1½ without tops
	18 to 20 (sliced or diced)	
Cauliflower	8 to 12 (separated)	2
	20 to 24 (whole)	
Celery	15 to 19 (cut-up)	1¼
Collards	15 to 20	1½ untrimmed
Corn	5 to 7 (on cob)	3 in husks
	6 to 8 (whole kernel)	
Kale	15 to 20	1¼ untrimmed
Okra	12 to 14	1¼
Onions, mature	11 to 15 (whole)	1¾
	10 to 14 (quartered)	
Parsnips	20 to 40 (whole)	1½
	8 to 15 (quartered)	
Peas	10 to 14	3 in pods
Potatoes	25 to 29 (whole, medium)	1½
	15 to 17 (quartered)	
Spinach	8 to 12	1½ prepackaged
Squash, acorn	18 to 20 (quartered)	2½
Squash, butternut	16 to 18 (cubed)	
Squash, yellow crookneck	11 to 13 (sliced)	1½
Squash, zucchini	13 to 15 (sliced)	
Sweetpotatoes	28 to 35 (whole)	2
Tomatoes	7 to 15 (cut-up)	1¼
Turnips	30 to 38 (whole)	1¾ without tops
	10 to 12 (cut-up)	

• Season vegetables in the same ways as plain boiled vegetables.

Baking

Potatoes or sweetpotatoes

Preheat oven to 425° F. (hot).

Wash and dry vegetables. Rub with a little fat to soften skin. Prick with a fork to allow steam to escape during baking and to prevent bursting.

Bake until tender—for medium-size potatoes, 50 to 60 minutes; for sweetpotatoes, 35 to 60 minutes.

If other foods are to be cooked at 350° or 375° F. (moderate), potatoes or sweetpotatoes may be baked along with them. Allow 10 to 20 minutes longer than times given above.

VARIATIONS

Remove baked potato from skin, mash with butter or margarine and milk, stuff back into skin, and sprinkle with grated cheese or spread with sour cream and chopped chives. Return to oven for 10 minutes or until lightly browned.

Scoop baked sweetpotato from the skin; mash with butter or margarine and milk. Or use 1 tablespoon peanut butter for each sweetpotato in place of butter or margarine, or orange juice and a little grated orange rind in place of the milk. Stuff sweetpotato mixture back into skins and return to oven for 10 minutes.

Carrots

Preheat oven to 375° F. (moderate).

Grease 1½-quart casserole.

Wash and scrape medium-size carrots; cut in half lengthwise.

TRY THESE VARIATIONS

Add a pinch of herbs or a tablespoon of minced onion, green pepper, or chives before cooking fresh vegetables. These add flavor, without calories.

Season after cooking with a flavorful fat—bacon drippings, butter, or margarine—or with salad oil to which a little lemon juice, horseradish, or garlic has been added.

Sprinkle lemon juice or herb vinegar on boiled vegetables for pleasantly tart touch.

Mash vegetables, beat in a little hot milk, add butter or margarine, and season with salt and pepper.

Serve with a tasty sauce.

Place in casserole. (For six servings, use about 1½ pounds medium-size carrots.

Add ¼ cup hot water. Dot with 2 to 3 tablespoons butter or margarine. Sprinkle with salt and pepper. Cover.

Bake until tender, about 45 minutes.

Onions

Preheat oven to 375° F. (moderate).

Grease 1½-quart casserole.

Peel onions; cut in half crosswise.

Arrange with cut side up in casserole. (For six servings, use 2 pounds of medium-size onions.)

Add just enough water to cover bottom of casserole. Sprinkle with salt and pepper. Cover.

Bake 30 minutes. Top with 1 cup buttered bread cubes and bake uncovered 15 to 20 minutes longer until cubes are brown and onions are tender.

Tomatoes

Preheat oven to 375° F. (moderate).

Wash tomatoes and cut off stem ends. (Use one medium-size tomato for each serving.)

Place tomatoes in a casserole. Sprinkle with salt and pepper. Top with buttered bread cubes (1 cup for six tomatoes). Add just enough water to cover bottom of casserole. Cover. Bake 15 minutes.

Uncover and bake 10 to 15 minutes longer until tomatoes are soft and bread cubes are browned.

VARIATIONS

Top tomatoes with onion slices and crisscross with green pepper strips before baking. Omit buttered bread cubes.

Winter squash

Preheat oven to 400° F. (hot).

Cut acorn squash in half or Hubbard squash into 3- or 4-inch cubes. (For six servings use three acorn squash, or 3 pounds Hubbard squash.) Arrange in a baking pan.

Brush squash with melted butter or margarine and sprinkle with salt and brown sugar. Add just enough water to cover bottom of baking pan. Cover the pan.

Bake acorn squash 30 minutes, uncover; bake Hubbard squash 45 minutes, uncover. Continue baking until squash is tender—20 to 30 minutes for acorn, about 30 minutes for Hubbard.

VARIATION

Sprinkle a little cinnamon or nutmeg on squash before baking.

Summer squash

Preheat oven to 400° F. (hot).

Slice squash into ½-inch slices. (Use 3 pounds squash for six servings.) Place squash in a casserole. Dot with butter or margarine, sprinkle with salt and 1 tablespoon finely chopped onion.

Add just enough water to cover bottom of casserole. Cover.

Bake 50 minutes to 1 hour until squash is tender.

French Frying

Vegetables that can be french fried successfully include: *potatoes; sweetpotatoes;* breaded *green pepper* rings; and batter-dipped *eggplant* sticks; *parsnips,* and *onion* rings. Before frying potatoes or sweetpotatoes, rinse them quickly in cold water to remove surface starch. Dry thoroughly.

Do not overload the fry basket when french frying. If too much food is put into the basket at one time, the temperature of the fat drops excessively, cooking slows down, and the vegetable absorbs more fat.

One-stage method:

- Fill kettle one-third full of fat or oil and heat to 370° to 385° F. Have fry basket in fat.
- Raise basket and add enough vegetable to cover bottom of basket.
- Lower basket gently into fat. If fat bubbles much, lift and lower basket several times until bubbling subsides.
- Fry until vegetable is cooked through and golden brown.
- Lift basket from fat. Drain a few seconds; then pour vegetable onto absorbent paper.
- Season. Spread fried vegetable on a cookie sheet and place in a warm oven to keep warm while frying additional vegetables.

Two-stage method:

You may prefer the two-stage method if you want to partially prepare french fried *potatoes* and *sweetpotatoes* ahead of time.

First stage—Proceed as for one-stage method except fry only until food is cooked, but not brown. Do not hold parfries longer than 1 or 2 hours at room temperature or 24 hours in covered container in refrigerator. To hold parfries longer than 24 hours, freeze them.

Second stage—

- Heat fat to 375° F. with fry basket in fat.

• Raise basket and add about two layers of parfries.

• Fry until golden brown.

• Lift basket from fat. Drain for a few seconds; then pour vegetable onto absorbent paper.

• Season and serve.

Frying

Fried cooked vegetables

Parsnips, potatoes, sweetpotatoes.—Use about 3 cups sliced or diced cooked vegetable for six servings (½ cup each).

Heat 2 or 3 tablespoons butter, margarine, or drippings in a heavy frypan over moderate heat.

Add vegetable and cook 5 to 10 minutes, or until lightly browned. Turn vegetable during cooking to insure even browning.

Add a little diced onion, crumbled bacon, or diced ham for variety.

Fried raw vegetables

Carrots, onions, or potatoes.—Use 3 cups sliced, raw vegetable to make six servings (½ cup each) of potatoes or carrots, or six servings (¼ cup each) of onions.

Heat 3 tablespoons fat or oil in a heavy frypan over moderate heat.

Add sliced vegetable and cook 15 to 25 minutes, or until vegetable is tender and lightly browned. Turn vegetable frequently.

Eggplant or tomatoes. — Use one medium eggplant or four medium-size, firm tomatoes for six servings.

Pare eggplant. Cut eggplant or tomatoes into ½-inch slices.

Dip vegetable slices into flour or fine dry breadcrumbs.

Heat ¼ cup fat or oil in a heavy frypan over moderate heat.

Add vegetable and cook over low heat 2 to 4 minutes, or until tender and lightly browned. Add more fat or oil if necessary during cooking to prevent sticking.

Panning

Panning—cooking shredded or sliced vegetables in a small amount of fat and water on top of the range—is a good way to prepare *snap beans, cabbage, carrots, corn, spinach,* and *summer squash.* See cooking guide below for length of time to cook and amounts of vegetable and other ingredients needed for six servings (½ cup each).

Directions for panning:

• Shred or slice vegetable.

• Heat fat (butter, margarine, or drippings) in heavy frypan over moderate heat.

• Add vegetable and sprinkle with salt.

• Add water and cover pan to hold in steam.

• Cook over low heat until vegetable is tender; stir occasionally to prevent sticking.

VARIATIONS

Add finely chopped onion or onion juice before cooking. Or add bits of crumbled crisp bacon or diced ham to cooked vegetable.

Creaming and Scalloping

Start with any cooked vegetable or combination of two or more vegetables that go well together. Besides the popular *peas-and-carrots* team, you can combine: *Cauliflower and peas, green beans and corn, lima beans and carrots, asparagus and celery, carrots and onions, and brussels sprouts and celery.*

Creamed vegetables

6 servings, ½ cup each

Add 3 cups cooked, drained vegetables to 1 cup hot white sauce; heat to serving temperature.

Scalloped vegetables

6 servings, ½ cup each

Guide for Cooking Panned Vegetables
6 servings (½ cup each)

Vegetable	Amount of—				Cooking time
	Vegetable	Fat	Salt	Water	
	Quarts	*Tablespoons*	*Teaspoons*		*Minutes*
Beans, snap (green or wax), sliced in 1-inch pieces	1	1½	½	⅔ cup	20 to 25.
Cabbage, finely shredded	1½	1½	¾	3 tablespoons	6 to 8.
Carrots, thinly sliced	1	2	½	3 tablespoons	10.
Corn, cut	1	1½	½	⅓ cup	15 to 18.
Spinach, finely shredded	3	2	½	-------------	6 to 8.
Summer squash, thinly sliced	1	1½	½	3 tablespoons	12 to 15.

Preheat oven to 350° F. (moderate).

Grease 1-quart casserole.

Combine 3 cups cooked, drained vegetables and 1½ cups medium white sauce (standard or low-fat recipe) in casserole.

Top with 3 tablespoons fine dry breadcrumbs (mixed with 2 teaspoons melted butter or margarine).

Bake 25 to 30 minutes.

For a special touch of flavor in scalloped vegetables, try one of the following:

- Add a pinch of an herb—marjoram, thyme, or oregano to white sauce before combining with vegetables.
- Alternate layers of vegetables and sauce.
- Sprinkle between layers with grated cheese, finely chopped onion or parsley, or cooked mushrooms.
- Use crushed ready-to-eat cereal in place of breadcrumbs on top.

Glazing

Carrots, parsnips, and sweetpotatoes are delicious when glazed. To prepare, cut the cooked vegetable into strips or large pieces. For six servings (½ cup each) you'll need about 3 cups cut cooked vegetable.

Blend 2 tablespoons butter or margarine with ¼ cup packed brown sugar and 1 tablespoon water in a heavy frypan over low heat.

Add 3 cups cooked vegetable.

Cook over low heat, turning vegetables several times until sirup is very thick and vegetables are well coated—takes from 5 to 10 minutes. Keep heat low to prevent scorching.

VARIATIONS

Substitute frozen orange juice concentrate for water. Or use honey or maple sirup instead of brown sugar and omit water.

COOKING FROZEN VEGETABLES

Frozen vegetables may be prepared by boiling in a small amount of water, or you can cook them in a moderate oven while you are baking other foods. Cooked frozen vegetables are seasoned and served like fresh vegetables. If you like, you can cream or scallop them or add them to souffles, soups, or salads.

Boiling

Thawing before cooking is not necessary for most frozen vegetables. Leafy vegetables, however, cook more evenly if thawed just enough to separate the leaves before you put them in boiling water. It is a good idea to partially thaw corn on the cob before cooking it so that the cob will be heated through by the time the corn is cooked.

Cook home-frozen vegetables as follows:

- Bring lightly salted water to a boil in a covered saucepan. The amount of water varies with kind of vegetable and size of package. For most vegetables, ½ cup of water is enough for a pint package. Use enough water to cover for corn-on-the-cob.

Boiling Guide for Home Frozen Vegetables

Vegetable	Cooking time after water returns to boil	Approximate amount of frozen vegetable for six servings (½ cup each)
	Minutes	*Ounces*
Asparagus, whole	8 to 10	24
Beans, lima	12 to 14	18
Beans, snap (green or wax), cut	7 to 9	16
Broccoli spears	6 to 8	22
Brussels sprouts	10 to 12	20
Carrots:		
Slices	6 to 8	18
Strips	7 to 9	18
Cauliflower	2 to 6	20
Corn:		
Whole kernel	7 to 9	20
On cob	4 to 8	32
Kale	8 to 10	25
Okra, whole	6 to 8	16
Peas	8 to 10	18
Spinach	2 to 6	25
Squash, summer, sliced	6 to 8	22

- Put frozen vegetable into boiling water, cover pan, and bring quickly back to a boil. To insure uniform cooking, it may be necessary to separate pieces with a fork.
- When water returns to boiling, reduce heat and start to count time (see boiling guide).

To cook commercially frozen vegetables, follow package directions.

Baking

Partially defrost vegetables to separate the pieces. Spread vegetables in a greased casserole, add seasonings as desired, and cover. Bake until just tender.

At 350° F. (moderate oven) most vegetables require approximately 45 minutes. Cooking time varies with the size of pieces and how much they were thawed before baking.

HEATING CANNED VEGETABLES

Commercially canned vegetables need reheating only. Cook gently just until heated through. Since some vitamins and minerals are in the cooking liquid, serve the cooking liquid with the vegetable whenever practicable, or use it in sauces, soups, or gravies.

Heat home-canned vegetables the same way if you are sure they have been processed correctly at the recommended temperature. If you are not absolutely sure, bring vegetables to a rolling boil in the liquid, then cover and boil for at least 10 minutes. Boil spinach and corn 20 minutes.

Do not use canned vegetables that show any sign of spoilage—bulging can ends, leakage, spurting liquid, off-odor, or mold. Do not even taste them. Destroy out of reach of children and pets.

COOKING DRIED VEGETABLES

Dehydrated Vegetables

Some of the newer dried vegetable products are quickly and easily prepared. Dehydrated potato products, for example, take less time than comparable products made from fresh potatoes. Dehydrated onions may be reconstituted with water, or added without reconstitution to foods high in liquid.

For best results with any quick-cooking vegetable product, follow package directions carefully.

Dry Beans and Whole Peas

Soaking.—Dry beans and whole peas require soaking before cooking. Use the amount of water recommended for the vegetable in the boiling guide.

Boil beans and peas 2 minutes, remove from heat, soak 1 hour, and then cook. Or soak overnight after the 2-minute boil, and then cook.

Long cooking times for beans can be shortened by adding small amounts of baking soda to water at beginning of soaking periods.

If tap water is of medium hardness, add 1/8 teaspoon soda to the water for each cup of dry beans to reduce cooking time about one-fourth. Measure soda exactly; excessive soda affects flavor and nutritive value of beans.

Boiling.—Cook in soaking water; add 1 teaspoon salt for each cup of the dry vegetable.

To reduce foaming during cooking, add 1 tablespoon meat drippings or other fat for each cup of dry beans or whole peas.

Boil gently, uncovered, for a few minutes until foaming has decreased. Then cover and boil gently until tender. See boiling guide for approximate boiling time.

Pressure cooking.—Most dry beans and whole peas can be fully cooked in a pressure cooker in less than 30 minutes after soaking. This length of time allows pressure to rise and fall slowly and cooks these vegetables evenly without breaking the skins.

Follow these directions for soaking and pressure cooking dry beans and whole peas:

- Add 2 cups water for each cup of beans or peas, boil 2 minutes, and soak 1 hour before cooking.
- Fill pressure cooker no more than one-third full of food and water. If cooker is too full, food may clog vent tube and cause an explosion.
- Add 1 tablespoon fat to reduce foaming, and 1 teaspoon salt per cup of dry beans or peas.
- Put lid on pressure cooker. Follow manufacturer's directions for exhausting cooker and bringing pressure up to 15 pounds.
- Cook vegetables at 15 pounds pressure as follows:

3 minutes — Great Northern beans, kidney beans, large lima beans, and whole peas.

5 minutes — black beans and cranberry beans.

5 to 10 minutes—navy (pea) beans.

10 minutes—pinto beans.

Boiling Guide for Dry Beans, Peas, and Lentils[1]

Vegetable (1 cup)	Amount of water	Approximate boiling time	Yield
	Cups	*Hours*	*Cups*
Black beans	3	2	2
Blackeye beans (blackeye peas, cowpeas)	2½	½	2½
Cranberry beans	3	2	2
Great Northern beans	2½	1 to 1½	2½
Kidney beans	3	2	2¾
Lentils	2	½	2½
Lima beans, large	2½	1	2½
Lima beans, small	2½	1	2
Navy (pea) beans	3	1½ to 2	2½
Peas, whole	2½	1	2½
Pinto beans	3	2	2½
Soybeans	4	2½	2½
Split peas	2	⅓	2½

[1] See soaking directions for each kind of vegetable before cooking.

- Remove cooker from heat. Let pressure drop gradually.

Yield of cooked vegetable will be the same as for boiled vegetable.

Lentils

Lentils may be cooked without soaking.

Add 1 teaspoon salt to the cooking water for each cup of lentils. Cover, boil gently until done. See boiling guide below.

Split Peas

Soaking.—Soaking split peas helps retain their shape. Follow the boiling guide below for amount of water to use. Boil for 2 minutes. Then soak ½ hour. Split peas used in soup do not need to be soaked before cooking.

Boiling.—Add ¾ teaspoon salt for each cup of split peas, cover, and boil gently without stirring for the time recommended in the guide.

Baking.—You can bake split peas after soaking. Add ¾ teaspoon salt for each cup of peas. Place in baking dish, cover, and bake at 350° F. (moderate oven) for 35 minutes.

NOTE: Pressure cooking is not advised for split peas because they may splatter and clog the cooker vent.

Tips

Cooked dry beans, peas, and lentils may be seasoned and eaten without further preparation, or they may be baked or combined with other foods.

If acid ingredients like tomatoes, catsup, or vinegar are included in the recipe, add them after the vegetables are tender. Acids prevent beans and peas from softening.

SEASONINGS AND SAUCES

Spices and Herbs

Discover how spices and herbs can lift humdrum vegetable dishes out of the ordinary.

Spices and herbs must be used sparingly or they overpower, rather than enhance, the natural flavor of vegetables. One-fourth to ½ teaspoon of most dried spices and herbs is enough for 2 cups of vegetable.

The term "spices," as generally used, includes the herbs as well as true spices. Herbs are leaves and sometimes the flowers of aromatic plants grown in the Temperate Zone; spices come from aromatic plants grown in the Tropics.

Dried herbs are more concentrated than fresh herbs. Use about ¼ teaspoon of a dried herb for 2 cups of vegetable and add it at beginning of cooking period. With fresh herbs, increase to about ¾ to 1 teaspoon for 2 cups of vegetable. Chop herbs very fine to allow some of the flavoring oils to escape. Heat chopped herbs in melted butter and add to vegetable after it has been cooked.

Sauces in Variety

It's simple to make sauces that add variety and distinction to vegetable dishes. Often the right sauce gives contrast in color, flavor, and texture. From a basic white sauce you can concoct many pleasing sauces to serve over cooked vegetables or in scalloped vegetables.

Thin white sauce is usually preferred with starchy vegetables like peas or lima beans; medium white sauce with other vegetables.

How to make white sauce

For a smooth white sauce, blend the flour with fat or cold liquid; then combine with remaining liquid, stirring constantly over low heat until thickened.

Fat may be omitted if white sauce is to be used in cream soups,

Give Vegetables a Gourmet Touch With

SPICES AND HERBS

Vegetable	Spice or herb[1]
Asparagus	Mustard seed, sesame seed, or tarragon.
Beans, lima	Marjoram, oregano, sage, savory, tarragon, or thyme.
Beans, snap	Basil, dill, marjoram, mint, mustard seed, oregano, savory, tarragon, or thyme.
Beets	Allspice, bay leaves, caraway seed, cloves, dill, ginger, mustard seed, savory, or thyme.
Broccoli	Caraway seed, dill, mustard seed, or tarragon.
Brussels sprouts	Basil, caraway seed, dill, mustard seed, sage, or thyme.
Cabbage	Caraway seed, celery seed, dill, mint, mustard seed, nutmeg, savory, or tarragon.
Carrots	Allspice, bay leaves, caraway seed, dill, fennel, ginger, mace, marjoram, mint, nutmeg, or thyme.
Cauliflower	Caraway seed, celery salt, dill, mace, or tarragon.
Cucumbers	Basil, dill, mint, or tarragon.
Eggplant	Marjoram or oregano.
Onions	Caraway seed, mustard seed, nutmeg, oregano, sage, or thyme.
Peas	Basil, dill, marjoram, mint, oregano, poppy seed, rosemary, sage, or savory.
Potatoes	Basil, bay leaves, caraway seed, celery seed, dill, chives, mustard seed, oregano, poppy seed, or thyme.
Salad greens	Basil, chives, dill, or tarragon.
Spinach	Basil, mace, marjoram, nutmeg, or oregano.
Squash	Allspice, basil cinnamon, cloves, fennel, ginger, mustard seed, nutmeg, or rosemary.
Sweetpotatoes	Allspice, cardamom, cinnamon, cloves, or nutmeg.
Tomatoes	Basil, bay leaves, celery seed, oregano, sage, sesame seed, tarragon, or thyme.

[1] Pepper and parsley may be added to any of the above vegetables. Curry powder is good with creamed vegetables.

casseroles, or other recipes where fat is not needed for flavor or texture.

Variations of white sauce

Certain vegetables are enhanced by special sauces. The following variations of white sauce taste particularly good with the vegetables mentioned.

Cheese sauce (asparagus, broccoli, cabbage, cauliflower, potatoes, and summer squash). Cook 1 cup of thin or medium white sauce. Remove sauce from heat; stir in 1 cup shredded Cheddar cheese. Blend well.

Mock hollandaise sauce (asparagus and broccoli). Make 1 cup of medium white sauce. Beat 2 egg yolks, stir a little hot white sauce into them, and stir mixture into rest of sauce. Stir in 2 tablespoons butter or margarine. Cook over hot water about 1 minute. Remove from heat and stir in 1 tablespoon lemon juice. Serve at once.

NOTE: *In this recipe use only clean eggs with no cracks in shell.*

Mushroom sauce (asparagus, green beans, and peas). Use proportions of fat and flour for 1 cup of medium white sauce. Cook 1 cup small whole or sliced fresh or canned mushrooms in fat. Add flour. Use liquid from canned mushrooms to replace part of milk.

Onion or celery sauce (carrots, green beans, and peas). Use proportions of fat and flour for 1 cup of thin white sauce. Cook ½ cup finely chopped onion or celery in the fat until tender, stir in flour and salt, and slowly blend in liquid. Cook over low heat stirring constantly until thickened. Add 1 teaspoon worcestershire sauce before serving.

LIVELY LEFTOVERS

A bit of imagination can transform leftover vegetables into new, interesting dishes. Try cold leftover vegetables in egg, meat, gelatin, or tossed green salads. Add them to soups or casseroles. Or combine yesterday's corn or snap beans with today's lima beans.

Actually, you can use leftover vegetables in any recipe that calls for cooked vegetables. Cream—scallop—glaze—or fry them as you would freshly cooked vegetables, or puree them to make cream soups.

Tomatoes add extra juiciness and flavor to meat loaves and ground meat patties. Dry beans extend meat proteins in money-saving combination dishes. And most families enjoy hearty vegetable soups and meat and vegetable stews.

Ingredients for 1 Cup of White Sauce

Ingredients	Measure			
	Thin sauce		Medium sauce	
	Standard	Low-fat	Standard	Low-fat
Butter or other fat	1 tablespoon	2 teaspoons	2 tablespoons	1 tablespoon.
All-purpose flour	1 tablespoon	1 tablespoon	2 tablespoons	2 tablespoons.
Salt	¼ teaspoon	¼ teaspoon	¼ teaspoon	¼ teaspoon.
Milk	1 cup[1]	1 cup[1,2]	1 cup[1]	1 cup.[1,2]
Calories in 1 cup white sauce	290	180	420	245.

[1] Vegetable liquid may be used in place of part of milk.

[2] Use skim milk or reconstituted nonfat dry milk for milk in low-fat white sauce.

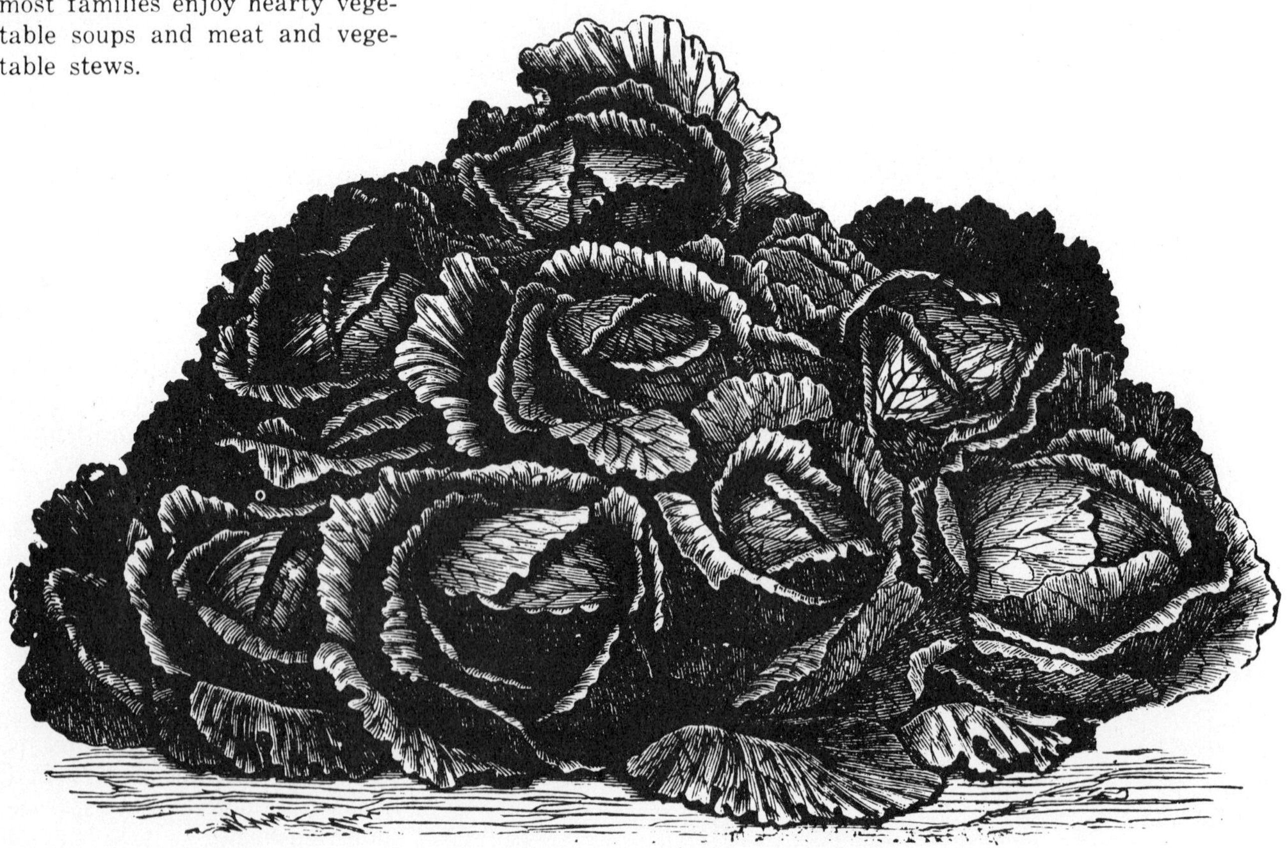

Keeping Food Safe to Eat

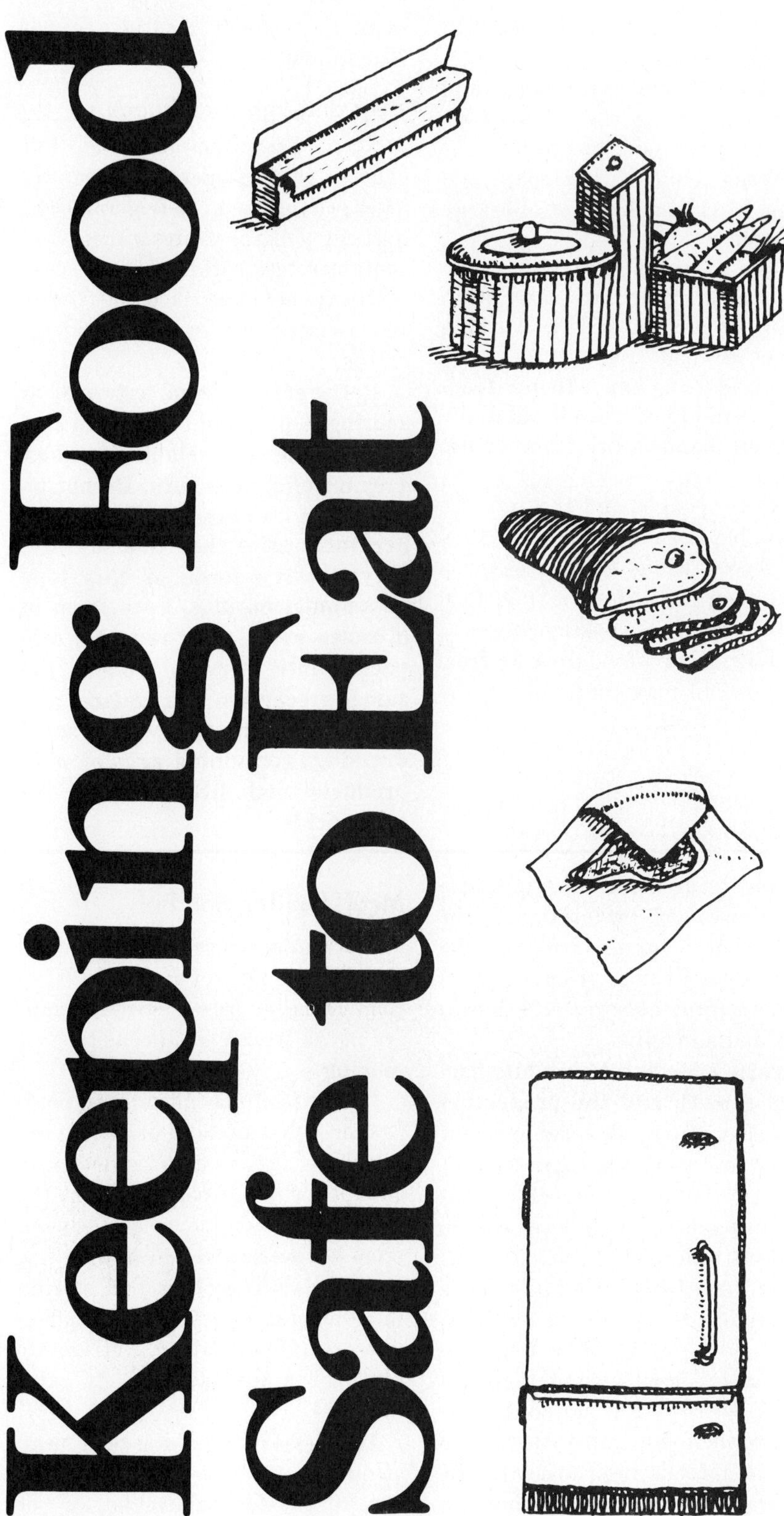

Poor food-handling practices in the home often cause illness in the family, even though the foods were safe to eat when purchased or first prepared.

Lack of sanitation, insufficient cooking, and improper storage can allow bacteria in food to increase to dangerous levels. Some bacteria produce poisonous substances called toxins that cause illness when the food is eaten.

Outbreaks of illness from food contaminated by harmful bacteria are especially common during hot summer months when perishable foods are carried on picnics and cookouts without proper refrigeration.

BACTERIA INVOLVED

Certain bacteria growing in food may cause illness in one of the following ways. Disease-producing bacteria may enter the body in contaminated food and set up infections in the digestive tract, and, in some cases, in the bloodstream. Other bacteria may form dangerous toxins in food. Eating food in which the bacteria have grown and produced toxin causes illness.

Foods containing Salmonellae can cause infection, called salmonellosis, in man. The disease is difficult to control because it spreads simply and easily. *Salmonella* infections result from eating food in which large numbers of Salmonellae are growing or from personal contact

with an infected person or a carrier of the infection.

Bacteria that can produce poisonous toxins in food are *Staphylococcus aureus* and *Clostridium botulinum*.

The first toxin, when eaten in food, results in so-called "staph" poisoning, probably the most common foodborne disease in the United States. The second toxin can cause botulism, the rarest and deadliest kind of food poisoning.

Another class of bacteria involved in foodborne illness is *Clostridium perfringens*. These bacteria often cause diarrheal upsets, which are rarely fatal.

WHAT YOU CAN DO

You can help protect your family from foodborne illness by—

- Stressing personal hygiene for all members of your household.
- Making sure all dishes, utensils, kitchen equipment, and work surfaces are clean.
- Taking simple precautions in storing, preparing, cooking, and preserving all foods.

PERSONAL HYGIENE

Strict cleanliness of person and surroundings is the best way to prevent the contamination of foods and the spread of foodborne illness in the home.

Any member of the household who has an infectious disease should be discouraged from handling, preparing, or serving food. Do not permit anyone with an infected cut or other skin infections to work with food because the bacteria causing the infection may also be the source of foodborne illness.

Anyone handling food should—

- Always work with clean hands, clean hair, clean fingernails, and wear clean clothing.
- Wash hands with soap and water after using the toilet or assisting anyone using the toilet.
- Wash hands with soap and water after smoking or blowing the nose.
- Wash hands with soap and water after touching raw meat, poultry, or eggs, before working with other food.
- Avoid using hands to mix foods when clean utensils can be used.
- Keep hands away from mouth, nose, and hair.
- Cover coughs and sneezes with disposable tissues.
- Avoid using the same spoon more than once for tasting food while preparing, cooking, or serving. Eating baby food directly from a jar or can may contaminate any remaining food.

STORING FOODS

Temperature and time influence the growth of bacteria and the production of toxins in foods. Like other livings things, bacteria need food, warmth, moisture, and time to grow and multiply.

Keeping foods cold inhibits bacterial growth and the production of toxins. In most cases, prompt cooling and proper refrigeration of foods can hold the number of bacteria in foods to a safe level and no ill effects follow.

The hazard lies in holding foods for any length of time at temperatures above refrigerator temperatures and below serving temperature of hot food. For more information, see the food temperature guide.

Certain foods need special care. For recommendations on how to store these foods see the sections that follow.

Eggs and Egg-Rich Foods

Keep eggs clean and cold. Put eggs in the refrigerator promptly after getting them. Refrigerate leftover egg yolks or whites in a covered container; use within a day or two.

Always hold uncooked and cooked foods containing eggs in the refrigerator.

Refrigerate cream, custard, or meringue pies and foods with custard fillings, including cakes, cream puffs, or eclairs. Do not allow them to stand at room temperatures after they cool slightly. If you carry foods of this type on summer outings, keep them in a cooler with ice or reusable cold packs until served. Follow the same precaution for salads and sandwiches made with salad dressings containing eggs or milk products and little vinegar or other acids.

Meat, Poultry, and Fish

Store unfrozen raw meat, poultry, and fish in the refrigerator. Keep commercially frozen stuffed poultry in the freezer until time to start cooking.

Do not stuff uncooked meat, poultry, or fish and hold it in the refrigerator. If stuffing is made in advance, store it separately in the refrigerator. Remove all stuffing from leftover cooked meat, poultry, or fish before cooling and storing in refrigerator; refrigerate stuffing in a separate container. Refrigerate broth or gravy immediately after the meal.

If necessary to hold cooked meat, poultry, or fish, keep the temperature of the food above 140° F or below 40° to prevent growth of bacteria or production of toxins. Promptly refrigerate cooked meat and fish to be eaten cold or after reheating. Store cold cuts in a refrigerator or cooler, never hold at room temperatures for more than 2 or 3 hours.

Freeze cooked meat, poultry, stuffing, and gravy if you want to keep them longer than a few days.

Store frozen cooked meat or poultry products in a freezer until they are reheated for serving or thawed for immediate use.

PREPARING AND COOKING FOODS

General Pointers

- Serve food soon after cooking—or refrigerate promptly. Hot foods may be refrigerated if they do not raise the temperature of the refrigerator above 45°F. Keep them in the refrigerator until served or reheated.
- Speed the cooling of large quantities of food by refrigerating in shallow containers.
- **Keep hot foods HOT (above 140° F) and cold foods COLD (below 40° F). Food may not be safe to eat if held for more than 2 or 3 hours at temperatures between 60° and 125° F, the zone where bacteria grow rapidly.** Remember to count all time during preparation, storage, and serving.
- Holding of foods for several hours in an automatic oven prior to cooking is not safe if the food is in the temperature zone of 60° to 125° F for more than 2 or 3 hours.
- Thoroughly clean all dishes, utensils, and work surfaces with soap and water after each use. It is especially important to thoroughly clean equipment and work surfaces that have been used for raw food before you use them for cooked food. This prevents the cooked food from becoming contaminated with bacteria that may have been present in the raw food. Bacteria can be destroyed by rinsing utensils and work surfaces with chlorine laundry bleach in the proportion recommended on the package. Cutting boards, meat grinders, blenders, and can openers particularly need this protection.
- Always wipe up spills with paper towels or other disposable material.

Eggs and Egg-Rich Foods

Use only fresh, clean, unbroken, and odor-free eggs in any recipe in which eggs are not thoroughly cooked, such as egg-milk drinks, soft-cooked eggs, poached eggs, scrambled eggs, omelets, uncooked salad dressings, ice cream, meringues, soft custards, or puddings cooked on the top of the range.

Cracked or soiled eggs may contain harmful bacteria. They should be used only in foods that are to be thoroughly cooked, such as baked goods or casseroles.

Cool hot foods containing a high proportion of eggs if they are not to be served hot. Set custards and puddings in ice water and stir large batches of pudding to speed cooling. Then refrigerate promptly until time to serve.

Meat, Poultry, and Fish

Thaw frozen raw meat or unstuffed raw poultry in the refrigerator, or for a quicker method, immerse the package in its watertight wrapper in cold water. Thaw until meat is pliable.

You can cook frozen meat, poultry, or fish without thawing, but you must allow more cooking time to be sure the center of the meat is properly cooked. Allow at least one and a half times as long to cook as required for unfrozen or thawed products of the same weight and shape. Undercooked foods may not be safe to eat.

Stuff fresh or thawed meat, poultry, or fish just before roasting. Put the stuffing in lightly—without packing—to allow heat to penetrate more quickly throughout the stuffing.

Cook meat, poultry, or fish as recommended in a reliable timetable.

Make sure that the stuffing reaches a temperature of at least 165° F during roasting. To check the temperature of the stuffing after roasting, insert a meat thermometer in the stuffing for about 5 minutes. Cook longer if necessary. Any stuffing cooked separately in the oven should also reach 165° F.

Do not partially cook meat or poultry one day and complete the cooking the next day. Keep cooked meat, fish, or poultry hot (above 140° F) until it is served.

Heat leftovers thoroughly. Boil broth and gravies several minutes when reheating them.

Heat frozen cooked meat, poultry, or fish without thawing or thaw in the refrigerator before using.

Directions on the package of all prepared and partially prepared frozen foods must be followed exactly. Heating for the specified time assures that the food will be safe to eat.

FREEZING FOODS

Maintain strict sanitation in preparing any food for the home freezer. Keep all food to be frozen—and everything that touches it—clean.

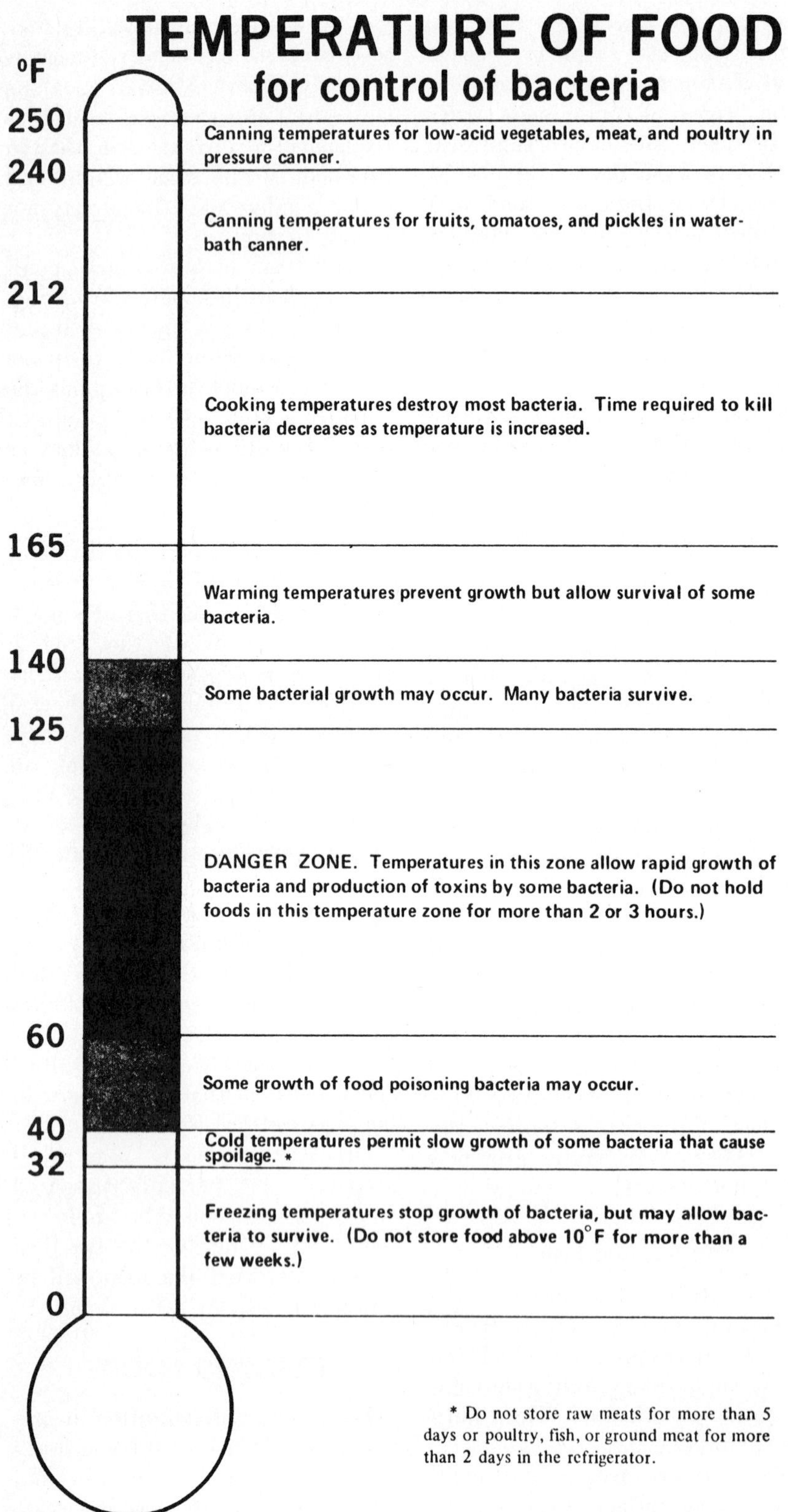

Freezing does not kill the bacteria in food; it simply stops their multiplication. They continue to multiply after the food is thawed. The number of bacteria in and on foods must be held at a minimum before food is frozen.

Freeze only high-quality food. Handle as little as possible all foods to be put in the home freezer. Bacteria are spread by handling. Be especially careful with cooked meats and poultry. Mixtures that contain sauces and gravies favor the growth of disease-causing bacteria.

Refreezing Foods

Occasionally frozen foods are partially or completely thawed before it is discovered that a freezer is not operating.

Whether or not these foods can be refrozen safely depends on the temperature at which these foods were held and the length of time they were held after thawing.

You may safely refreeze frozen foods that have thawed if they still contain ice crystals or if they are still cold—about 40° F—and have been held no longer than 1 or 2 days at refrigerator temperature after thawing. In general, if a food is safe to eat, it is safe to refreeze.

Thawed ground meats, poultry, or fish that have any off-odor or off-color should not be refrozen and should not be eaten. Thawed ice cream should not be refrozen. *If the odor or color of any food is poor or questionable, do not taste it. Throw it out. The food may be dangerous.*

Even partial thawing and refreezing reduce the eating quality of foods, particularly fruits, vegetables, and prepared foods. The eating quality of red meats is reduced less than that of other foods.

Foods that have been frozen and thawed require the same care as foods that have not been frozen.

Use refrozen foods as soon as possible to save as much of their eating quality as you can.

In Case of Emergency

If power fails or the freezer stops operating normally, try to determine how long it will be before the freezer is back in operation.

A fully loaded freezer usually will stay cold enough to keep foods frozen for 2 days if the door is not opened. In a cabinet with less than half a load, food may not stay frozen more than 1 day.

If normal operation cannot be resumed before the food will start to thaw, use dry ice. If dry ice is placed in the freezer soon after the power is off, 25 pounds should keep the temperature below freezing for 2 to 3 days in a 10-cubic-foot cabinet with half a load, 3 to 4 days in a fully loaded cabinet.

Handle dry ice with care. Be sure the room is well ventilated when you use it. Never touch dry ice with bare hands.

Place the dry ice on cardboard or small boards on top of packages and do not open freezer again except to put in more dry ice or to remove it when normal operation is resumed.

Or move food to a locker plant, using insulated boxes or thick layers of paper to prevent thawing.

CANNING FOODS

Commercially canned foods are considered safe because they are processed under carefully controlled conditions. ***However, if a canned food shows any sign of spoilage—bulging can ends, leakage, spurting liquid, off-odor, or mold—do not use it. Do not even taste it.***

If home-canned vegetables, meat, and poultry are not properly processed, they may contain the toxin that causes botulism.

It is not safe to can vegetables, meat, or poultry in a boiling-water bath, an oven, a steamer without pressure, or an open kettle. None of these methods will heat these products enough to kill the dangerous bacterial spores of *Clostridium botulinum* within a reasonable time.

There is no danger of botulism, however, if these foods are canned properly in a pressure canner. ***Be sure that the pressure canner is in perfect order and that each step of the canning process—including time and temperature directions—is followed exactly.***

Tomatoes, pickled vegetables, and fruits can be processed safely in a boiling-water bath because they are more acid than other vegetables, meat, and poultry. However, do not use overripe tomatoes for canning, since tomatoes lose acidity as they mature.

Boil all home-canned vegetables and home-canned meats as described below, after opening and **before tasting. Heating usually makes any odor of spoilage more noticeable.**

Bring home-canned vegetables to a rolling boil, then cover and boil for at least 10 minutes. Boil spinach and corn 20 minutes. If the food looks spoiled, foams, or has an off-odor, ***do not taste it;*** **destroy it.**

Boil home-canned meat or poultry 20 minutes in a covered pan before tasting. If meat develops the characteristic odor of spoiled meat, destroy it without tasting.

Keep Household Insects Under Control

Certain household insects, particularly house flies and cockroaches, can carry some of the bacteria discussed in this bulletin. It is easier to prevent these pests from infesting your home than it is to get rid of them after they get indoors.

Keep all windows and doors tightly screened. Make sure screen doors swing outward. These simple measures will keep out most flies.

Sanitation measures, including prompt disposal of garbage, will help control cockroaches. Caulk openings and cracks around wash basins, drain pipes, water pipes, and radiator pipes. Make sure that cockroaches are not entering your home in containers and cardboard cartons brought in from the outside. Get rid of any infested containers at once.

If you need an insecticide to supplement these sanitation measures, buy a product specifically labeled for control of the kind of insect you want to kill. Read the label before you buy. Read the label before each use, and follow the directions.

Observe all precautions listed on the product label. Used improperly, many household insecticides can be injurious to humans or to household pets. Be careful not to get insecticide on food, dishes, or cooking utensils.

Bacterial Foodborne Illness:

Name of illness	What causes it	Symptoms
Salmonellosis. Examples of foods involved: Poultry, red meats, eggs, dried foods, dairy products.	Salmonellae. Bacteria widespread in nature, live and grow in intestinal tracts of human beings and animals.	Severe headache, followed by vomiting, diarrhea, abdominal cramps, and fever. Infants, elderly, and persons with low resistance are most susceptible. Severe infections cause high fever and may even cause death.
Perfringens poisoning. Examples of foods involved: Stews, soups, or gravies made from poultry or red meat.	*Clostridium perfringens.* Spore-forming bacteria that grow in the absence of oxygen. Temperatures reached in thorough cooking of most foods are sufficient to destroy vegetative cells, but heat-resistant spores can survive.	Nausea without vomiting, diarrhea, acute inflammation of stomach and intestines.
Staphylococcal poisoning (frequently called staph). Examples of foods involved: Custards, egg salad, potato salad, chicken salad, macaroni salad, ham, salami, cheese.	*Staphylococcus aureus.* Bacteria fairly resistant to heat. Bacteria growing in food produce a toxin that is extremely resistant to heat.	Vomiting, diarrhea, prostration, abdominal cramps. Generally mild and often attributed to other causes.
Botulism. Examples of foods involved: Canned low-acid foods, smoked fish.	*Clostridium botulinum.* Spore-forming organisms that grow and produce toxin in the absence of oxygen, such as in a sealed container.	Double vision, inability to swallow, speech difficulty, progressive respiratory paralysis. Fatality rate is high, in the United States about 65 percent.

Causes, Symptoms, and Prevention

Characteristics of illness	Preventive measures
Transmitted by eating contaminated food, or by contact with infected persons or carriers of the infection. Also transmitted by insects, rodents, and pets. Onset: Usually within 12 to 36 hours. Duration: 2 to 7 days.	**Salmonellae in food are destroyed by heating the food to 140° F and holding for 10 minutes or to higher temperatures for less time; for instance, 155° F for a few seconds. Refrigeration at 40° F inhibits the increase of Salmonellae, but they remain alive in foods in the refrigerator or freezer, and even in dried foods.**
Transmitted by eating food contaminated with abnormally large numbers of the bacteria. Onset: Usually within 8 to 20 hours. Duration: May persist for 24 hours.	To prevent growth of surviving bacteria in cooked meats, gravies, and meat casseroles that are to be eaten later, cool foods rapidly and refrigerate promptly at 40° F or below, or hold them above 140° F.
Transmitted by food handlers who carry the bacteria and by eating food containing the toxin. Onset: Usually within 3 to 8 hours. Duration: 1 to 2 days.	Growth of bacteria that produce toxin is inhibited by keeping hot foods above 140° F and cold foods at or below 40° F Toxin is destroyed by boiling for several hours or heating the food in a pressure cooker at 240° F for 30 minutes.
Transmitted by eating food containing the toxin. Onset: Usually within 12 to 36 hours or longer. Duration: 3 to 6 days.	Bacterial spores in food are destroyed by high temperatures obtained only in the pressure canner.[1] More than 6 hours is needed to kill the spores at boiling temperature (212° F). The toxin is destroyed by boiling for 10 to 20 minutes; time required depends on kind of food.

A Buyer's Guide to:

Fresh Vegetables
Fresh Fruits
Cheese
Dairy Products

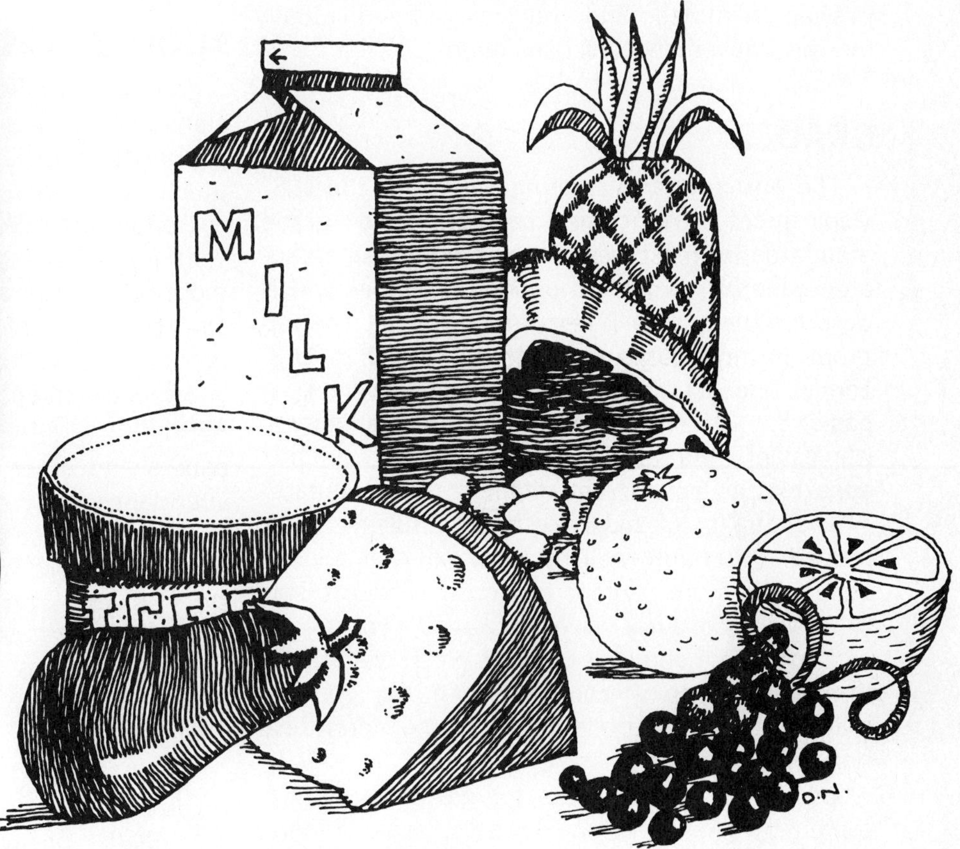

Fresh Vegetables

Fresh vegetables not only are packed with good-for-you ingredients like vitamins and minerals, but they also add color and variety to your meals.

Properly cooked vegetables add interest and enjoyment as well as nutrition to a meal. Cooking only long enough to make the vegetable tender tends to preserve more flavor and better texture than prolonged cooking.

Thanks to the increased efficiency of marketing and the great strides made in recent years in the produce industry, most of the fresh vegetables on today's market are of good quality. Advanced technology of production methods, mechanical precooling, better shipping and storage methods, and refrigerated displays make possible an abundance of vegetables.

In food stores, many fresh vegetables come washed, trimmed, and prepackaged individually for the convenience of consumers.

GRADES

The Agricultural Marketing Service of the U.S. Department of Agriculture has established grade standards for most fresh vegetables. These standards generally provide two or more grades which describe the quality of vegetables in a lot. The top grade in most cases is either U.S. No. 1 or U.S. Fancy. The standards are used extensively as a basis for trading between growers, shippers, wholesalers and retailers. They are used to a limited extent in sales from retailers to consumers.

The quality of most fresh vegetables can be judged reasonably well by their external appearance. Therefore, except for those products sold in closed consumer-size packages, consumers can make a good selection of fresh vegetables from retail display counters even though they may not bear any grade mark or other identification of quality at this stage of sale.

Use of USDA standards for grades is not required by Federal law. However, some Federal marketing programs set minimum quality levels based on U.S. grades and require official inspection. In addition, a few States require that some products packed for marketing be graded and labeled on the basis of either Federal or State grade standards.

In retail stores, grade designations are often found on packages of potatoes, onions, carrots, and occasionally on other vegetables. Such terms in themselves give little assurance of the quality of the contents of the package. However, if the package also bears the official USDA grade shield or the statement, "Packed under Continuous Inspection of the U.S. Department of Agriculture," or "USDA Inspected," the shopper can buy with a much greater degree of confidence. She has assurance that the product was officially inspected during the packing operation and that, at the time of packing, it met the requirements of the grade shown on the package.

FOOD BUYING TIPS

Demand freshness! Check the characteristic signs of freshness such as bright, lively color and crispness. Vegetables are usually at their best quality and price at the peak of the season.

Handle with care. Use thoughtful care to prevent injury to vegetables. Some vegetables are more hardy than others, but bruising and damage can be prevented by just being careful. The consumer pays for carelessness in the long run.

Shop the plentifuls. The U.S. Department of Agriculture notifies consumers through newspapers and other media when vegetables are in abundant supply across the country.

Don't buy just because of low price. It doesn't pay to buy more vegetables than you can properly store in your refrigerator, or than you can use without waste. Most fresh vegetables can be stored for two to five days, except for root vegetables which can be stored from one to several weeks.

Avoid decay. It's "penny foolish" to buy fresh vegetables affected by decay. Even if you do trim off the decayed area, rapid deterioration is likely to spread to the salvaged area. A few cents extra for vegetables in good condtion is a good investment.

A CONSUMER'S GUIDE TO BUYING FRESH VEGETABLES

There are no set rules in buying vegetables because they all have individual characteristics and values. Experience in personal selection is the best teacher. The following alphabetical list is designed as a handy reference to help you make your selection.

ARTICHOKES

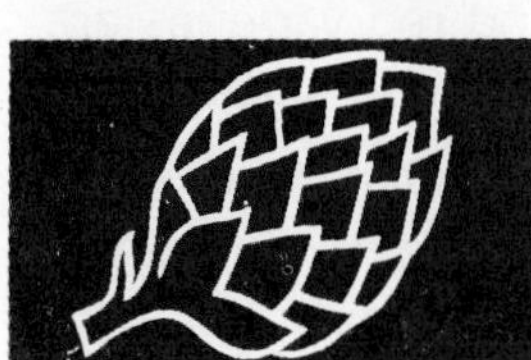

The globe artichoke is the large, unopened flower bud of a plant belonging to the thistle family. The many leaf-like parts making up the bud are called "scales." Produced only in Califorina, artichokes are shipped in limited amounts most of the year, but the peak of the crop comes in April and May.

Look for: Plump, globular artichokes that are heavy in relation to size, and compact with thick, green, fresh-looking scales. Size is not important in relation to quality.

Avoid: Artichokes with large areas of brown on the scales and with spreading scales (a sign of age, indicating drying and toughening of the edible portions), grayish-black discoloration (caused by bruises), mold growth on the scales, and worm injury.

ASPARAGUS

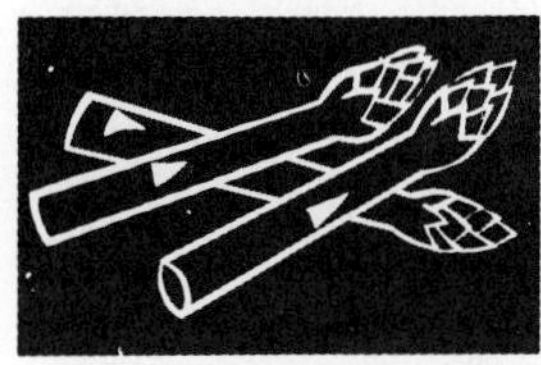

California, New Jersey, Washington, and Michigan are the chief sources of asparagus, available from mid-February through June, with peak supplies from April to June. Very little is available after the end of June.

Look for: Closed, compact tips, smooth, round spears and a fresh appearance. A rich green color should cover most of the spear. Stalks should be tender almost as far down as the green extends.

Avoid: Tips that are open and spread out, moldy or decayed tips, or ribbed spears (spears with up-and-down ridges, or that are not approximately round). These are all signs of aging, and mean tough asparagus and poor flavor. Also avoid excessively sandy asparagus, because sand grains can lodge beneath the scales or in the tips of the spears and are difficult to remove in washing.

BEANS (Snap Beans)

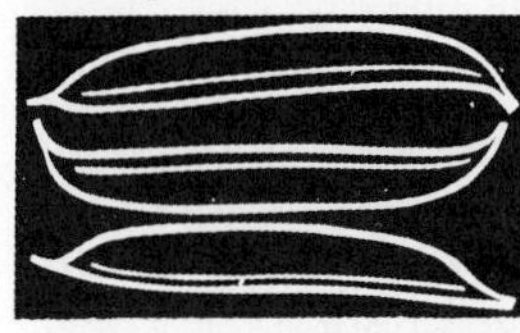

Snap beans, produced commercially in many States, are available throughout the year. Most beans found in the food store will be the common green podded varieties, but large green pole beans and yellow wax beans are occasionally available.

Look for: A fresh, bright appearance with good color for the variety. Get young, tender beans with pods in a firm, crisp condition.

Avoid: Wilted or flabby bean pods, serious blemishes, and decay. Thick, tough, fibrous pods indicate overmaturity.

BEETS

Beets, available year-round, are grown in most parts of the nation, but major growing areas are California, Texas, New Jersey, Ohio, New York, and Colorado. Many beets are sold in bunches with the tops still attached, while others are sold on the basis of weight with the tops removed.

Look for: Beets that are firm, round, with a slender tap root (the large main root), a rich, deep red color, and smooth over most of the surface. If beets are bunched, you can judge their freshness fairly accurately by the condition of the tops. Badly wilted or decayed tops indicate a lack of freshness, but the roots may be satisfactory if they are firm.

Avoid: Elongated beets with round, scaly areas around the top surface—these will be tough, fibrous, and strong-flavored. Also avoid wilted, flabby beets—which have been exposed to the air too long.

BROCCOLI

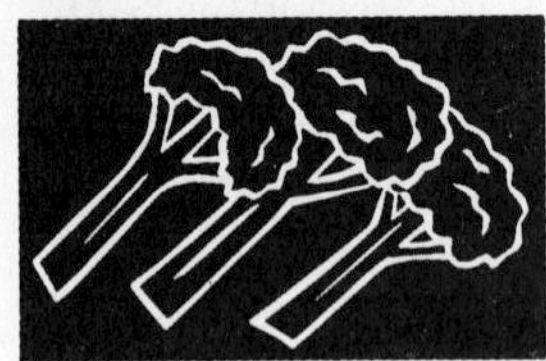

A member of the cabbage family, and a close relative of cauliflower, broccoli is available throughout the year but—because broccoli grows better in cool weather—is least abundant in July and August.

California is the heaviest producer, but Texas, New Jersey, Oregon, Florida, Pennsylvania, and other States produce large amounts of broccoli.

Look for: A firm, compact cluster of small flower buds, with none opened enough to show the bright yellow flower. Bud clusters should be dark green or sage green—or even green with a decidedly purplish cast. Stems should not be too thick or tough.

Avoid: Broccoli with spread bud clusters, enlarged or open buds, yellowish green color, or wilted condition—signs of overmaturity and overlong display. Also avoid broccoli with soft, slippery, watersoaked spots on the bud cluster. These are signs of decay.

BRUSSELS SPROUTS

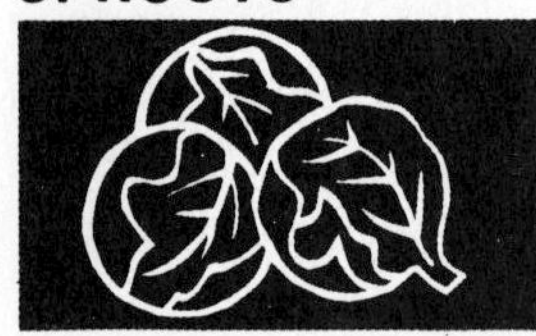

Another close relative of the cabbage, Brussels sprouts develop as enlarged buds on a tall stem, one sprout appearing where each main leaf is attached. The "sprouts" are cut off, and in most cases are packed in small containers. Most Brussels sprouts are produced in California, New York, and Oregon, and some are imported. Although they are often available about 10 months of the year, peak supplies are from October through December.

Look for: A fresh, bright-green color, tight fitting outer leaves, firm body, and freedom from blemishes.

Avoid: Brussels sprouts with yellow or yellowish-green leaves, or leaves which are loose, soft, or wilted. Small holes or ragged leaves may indicate worm injury.

CABBAGE

Three major groups of cabbage varieties are available: smooth-leaved green cabbage, crinkly-leaved green Savoy cabbage, and red cabbage. All types are suitable for any use, although the Savoy and red varieties are more in demand for use in slaws and salads.

Cabbage may be sold fresh (called "new" cabbage) or from storage (called "old" cabbage). New cabbage is available throughout the year, since it is grown in many States. In winter, California, Florida, and Texas market most new cabbage. Many northern States grow cabbage for late summer and fall shipment or to be held in storage for winter sale.

Look for: Firm or hard heads of cabbage that are heavy for their size. Outer leaves should be a good green or red color (depending on type), reasonably fresh, and free from serious blemishes. The outer leaves (called "wrapper" leaves) fit loosely on the head and are usually discarded, but too many loose wrapper leaves on a head cause extra waste.

Some early-crop cabbage may be soft or only fairly firm—but is suitable for immediate use if the leaves are fresh and crisp. Cabbage out of storage is usually trimmed of all outer leaves and lacks green color, but is satisfactory if not wilted or discolored.

Avoid: New cabbage with wilted or decayed outer leaves or with leaves turning decidedly yellow. Worm-eaten outer leaves often indicate that the worm injury penetrates into the head.

Storage cabbage with outer leaves badly discolored, dried, or decayed probably is over-aged. Separation of the stems of leaves from the central stem at the base of the head also indicates over-age.

CARROTS

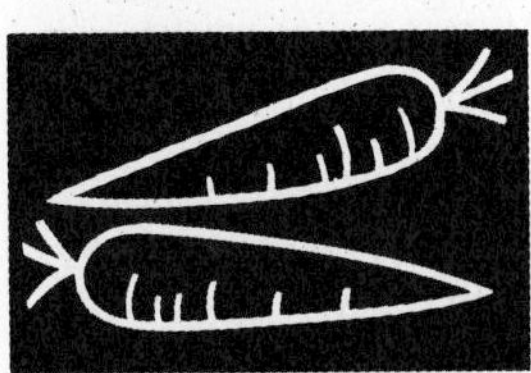

Freshly harvested carrots are available the year round. Most of them are marketed when relatively young, tender, well-colored, and mild-flavored—an ideal stage for use as raw carrot sticks. Larger carrots are packed separately and are used primarily for cooking or shredding. California and Texas market most carrots, but many other States produce large quantities.

Look for: Carrots which are well formed, smooth, well-colored, and firm.

Avoid: Roots with large green "sunburned" areas at the top (which must be trimmed) and roots which are flabby from wilting or show spots of soft decay.

CAULIFLOWER

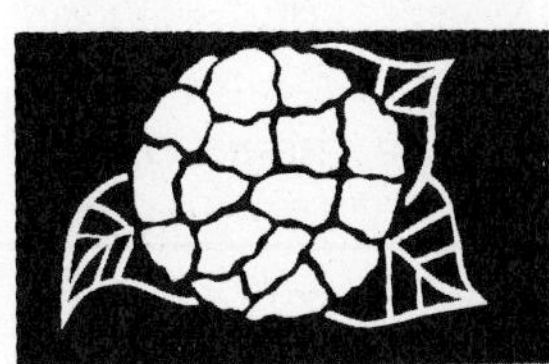

Though most abundant from September through January, cauliflower is available during every month of the year. California, New York, Oregon, Texas, and Michigan are major sources. The white, edible portion is called the curd and the heavy outer leaf covering, the jacket leaves. Cauliflower is generally sold with most of the jacket leaves removed, and is wrapped in clear plastic film.

Look for: White to creamy-white, compact, solid and clean curds. A slightly granular or "ricey" texture of the curd will not hurt the eating quality if the surface is compact. Ignore small green leaflets extending through the curd. If jacket leaves are attached, a good green color is a sign of freshness.

Avoid: A spreading of the curd—a sign of aging or overmaturity. Also avoid severe wilting or many discolored spots, on the curd. A smudgy or speckled appearance of the curd is a sign of insect injury, mold growth or decay and should be avoided.

CELERY

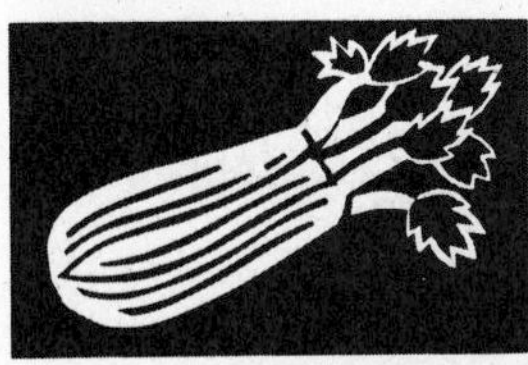

Celery, a popular vegetable for a variety of uses, is available throughout the year. Production is concentrated in California, Florida, Michigan, and New York. Most celery is of the so-called "Pascal" type which includes thick-branched, green varieties.

Look for: Freshness and crispness in celery. The stalk should have a solid, rigid feel and leaflets should be fresh or only slightly wilted. Also look for a glossy surface, stalks of light green or medium green, and mostly green leaflets.

Avoid: Wilted celery and celery with flabby upper branches or leaf stems. You can freshen celery somewhat by placing the butt end in water, but badly wilted celery will never become really fresh again.

Also avoid celery with pithy, hollow, or discolored centers in the branches. Celery with internal discoloration will show some gray or brown on the inside surface of the larger branches near where they are attached to the base of the stalk.

Avoid celery with: 1. "Blackheart," a brown or black discoloration of the small center branches; 2. Insect injury in the center branches or the insides of outer branches; 3. Long, thick seedstem in place of the usually small, tender heart branches.

CHARD (See Greens)

CHINESE CABBAGE

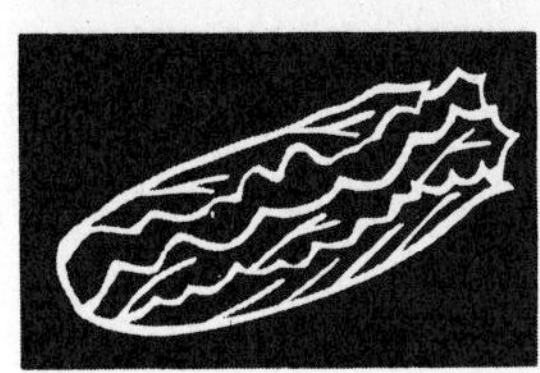

Primarily a salad vegetable, Chinese cabbage plants are elongated, with some varieties developing a firm head and others an open, leafy form.

Look for: Fresh, crisp, green plants that are free from blemishes or decay.

Avoid: Wilted or yellowed plants.

CHICORY, ENDIVE, ESCAROLE

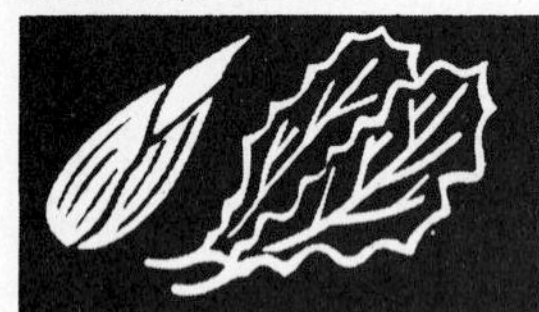

These vegetables, used mainly in salads, are available practically all year round—but primarily in the winter and spring. Chicory or endive has narrow, notched edges, and crinkly leaves resembling the dandelion leaf. Chicory plants often have "blanched" yellowish leaves in the center which are preferred by many persons. Escarole leaves are much broader and less crinkly than those of chicory.

Look for: Freshness, crispness, tenderness, and a good green color of the outer leaves.

Avoid: Plants with leaves which have brownish or yellowish discoloration or which have insect injury.

Note: Witloof or Belgian endive is a compact, cigar-shaped plant which is creamy white from blanching. The small shoots are kept from becoming green by being grown in complete darkness.

COLLARDS (See Greens)

CORN

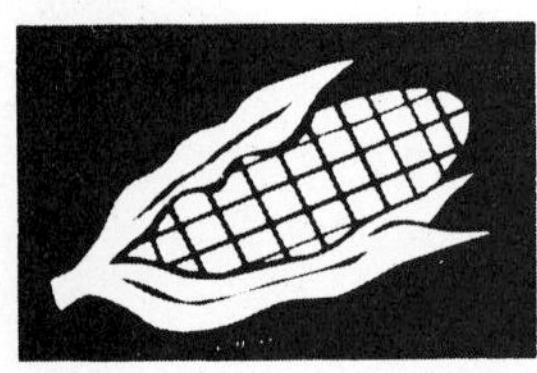

Sweet corn is available practically every month of the year, but is most plentiful from early May until mid - September. Most supplies are yellow-kernal corn, but some white corn is sold. Sweet corn is produced in a large number of States during the spring and summer, but most mid-winter supplies come from south Florida.

For best quality, corn should be refrigerated immediately after being picked. Corn will retain fairly good quality for a number of days, if it has been kept cold and moist since harvesting. For the same reason, it should be placed in the home refrigerator as soon as possible and kept moist until used.

Look for: Fresh, succulent husks with good green color, silk-ends that are free from decay or worm injury, and stem ends (opposite from the silk) that are not too discolored or dried.

Select ears that are well covered with plump, not-too-mature kernels.

Avoid: Ears with under-developed kernels which lack yellow color (in yellow corn), old ears with very large kernels, and ears with dark yellow kernels with depressed areas on the outer surface.

Also avoid ears of corn with yellowed, wilted, or dried husks, or discolored and dried-out stem ends.

CUCUMBERS

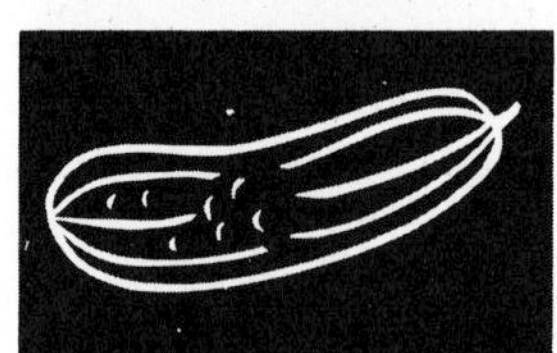

Although cucumbers are produced at various times in many States—and imported during the colder months — the supply is most plentiful in the summer months.

Look for: Cucumbers with good green color which are firm over their entire length. They should be well-shaped and well-developed, but should not be too large in diameter. Good cucumbers typically have many small lumps on their surfaces. They may also have some white or greenish-white color and still be of top quality.

Avoid: Overgrown cucumbers which are large in diameter and have a dull color, turning yellowish. Also avoid cucumbers with withered or shriveled ends—signs of toughness and bitter flavor.

EGGPLANT

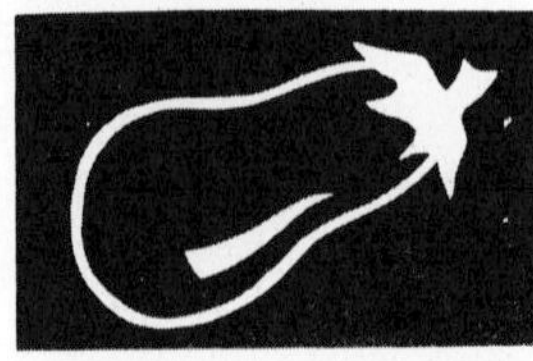

Eggplant is most plentiful during the late summer, but is available all year to some extent.

Look for: Firm, heavy, smooth, and uniformly dark purple eggplants.

Avoid: Those which are poorly colored, soft, shriveled, cut, or which show decay in the form of irregular dark-brown spots.

ENDIVE, ESCAROLE (See Chicory)

GREENS

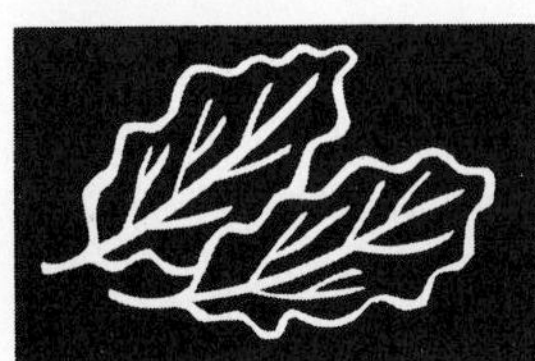

A large number of widely differing species of plants are grown for uses as "greens." The better known kinds are spinach, kale, collards, turnips, beets, chard, mustard, broccoli leaves, chicory, endive, escarole, dandelion, cress, and sorrel. Many others, some of them wild, are also used to a limited extent as greens.

Look for: Leaves that are fresh, young, tender, free from blemishes, and which have a good, healthy green color. Beet tops and ruby chard show reddish color.

Avoid: Leaves with coarse, fibrous stems, yellowish-green color, softness (a sign of decay), or a wilted condition. Also avoid greens with evidence of insects—especially aphids—which are sometimes hard to see, and equally hard to wash away.

KALE (See Greens)

LETTUCE

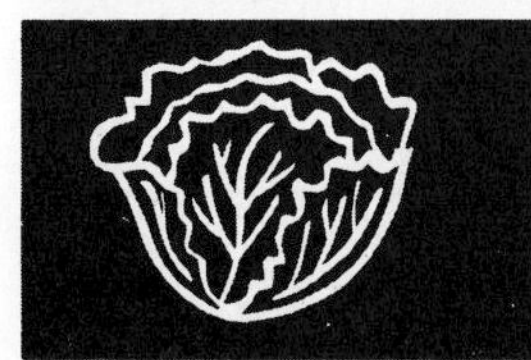

Among the Nation's leading vegetables, lettuce owes its prominence to the growing popularity of salads in our diet. It's available throughout the year, at various seasons, from California, Arizona, New York, New Jersey, Texas, Colorado, New Mexico, Wisconsin, and other States. Four types of lettuce are generally sold: iceburg, butter-head, Romaine, and leaf.

Iceberg lettuce is the major group. Heads are large, round, and solid, with medium-green outer leaves and lighter green or pale-green inner leaves.

Butter-head lettuce, including the Big Boston and Bibb varieties, has a smaller head than Iceberg. This type will be slightly flat on top and have soft, succulent, light-green leaves in a rosette pattern in the center.

Romaine lettuce plants are tall and cylindrical with crisp, dark-green leaves in a loosely folded head.

Leaf Lettuce includes many varieties—none with a compact head. Leaves are broad, tender, succulent, fairly smooth and vary in color according to variety. It is grown mainly in greenhouses or on truck farms and sold locally.

Look for: Signs of freshness in lettuce. For Iceberg lettuce and Romaine, the leaves should be crisp. Other lettuce types will have a softer texture, but leaves should not be wilted. Look for a good, bright color—in most varieties, medium to light green.

Avoid: Heads of iceberg type which are very hard and which lack green color (signs of overmaturity). Such heads sometimes develop discoloration in the center of the leaves (the "midribs"), and may have a less attractive flavor. Also avoid heads with irregular shapes and hard bumps on top, which indicates the presence of overgrown central stems.

Check the lettuce for tipburn, a tan or brown area (dead tissue) around the margins of the leaves. Look for tipburn on the edges of the head leaves. Slight discoloration of the outer or wrapper leaves will usually not hurt the quality of the lettuce, but serious discoloration or soft decay definitely should be avoided.

MUSHROOMS

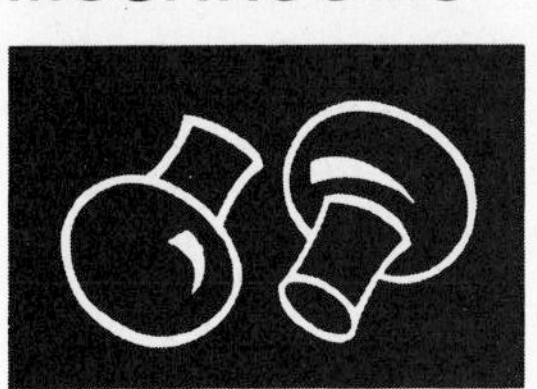

Grown in houses, cellars, or caves, mushrooms are available the year round in varying amounts. Most come from Pennsylvania, but many are produced in California, New York, Ohio, and Illinois and other States.

We usually describe mushrooms as having caps—the wide portion on top, gills—the numerous rows of paper-thin tissue seen underneath the cap when it opens, and a stem.

Look for: Young mushrooms that are small to medium in size. Caps should be either closed around the stem or moderately open with pink or light-tan gills. The surface of the cap should be white or creamy—or light brown from some producing areas.

Avoid: Overripe mushrooms (shown by wide-open caps and dark, discolored gills underneath) and those with pitted or seriously discolored caps.

OKRA

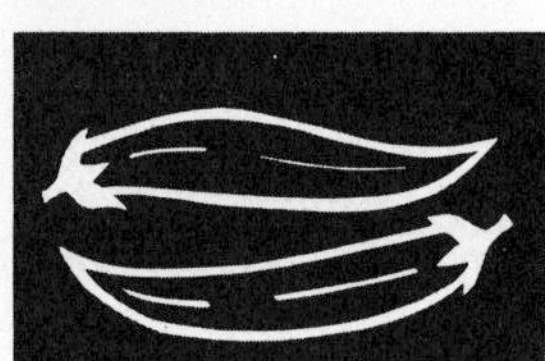

Okra is the immature seed pod of the okra plant, grown and marketed locally in the southern states.

Look for: Tender pods (the tips will bend with very slight pressure) under 4-½ inches long. They should have a bright green color and be free from blemishes.

Avoid: Tough, fibrous pods, indicated by tips which are stiff and resist bending, or by a very hard body of the pod, or by pale, faded green color.

ONIONS

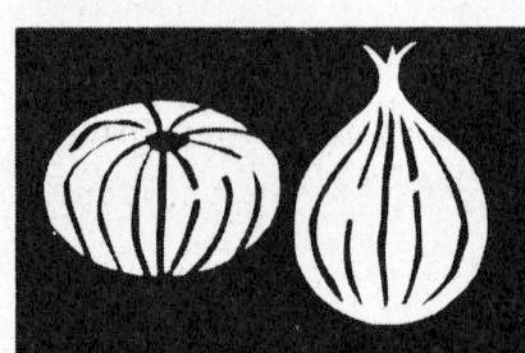

The many varieties of onions grown commercially fall into three general classes:

Globe onions are the most common group, and are considered primarily cooking onions. There are many varieties, mostly with yellow skins, but also some white and red-skinned types. Globe onions are predominantly round to oval, and have rather pungent flavor. They are available in quantity during the late summer, fall, and winter. Most fall in the medium size range, but in some cases the smaller onions are packed and sold separately.

Granex-Grano onions are available during the spring and summer, coming from the warmer growing areas. Most are yellow-skinned; a few are white. The shape tends to be less round and less symmetrical than the globes, ranging from somewhat flattened to top shaped. Rather mild in flavor, they are considered ideal for slicing and eating raw and good for cooking. In size they range from medium to large.

Spanish onions resemble globe onions in shape, but they are generally much larger. Most varieties are yellow, but some are white-skinned. They are mild in flavor, often called "sweet Spanish," and are ideal for slicing or for salads. Sometimes the medium sizes are packed separately from the large ones (3 inches or more in diameter). Spanish type onions are generally available in moderate supply during fall and winter.

Major onion growing areas are California, New York, Texas, Michigan, Colorado, Oregon, and Idaho.

Look for: Hard or firm onions which are dry and have small necks. They should be covered with papery outer scales and reasonably free from green sunburn spots, and other blemishes.

Avoid: Onions with wet or very soft necks, which usually are immature or affected by decay. Also avoid onions with thick, hollow, woody centers in the neck or with fresh sprouts.

ONIONS, (GREEN), SHALLOTS, LEEKS

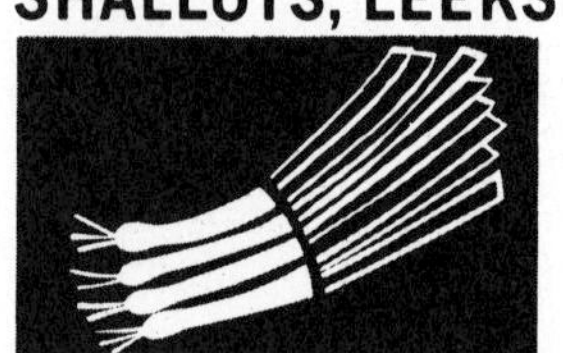

All three of these (sometimes called scallions) are similiar in appearance, but are somewhat different in nature.

Green onions are ordinary onions harvested very young. They have very little or no bulb formation, and their tops are tubular.

Shallots are similar to green onions, but grow in clusters and have practically no swelling at the base.

Leeks are larger than shallots, and have slight bulb formation and broad, flat, dark-green tops.

Sold in small, tied bunches, they are all available to some extent throughout the entire year, but are most plentiful in the spring and summer.

Look for: Bunches with fresh, crisp, green tops. They should have well-blanched (white) portions extending two or three inches up from the root end.

Avoid: Yellowing, wilted, discolored, or decayed tops (indicating flabby, tough, or fibrous condition of the edible portions). Bruised tops will not affect the eating quality of the bulbs, if the tops are removed.

PARSLEY

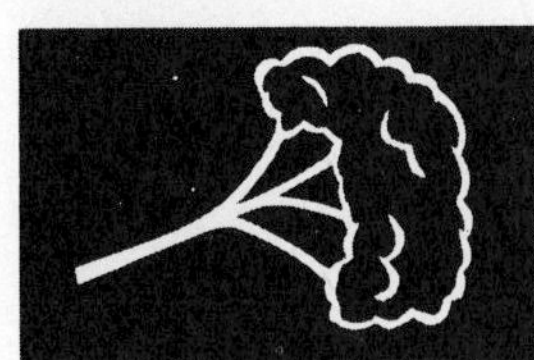

Parsley, which ranks at the top among vegetables in vitamin A content, can be a valuable addition to your diet as well as a taste treat if you consider it as a food instead of just a decorative garnish. It is generally available the year round.

Look for: Fresh, crisp, bright-green leaves, for both the curled-leaf and the flat-leaf types of parsley. Slightly wilted leaves can be freshened by trimming off the ends of the stems and placing them in cold water.

PARSNIPS

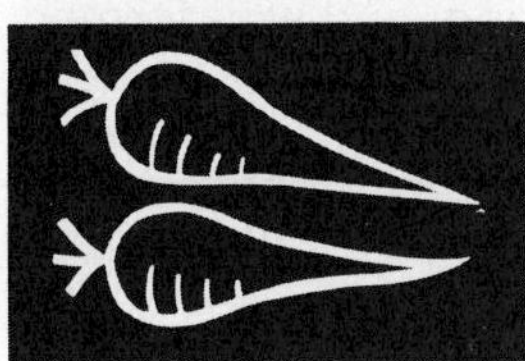

Although available to some extent throughout the year, parsnips are primarily a late winter vegetable. This is because the flavor becomes sweeter and more desirable after long exposure to cold temperatures (below 40° F).

Look for: Parsnips of small or medium width that are well formed, smooth, firm, and free from serious blemishes or decay.

Avoid: Large, coarse roots (which probably have woody, fibrous, or pithy centers), and badly wilted and flabby roots (which will be tough when cooked).

PEPPERS

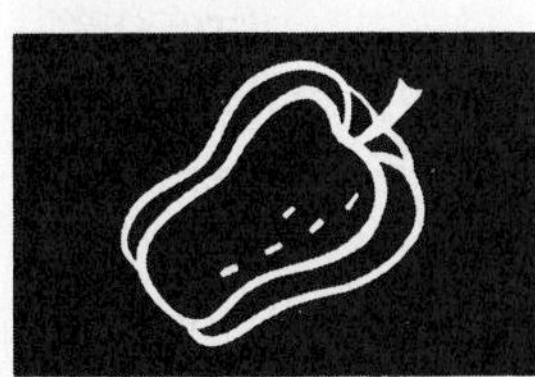

Most of the peppers you'll find are the sweet green peppers, available in varying amounts throughout the year, but most plentiful during the late summer. (Fully matured peppers of the same type have a bright red color.)

Look for: Medium to dark green color, glossy sheen, relatively heavy weight, and firm walls or sides.

Avoid: Peppers with very thin walls (shown by light weight and flimsy sides), peppers that are wilted or flabby with cuts or punctures through the walls, and peppers with soft watery spots on the sides (evidence of decay).

POTATOES

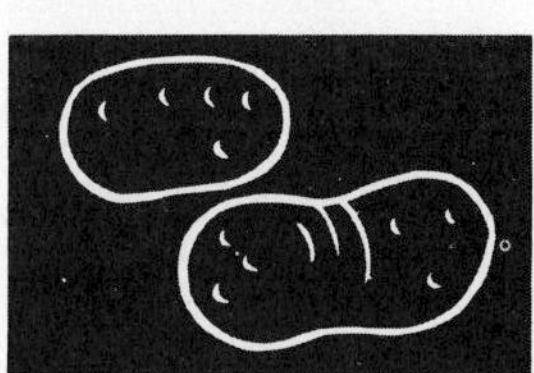

For practical purposes, potatoes can be put into three groups, although the distinctions between them are not clear-cut, and there is much overlapping.

"New" potatoes is a term most frequently used to describe those freshly harvested and marketed during the late winter or early spring. The name is also widely used in later crop producing areas to designate freshly dug potatoes which are not quite fully matured. Best use of new potatoes is boiling or creaming. They vary widely in size and shape, depending upon variety, but are likely to be affected by "skinning" or "feathering" of the outer layer of skin. This skinning usually affects only their appearance.

General purpose potatoes include the great majority of supplies offered for sale in the markets, both round and long types. With the aid of air-cooled storages, they are amply available throughout the year. As the term implies, they are used for boiling, frying and baking, although many of the common varieties are not considered to be best for baking.

Baking Potatoes. Both the variety and the area where grown are important factors affecting baking quality. The Russet Burbank, a long variety with fine, scaly netting on the skin is the most widely grown and best known among this group.

Look for: (in new potatoes) Well-shaped, firm potatoes that are free from blemishes and sunburn (a green discoloration under the skin). Some amount of skinned surface is normal, but potatoes with large skinned and discolored areas are undesirable.

Look for: (in general purpose and baking potatoes) Reasonably smooth, well-shaped, firm potatoes free from blemishes, sunburn, and decay. These potatoes should be relatively free from skinned surfaces.

Avoid: Potatoes with large cuts or bruises (they'll mean waste in peeling), those with a green color (probably caused by sunburn or exposure to light in the store), and potatoes showing any signs of decay.

Also avoid sprouted or shriveled potatoes.

RADISHES

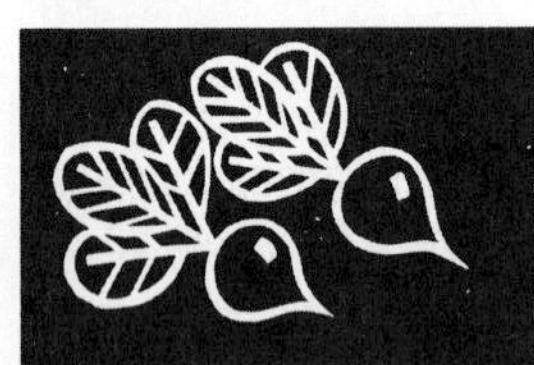

Radishes, available the year round, are most plentiful from May through July. California and Florida produce most of our winter and spring supplies, while several Northern States provide radishes the rest of the year.

Look for: Medium size radishes (¾ to 1-⅛ inches in diameter) that are plump, round, firm, and of a good red color.

Avoid: Very large or flabby radishes (likely to have pithy centers). Also avoid radishes with yellow or decayed tops (sign of over-age).

RHUBARB

This highly specialized vegetable is used like a fruit in sweetened sauces and pies. Very limited supplies are available during most of the year, with most supplies available from January to June.

Look for: Fresh, firm rhubarb stems with a bright, glossy appearance. Stems should have a large amount of pink or red color, although many good-quality stems will be predominantly light green. Be sure the stem is tender and not fibrous.

Avoid: Either very slender or extremely thick stems, which are likely to be tough and stringy. Also avoid rhubarb that is wilted and flabby.

RUTABAGAS (See Turnips)

SPINACH (See Greens)

SQUASH (Summer)

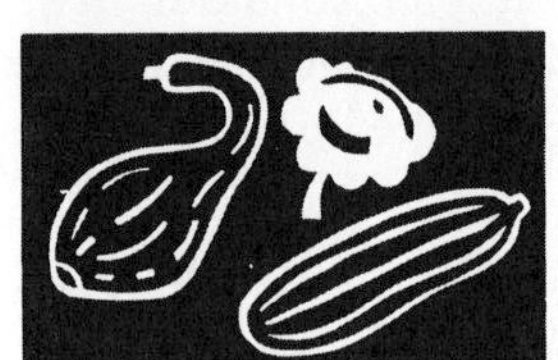

Summer squash includes those varieties which are harvested while still immature and when the entire squash is tender and edible. They include the yellow *Crookneck,* the large yellow *Straightneck,* the greenish-white *Patty Pan,* and the slender green *Zucchini* and *Italian Marrow.* Some of these squash are available at all times of the year.

Look for: Squash that are tender and well developed, firm, fresh-appearing, and well formed. You can identify a tender squash because the skin is glossy instead of dull, and it is neither hard nor tough.

Avoid: Stale or overmature squash, which will have a dull appearance and a hard, tough surface. Such squash usually have enlarged seeds and dry, stringy flesh.

SQUASH (Fall and Winter)

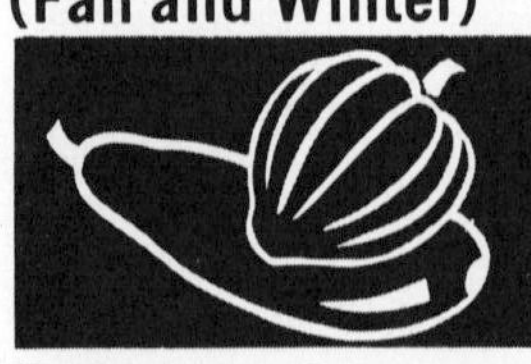

Winter squashes are those varieties which are marketed only when fully mature. Some of the most important varieties are the small corrugated *Acorn* (available all year round), *Butternut, Buttercup,* green and blue *Hubbard,* green and gold *Delicious,* and *Banana.* Winter squash is most plentiful from early fall until late winter.

Look for: Full maturity, indicated by a hard, tough rind. Also look for squash that is heavy for its size (meaning a thick wall, and more edible flesh). Slight variations in skin color do not affect flavor.

Avoid: Squash with cuts, punctures, sunken spots, or moldy spots on the rind—all indications of decay. A tender rind indicates immaturity which is a sign of poor eating quality in winter squash varieties.

SWEETPOTATOES

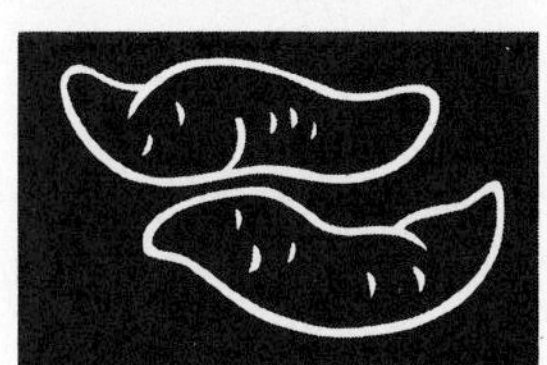

Two types of sweetpotatoes are available in varying amounts the year round.

Moist sweetpotatoes, sometimes called yams, are the most common type. They have orange colored flesh and are very sweet. The true yam is the root of a tropical vine which is not grown commercially in the U.S.

Dry sweetpotatoes have a pale colored flesh, low in moisture. Their production has dwindled rapidly.

Most sweetpotatoes are grown in the Southern tier and some Eastern States, in an area from Texas to New Jersey. California is also a heavy producer.

Look for: Well-shaped, firm sweet potatoes with smooth, bright, uniformly colored skins, free from signs of decay. Because they are more perishable than Irish potatoes, extra care should be used in selecting sweetpotatoes.

Avoid: Sweetpotatoes with worm holes, cuts, grub injury, or any other defects which penetrate the skin; this causes waste and can readily lead to decay. Even if you cut away the decayed portion, the remainder of the potato flesh which looks normal may have a bad taste.

Decay is the worst problem with sweetpotatoes and is of three types: wet, soft decay, dry firm decay which begins at the end of the potato, making it discolored and shriveled; and dry rot in the form of sunken, discolored areas on the sides of the potato.

Sweetpotatoes should not be stored in the refrigerator.

TOMATOES

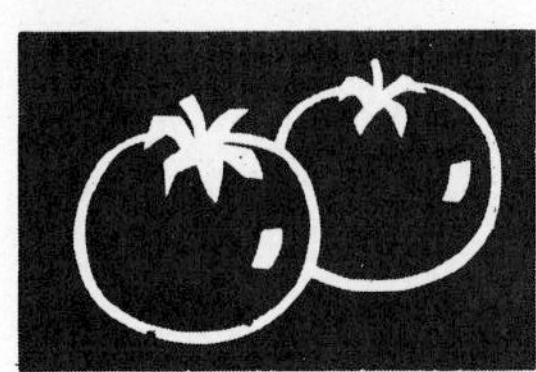

Extremely popular and nutritious, tomatoes are in moderate to liberal supply throughout the year. Florida, California, Texas, and a number of other States are major producers, but imports supplement domestic supplies from late winter to early spring.

Best flavor usually comes from "home grown" tomatoes produced on nearby farms. This type of tomato is allowed to ripen completely before being picked. Many areas, however, now ship tomatoes which are picked after the color has begun to change from green to pink. These tomatoes have flavor almost as satisfying as the home-grown ones.

If your tomatoes need further ripening, keep them in a warm place. Unless they are fully ripened, do not store tomatoes in a refrigerator—the cold temperatures might keep them from ripening later on. Once tomatoes are ripe, however, you may keep them in the refrigerator for some time.

Look for: Tomatoes which are well formed, smooth, well ripened, and reasonably free from blemishes.

For fully ripe fruit, look for an overall rich red color and a slight softness. Softness is easily detected by gentle handling.

For tomatoes slightly less than fully ripe, look for firm texture and color ranging from pink to light red.

Avoid: Overripe and bruised tomatoes (they're both soft and watery) and tomatoes with sunburn (green or yellow areas near the stem scar) and growth cracks (deep cracks around the stem scar). Also avoid decayed tomatoes which will have soft, water-soaked spots, depressed areas, or surface mold.

TURNIPS

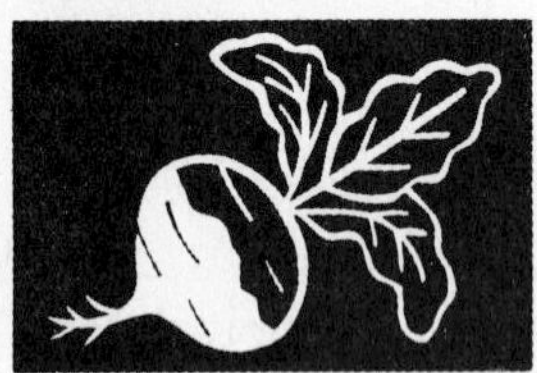

The most popular *turnip* has white flesh and a purple top (reddish-purple tinting of upper surface). It may be sold "topped" (with leaves removed) or in bunches with tops still on, and is available in some food stores most of the year.

Rutabagas are distinctly yellow-fleshed, large-sized relatives of turnips. They are available generally in the fall and winter, but cold-storage rutabagas are often available in the spring. Late winter storage rutabagas are sometimes coated with a thin layer of paraffin in order to prevent loss of moisture and shriveling. The paraffin is readily removed with the peeling before cooking.

Look for: (in turnips) Small or medium size, smooth, fairly round, and firm vegetables. If sold in bunches, the tops should be fresh and should have a good green color.

Avoid: Large turnips with too many leaf scars around the top and with obvious fibrous roots.

Look for: (in rutabagas) Heavy weight for their size, generally smooth, round or moderately elongated shape, and firmness.

Avoid: Rutabagas with skin punctures, deep cuts or decay.

WATERCRESS

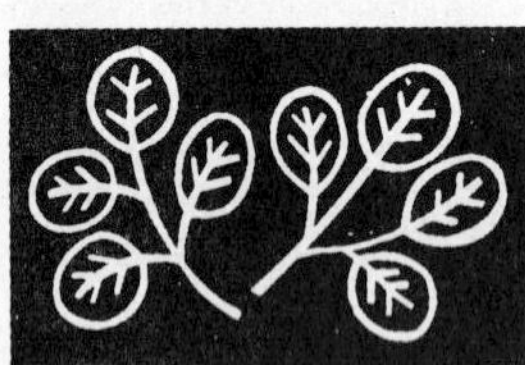

Watercress is a small, round-leaved plant that grows naturally (or may be cultivated) along the banks of freshwater streams and ponds. It is prized as an ingredient of mixed green salads and as a garnish, because of its spicy flavor. Also its very high vitamin A content makes it a valuable addition to the diet. Watercress is available in limited supply through most of the year.

Look for: Watercress that is fresh, crisp, and rich green.

Avoid: Bunches with yellow, wilted, or decayed leaves.

Fresh Fruits

Walk into today's food store and look at the luscious displays of fresh fruits available in fairly constant supply during the entire year.

This year-round abundance can be credited to the great strides made by growers, shippers and distributors—including improved varieties, more efficient methods of production, and advanced techniques of packaging, precooling, shipping, storing and refrigerated displaying of fruits.

GRADES FOR FRUIT

The Agricultural Marketing Service of the U.S. Department of Agriculture has established grade standards for most fresh fruits. These standards generally provide two or more grades which describe the quality of the fruit in a package. The top grade in most cases is either U.S. Fancy or U.S. No. 1. Official USDA standards define the quality each product should be to permit the USDA grade.

Use of USDA standards for grades is voluntary. Sometimes, however, under State or Federal regulations products must be graded and labeled on the basis of grade standards.

Most packers of fruits grade their products and some mark the containers with one of the established grades. If packages are so labeled, the packer is then legally obligated to make the contents measure up to official grade requirements. The shopper may purchase with a greater measure of confidence if he selects packages of fruit labeled with a grade.

Also, a few fruit dealers who pack consumer-size packages operate under the Federal or Federal-State continuous inspection service. This voluntary program—paid for by the dealer—provides for continuous inspection of the entire packing operation, including frequent inspection and grade analysis of the product. Products packed and certified under this service may be labeled with an official USDA grade shield or with one of the following statements "Packed Under Continuous Inspection of the U.S. Department of Agriculture" or "Packed By __________ Under Continuous Federal-State Inspection."

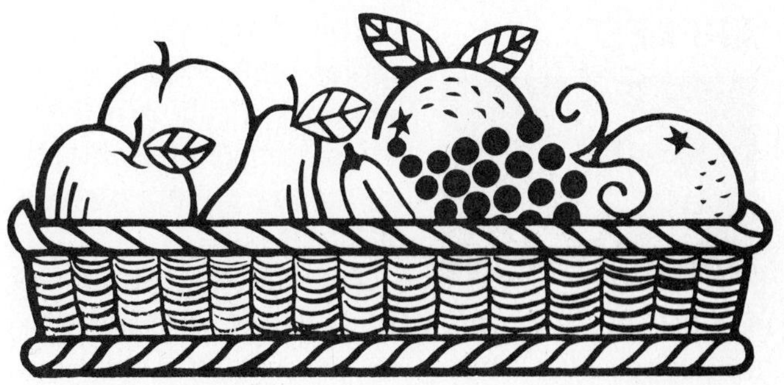

FOOD-BUYING TIPS

Do it yourself—There is no substitute for your own experience in choosing the right quality of fresh fruit for different uses.

Don't buy just because of low price—It seldom pays to buy perishable fruits merely because the price is low. Unless the lower price is a result of overabundance of the fruit at the time, the so-called bargain may be undesirable.

Buy only what you need—Modern home refrigeration makes it possible to keep an adequate supply of most perishable fruits on hand, but never buy more than you can properly refrigerate and use without waste—even if the product is cheaper in quantity.

Keep a lookout for deterioration—Even with the most modern handling methods, some products decline rapidly in quality while on display. Frequently such off-quality fruit can be bought at a reduced price, but the waste in preparation may offset the price reduction.

Don't buy on size alone—Large sized fruits are not necessarily the best quality, nor are they always economical. They may appear to be bargains, but may be entirely unsuited to the purpose you have in mind.

Appearance isn't everything—Select your fruit for best eating quality rather than outer appearance, if you want to shop economically. Appearance and quality are closely associated in many respects, but fine appearance does not always denote fine quality. Often a fruit with a very attractive appearance may have relatively poor eating quality because of a varietal characteristic or because of some internal condition such as overmaturity. On the other hand, a fruit with poor appearance due to poor color or superficial blemishes may have excellent eating quality.

Buy in season—Quality is usually higher, and prices more reasonable, when you buy fruit in season. Out-of-season produce is generally more expensive.

Shop for plentifuls—Through newspapers, radio, and television, the U.S. Department of Agriculture tells you each month which fruits are in greatest supply and worthy of your special attention. Such plentiful foods are usually good choices and reasonably priced.

Don't pinch!—Rough handling of fruits while you are selecting them causes spoilage and waste. Such loss to the grocer usually is passed on to the consumer, so your costs go up when fruit is carelessly handled. When you must handle a fruit to judge its quality, use thoughtful care to prevent injury.

A CONSUMER'S GUIDE TO BUYING FRUIT

The following alphabetical list of fruits is designed as a reference to help you shop more intelligently. Some of the terms used (such as "mature" and "ripe") have special meanings in the produce field. A brief glossary in the back will help you understand these terms.

APPLES

The many varieties of apples differ widely in appearance, flesh characteristics, seasonal availability, and suitability for different uses.

For good eating as fresh fruit, the commonly available varieties are: Delicious, McIntosh, Stayman, Golden Delicious, Jonathan, and Winesap. For making pies and applesauce, use tart or slightly acid varieties such as Gravenstein, Grimes Golden, Jonathan, and Newtown.

For baking, the firmer-fleshed varieties—Rome Beauty, Northern Spy, Rhode Island Greening, Winesap, and York Imperial—are widely used.

Look for: Firm, crisp, well-colored apples. Flavor varies in apples and depends on the stage of maturity at the time the fruit is picked. Apples must be mature when picked to have a good flavor, texture, and storing ability. Immature apples lack color and are usually poor in flavor. They may have a shriveled appearance after being held in storage.

Most apples are marketed by grade, and many consumer packages show the variety, the grade, and the size. U.S. grades for apples are U.S. Extra Fancy, U.S. Fancy, U.S. No. 1, and combinations of these grades. U.S. No. 2 is a less desirable grade. Apples from the far western States are usually marketed under State grades which are similar to Federal grades. The qualities of color, maturity, and lack of defects—appearance in general—determine the grade.

Avoid: Overripe apples (indicated by a yielding to slight pressure on the skin and soft, mealy flesh) and apples affected by freeze (indicated by internal breakdown and bruised areas). Scald on apples (irregular shaped tan or brown areas) may not seriously affect the eating quality of the apple.

APRICOTS

Most fresh apricots are marketed in June and July, but a limited supply of imported apricots are available in the larger cities during December and January. Domestic apricots are grown principally in California, Washington, and Utah.

Apricots develop their flavor and sweetness on the tree, and should be mature—but firm—at the time they are picked.

Look for: Apricots that are plump and juicy looking, with a uniform, golden-orange color. Ripe apricots will yield to gentle pressure on the skin.

Avoid: Dull-looking, soft, or mushy fruit, and very firm, pale yellow, or greenish-yellow fruit. These are indications of overmaturity or immaturity respectively.

AVOCADOS

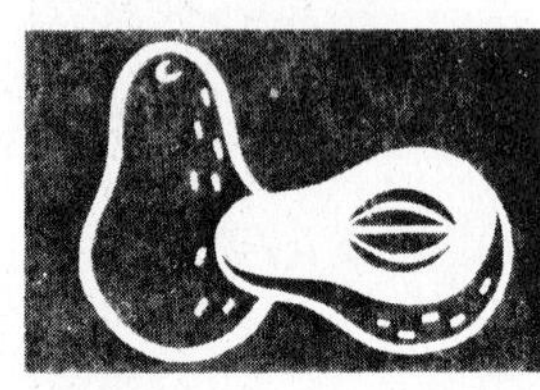

Avocados — grown in California and Florida—are available all year. Two general types and a number of varieties of each are grown. Depending upon type and variety, avocados vary greatly in shape, size and color. Most tend to be pear shaped, but some are almost spherical. Fruits weighing under one-half pound are most commonly available. Some have a rough or leathery textured skin, while others have a smooth skin. The skin color of most varieties is some shade of green, but certain varieties turn maroon, brown or purplish-black as they ripen.

Despite this variation in appearance, avocados are of good eating quality when they are properly ripened—becoming slightly soft. This ripening process normally takes from three to five days at room temperature, for the quite firm avocados usually found in the food store. Ripening can be slowed down by refrigeration.

Look for: For immediate use, slightly soft avocados which yield to a gentle pressure on the skin.

For use in a few days, firm fruits that do not yield to the squeeze test. Leave them at room temperature to ripen.

Irregular light brown markings are sometimes found on the outside skin. These markings have no effect on the flesh of the avocado.

Avoid: Avocados with dark sunken spots in irregular patches or cracked or broken surfaces. These are signs of decay.

An extra tip: When preparing avocados—to avoid the brownish color of avocado flesh when exposed to air—immediately place the peeled fruit in lemon juice until you are ready to use it.

BANANAS

Unlike most other fruits, bananas develop their best eating quality after they are harvested. This allows bananas to be shipped great distances, and almost our entire supply of bananas—available the year round—is imported from Central and South America. Bananas are sensitive to cool temperatures and will be injured in temperatures below 55 degrees. For this reason they should never be kept in the refrigerator. The ideal temperature for ripening bananas is between 60 and 70 degrees; higher temperatures cause them to ripen too rapidly.

Look for: Bananas which are firm, bright in appearance, and free from bruises or other injury. The stage of ripeness is indicated by the skin color: best eating quality has been reached when the solid yellow color is specked with brown. At this stage, the flesh is mellow and the flavor is fully developed. Bananas with green tips or with practically no yellow color have not developed their full flavor potential.

Avoid: Bruised fruit (which means rapid deterioration and waste); discolored skins (a sign of decay); a dull, grayish, aged appearance (showing the bananas have been exposed to cold and will not ripen properly).

Occasionally, the skin may be entirely brown and yet the flesh will still be in prime condition.

BLUEBERRIES

Fresh blueberries are on the market from May through September. Generally, the large berries are cultivated varieties and the smaller berries are the wild varieties.

Look for: A dark blue color with a silvery bloom, your best indication of quality. This silvery bloom is a natural, protective waxy coating. Buy blueberries that are plump, firm, uniform in size, dry, and free from stems or leaves.

CHERRIES

Excellent as dessert fruit, most sweet cherries found in the food store are produced in our Western States and are available from May through August. Red tart cherries—also called sour or pie cherries and used mainly in cooked desserts—have a softer flesh, lighter red color, and a tart flavor. They generally are shipped to processing plants and are sold frozen or canned.

Look for: A very dark color, your most important indication of good flavor and maturity in sweet cherries. Bing, Black Tartarian, Schmidt, Chapman, and Republican varieties should range from deep maroon or mahogany red to black, for richest flavor. Lambert cherries should be dark red. Good cherries have bright, glossy, plump-looking surfaces and fresh-looking stems.

Avoid: Overmature cherries lacking in flavor, indicated by shrivelling, dried stems, and a generally dull appearance. Decay is fairly common at times on sweet cherries, but because of the normal dark color, decayed areas are often inconspicuous. Soft, leaking flesh, brown discoloration, and mold growth are indications of decay.

CRANBERRIES

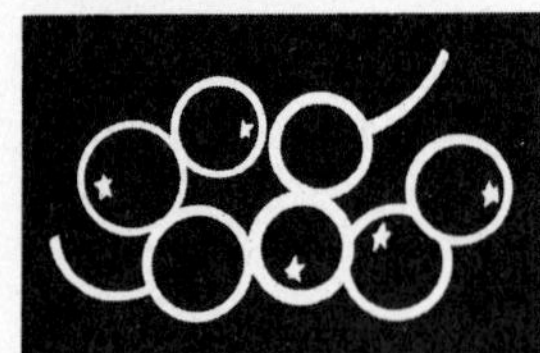

A number of varieties of fresh cranberries are marketed in large volume from September through January. They differ considerably in size and color, but are not identified by variety names in your food store.

Look for: Plump, firm berries with a lustrous color, for the best quality. Duller varieties should at least have some red color. Occassional soft, spongy, or leaky berries should be sorted out before cooking, because they may produce an off-flavor.

GRAPEFRUIT

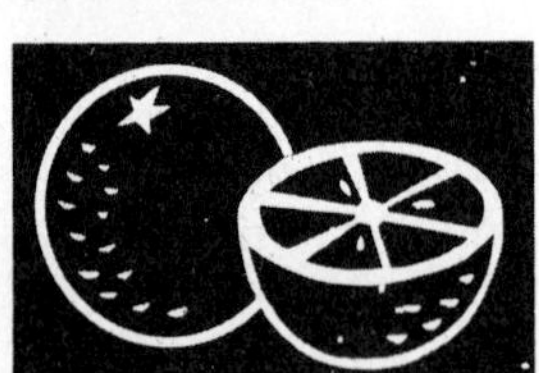

Grapefruit is available all year, with most abundant supplies from January through May. While Florida is the major source of fresh grapefruit, there also is substantial production in Texas, California, and Arizona. Several varieties are marketed, but the principal distinction at retail is between those which are "seedless" (having few or no seeds) and the "seeded" type. Another distinction is color of flesh; white fleshed fruit is most common, but pink or red fleshed varieties are becoming increasingly available.

Grapefruit is picked "tree ripe" and is always ready to eat when you buy it in the store.

Look for: Firm, well-shaped fruits–heavy for their size, which are usually the best eating. Thin-skinned fruits have more juice than coarse-skinned ones. If a grapefruit is pointed at the stem end, it is likely to be thick-skinned. Rough, ridged, or wrinkled skin can also be an indication of thick skin, pulpiness, and lack of juice.

Grapefruit often has skin defects—such as scale, scars, thorn scratches, or discoloration—which usually do not affect the eating quality of the fruit.

Avoid: Soft, discolored areas on the peel at the stem end; water-soaked areas; loss of bright color, and soft and tender peel that breaks easily with finger pressure. These are all symptoms of decay—which has an objectionable effect on flavor.

GRAPES

Most table grapes available in food stores are of the European type, grown principally in California. Only small quantities of Eastern-grown American-type grapes are sold for table use.

European types are firm-fleshed and generally have high sugar content. Common varieties are Thompson seedless (an early green grape), Tokay and Cardinal (early bright red grapes), and Emperor (late, deep red grape). These all have excellent flavor when well matured.

American-type grapes have softer flesh and are more juicy than European types. The outstanding variety—for flavor—is the Concord, which is blue-black when fully matured. Delaware and Catawba are also popular.

Look for: Well colored, plump grapes that are firmly attached to the stem. White or green grapes are sweetest when the color has a yellowish cast or straw color, with a tinge of amber. Red varieties are better when good red predominates on all or most of the berries. Bunches are more likely to hold together if the stems are predominantly green and pliable.

Avoid: Soft or wrinkled grapes (showing effects of freezing or drying), grapes with bleached areas around the stem end (indicating injury and poor quality), and leaking berries (a sign of decay).

LEMONS

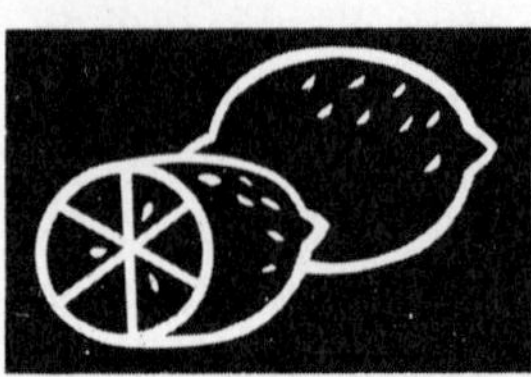

Most of the Nation's commercial lemon supply comes from California and Arizona, and is available the year round.

Look for: Lemons with a rich yellow color, reasonably smooth-textured skin with a slight gloss, and those which are firm and heavy. A pale or greenish yellow color means very fresh fruit with slightly higher acidity. Coarse or rough skin texture is a sign of thick skin and not much flesh.

Avoid: Lemons with a darker yellow or dull color, or with hardening or shriveling of the skin (signs of age), and those with soft spots, mold on the surface, and punctures of the skin (signs of decay).

LIMES

Most green limes sold at retail (sometimes called Persian or Tahitian limes) are produced in Florida and are marketed when mature. Imported limes are mostly the smaller yellow (or Key) lime.

Look for: Limes with glossy skin and heavy weight for the size.

Avoid: Limes with dull, dry skin (a sign of aging and loss of acid flavor), and those showing evidence of decay (soft spots, mold, and skin punctures).

Purplish or brownish irregular mottling of the outer skin surface is a condition called "scald," which in its early stages does not damage the flesh of the lime itself.

MELONS

Selection of melons for quality and flavor is difficult—challenging the skill of even the most experienced buyer. No absolute formula exists, but the use of several factors in judging a melon will increase the likelihood of success.

CANTALOUPS (Muskmelons)

Cantaloups, generally available from May through September, are produced principally in California, Arizona, and Texas, and some are imported early in the season.

Look for: The three major signs of full maturity —1. The stem should be gone, leaving a smooth, symmetrical, shallow basin called a "full slip." (If all or part of the stem base remains or if the stem scar is jagged or torn, the melon is probably not fully matured.) 2. The netting, or veining, should be thick, coarse, and corky—and should stand out in bold relief over some part of the surface. And 3. The skin color (ground color) between the netting should have changed from green to a yellowish-buff, yellowish gray, or pale yellow.

But also look for signs of ripeness, for a cantaloup might be mature, but not ripe. A ripe cantaloup will have a yellowish cast to the rind, have a pleasant cantaloup odor when held to the nose, and will yield slightly to light thumb pressure on the blossom end of the melon.

Most cantaloups are quite firm when freshly displayed in retail stores. While some may be ripe, most have not yet reached their best eating stage. Hold them for two to four days at room temperature to allow completion of ripening. After conditioning the melons, some people like to place them in the refrigerator for a few hours before serving.

Avoid: Overripeness, shown by a pronounced yellow rind color, a softening over the entire rind, and soft, watery, and insipid flesh. Small bruises normally will not hurt the fruit, but large bruised areas should be avoided, since they generally cause soft, watersoaked areas underneath the rind. Mold growth on the cantaloup—particularly in the stem scar, or if the tissue under the mold is soft and wet—is a sign of decay.

CASABA

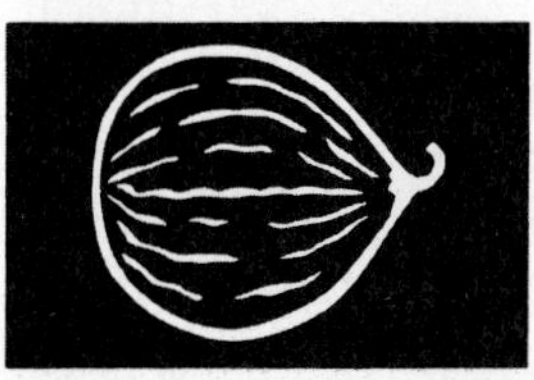

This sweet, juicy melon is normally pumkin-shaped with a very slight tendency to be pointed at the stem end. It is not netted, but has shallow, irregular furrows running from stem end toward the blossom end. The rind is hard with a light green or yellow color. The stem does not separate from the melon, and must be cut in harvesting. The casaba melon season is from July to November; they are produced in California and Arizona.

Look for: Ripe melons with a gold yellow rind color and a slight softening at the blossom end. Casabas have no odor or aroma.

Avoid: Decayed melons, shown by dark, sunken water-soaked spots.

CRENSHAW

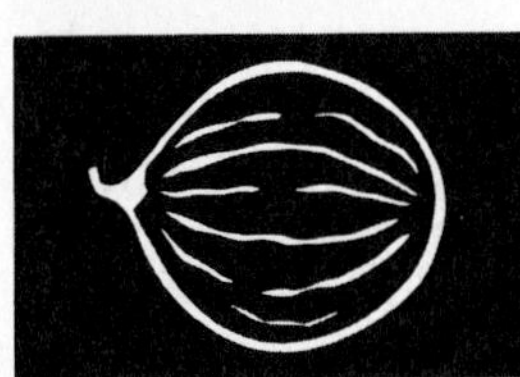

The large size and distinctive shape make this melon easy to identify. It is rounded at the blossom end and tends to be pointed at the stem end. The rind is relatively smooth with only very shallow lengthwise furrowing. The flesh is pale orange, juicy, and delicious—and generally considered outstanding in the melon family. Crenshaws are grown in California from July through October, with peak shipments in August and September.

Look for: These signs of ripeness—1. The rind should be generally a deep golden yellow, sometimes with small areas having a lighter shade of yellow. 2. The surface should yield slightly to moderate pressure of the thumb, particularly at the blossom end. 3. It should have a pleasant aroma.

Avoid: Slightly sunken, watersoaked areas on the rind (a sign of decay, which spreads quickly through the melon).

HONEY BALL

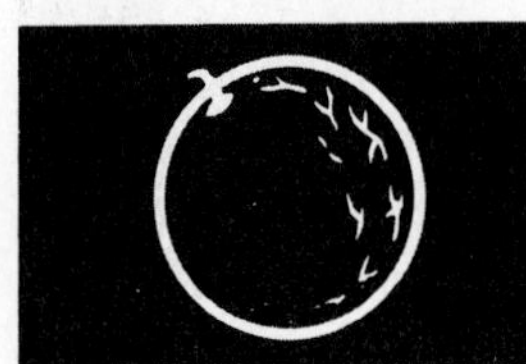

The honey ball melon is very similar to the honey dew melon, except that it is much smaller, is very round, and is slightly and irregularly netted over the surface. Use the same buying tips for this melon as for the honey dew melon.

HONEYDEW

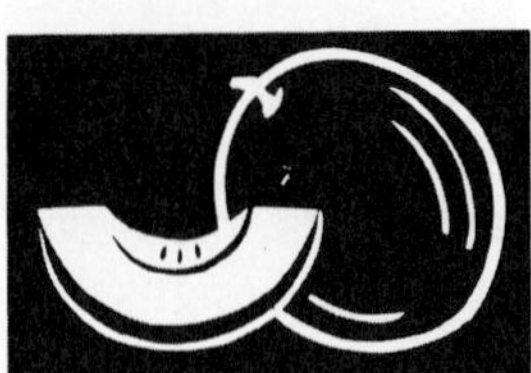

The outstanding flavor characteristics of honeydews make them highly prized as a dessert. The melon is large (4 to 8 pounds), bluntly oval in shape, and generally very smooth with only occasional traces of surface netting. The rind is firm and ranges from creamy white to creamy yellow, depending on the stage of ripeness. The stem does not separate from the fruit, and must be cut for harvesting.

Honeydews are available to some extent almost all year round, due in part to imports during the winter and spring. Chief sources, however, are California, Arizona, and Texas—with the most abundant supplies available from July through October.

Look for: Maturity, shown by a soft, velvety feel, and for ripeness, shown by a slight softening at the blossom end, a faint pleasant fruit aroma, and a yellowish white to creamy rind color.

Avoid: Melons with a dead-white or greenish-white color and hard, smooth feel (which are signs of immaturity), large, watersoaked bruised areas (signs of injury), and cuts or punctures through the rind (which usually lead to decay). Small, superficial, sunken spots do not damage the melon for immediate use, but large decayed spots will.

PERSIAN

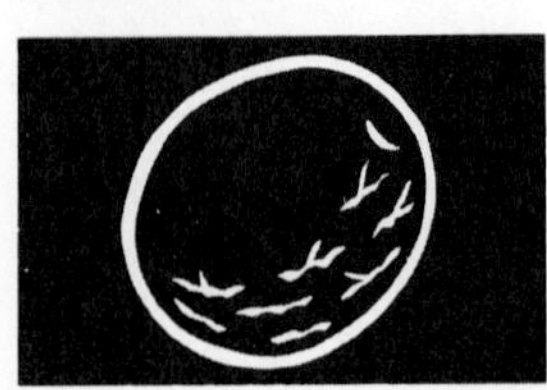

Persian melons resemble cantaloups, but are more nearly round, have finer netting, and are about the same size as honey dews. The flesh is thick, fine-textured, and orange colored. Grown primarily in California, they are available in fair supply in August and September.

Look for: The same factors of quality and ripeness listed for cantaloups.

WATERMELONS

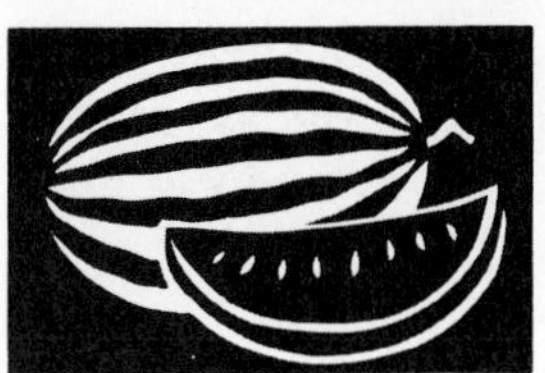

Although watermelons are available to some degree from early May through September, peak supplies come in June, July, and August. Judging the quality of a watermelon is very difficult unless it is cut in half or quartered.

Look for: (in cut melons) Firm, juicy flesh with good red color, free from white streaks; seeds which are dark brown or black.

Avoid: Melons with pale colored flesh, and white streaks or "white heart," whitish seeds (indicating immaturity). Dry, mealy flesh or watery, stringy flesh are signs of overmaturity or aging after harvest.

If you want to buy an uncut watermelon, here are a few appearance factors which may be helpful (though not totally reliable) in guiding you to a satisfactory selection. The watermelon surface should be relatively smooth; the rind should have a slight dullness (neither shiny nor dull); the ends of the melon should be filled out and rounded; and the underside, or "belly," of the melon should have a creamy color.

NECTARINES

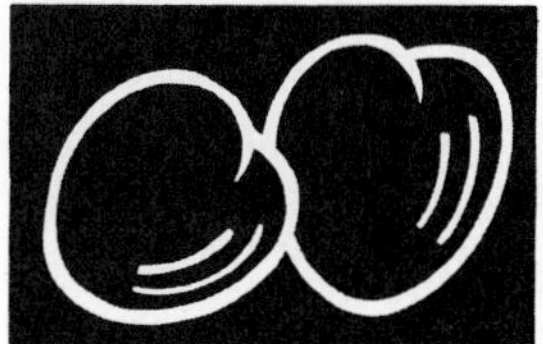

This fruit, available from June through September from California, combines characteristics of both the peach and the plum.

Look for: Rich color and plumpness and a slight softening along the "seam" of the nectarine. Most varieties have an orange-yellow color (ground color) between the red areas, but some varieties have a greenish ground color. Bright-looking fruits which are firm to moderately hard will probably ripen normally within two or three days at room temperature.

Avoid: Hard, dull fruits or slightly shriveled fruits (which may be immature—picked too soon—and of poor eating quality), and soft or overripe fruits or those with cracked or punctured skin or other signs of decay.

Russeting or staining of the skin may affect the appearance but not detract from the internal quality of the nectarine.

ORANGES

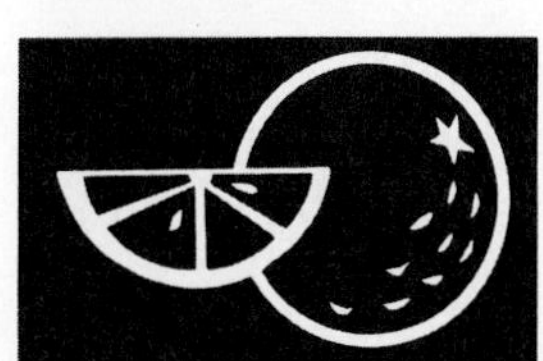

California, Florida, Texas, and Arizona produce our year-round supply of oranges.

Leading varieties from California and Arizona are the Washington Navel and the Valencia, both characterized by a rich orange skin color. The Navel orange, available from November until early May, has a thicker, somewhat more pebbled skin than the Valencia, the skin is more easily removed by hand, and the segments separate more readily. It is ideally suited for eating as whole fruit or as segments in salads. The western Valencia orange, available from late April through October, is excellent either for juicing or for slicing in salads.

Florida and Texas orange crops are marketed from early October until late June. Parson Brown and Hamlin are early varieties, while the Pineapple orange—an important, high-quality orange good for hand eating—is available from late November through March. Florida and Texas Valencias are marketed from late March through June. The Florida Temple orange is available from early December until early March. Somewhat like the California Navel, it peels easily, separates into segments readily, and has excellent flavor.

Oranges are required by strict State regulations to be well matured before being harvested and shipped out of the producing State. Thus skin color is not a reliable index of quality, and a greenish cast or green spots do not mean that the orange is immature. Often fully matured oranges will turn greenish (called "regreening") late in the marketing season. Some oranges are artificially colored to improve the appearance of the fruits. This practice has no effect on eating quality, but artificially colored fruits must be labeled "color added."

"Russeting" is often found on Florida and Texas oranges (but not on California oranges). This is a tan, brown, or blackish mottling or specking over the skin. It has no effect on eating quality, and in fact often occurs on oranges with thin skin and superior eating quality.

Look for: Firm and heavy oranges with fresh, bright-looking skin which is reasonably smooth for the variety.

Avoid: Light-weight oranges, which are likely to lack flesh content and juice. Very rough skin texture indicates abnormally thick skin and less flesh. Dull, dry skin and spongy texture indicate aging and deteriorated eating quality. Also avoid decay—shown by cuts or skin punctures, soft spots on the surface, and discolored, weakened areas of skin around the stem end or button.

PEACHES

A great many varieties of peaches are grown, but only an expert can distinguish one from another. These varieties fall into two general types: freestone (flesh readily separates from the pit) and clingstone (flesh clings tightly to the pit). Freestones are usually preferred for eating fresh or for freezing, while clingstones are used primarily for canning, although sometimes sold fresh.

Look for: Peaches which are fairly firm or becoming a trifle soft. The skin color between the red areas (ground color) should be yellow or at least creamy.

Avoid: Very firm or hard peaches with a distinctly green ground color, which are probably immature and won't ripen properly. Also avoid very soft fruits, which are overripe. Don't buy peaches with large flattened bruises (they'll have large areas of discolored flesh underneath) or peaches with any sign of decay. Decay starts as a pale tan spot which expands in a circle and gradually turns darker in color.

PEARS

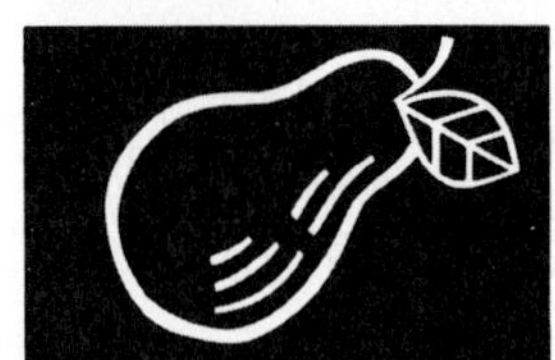

Most popular variety of pear is the Bartlett, which is produced in great quantities (in California, Washington, and Oregon) both for canning and for sale as a fresh fruit. With the aid of cold storage, Bartlett pears are available from early August through November.

Several fall and winter varieties of pear are grown in Washington, Oregon, and California—and shipped to fresh fruit markets. These varieties—Anjou, Bosc, Winter Nellis, and Comice—keep well in cold storage and are available over a long period, from November until May.

Look for: Firm pears of all varieties. The color depends on variety. For Bartletts, look for a pale yellow to rich yellow color; Anjou or Comice—light green to yellowish green; Bosc—greenish yellow to brownish yellow (the brown cast is caused by skin russeting, a characteristic of the Bosc pear); Winter Nellis—medium to light green.

Pears which are hard when you find them in the food store will probably ripen if kept at room temperature, but it is wise to select pears that have already begun to soften—to be reasonably sure that they will ripen satisfactorily.

Avoid: Wilted or shriveled pears with dull-appearing skin and slight weakening of the flesh near the stem—which indicates immaturity. These pears will not ripen. Also avoid spots on the sides or blossom ends of the pear, which means that corky tissue may be underneath.

PINEAPPLES

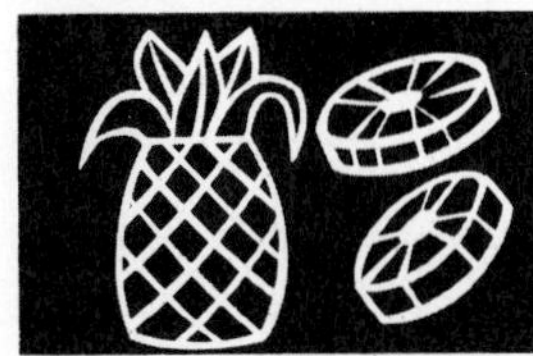

Pineapples, which are available the year round but are at peak supply in April and May, come principally from Puerto Rico, Hawaii, and Mexico. Because pineapples must be picked when still hard (but mature), they must be allowed to ripen before they can be eaten. They will normally ripen within a few days at room temperature, but many are already ripe when you find them in the food store.

Look for: The proper color, the fragrant pineapple odor, a very slight separation of the eyes or pips, and the ease with which the "spike" or leaves can be pulled out from the top. Pineapples are usually dark green in mature hard stage. As the more popular varieties (such as Red Spanish and Smooth Cayenne) ripen, the green color fades and orange and yellow take its place. When fully ripe, the pineapples are golden yellow, orange yellow, or reddish brown—depending on the variety, although one seldom-seen pineapple (the Sugar Loaf) remains green even when ripe.

Also look for the maturity, shown by plump, glossy eyes or pips, firmness, a lively color, and fruits which are heavy for their size.

Avoid: Pineapples with sunken or slightly pointed pips, dull yellowish-green color, and dried appearance (all signs of immaturity). Also avoid bruised fruit—shown by discolored or soft spots—which are susceptible to decay. Other signs of decay (which spreads rapidly through the fruit) are: traces of mold, an unpleasant odor, and eyes which turn watery and darker in color.

PLUMS AND PRUNES

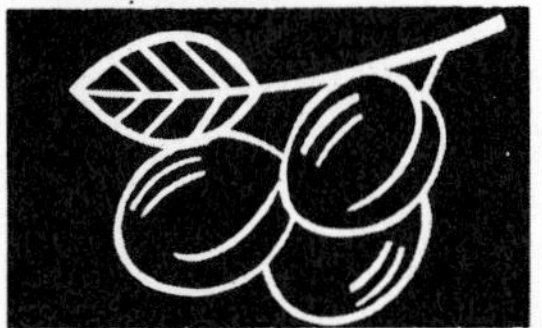

Quality characteristics for both are very similar and the same buying tips apply to both.

Plums—A number of varieties of plums are produced in California and are available from June to September. Varieties differ widely in appearance and flavor, so you should buy and taste one to see if that variety appeals to you.

Prunes—Only a few varieties of prunes are commonly marketed and they are all very similar. Prunes are purplish-black or bluish-black, with a moderately firm flesh which separates freely from the pit. Most commercial production is in the Northwestern States. Fresh prunes are available in food stores from August through October.

Look for: Plums and prunes with a good color for the variety, in a fairly firm to slightly soft stage of ripeness.

Avoid: Fruits with skin breaks, punctures, or brownish discoloration. Also avoid immature fruits (relatively hard, poorly colored, very tart, sometimes shriveled) and overmature fruits (excessively soft, possibly leaking or decaying).

RASPBERRIES, BOYSENBERRIES, ETC.

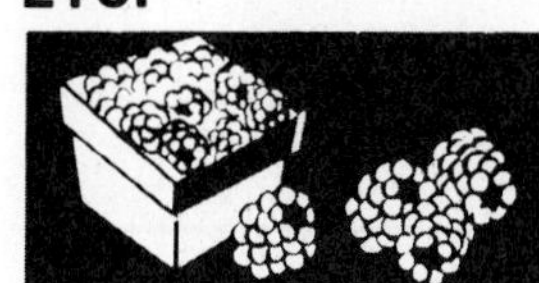

Blackberries, raspberries, dewberries, loganberries, and youngberries are similar in general structure. They differ from one another in shape or color, but quality factors are about the same for all.

Look for: A bright clean appearance and a uniform good color for the species. The individual small cells making up the berry should be plump and tender but not mushy. Look for berries that are fully ripened—with no attached stem caps.

Avoid: Leaky and moldy berries. You can usually spot them through the openings in ventilated plastic containers. Also look for wet or stained spots on wood or fiber containers, as possible signs of poor quality or spoiled berries.

STRAWBERRIES

First shipments of strawberries come from southern Florida in January, and then production increases, gradually spreading north and west into many parts of the country before tapering off in the fall. Strawberries are in best supply in May and June.

Look for: Berries with a full red color and a bright luster, firm flesh, and the cap stem still attached. The berries should be dry and clean, and usually medium to small strawberries have better eating quality than large ones.

Avoid: Berries with large uncolored areas or with large seedy areas (poor in flavor and texture), a dull shrunken appearance or softness (signs of overripeness or decay), or those with mold, which can spread rapidly from one berry to another.

Note: In most containers of strawberries you will likely find a few that are less desirable than others. Try to look at some of the berries down in the container to be sure that they are reasonably free from defects or decay.

TANGERINES

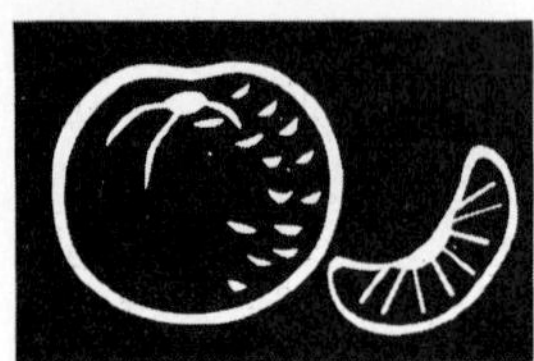

Florida is the chief source of tangerines. Considerable quantities of tangerines and similar types of oranges are produced in California and Arizona, some in Texas, and a few are imported. Tangerines are available from late November until early March, with peak supplies in December and January. The Murcott, a large, excellent variety of orange resembling the tangerine, is available from late February through April.

Look for: Deep yellow or orange color and a bright luster as your best sign of fresh, mature, good-flavored tangerines. Because of the typically loose nature of the tangerine skin, they will frequently not feel firm to the touch.

Avoid: Very pale yellow or greenish fruits, likely to be lacking in flavor (although small green areas on otherwise high-colored fruit are not bad) and tangerines with cut or punctured skins or very soft spots (all signs of decay, which spreads rapidly).

A CONSUMER'S GLOSSARY OF FRUIT TERMS

Blossom end—The opposite end from the stem end. The stem end will have a scar or remains of the stem to identify it. The blossom end is often more rounded than the stem end.

Breakdown of tissue—Decomposition or breaking down of cells due to pressure (bruise) or age (internal breakdown).

Decay—Decomposition of the fruit due to bacteria or fungus infection.

Ground color—The basic or background color of a fruit before the sun's rays cause the skin to redden. The ground color may be seen beneath and between the red blush of the fruit.

Hard—The terms "hard," "firm," and "soft" are subjective terms used to describe the degrees of maturity or ripeness of a fruit. A "hard" texture will not give when pressed. A "firm" texture will give slightly to pressure. A "soft" texture is, of course, soft to the touch. The term "mature green" is sometimes used instead of "hard."

Mature—Describes a fruit that is ready to be picked, whether or not it is ripe at this time. If a fruit is picked when mature, it is capable of ripening properly, but if picked when immature, it will not ripen properly.

Netting—The vein-like network of lines running randomly across the rind of some melons.

Ripe—Describes a fruit that is ready to be eaten.

Russeting—A lacy, brownish, blemish-type coating on top of the skin.

Scald—A blemish, or brownish discoloration, which occasionally develops in the skin of apples or other fruits in cold storage.

Cheese

MAKING NATURAL CHEESE

The making of natural cheese is an art centuries old. It consists of separating most of the milk solids from the milk by curdling with rennet or bacterial culture or both and separating the curd from the whey by heating, stirring, and pressing. Most cheeses in this country are made from whole milk. For certain types of cheese both milk and cream are used and for other types, skim milk, whey or mixtures of all of these are used.

The distinctive flavor and body and texture characteristics of the various cheeses are due to: (1) the kind of milk used, (2) the method used for curdling the milk and for cutting, cooking, and forming the curd, (3) the type of bacteria or molds used in ripening, (4) the amount of salt or other seasonings added and (5) the conditions of ripening such as temperature, humidity and length of time. Sometimes only minor differences in the procedures followed may make the difference between one variety of cheese and another.

After the cheese has been formed into its characteristic shape it is given a coating of wax or other protective coating or wrapping and allowed to cure or age for varying lengths of time depending upon the kind or variety of cheese being made.

When the cheese has reached its proper curing stage it is often cut or sliced from larger blocks or wheels into more suitable sizes for consumer use. The refrigerated showcase in a modern food market is most enticing with its display of various shapes and sizes of cheese packages such as wedges, oblongs, segments, cubes, slices, blocks and cut portions.

CARE IN THE HOME

All natural cheese should be kept refrigerated. Soft unripened cheeses, such as cottage, cream or Neufchatel, are quite perishable and should be used within a few days after purchase. Ripened or cured cheeses keep well in the refrigerator for several weeks if protected from mold contamination and drying out. When possible the original wrapper or covering should be left on the cheese. The cut surface of cheese should be covered with wax paper, foil, or plastic wrapping material to protect the surface from drying. If large pieces are to be stored for any extended length of time, the cut surface may be dipped in hot paraffin. Small pieces may be completely rewrapped. Mold which may develop on natural cheeses is not harmful, and it is easily scraped or cut from the surface of the cheese. The particular mold in the interior of such cheeses as Blue, Gorgonzola, Roquefort or Stilton has been carefully developed to produce the characteristic color and distinctive flavor of those varieties and is consumed as part of the cheese.

Ends or pieces of cheese that have become dried out and hard may be grated and kept refrigerated in a clean, tightly covered glass jar, and used for garnishing or accenting.

Cheese with an aromatic or a strong odor such as Limburger should be stored in a tightly covered jar or container. Such cheeses are fast curing and are best when used within a reasonable time after purchase.

Normally cheese should not be allowed to freeze as this may damage the characteristic body and texture and cause the cheese to become crumbly and mealy. However, small pieces (1 pound or less) not over 1 inch thick of certain varieties may be frozen satisfactorily for as long as 6 months if handled and stored properly. Since it is necessary that the cheese be frozen quickly, the temperature of the freezer should be 0° F. or lower. Cut cheese should be carefully wrapped (foil or other moistureproof freezer wrapping should be pressed tightly against surfaces to eliminate air, and to prevent evaporation), then frozen immediately. Among the varieties of cheese which can be successfully frozen in small pieces are: Brick, Cheddar, Edam, Gouda, Muenster, Port du Salut, Swiss, Provolone, Mozzarella, and Camembert. Small sizes as in the case of Camembert can be frozen in their original package. When removed from the freezer, cheese should be thawed in the refrigerator and used as soon as possible after thawing.

Except for soft unripened cheeses such as cottage and cream cheese, all cheese should be served unchilled in order to help bring out its distinctive flavor and texture characteristics. This usually requires 20 minutes to 1 hour or more at room temperature.

USES

Cheese is one of the most nutritious and versatile foods. Because it is an excellent source of many important nutrients in the diet and because it is a well-liked food, cheese is used freely by nutritionists and homemakers in planning meals and in the preparation of many flavorful dishes. With the wide variety of flavors, colors, and consistencies to choose from, natural cheeses are suitable for any meal of the day, from appetizers to desserts, and between-meal snacks as well. Whether served separately or in combination dishes, cheese adds zest and flavor to other foods. There is a cheese to suit every taste, mood or occasion.

Some of the many ways of using different kinds of cheese are as follows:

(a) Main dish in the form of fondue, soufflé, Welsh rabbit, omelet, pizza, or in combination with potatoes, other vegetables, rice, macaroni, noodles or spaghetti.

(b) Salads and salad dressings.

(c) Assorted cheeses on trays with fruit, nuts and crackers or chips.

(d) Appetizers in the form of cut cheese or as spreads and dips.

(e) Sliced in toasted or cold sandwiches or as an ingredient in sandwich spreads and sauces.

(f) Grated as a garnish for soups, sauces and hot dishes.

(g) Desserts, as cheese and crackers, cheese cakes, cheese pies, or fruit pies with cheese.

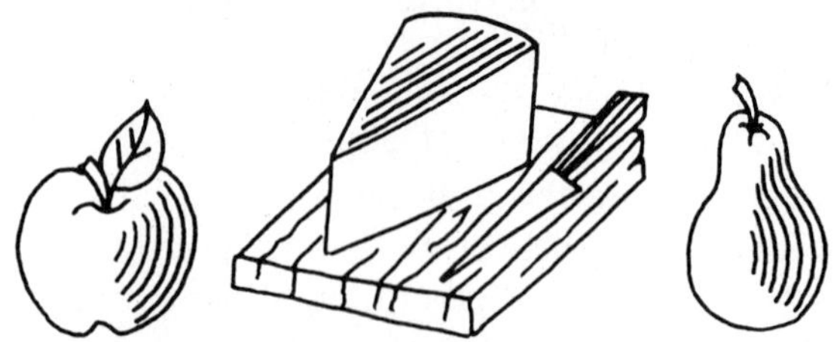

RIPENING CLASSIFICATIONS

Unripened

The soft unripened varieties such as cottage cheese contain relatively high moisture and do not undergo any curing or ripening. They are consumed fresh—soon after manufacture. The firm unripened cheeses such as Gjetost and Mysost also may be used soon after manufacture but because they contain very low moisture may be kept for several weeks or months.

Soft Ripened

In the soft ripened cheeses, curing progresses from the outside or rind of the cheese, towards the center. Particular molds or culture of bacteria or both, which grow on the surface of the cheese aid in developing the characteristic flavor and body and texture during the curing process. Curing continues as long as the temperature is favorable. These cheeses usually contain more moisture than semi-soft ripened varieties.

Semisoft Ripened

Unlike the soft ripened varieties, these cheeses ripen from the interior as well as from the surface. This ripening process begins soon after the cheese is formed, with the aid of a characteristic bacterial or mold culture or both. Curing continues as long as the temperature is favorable. These cheeses contain higher moisture than the firm ripened varieties.

Firm Ripened

These cheeses ripen with the aid of a bacterial culture, throughout the entire cheese. Ripening continues as long as the temperature is favorable. The rate and degree of curing is also closely related to the moisture content. Therefore, these cheeses, being lower in moisture than the softer varieties, usually require a longer curing time.

Very Hard Ripened

These cheeses also are cured with the aid of a bacterial culture and enzymes. The rate of curing however is much slower because of the very low moisture and higher salt content.

Blue-Vein Mold Ripened

Curing is accomplished by the aid of bacteria but more particularly by the use of a characteristic mold culture that grows throughout the interior of the cheese to produce the familiar appearance and characteristic flavor.

KINDS OF CHEESE

The charts in this pamphlet will help you in learning some of the more popular and generally available varieties of natural cheese, their general classification, principal characteristics, and some of their uses.

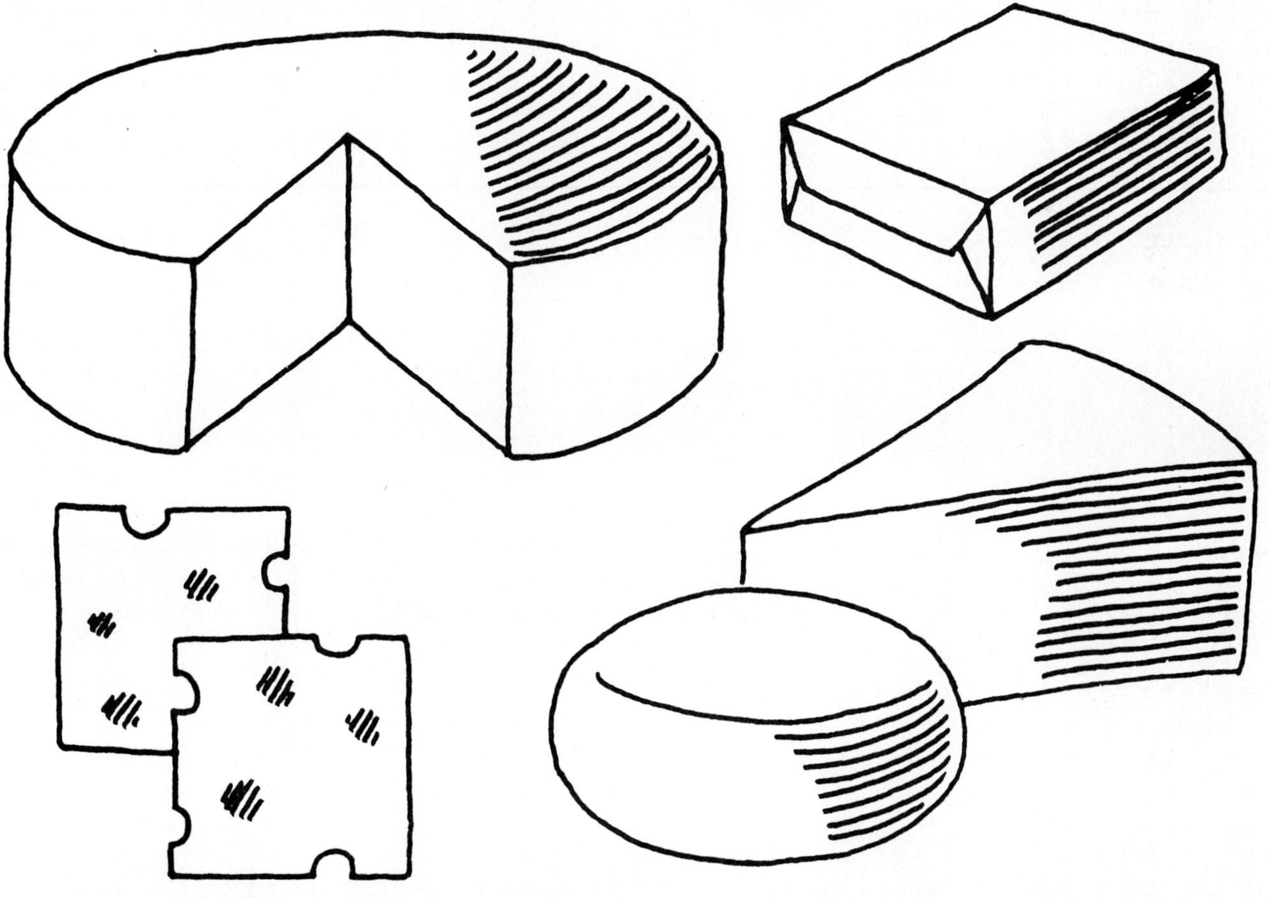

CHARACTERISTICS OF SOME POPULAR VARIETIES OF NATURAL CHEESES

Kind or name Place of origin	Kind of milk used in manufacture	Ripening or curing time	Flavor	Body and texture	Color	Retail packaging	Uses
			SOFT, UNRIPENED VARIETIES				
Cottage, plain or creamed. (Unknown)	Cow's milk skimmed; plain curd, or plain curd with cream added.	Unripened..	Mild, acid...	Soft, curd particles of varying size.	White to creamy white.	Cup-shaped containers, tumblers, dishes.	Salads, with fruits, vegetables, sandwiches, dips, cheese cake.
Cream, plain (U.S.A.)	Cream from cow's milk.	Unripened..	Mild, acid...	Soft and smooth....	White............	3- to 8-oz. packages	Salads, dips, sandwiches, snacks, cheese cake, desserts.
Neufchatel (Nû-shă-tĕl'). (France)	Cow's milk..........	Unripened..	Mild, acid...	Soft, smooth similar to cream cheese but lower in milkfat.	White............	4- to 8-oz. packages.	Salads, dips, sandwiches, snacks. cheese cake, desserts.
Ricotta (Rĭ-cō'-ta) (Italy)	Cow's milk, whole or partly skimmed, or whey from cow's milk with whole or skim milk added. In Italy, whey from sheep's milk.	Unripened..	Sweet, nutlike.	Soft, moist or dry...	White............	Pint and quart paper and plastic containers, 3 lb. metal cans.	Appetizers, salads, snacks, lasagne, ravioli, noodles and other cooked dishes, grating, desserts.

Kind or name Place of origin	Kind of milk used in manufacture	Ripening or curing time	Flavor	Body and texture	Color	Retail packaging	Uses
			FIRM, UNRIPENED VARIETIES				
Gjetost,[1] (Yĕt'ôst). (Norway)	Whey from goat's milk or a mixture of whey from goat's and cow's milk.	Unripened..	Sweetish, caramel.	Firm, buttery consistency.	Golden brown.....	Cubical and rectangular.	Snacks, desserts, served with dark breads, crackers, biscuits or muffins.
Mysost (Müs-ôst) also called Primost (Prēm'-ôst). (Norway)	Whey from cow's milk.	Unripened..	Sweetish, caramel.	Firm, buttery consistency.	Light brown.......	Cubical, cylindrical, pie-shaped wedges.	Snacks, desserts, served with dark breads.
Mozzarella (Mō-tsa-rel'la) also called Scamorza. (Italy)	Whole or partly skimmed cow's milk. In Italy, originally made from buffalo's milk.	Unripened	Delicate, mild.	Slightly firm, plastic.	Creamy white.....	Small round or braided form, shredded, sliced.	Snacks, toasted sandwiches, cheeseburgers, cooking, as in meat loaf, or topping for lasagne, pizza, and casseroles.

[1] Imported only.

Kind or name Place of origin	Kind of milk used in manufacture	Ripening or curing time	Flavor	Body and texture	Color	Retail packaging	Uses
SOFT, RIPENED VARIETIES							
Brie (Brē) (France)	Cow's milk..........	4 to 8 weeks.	Mild to pungent.	Soft, smooth when ripened.	Creamy yellow interior; edible thin brown and white crust.	Circular, pie-shaped wedges.	Appetizers, sandwiches, snacks, good with crackers and fruit, dessert.
Camembert (Kăm'ĕm-bâr). (France)	Cow's milk..........	4 to 8 weeks.	Mild to pungent.	Soft, smooth; very soft when fully ripened.	Creamy yellow interior; edible thin white, or gray-white crust.	Small circular cakes and pie-shaped portions.	Appetizers, sandwiches, snacks, good with crackers, and fruit such as pears and apples, dessert.
Limburger (Belgium)	Cow's milk..........	4 to 8 weeks.	Highly pungent, very strong.	Soft, smooth when ripened; usually contains small irregular openings.	Creamy white interior; reddish yellow surface.	Cubical, rectangular.	Appetizers, snacks, good with crackers, rye or other dark breads, dessert.

Kind or name Place of origin	Kind of milk used in manufacture	Ripening or curing time	Flavor	Body and texture	Color	Retail packaging	Uses
SEMISOFT, RIPENED VARIETIES							
Bel Paese [2] (Bĕl Pă-ā-zĕ). (Italy)	Cow's milk..........	6 to 8 weeks.	Mild to moderately robust.	Soft to medium firm, creamy.	Creamy yellow interior; slightly gray or brownish surface sometimes covered with yellow wax coating.	Small wheels, wedges, segments.	Appetizers, good with crackers, snacks, sandwiches, dessert.
(Brick) (U.S.A.)	Cow's milk..........	2 to 4 months.	Mild to moderately sharp.	Semisoft to medium firm, elastic, numerous small mechanical openings.	Creamy yellow....	Loaf, brick, slices, cut portions.	Appetizers, sandwiches, snacks, dessert.
Muenster (Mün' stĕr). (Germany)	Cow's milk..........	1 to 8 weeks.	Mild to mellow.	Semisoft, numerous small mechanical openings. Contains more moisture than brick.	Creamy white interior; yellow tan surface.	Circular cake, blocks, wedges, segments, slices.	Appetizers, sandwiches, snacks, dessert.
Port du Salut (Por dü Sȧ-lü"). (France)	Cow's milk..........	6 to 8 weeks.	Mellow to robust.	Semisoft, smooth, buttery, small openings.	Creamy yellow....	Wheels and wedges.	Appetizers, snacks, served with raw fruit, dessert.

[2] Italian trademark—licensed for manufacture in U.S.A.; also imported.

CHARACTERISTICS OF SOME POPULAR VARIETIES OF NATURAL CHEESES—Continued

Kind or name Place of origin	Kind of milk used in manufacture	Ripening or curing time	Flavor	Body and texture	Color	Retail packaging	Uses
				FIRM RIPENED VARIETIES			
Cheddar (England)	Cow's milk..........	1 to 12 months or more.	Mild to very sharp.	Firm, smooth, some mechanical openings.	White to medium-yellow-orange.	Circular, cylindrical loaf, pie-shaped wedges, oblongs, slices, cubes, shredded, grated.	Appetizers, sandwiches, sauces, on vegetables, in hot dishes, toasted sandwiches, grating, cheeseburgers, dessert.
Colby (U.S.A.)	Cow's milk..........	1 to 3 months.	Mild to mellow.	Softer and more open than Cheddar.	White to medium-yellow-orange.	Cylindrical, pie-shaped wedges.	Sandwiches, snacks cheeseburgers.
Caciocavallo (Kä' chō-kä-val'lō). (Italy)	Cow's milk. In Italy, cow's milk or mixtures of sheep's, goat's, and cow's milk.	3 to 12 months.	Piquant, similar to Provolone but not smoked.	Firm, lower in milkfat and moisture than Provolone.	Light or white interior; clay or tan colored surface.	Spindle or ten-pin shaped, bound with cord, cut pieces.	Snacks, sandwiches, cooking, dessert; suitable for grating after prolonged curing.
Edam (Ē'dăm) (Netherlands.)	Cow's milk, partly skimmed.	2 to 3 months.	Mellow, nut-like.	Semisoft to firm, smooth; small irregularly shaped or round holes; lower milkfat than Gouda.	Creamy yellow or medium yellow-orange interior; surface coated with red wax.	Cannon ball shaped loaf, cut pieces, oblongs.	Appetizers, snacks, salads, sandwiches, seafood sauces, dessert.
Gouda (Gou'-dá) (Netherlands)	Cow's milk, whole or partly skimmed.	2 to 6 months.	Mellow, nut-like.	Semisoft to firm, smooth; small irregularly shaped or round holes; higher milkfat than Edam.	Creamy yellow or medium yellow-orange interior; may or may not have red wax coating.	Ball shaped with flattened top and bottom.	Appetizers, snacks, salads, sandwiches, seafood sauces, dessert.
Provolone (Prō-vō-lō'-nĕ) also smaller sizes and shapes called Provolette, Provoloncini. (Italy)	Cow's milk.........	2 to 12 months or more	Mellow to sharp, smoky, salty.	Firm, smooth.......	Light creamy interior; light brown or golden yellow surface.	Pear shaped, sausage and salami shaped, wedges, slices.	Appetizers, sandwiches, snacks, souffle, macaroni and spaghetti dishes, pizza, suitable for grating when fully cured and dried.
Swiss, also called Emmentaler. (Switzerland)	Cow's milk..........	3 to 9 months.	Sweet, nut-like.	Firm, smooth with large round eyes.	Light yellow.......	Segments, pieces, slices.	Sandwiches, snacks, sauces, fondue, cheeseburgers.

Kind or name Place of origin	Kind of milk used in manufacture	Ripening or curing time	Flavor	Body and texture	Color	Retail packaging	Uses
VERY HARD RIPENED VARIETIES							
Parmesan (Pär´ mē-zăn´) also called Reggiano. (Italy)	Partly skimmed cow's milk.	14 months to 2 years.	Sharp, piquant.	Very hard, granular, lower moisture and milkfat than Romano.	Creamy white.....	Cylindrical, wedges, shredded, grated.	Grated for seasoning in soups, or vegetables, spaghetti, ravioli, breads, popcorn, used extensively in pizza and lasagne.
Romano (Rō-mä´-nō) also called Sardo Romano Pecorino Romano. (Italy)	Cow's milk. In Italy, sheep's milk (Italian law).	5 to 12 months.	Sharp, piquant.	Very hard granular..	Yellowish-white interior, greenish-black surface.	Round with flat ends, wedges, shredded, grated.	Seasoning in soups, casserole dishes, ravioli, sauces, breads, suitable for grating when cured for about one year.
Sap Sago [1] (Săp´-sä-gō). (Switzerland)	Skimmed cow's milk.	5 months or more.	Sharp, pungent clover-like.	Very hard...........	Light green by addition of dried, powdered clover leaves.	Conical, shakers..	Grated to flavor soups, meats, macaroni, spaghetti, hot vegetables; mixed with butter makes a good spread on crackers or bread.

Kind or name Place of origin	Kind of milk used in manufacture	Ripening or curing time	Flavor	Body and texture	Color	Retail packaging	Uses
BLUE-VEIN MOLD RIPENED VARIETIES							
Blue, spelled Bleu on imported cheese. (France)	Cow's milk..........	2 to 6 months.	Tangy, peppery.	Semisoft, pasty, sometimes crumbly.	White interior, marbled or streaked with blue veins of mold.	Cylindrical, wedges, oblongs, squares, cut portions.	Appetizers, salads, dips, salad dressing, sandwich spreads, good with crackers, dessert.
Gorgonzola (Gôr-gŏn-zō´-lâ). (Italy)	Cow's milk. In Italy, cow's milk or goat's milk or mixtures of these.	3 to 12 months.	Tangy, peppery.	Semisoft, pasty, sometimes crumbly, lower moisture than Blue.	Creamy white interior, mottled or streaked with blue-green veins of mold. Clay colored surface.	Cylindrical, wedges, oblongs.	Appetizers, snacks, salads, dips, sandwich spread, good with crackers, dessert.
Roquefort [1] (Rōk´-fẽrt) or (Rôk-fôr´). (France).	Sheep's milk........	2 to 5 months or more.	Sharp, slightly peppery.	Semisoft, pasty, sometimes crumbly.	White or creamy white interior, marbled or streaked with blue veins of mold.	Cylindrical, wedges.	Appetizers, snacks, salads, dips, sandwich spreads, good with crackers, dessert.
Stilton [1] (England).	Cow's milk..........	2 to 6 months.	Piquant, milder than Gorgonzola or Roquefort.	Semisoft, flaky; slightly more crumbly than Blue.	Creamy white interior, marbled or streaked with blue-green veins of mold.	Circular, wedges, oblongs.	Appetizers, snacks, salads, dessert.

[1] Imported only.

PASTEURIZED PROCESS CHEESE

Pasteurized process cheese is a blend of fresh and aged natural cheeses which have been shredded, mixed and heated (pasteurized), after which no further ripening occurs. It melts easily when reheated. The blend may consist of one or two or more varieties of natural cheese and may contain pimentos, fruits, vegetables, or meats. Smoked cheese or smoke flavor may also be added.

The flavor of pasteurized process cheese depends largely upon the flavor of the cheese used which may be modified by flavoring materials added. Pasteurized Gruyere cheese has a nut-sweet flavor, somewhat similar to Swiss.

Some other available varieties are: pasteurized process American cheese, pasteurized process Swiss cheese, pasteurized process Swiss cheese blended with American, and pasteurized process Brick cheese.

Process cheese is packaged in slices, ½-, 1- and 2-pound loaves and cut portions.

It may be used in main dishes, for snacks and cheeseburgers, with cold cuts and salads, on grilled or toasted sandwiches, in numerous sandwich combinations and in casseroles.

PASTEURIZED PROCESS CHEESE FOOD

Pasteurized process cheese food is prepared in much the same manner as process cheese except that it contains less cheese, with nonfat dry milk, or whey solids and water added. This results in a lower milk fat content and more moisture than in process cheese. Pasteurized process cheese food also may contain pimentos, fruits, vegetables or meats or may have a smoked flavor.

Cheese food is milder in flavor, has a softer texture, spreads more easily and melts quicker than process cheese due to the higher moisture.

The most popular variety is pasteurized process American cheese food and is packaged in slices, rolls, links and loaves.

It may be used in any place where process cheese is used though it is not likely to add as much cheese flavor.

PASTEURIZED PROCESS CHEESE SPREAD

Pasteurized process cheese spread is made in much the same manner as pasteurized process cheese food but generally contains higher moisture, and the milk fat content is usually lower. A stabilizer is used in the preparation of this product to prevent separation of ingredients. It is normally more spreadable than cheese food. Cheese spread also may contain pimentos, fruits, vegetables or meats or may have a smoked flavor.

The flavor of pasteurized process cheese spread depends largely upon the flavor of the cheese used which may be modified by flavoring materials added.

Some available varieties are: pasteurized process American cheese spread, pasteurized process pimento cheese spread, pasteurized process pineapple cheese spread and pasteurized process Blue cheese spread.

Spreads are packaged in jars and loaves convenient for use as snacks, in stuffing celery stalks, and in deviled eggs, noodle casseroles, meat balls, hot vegetables, sandwiches, sauces, and dressings.

COLDPACK CHEESE

Coldpack cheese or Club cheese is a blend of the same or two or more varieties of fresh and aged natural cheese, as in process cheese, except that the cheese is mixed into a uniform product without heating. It may have a smoked flavor.

The principal varieties are coldpack American cheese and cold pack Swiss cheese.

The flavor is the same as the natural cheese used and usually is aged or sharp. The body is softer than the natural cheese and it spreads easily.

Coldpack cheese is packed in jars, rolls, or links and it is especially good as an appetizer, snack, or dessert.

COLDPACK CHEESE FOOD

Coldpack cheese food is prepared in the same manner as Coldpack cheese but includes other dairy ingredients as used in process cheese food. In addition, sweetening agents such as sugar and corn sirup may be added.

Coldpack cheese food may contain pimentos, fruits, vegetables or meats or may have a smoked flavor.

The flavor resembles the cheese from which it is made but is milder. It is softer than the natural cheese and spreads more easily due to the other ingredients added and the higher moisture content.

It is packaged in the same way as Coldpack cheese and may be served in the same manner.

BUYING CHEESE

CHECK THE LABEL

The labels of natural cheese, pasteurized process cheese, and related products carry important descriptive information. The name of a natural cheese will appear as the variety such as "Cheddar cheese", "Swiss cheese", or "Blue cheese."

Pasteurized process cheese labels will always include the words "pasteurized process", together with the name of the variety or varieties of cheese used, for instance, "pasteurized process American cheese" or "pasteurized process Swiss and American cheese".

Cheese food also contains ingredients other than cheese and therefore is labeled as "pasteurized process cheese food". Cheese spreads have a different composition from cheese foods and are labeled as "pasteurized process cheese spread". All the ingredients used in the preparation of these products are listed on the respective label along with the kinds or varieties of cheese used in the mixture. Also the milkfat and moisture content may be shown.

Coldpack cheese and coldpack cheese food are labeled in the same manner as other cheese and cheese foods except that "club cheese" or "comminuted cheese" may be substituted for the name "coldpack cheese".

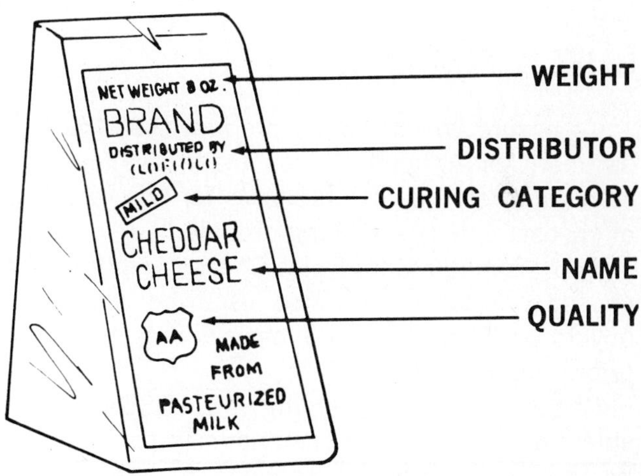

CHECK THE CURE

A very important bit of information on the label of certain varieties of natural cheese pertains to the age or degree of curing. For instance, Cheddar cheese may be labeled as "mild", "medium" or "mellow", or "aged" or "sharp". In some cases pasteurized process cheese may be labeled to indicate a sharp flavor when a much higher proportion of sharp or aged cheese was used in its preparation.

CHECK THE NAME

Look for the name of the article. Do not confuse the brand name with the name of the cheese. For some purposes you may want natural cheese, for others, process cheese or cheese food, and for still others, pasteurized process cheese spread or coldpack cheese may best serve your needs. In many cases they may be packaged alike but the names on the labels will be different.

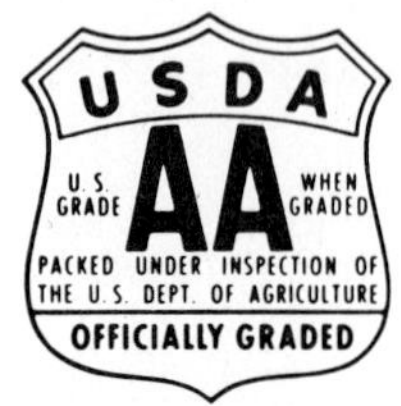

CHECK FOR QUALITY

To assure you a quality product the U.S. Department of Agriculture has made available to manufacturers quality standards for two varieties of cheese. Others are being prepared.

Grade standards for Swiss Cheese and Cheddar cheese are available to be used by wholesale buyers and handlers as a basis for establishing price/quality terms.

Cheddar cheese carrying the USDA grade shield on the label of consumer-size packages is being used in several sections of the United States.

The USDA grade shield means that the Cheddar cheese has been inspected and graded by an experienced and highly trained Government grader. And it means the cheese was produced in a USDA inspected and approved plant, under sanitary conditions. It is your guarantee of consistent and dependable quality.

Cheddar cheese carrying the U.S. Grade AA shield is the highest quality. It meets exacting USDA standards, has a fine, highly pleasing Cheddar flavor, a smooth compact texture, uniform color, and attractive appearance.

To earn this grade, cheese must be produced with special care—in the quality of the milk, cheese-making skill, curing or ripening process, and packaging.

The AA shield is assurance of consistently fine Cheddar flavor and texture in every package.

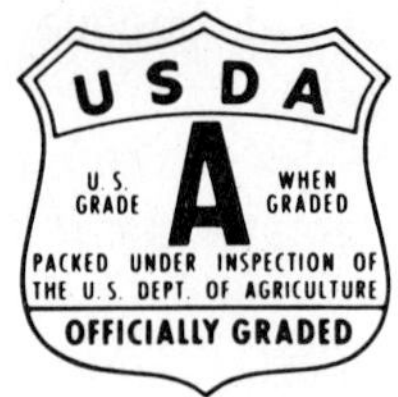

Cheddar cheese bearing the U.S. Grade A shield on the package is also of good quality—but not as high as AA. The flavor is pleasing; however, there may be more variation in flavor and texture between packages. Cheese and cheese products not covered by a U.S. grade standard may be inspected and bear the USDA "Quality Approved" inspection shield on the container. Pasteurized Process Cheese, Cheese Food and Spreads, and Cottage cheese are current examples of cheese products being inspected by the U.S. Department of Agriculture.

To carry the "Quality Approved" shield, the product must be manufactured in a plant meeting the USDA sanitary specifications for plant and equipment as well as the quality specifications for the cheese itself.

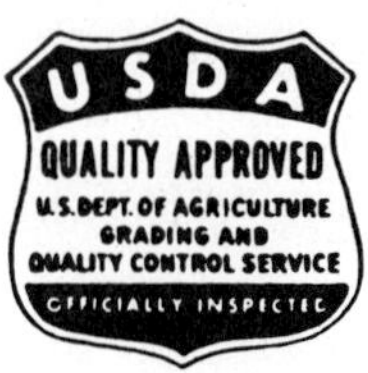

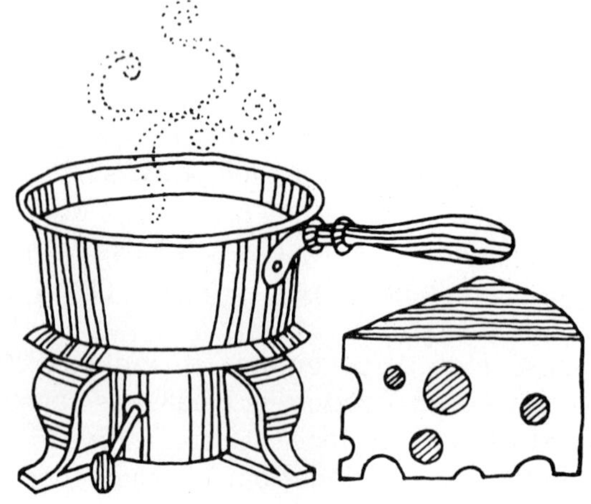

Dairy Products

Milk is an excellent source of calcium, protein, and riboflavin, and contains many other vitamins and minerals as well. It also supplies fat and sugar. Getting enough milk should be a pleasure.

DAIRY DICTIONARY

Dairy products include not only milk and cream, but also products such as butter, cheese, and frozen desserts. The following dictionary defines the dairy products you use, and offers buying and using tips where applicable.

MILK AND CREAM

MILK

Fresh Fluid Whole Milk

Fresh whole milk is usually homogenized and fortified with vitamins. Sometimes it's also fortified with minerals. It must meet the requirements for minimum milkfat content set by the State or municipality where it is sold. The milkfat content is usually about 3.25 percent, the minimum recommended by the Public Health Service "Grade A Pasteurized Milk Ordinance."

All Grade A milk and milk products sold today are pasteurized—heated to kill harmful bacteria. Grade A pasteurized milk, according to the standards recommended in the Pasteurized Milk Ordinance, must come from healthy cows and be produced, pasteurized, and handled under strict sanitary control enforced by State and local milk sanitation officials. Requirements may vary in different localities. The "Grade A" rating designates wholesomeness rather than a level of quality.

Homogenized milk has been treated to reduce the size of the milkfat globules. In homogenized milk, the cream does not separate and the product stays uniform throughout.

In Vitamin D milk, the vitamin D content has been increased to at least 400 U.S.P. units per quart. This is the minimum daily requirement for children, pregnant women, and nursing mothers.

Tips on Fresh Whole Milk:

- Get enough milk. Children under 9 need the equivalent of two to three 8-ounce glasses each day; children 9 to 12 and pregnant women need three or more; teenagers and nursing mothers need four or more; adults need two or more. See the Milk Equivalencies Chart to find out what foods can be substituted for fresh whole milk to meet these requirements.

Chocolate Flavored Milk and Chocolate Flavored Milk Drink

Chocolate flavored milk is made from pasteurized whole milk with sugar and chocolate sirup or cocoa added. In most States, regulations require that to be labeled chocolate flavored milk, the product must be made from whole milk; to be labeled chocolate flavored milk drink, it must be made from skim or partially skimmed milk.

Strawberry, coffee, or maple flavorings are sometimes used for other flavored milk and milk drinks.

Tips on Chocolate Flavored Milk:

- Chocolate flavored milk (or milk drink) can be heated for quick and easy hot chocolate.
- It can also be used in cookie or cake recipes that call for both milk and chocolate or cocoa.

Cultured Buttermilk

Cultured buttermilk is made by adding a lactic acid-producing bacterial culture to fresh pasteurized skim or partially skimmed milk. The resulting buttermilk is much thicker than skim milk with the same nutritive value. It has an acid flavor and it's a good thirst quencher. Almost all commercially marketed buttermilk is cultured. There is, however, a natural type which is a by-product of buttermaking.

Tips on Buttermilk:

•Always keep cultured buttermilk chilled. If allowed to warm, it may separate. If your buttermilk should separate, just stir it.

• Natural buttermilk is not sold in consumer packages. It's dried and used in pancake mixes and bakery products.

Dry Whole Milk

Dry whole milk is pasteurized whole milk with the water removed. It has only limited retail distribution. Where it is distributed, it's used mostly for infant feeding and by persons such as campers who don't have access to fresh milk. Dry whole milk is distributed mostly to manufacturers of chocolate and other candy.

Tip on Dry Whole Milk:

• Because of its fat content, dry whole milk doesn't keep as well as nonfat dry milk. If it is not used soon after the package is opened, it develops an off-flavor.

Nonfat Dry Milk

Nonfat dry milk is made by removing nearly all the fat and water from pasteurized milk. "Instant" nonfat dry milk is made of larger particles which are more easily dissolved in water. Nonfat dry milk has about half the calories of whole milk and the same nutritive value as fresh skim milk. Some instant nonfat dry milk contains added vitamins A and D.

Tips on Nonfat Dry Milk:

• Nonfat dry milk needs no refrigeration and can be stored for several months in a cool dry place. After it is reconstituted, however, it should be refrigerated and handled like fresh milk.

• Nonfat dry milk can be used both as a beverage and in cooking. When using as a beverage, reconstitute it several hours before serving to allow time to chill. Use cool water.

• Nonfat dry milk is very economical. A family of four that has 21 quarts of whole milk delivered each week could save more than $3.00 each week by using nonfat dry milk instead.

Skim Milk

Fresh skim (or nonfat) milk usually has less than 0.5 percent milkfat, the percentage recommended to States under the Pasteurized Milk Ordinance. It is often fortified with vitamins A and D.

Tips on Skim Milk:

• Skim milk contains all the nutrients of whole milk except the fat.

• The flavor and food value of skim milk can be improved by adding a teaspoonful of instant nonfat dry milk to each glass.

Lowfat Milk

Lowfat milk usually has between 0.5 and 2 percent milkfat, depending on State regulations.

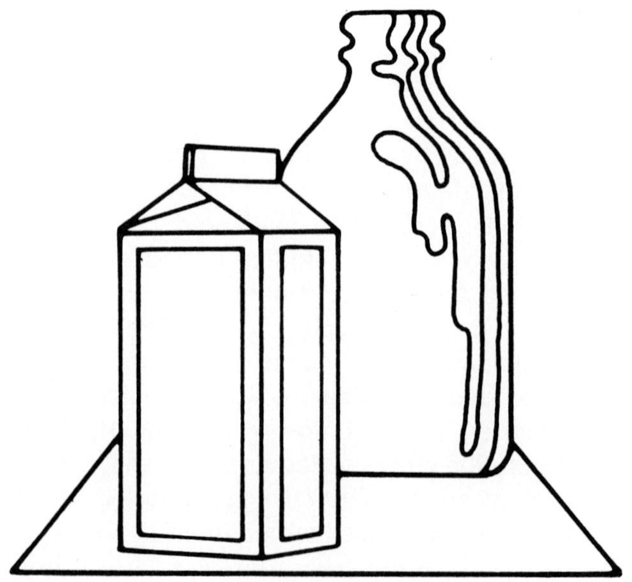

Tips on Lowfat Milk:

- This kind of milk may also be labeled "2%" or "2-10" milk in the store.
- Lowfat milk can be "made" at home by using half whole milk and half skim or instant nonfat dry milk.

Evaporated Milk

This type of milk is prepared by heating homogenized whole milk under a vacuum to remove half of its water, then sealing it in cans and sterilizing it. When mixed with an equal amount of water, its nutritive value is about the same as whole milk. Evaporated skim milk is also available.

Tips on Evaporated Milk:

- Refrigerate after opening.
- Evaporated milk is handy to store and is usually less expensive than fresh whole milk.
- A mixture of water and evaporated milk makes an inexpensive infant formula.
- Evaporated milk, with an equal amount of water added, may replace fresh milk in recipes. (Used full-strength, evaporated milk adds extra nutritive value.) It also can be used in coffee or on hot or cold cereal.

Sweetened Condensed Milk

Sweetened condensed milk is a concentrated milk with at least 40 percent sugar added to help preserve it. This canned milk is prepared by removing about half the water from whole milk. It is often used in candy and dessert recipes.

CREAM

The U.S. Food and Drug Administration has standards of identity for many of the different types of cream if they are shipped in interstate commerce. These standards give minimum milkfat requirements for each type of cream.

Light Cream (Coffee or Table Cream)

Light cream must have at least 18 percent milkfat according to Federal standards of identity and most State standards.

Tip on Light Cream:

- For maximum shelf life, do not return unused cream from a pitcher to its original container. Store it separately in the refrigerator, or better, pour only the amount to be used at one time.

Half-and-Half

Half-and-half is a mixture of milk and cream, homogenized. Under State requirements, it must have between 10 and 12 percent milkfat.

Tips on Half-and-Half:

- Half-and-half can be mixed at home using half homogenized whole milk and half table cream.
- As with light cream, do not return unused half-and-half to its original container.

Light Whipping Cream

Light whipping cream must have at least 30 percent milkfat under Federal standards of identity.

Tip on Light Whipping Cream:

- To whip this kind of cream, have both the bowl and the cream well chilled.

Heavy Whipping Cream

Heavy whipping cream must have at least 36 percent milkfat.

Tips on Heavy Whipping Cream:

- Although heavy whipping cream is more easily whipped than light whipping cream, it is still good to have the cream and the bowl well chilled.
- Don't overwhip heavy cream. It may get grainy.

Sour Cream

Sour cream is made by adding lactic acid bacteria culture to light cream. It is smooth and thick and contains at least 18 percent milkfat.

Tips on Sour Cream:

- Sour cream is sometimes called "salad cream" or "cream dressing" in the supermarket.
- It's great on vegetables or baked potatoes.

Sour Half-and-Half

Sour half-and-half is the same as half-and-half except that a culture is added.

Tip on Sour Half-and-Half:

- This can replace sour cream, if you prefer less fat.

OTHER DAIRY PRODUCTS

BUTTER

Butter is made by churning pasteurized cream. It must have at least 80 percent milkfat, according to Federal law. Salt and coloring may be added. Whipped butter is regular butter that has been whipped for easier spreading. Whipping also increases the volume of butter.

Tips on Butter:

- Unsalted butter may be labeled **sweet butter** or **unsalted butter.** Some people prefer its flavor.
- Nothing beats butter for flavor in baking, or basting turkey or chicken.
- When using whipped butter in place of regular butter in recipes, use ⅓ to ½ more than the recipe calls for if the measurement is by volume (one cup, one half cup, etc.). If the measurement is by weight (¼ pound, ½ pound, etc), then use the same amount.
- Store butter in its original wrapping or container so it won't pick up odor from other foods.
- Butter can be kept frozen for up to a month.
- Butter is sold in 1-pound, ½-pound, and ¼-pound packages. It may be less expensive in the larger packages, and the reserve can be frozen.
- For easier spreading, let butter warm to room temperature. (This isn't necessary for whipped butter.)
- Make butter the first ingredient on sandwiches. It adds moisture and flavor and keeps the filling from soaking into the bread.

CHEESE

Natural cheese is cheese made directly from milk. There are virtually hundreds of varieties of natural cheese.

Process cheese is a blend of natural cheeses which have been shredded, mixed, and heated. This cheese may contain pimentos, fruits, vegetables, or meats.

If the label says "process cheese food," other ingredients such as nonfat dry milk have been mixed in.

"Process cheese spread" has higher moisture content and lower milkfat content than process cheese and cheese food. It's more spreadable.

Process cheese products usually come packed in slices, loaves, and jars.

Cottage cheese is a soft unripened natural

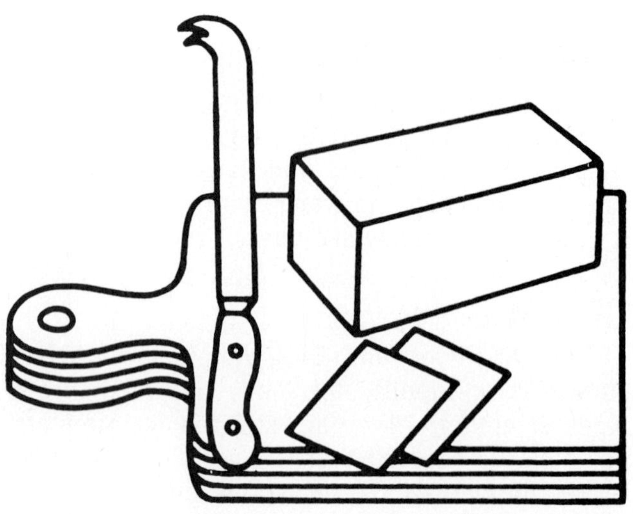

cheese that can be bought in cup-shaped containers or tumblers. It may be bought plain or creamed and in different curd sizes. Federal standards require that it have no more than 80 percent moisture. Creamed cottage cheese contains a minimum of 4 percent fat. Cottage cheese should be used within a few days of purchase.

YOGURT

Yogurt is a custard-like product made by fermenting milk with a special culture. It is usually made from homogenized, pasteurized whole milk, but may be made from skim or partly skimmed milk. Yogurt has the same nutritive value as the milk from which it is made. Often yogurt is sweetened and fruit flavored.

Tips on Yogurt:

Yogurt can be served at any meal or as a snack. A fruit-flavored yogurt is good for breakfast, or for dessert.

- Yogurt should be kept cold, but not frozen. If allowed to warm to room temperature, it might separate slightly.

FROZEN DESSERTS

Frozen desserts include ice cream, ice milk, sherbets, and ices in their various forms (cartoned, cones, popsicles, etc.) If they are shipped in interstate commerce, they must meet U.S. Food and Drug Administration standards of identity. In addition, the U.S. Department of Agriculture has issued recommended standards for the manufacture of frozen desserts. These can be adopted voluntarily by any State. They set minimum quality requirements for the product as well as for its dairy ingredients. The standards also provide criteria for plant sanitation.

Ice Cream

Ice cream is made from cream, milk, sugar, flavorings, and stabilizers. It must contain at least 10 percent milkfat.

Tips on Ice Cream:

- Keep ice cream in a tightly closed carton and try to use it within a week if you store it in your refrigerator frozen food compartment. If you store it in a deep freezer, it will keep for a month or two (so long as the temperature is kept below zero). It should be kept hard frozen to prevent it from becoming "icy."

Ice cream is easier to serve if it is transferred from the frozen food compartment to the refrigerator section a short time before serving—about 10 minutes for a pint and 20 minutes for a half gallon.

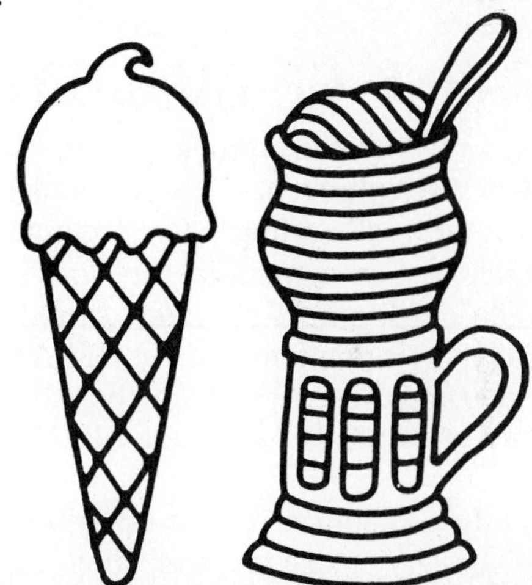

Frozen Custard (French Ice Cream)

Some ice cream has egg yolks added. This may be called frozen custard, French ice cream, or New York ice cream.

Ice Milk

Ice milk is made from milk, stabilizers, sugar, and flavorings. It must contain between 2 and 7 percent milkfat if it is sold in interstate commerce. The soft-serve frozen dessert you can buy at the roadside stand is like ice milk except that it's specially processed to be served soft.

Tip on Ice Milk:

• Treat ice milk as you do ice cream. (See "Tips for Ice Cream.")

Sherbet

Sherbet is made from milk, fruit or fruit juice, stabilizers, and sugars. Sherbet has a high level of sugar—about twice as much as ice cream. It must have 1 to 2 percent milkfat.

Tip on Sherbet:

• Handle sherbet like ice cream. (See "Tips for Ice Cream.")

Water Ice

Water ice is like sherbet except that it contains no milk solids.

MARKS OF QUALITY

To help you buy dairy products, the U.S. Department of Agriculture has quality grades, or a "Quality Approved" rating, for manufactured dairy products. For a manufacturer to use the USDA grade or "Quality Approved" shield on his product labels, his plant must meet USDA's specifications and must operate under the continuous inspection of USDA's Agricultural Marketing Service.

To qualify, a plant must pass an initial survey by a USDA dairy inspector and subsequent inspections made a number of times a year. The inspector checks the plant and surrounding areas to see if they are clean, orderly, soundly constructed, and in good repair. Processing and packaging techniques must be sanitary. Incoming raw products are checked regularly, and the plant must have a laboratory testing program to maintain proper quality control. Even the labels must be approved by USDA before the packages can carry the shield. The labels may carry no conflicting or misleading statements.

During processing, a USDA inspector keeps constant check on all aspects of product quality, right down to a final check on the product in consumer packages. Some brands of the following products bear a USDA shield.

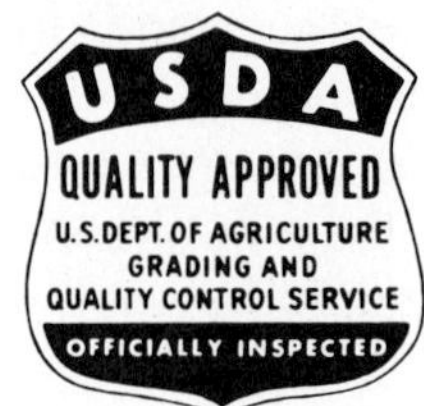

COTTAGE CHEESE AND PASTEURIZED PROCESS CHEESE

Cottage cheese and pasteurized process cheese may bear the USDA "Quality Approved" shield if they are of good quality and are made under USDA supervision.

BUTTER

One way to be assured of high quality butter is to look for the USDA grade shield on the package. The grade shield (AA, A, or B) means that the butter has been tested and graded by experienced government graders. Butter graders judge quality by U.S. grade standards that set forth the requirements for each grade. They also test the keeping quality of butter.

USDA
U.S. GRADE AA WHEN GRADED
PACKED UNDER INSPECTION OF THE U.S. DEPT. OF AGRICULTURE
OFFICIALLY GRADED

U.S. Grade AA Butter:

• has delicate sweet flavor, with a fine highly pleasing aroma;

• is made from high-quality fresh sweet cream;

• has a smooth, creamy texture with good spreadability;

• has salt completely dissolved and blended in just the right amount.

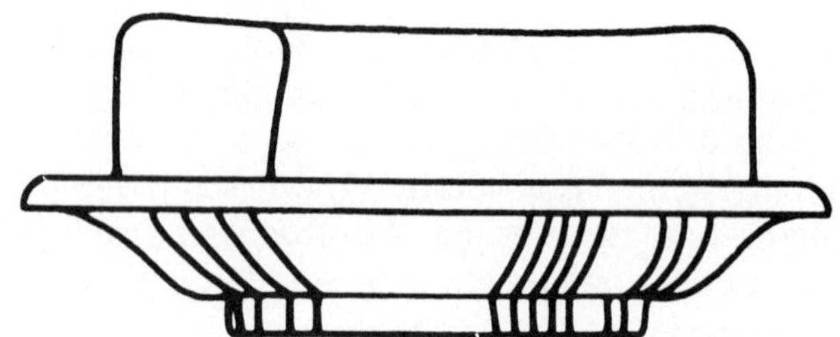

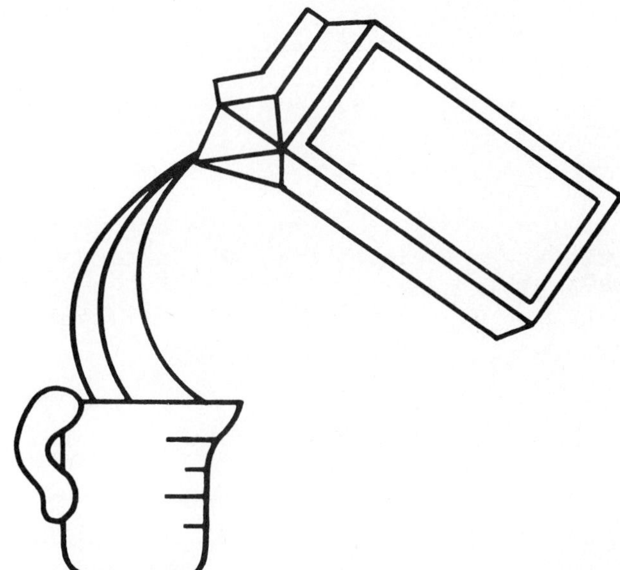

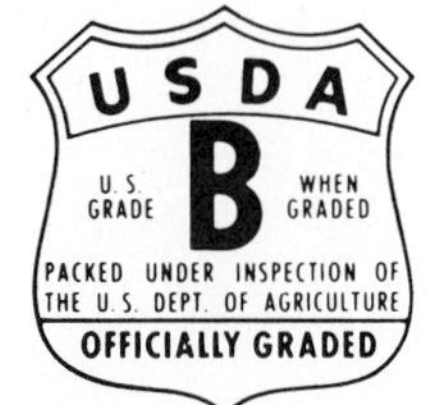

U.S. Grade A Butter

- has a pleasing flavor;
- is made from fresh cream;
- is fairly smooth in texture;
- rates close to the top grade.

USDA
U.S. GRADE B WHEN GRADED
PACKED UNDER INSPECTION OF THE U.S. DEPT. OF AGRICULTURE
OFFICIALLY GRADED

U.S. Grade B Butter:

- may have a slightly acid flavor;
- generally is made from selected sour cream;
- is readily acceptable to many consumers.

CHEDDAR CHEESE

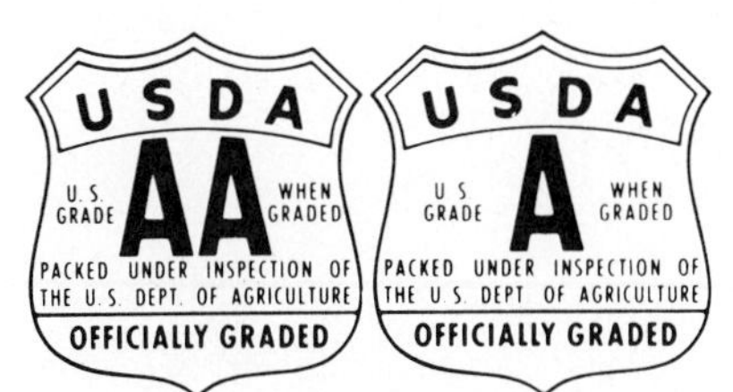

USDA Grades AA and A are used on Cheddar cheese. As with butter, U.S. Grade AA is the best and Grade A is almost as good.

INSTANT NONFAT DRY MILK

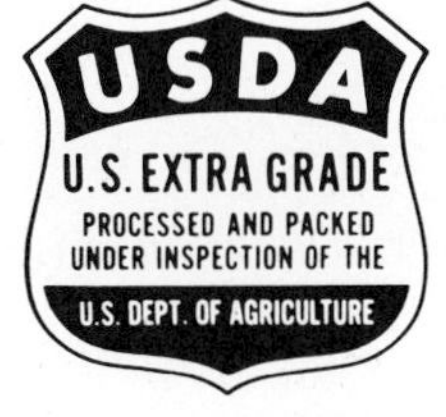

To earn the "U.S. Extra Grade" shield, instant nonfat dry milk must have a sweet and pleasing flavor and a natural color. It must also dissolve immediately when mixed with water.

MILK EQUIVALENCIES

On the basis of the calcium they provide, the following are alternatives for 1 cup of fresh whole milk:

1⅓ ounces natural Cheddar cheese

1½ ounces process Cheddar cheese

1⅓ cups creamed cottage cheese

1 cup cocoa made with milk

1 cup custard

1⅓ cups ice cream

1 cup ice milk, soft serve

¾ cup homemade macaroni and cheese

1 milkshake (made with ⅔ cup milk and ½ cup ice cream)

1 cup oyster stew

⅕ of 15-inch-diameter round pizza, made with cheese topping

1 cup pudding, made with milk and cornstarch

1⅓ cups canned cream soup, prepared with equal volume of milk

1 cup yogurt

HEALTH AND PHYSICAL FITNESS

Part 2

Protect Your Lifeline

Fight High Blood Pressure

WHAT IS BLOOD PRESSURE?

Everyone has blood pressure. It is the amount of force required to circulate the blood through the body. As your heart pumps the blood through the arteries (vessels) the push of this blood on the walls of these vessels determines the amount of pressure.

The arterial walls are elastic and muscular. They stretch and contract to take the ups and downs of blood pressure. Each time the heart contracts, or beats - some 70 to 90 times a minute the blood pressure in the arteries increase; each time the heart relaxes between beats the blood pressure goes down. Thus there is an "upper" and a "lower" blood pressure. Both pressures are measured when you are examined.

These two pressures are known as SYSTOLIC and DIASTOLIC. The systolic - the first and highest reading is the pressure in the arteries when the heart contracts (empties) in order to pump blood through the body. The diastolic - the second and lower reading - is the pressure in the arteries when the heart relaxes and rests between beats in order to fill again with blood. When your pressure is recorded the highest number is written first (systolic) and then the lowest number (diastolic). An example would be 120/80. The 120 is the high or systolic pressure and the 80 is the low or diastolic pressure.

HOW IS BLOOD PRESSURE MEASURED (READ)?

Your blood pressure is measured by using a gauge or machine which consists of several parts: A cuff, a rubber bulb, and a glass mercury tube or dial. The cuff is like a wide band. It is placed snugly around your arm just above your elbow. It has two rubber hoses attached. One of these has a bulb connected at the end and the other is attached to the mercury pressure indicator.

The cuff is inflated with air when the bulb is squeezed. As the cuff gets tighter, it compresses or closes a large artery in your arm. This temporarily shuts off the flow of blood through the artery because the squeeze from the air pressure in the cuff is greater than the push of the blood in the artery. At this point the mercury is high in the glass tube and the numbers alongside the column of mercury show the height of air pressure in the cuff.

A stethoscope is applied to your arm over the compressed artery just below the cuff. The air is then slowly let out. When the air pressure in the cuff is slightly lower than the blood pressure in the artery, blood begins to flow through the artery with each heart beat. This escape of blood in the artery produces a distinct sound or beat which can be heard through the stethoscope. As soon as this sound appears the height of the mercury is noted. The air continues to be let out of the cuff until this distinct beat disappears as the blood is flowing steadily through the artery. At this point, the height of the mercury shows the least amount of pressure in the artery. By matching the sounds with the numbers indicated on the dial your blood pressure is read. The beginning sound is recorded as the systolic pressure and the last beat as the diastolic pressure.

WHAT IS HIGH BLOOD PRESSURE?

There is no blood pressure reading that is normal for everyone. Your age, sex and overall health determine what is "normal" for you. Blood pressure not only varies among people but it varies in the same person at different times. It decreases during sleep and increases during exertion or excitement. There is a normal pressure range from a systolic reading of 90 over a diastolic reading of 60 (90/60) to systolic of 139 over a diastolic of 89 (139/89). When pressure goes above that and remains elevated (up) it becomes the disease called high blood pressure (hypertension).

Over a period of time, the constant impact of hypertension, even when slight, takes its toll in several ways. Complications resulting from untreated hypertension affect vital areas of the body, particularly the heart, brain and kidneys. Here's what happens.

High blood pressure can make your heart pump harder than normal and the arteries become less elastic. After a while the heart may get larger, then weaken and stop pumping effectively. This alone kills about 50, 000 Americans each year. Or hypertension can speed up the progression of atherosclerosis, a kind of hardening of the arteries in which the inner layer of artery walls thickens and deposits of a fatty substance are formed. Atherosclerosis is involved in coronary heart attacks which every year kills some 400, 000 in the United States.

In the eyes, wear and tear on the retina's blood vessels may bring on swelling, tiny hemorrhages, and eventually blindness. Vessels of the kidneys are often hardest hit, and eventually the kidneys are no longer able to perform their task of clearing wastes from the blood stream.

While a stroke (hemorrhage of a brain blood vessel) is not inevitable if you are hypertensive, it is another possible complication and the risk of stroke is much higher than among persons with normal blood pressure. As deposits build up in the arteries they narrow. Thus their capacity to carry blood is reduced or sometimes completely blocked. When this happens to an artery feeding the brain, a stroke is suffered. Some 200, 000 persons die of stroke each year in this Country.

WHAT CAUSES HIGH BLOOD PRESSURE?

The main artery leaving the heart is the aorta. It is the largest of the body's arteries. It can be thought of as a tree trunk, with smaller and smaller arteries branching out from it. The smallest twigs of this arterial tree, the arteriolies, regulates your blood pressure. They control blood pressure by making it hard - or - easy - for the blood to get through to the capillaries those blood vessels which actually deliver the blood and its nutrients to all body tissue.

If the arterioles clamp or close down, the blood cannot easily pass through them to the capillaries. When this happens, the heart must pump harder to push the blood through. This increases the blood pressure in the arteries. The way arterioles control blood pressure is sometimes compared to the way a nozzle regulates water pressure in a hose. If you turn the hose nozzle to make its opening narrower, the pressure of the hose increases. With a larger opening, less pressure is needed to force the water through the hose.

It is known that if for some reason the arterioles clamp down all over the body, blood pressure will rise and stay up, the result is high blood pressure. Why does this happen?

In a small percentage of individuals high blood pressure can be traced to a specific disease or condition which is called Secondary Hypertension. More than 50 conditions that can cause "secondary" hypertension have been described and have been roughly placed in seven groups. Many of these can be specifically cured by surgery or treated by a special medicine. The seven groups are as follows:

1. Kidney Defects: The most common cause for correctable secondary hypertension is obstruction of blood flow to the kidney.

2. Adrenal Cortex Defects: Such defects may cause secretion of excessive quantities of a hormone, usually aldosterone, which causes the body to hang on to too much sodium. This excessive amount of hormone can come from a small non-cancerous tumor or from an inherited defect in hormone formation.

3. Defects of Adrenaline Hormones: Adrenaline chemicals come from nerve endings and from the inner part of the adrenal gland. Some people develop a tumor, called a pheochromocytoma, that produces excessive amounts of the adrenaline compounds. Others have an inherited lack of an enzyme that inactivates adrenaline, or they may be taking a monoamine oxidase inhibitor medicine that may prevent the working of that enzyme. These persons may develop severe high blood pressure from dexedrine sulfate ("bennies") used for weight reduction or from "cold" tablets, or after eating fermented foods such as yellow cheese, or after drinking wine.

4. Other Hormone and Regulation Defects: Certain diseases of the petuitary, thyroid, or parathyroid glands may also cause hypertension.

5. Defects of Blood and Blood Vessels:

6. Nervous System Disorders:

7. Chemicals and Drugs: There are several specific chemicals that can cause high blood pressure. Eating too much salt over a period of years is one example. Heavy metals, such as lead, mercury or cadmium are also known to elevate blood pressure but these usually cause other symptoms that tip off the doctor that they may be the cause.

The most common (approximately 80 to 85%) kind of high blood pressure is Primary Hypertension (also known as Essential Hypertension). This condition does not seem to be related to any other disease. At present its cause is unknown. Researchers are working hard to find its cause, or causes. Although they do not have the final answer yet, they do have a few good leads:

1. Heredity: Experts who studied high blood pressure report that a tendency towards this condition is often inherited. Therefore, individuals whose parents had high blood pressure are more likely to develop it than those whose parents did not. Consequently, if there is someone in your family who has high blood pressure, all members of the family should be checked periodically to see whether their blood pressure is elevated.

2. Body Chemistry: In high blood pressure as in any other disorder something may have gone wrong with the way some body part or organ works. The kidneys or the adrenal glands, located just above the kidneys, may send substances into the blood stream which start a chain of chemical events. These events raise blood pressure. Moreover, the kidney's handling of water, sodium, and other electolytes may often be abnormal in people with primary hypertension. However, current evidence favors the view that abnormalities in the kidneys are probably a result of high blood pressure rather than a cause.

3. Emotions: When you're angry or fearful, your blood pressure goes up, that's natural. But as the American Heart Association points out, some people who are "hyper-reactors" or "pre-hypertensive" tend to develop hypertension in time. Their bodies simply get accustomed to responding to events in daily life as if they were a series of emergencies. As we all know with the complexity of todays living, it is almost impossible to avoid stress. For this reason, individuals with high blood pressure should consistently be on the alert and those on medicine must take it regularly so that the increases in pressure due to emotional tension may be minimized.

4. Smoking: Heavy cigarette smoking is implicated. Nicotine is known to raise blood pressure.

5. Diet: High-fat and high-salt foods may contribute to hypertension. Chemically, fats and salts help accelerate the development of atherosclerosis (narrowing of the large and medium size arteries due to de-

posits forming on the inside walls). This in turn can lead to heart attacks and strokes.

6. The above leads are some of the ones advanced by medical researchers. However, probably the most widely accepted theory is the Mosaic Hypotheses. This is the view which holds that any of a number of factors may be involved in hypertension and its various phases. The factors that launch the hypertension state may not necessarily be responsible for maintaining it, and those of greatest importance at one stage of the disease may not be the main ones during other stages.

It is important to note that Primary Hypertension cannot be cured, but it can be controlled.

A third type of hypertension is -

Severe and Malignant Hypertension.

In a "severe" case of hypertension, readings may jump to 200/115. In the grave, accelerating type (240/140-150), which physicians term "malignant", the course of the disease is steadily downhill as patients get progressively worse.

"Malignant", in this sense, has no relation to cancer. This worst type of hypertension is often fatal unless vigorous treatment has been provided.

WHAT ARE THE SYMPTOMS OF HIGH BLOOD PRESSURE?

In most cases individuals with high blood pressure have no unusual symptoms and only find they have it when it is checked. When a sign does crop up, it may be bothersome headaches now and then, characteristically in the back of the head and upper part of the neck; they seem to strike most acutely when blood pressure is relatively low in the early morning. Other symptoms might be fatigue or insomnia, tension or excessive flushing of the face. It must be noted however, that these symptoms are also common in our general population and may result from other disorders.

It is thus unwise to try and rely on symptoms, or to try to diagnose and treat them yourself. Usually, high blood pressure creates symptoms only after it has produced disease in some organ, such as the kidney or heart and that can take years.

So it is up to you to see your physician or go to a clinic to have your blood pressure checked. If you have some symptoms tell the doctor who will do the detective work for a diagnosis.

ARE SOME GROUPS OF PEOPLE MORE AFFECTED BY HIGH BLOOD PRESSURE?

One out of every ten Americans has high blood pressure. Or twenty-three million people in this Country have high blood pressure that if untreated can take fifteen years off their lives. To put these numbers in to perspective, the number of deaths directly or indirectly linked to high blood pressure exceeds the combined total of all deaths due to accidents in the entire U. S. including highway deaths.

In the above there are groups of individuals who are more affected by high blood pressure. they are as follows:

1. Blacks are more affected by high blood pressure than whites. One in four has the disease. It is the single biggest cause of deaths among blacks. Generally, the hypertensive death rates among blacks in young adult-hood and in middle age are from three to twelve times greater than those among whites.

High blood pressure seems to be different among black people. Developing earlier in their life, it is frequently more severe and results in a greater number of deaths at a younger age - more commonly from stroke than from coronary artery disease.

No one knows why blacks get high blood pressure more often than whites. Some researchers noted that many blacks live in cities and that the stress of city living may lead to high blood pressure, although blacks in the Bahamas and West Indies have a high incident of high blood pressure. Others link high blood pressure to the amount of salt a person eats and point out the high salt content in a normal black diet.

2. High blood pressure can present special problems for women in the following ways:

Statistics have shown that women who have never had high blood pressure may develop it rapidly during pregnancy. Sometimes it disappears after delivery. If it does not, it is important for the woman to follow her doctor's advice and treatment. It has also been noted that as a woman grows older her chances of having high blood pressure increases. Doctors don't know the reason yet, but they think that if a woman is overweight her chances of developing high blood pressure as she grows older increases further.

There is also a link between contraceptives and high blood pressure. Estrogen causes an increase in blood pressure in perhaps one out of five women. It is thus a good idea for a woman to ask her doctor to take her blood pressure before prescribing the pill and then have it checked every six months or so. Special caution should be observed in prescribing oral contraceptives for a woman with a history of high blood pressure and excessive weight gain and edema during menstruation.

3. If high blood pressure runs in your family you are probably in a higher risk group of developing hypertension.

4. Age is also a factor in that most cases of primary hypertension have their onset before the age of 40. When a high level of blood pressure is detected in the 15 - 30 age group, the prognosis is poor unless it's treated as early as possible.

Blood pressure levels increase as we grow older, and systolic hypertension is one of the most familiar findings in the elderly. As blood vessels get less elastic, the systolic hypertension is one of the most familiar findings in the elderly. As blood vessels get less elastic, the systolic pressure may increase, while the diastolic remains relatively normal. But after 65 the rise is not as consistant as it was before that age.

WHAT SHOULD YOU DO IF YOU HAVE HIGH BLOOD PRESSURE?

Your physician can do much to help control your high blood pressure. When it is definitely diagnosed, whether mild or very severe, it's wise to start treatment as soon as it is prescribed.

Whatever the treatment, the dual purpose is not only to keep your blood pressure down but also to avoid possible complications. The following are some of the ways high blood pressure can be treated and/or reduced:

Sometimes hypertension can be controlled without medication. In people who are overweight, losing excess weight may be enough to lower blood pressure. As you are probably aware, obesity imposes an added circulatory burden on your heart, blood volume increases with body weight, and the body's fat reserves must be supplied with blood. Thus the heart of an overweight person is forced to pump more blood through a much larger system of blood vessels. The diet prescribed would limit the amount and type of fat in your food, as well as your total calorie intake. The diet would also reduce the amount of salt. Your doctor may tell you to avoid salty foods and not to add salt at the table or you may have your salt intake limited more severely. The reduction in salt helps the body curb retention of fluids.

Many physicians believe that drug therapy treatment of mild hypertension is warranted, medical opinion is not unanimous on this point. Some specialists recommend that drug therapy for mild cases be reserved for individuals with additional risk factors such as high cholesterol levels, heart or kidney involvement, or a family history of vascular disease. Severe primary hypertension invariable does call for medication and only rarely does it prove impossible to bring a rampaging blood pressure under some control.

Your physician knows how to choose medicines best suited to your needs. However, since people respond to medicine in different ways, you may find your doctor trying out a variety of drugs or a combination of them in order to see what's going to work best for you.

It is good to remember once a program of treatment has been decided upon for you it is usually easier and less complicated than you thought it would be. Even more important is to know that effective control of your blood pressure may be expected to prolong your life and reduce the threat of the dreaded complications: stroke, heart attack, kidney failure and heart failure.

A last comment on this area of therapy is that even though most patients can achieve effective blood pressure control through the now available anti-hypertensive drugs as well as other measures, the goal of developing a uniformly effective, completely non-toxic, inexpensive single drug has of yet not been reached. The research in this area continues.

There are some general health habits which when practiced can help you in your battle with high blood pressure.

REST AND RECREATION:

Having high blood pressure doesn't mean you should make an invalid or even simi-invalid out of yourself. Many individuals whose condition has been adequately controlled carry on their usual activities. Recreation should be a part of your regular schedule. Your physician can recommend the amount and kind of exercise best suited for you.

Getting plenty of sleep is important because blood pressure is lowest during sleep and rises during waking hours. If feasible, make a habit of taking a short nap during the day. Whatever else relaxes you, whether it's watching a movie or TV, reading a book or taking a warm bath, is good therapy.

If you have been overly tense or perhaps worrying too much you can do much to ease this nervous tension by reviewing the way you've been living. Then apply moderation whenever and wherever possible.

TOBACCO:

Research reports on cigarette smoking have been widely published. Thus the dangers to one's health is well known. Its relation to high blood pressure is serious because if you smoke there is a constriction of the blood vessels which boosts your blood pressure.

ALCOHOL

Alcohol consumption does not raise blood pressure, but some people react poorly to it. Therefore, it is wise to discuss the advisability of drinking of alcoholic beverages with your physician. This is especially true if you are taking any kind of medications because alcohol is a drug (depressant) and the mixing of drugs can be dangerous.

The question is always raised as to why some people don't get or keep taking treatment for their high blood pressure. First of all, treatment is not a cure in primary hypertension. A person who has high blood pressure must treat it for the rest of their life. Second, treatment sometimes involves drugs that cause drowsiness and other side effects that may impair daily activities. Unfortunately, this is the treatment people hear about. In eight out of ten cases, changes in diet, moderate exercise, a simple pill, or perhaps abstinence from smoking is enough to control the disease.

Nevertheless, it is often hard for a person who looks and feels fine to adhere to even the simple treatment. Such individuals need constant reminding. Often times they do not see a doctor regularly or when they do the doctor may not have the time and initiative to deal with people whose blood pressure is "a few points above normal" - the "few points" that over the years may eventually kill or cripple.

The regimen and expense of daily pills and regular blood pressure tests often does not seem worth it to an individual who participates in a clinic and finds himself faced with long waiting periods and possibly unfamiliar doctors just to get another prescription for a disease he or she doesn't see or feel. Thus they become one of the "dropouts" hypertensives who are no longer receiving the treatment they so desperately need.

In summary taking your medicine, and carefully adhering to a prescribed diet, may become a lifelong routine. Such a routine will involve seeing your physician regularly to check your blood pressure and the effects of your treatment program. Remember, however, your doctor cannot lower your blood pressure without your full cooperation. So it's really up to you whether or not you want to feel better and possibly live longer.

DIET AND YOUR HYPERTENSION:

Much can be done with diet to assist in the treatment of high blood pressure and its complications. It's best to eat foods with a minimal amount of salt, sugar, and grease (saturated fats) for the following reasons:

1. Saturated fats play a very significant role in the development of cholesterol deposits in the arteries. The formation of these deposits proceeds at a more rapid pace in people who have hypertension than in those with normal blood pressure. A diet low in saturated fats will decrease the rate at which the cholesterol is deposited in the arteries and help avoid the strokes and heart attacks that may result.

A person with hypertension should avoid greases, such as animal fats, shortening, hydrogenated (partially hardened) oils. Oils which are liquid at room temperature (polyunsaturated oils) should be substituted in their place, but even these should be used in moderation. Since the body can convert table sugar into saturated fats, intake of this should also be limited.

2. One of the medications prescribed by your physician may be a diuretic which is a drug that lowers blood pressure in some people with high blood pressure. The diuretic helps the body remove excess salt and water however, it also removes another mineral, potassium, but usually severe potassium loss can be prevented by eating the right foods. Sometimes too much potassium is lost

though, most often in older people, people with kidney disease or people who are taking another medication, Digitalis. For these people, potassium may be given in a pill or liquid form.

The diuretic will do the best possible job for your hypertension if you eat foods that are low in salt and high in potassium. The foods (see list below) are not exotic - you are probably eating them now. Foods very high in salt are also listed. Try to eat less of them. Remember, an important source of salt in anyones diet is the salt they sprinkle on their food at the table. Taste your food, first, before you salt it, and maybe you'll decide not to add any at all.

FOODS FOR YOU TO WATCH FOR:

These foods are good for you. (They have the perfect combination: high in potassium and low in salt.)

Fruits:
- apples
- apricots
- avocados
- bananas**
- cantaloupes
- dates
- grapefruits
- nectarines
- melons (casaba or honeydew)
- prunes
- raisins**
- watermelon
- peaches
- (Dried fruit is usually good, but make sure to read the label on the package.)

Vegetables:
- asparagus
- beans (white, green, snap, etc.)
- brussels sprouts
- cabbage
- cauliflower
- corn on the cob
- lima beans (not frozen)
- mushrooms
- green peppers
- potatoes (sweet, white, raw, baked,** boiled without skin)
- **radishes**
- **squash**
- **tomatoes**

Fruit Juices:
- **apple**
- **grapefruit**
- **prune**
- **orange****

Unsalted nuts (peanuts, pecan halves)

****especially good**

Try to avoid these foods. (They all have a great deal of salt or sodium).

- **buttermilk**
- **cheese (except unsalted cottage or pot)**
- **dried, salted, smoked or canned meats (bacon, ham, bologna, etc.)**
- **canned tuna, or salmon (unless unsalted)**
- **mayonnaise**
- **relished**
- **sauces (soy, Worcestershire, ketchup, chili, bar-b-q)**
- **bottled dressings**
- **crackers (soda and graham)**
- **pretzels**
- **potato chips**
- **packaged snack foods**
- **instant potatoes**
- **commercially prepared desserts**
- **frozen dinners**
- **foods made with baking powder or baking soda**
- **soups (except homemade)**

Foods that might fool you. (These have a great deal of potassium but also have a high salt content.)

- canned tomato juice
- clams, raw
- pickles
- olives
- frozen peas
- frozen lima beans
- celery
- sauerkraut
- most canned vegetables (read the labels)

In order to assist you in using less or no salt the following chart on "Where To Use Herbs" is offered as a cooking guide:

WHERE TO USE HERBS

	BASIL	BAY LEAF	CAYENNE	CELERY SEED	GINGER	MARJORAM	SAGE	THYME	OREGANO	ROSEMARY	TARRAGON	SAVORY
APPETIZERS	tomato juice	tomato juice						tomato juice	guacamole	fruit cup		
SOUP	tomato spinach	stock			cold tomato	spinach onion	cream	borscht vegetable	tomato	pea spinach chicken	consomme chicken mushroom tomato	
MEAT	lamb	roast stew fricassee	beef veal lamb			pot roast lamb veal		meatloaf veal	meatloaf pork lamb	lamb stews	veal	veal
FISH	all			all		broiled baked creamed		all		salmon	broiled	broiled baked
GAME FOWL	duck						poultry game stuffing	poultry	stuffing	stuffing	poultry	chicken
EGGS DAIRY	scramb. eggs		all eggs			cottage cheese omelet scramb.	scramb. eggs cottage cheese	cottage cheese	boiled or poached eggs		all eggs	scramb. eggs
SAUCES GRAVIES	tomato					cream	chicken gravy	tomato	spaghetti sauce spanish		vinegar	
VEGETABLES	tomato peas squash beans	boiled potato carrots tomato		tomato potato	squash	carrots zucchini peas spinach	eggplant tomato	onions carrots beets	tomato	peas spinach	baked potato	rice
SALADS	tomato greens					greens		tomato			greens	greens green-beans

The following items should NOT be used for seasoning on a 1000 mg. Sodium Diet:

- Salt
- Seasoned Salts
- Catsup
- Chili Sauce
- Worcestershire Sauce and other steak sauces
- Pickles
- Relish
- Olives
- Salt Pork
- Ham Hocks
- Soy Sauce
- Accent (monosodium glutamate)
- Bouillon Cubes or Granules
- Cheeses

The following items may be used for seasoning on a 1000 mg. Sodium Diet:

- Tabasco Sauce
- Garlic Powder
- Vinegar
- Pepper and all other dry spices such as curry, paprika, cinnamon, etc.
- All herbs listed on this page
- Special dietetic **Low** Sodium **Catsup** and Chili Sauce. Low Sodium Mustard
- Special dietetic Low Sodium Bouillon Cubes
- Salt Substitutes
- Dry Mustard

SUMMARY

There are an estimated 23 million Americans with hypertension. Less than 15 per cent of these are receiving adequate anti-hypertensive treatment.

Because this condition can be so readily detected and because certain types can be cured and others controlled, it is of utmost importance that persons with high blood pressure learn of their condition and secure proper treatment.

Your doctor is the only one who can decide if you have hypertension that needs to be treated. It is important to know that blood pressure changes in every person - when you are sleeping it is lower, when you are smoking it rises, it is different if you are sitting or standing. People with hypertension have too much blood pressure most of the time - it is almost always elevated.

Your doctor will work with you to find a treatment that is best for your hypertension. During the first few months, this may require changes in the treatment. Remember - you have an important part in this treatment. Call your doctor with any questions or problems.

more potassium-rich foods

Foods	Average Portion	Potassium (in mg.)	Calories
Fruits			
Orange	1 medium	360 mg.	95
Grapefruit	1 cup	380 mg.	75
Banana	1 medium	630 mg.	130
Strawberries	1 cup	270 mg.	55
Avocado	one half	380 mg.	275
Apricots	3 medium	500 mg.	55
Dates	1 cup	1390 mg.	500
Watermelon	one half slice	380 mg.	95
Cantaloupe	one half melon	880 mg.	75
Raisins	1 cup	1150 mg.	425
Prunes	4 large	240 mg.	90
Juices			
Orange	8 oz. glass	440 mg.	105
Grapefruit	8 oz. glass	370 mg.	130
Prune	8 oz. glass	620 mg.	170
Pineapple	8 oz. glass	340 mg.	120
Meats			
Hamburger	3 ounces	290 mg.	310
Beef Chuck	3 ounces	310 mg.	260
Beef Round	3 ounces	340 mg.	200
Rib Roast	3 ounces	290 mg.	270
Turkey	4 ounces	350 mg.	300
Vegetables			
Tomato	1 medium	340 mg.	30
Artichoke	1 medium	210 mg.	30
Brussels sprouts	1 cup	300 mg.	35

What You Should Know About Stroke and Stroke Prevention

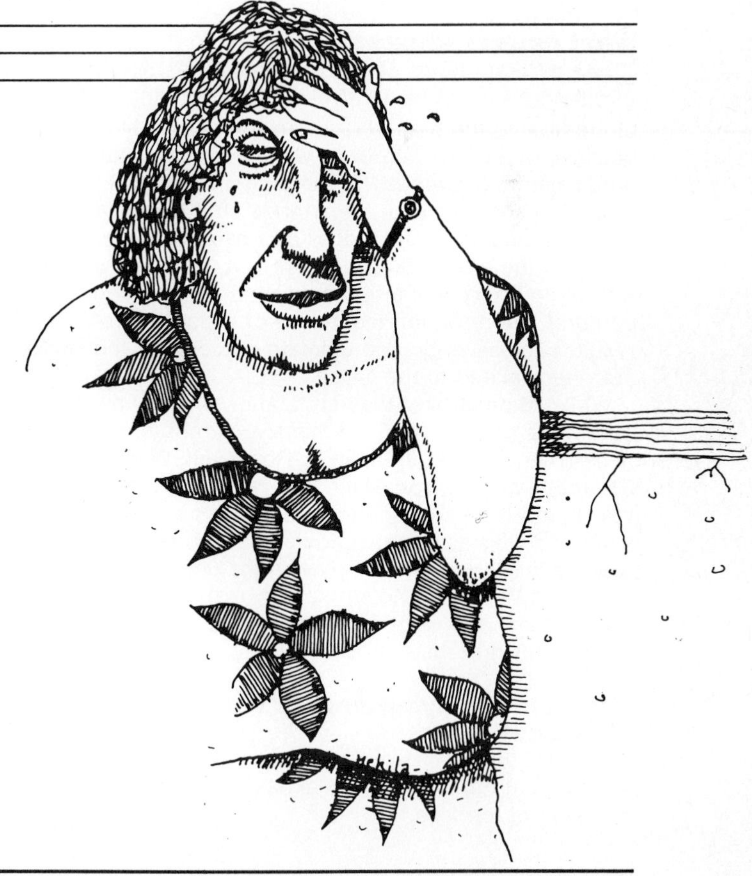

What is a stroke?
A computer with its wires and data or memory bank is an electrical brain. When the computer is deprived of electricity, its "fuel," it falters—which is similar to what happens in a stroke.

The brain, however, is a far more complex and marvelous computer. It not only "computes" the body's functions, actions, and reactions, but also is capable of thinking and creativity. Nerves are the computer-brain's wires, carrying impulses back and forth to the body and the brain, with arteries providing the brain's power by furnishing it with its fuel—blood containing oxygen and glucose. When the brain is deprived of blood because of a disturbance in the circulatory system, a stroke results. The important point to remember is that most strokes affect relatively small areas of the brain.

A stroke, therefore, is a loss of functioning brain tissue, with the loss resulting in a disability. Disability can take many forms, although a typical victim of stroke is one who cannot move the right or left side of the body as easily as the normal side and who may have difficulty speaking (aphasia). When one side of the brain is injured, the opposite side of the body is affected; that is, a stroke on the right side of the brain affects the left side of the body, with the amount of paralysis and the loss of particular function (aphasia, for example) depending on the site of the brain damage and the extent. Different areas of the brain, moreover, control distinct functions, which is why not every stroke will result in aphasia. One stroke, then, is not the same as another stroke. In addition, disabilities may fade. Thus, the sooner therapy is started, the better the chances for recovery.

What causes strokes?

Three different types of disturbances in the brain's circulatory system cause strokes by interfering with blood flow to the brain: (1) An artery may be blocked because of a narrowing of its walls and the buildup of a plug called a *thrombus;* (2) the plug, instead of being stationary, can travel in the arteries until this traveling plug or *embolus* finally lodges at a particular site, blocking the artery; or (3) if there is a weakness in the wall of an artery, the artery may rupture, resulting in a *cerebral hemorrhage.* Regardless of cause, a stroke results. The severity and ultimate outcome of the stroke are often related to the cause.

While some strokes may be fatal or severely disabling, others are not. It's true that massive cerebral hemorrhages killed Franklin D. Roosevelt, Winston Churchill, and Joseph Stalin, the famous trio of World War II and the Yalta Conference. But it's also true that such geniuses as scientist Louis Pasteur, composer George Frederick Handel, playwright Henrik Ibsen, and poet Walt Whitman had strokes (probably due to thromboses) and went on afterwards to gather even more renown in their chosen fields.

What are the symptoms or warning signs of stroke?

There are three major warning symptoms of stroke:

- Transient numbness or weakness of an arm, a leg, or one side of the face.
- Transient visual disturbances or blindness.
- Transient speech disturbances.

These symptoms are caused by TIA, a medical term standing for *transient ischemic attacks,* ischemic meaning lack of sufficient blood.

The symptoms may last only a few seconds or minutes. They may occur only infrequently, or several times a day. In any case, because symptoms go away does not mean they can be ignored. Any of these symptoms must be reported to your physician as soon as they occur in order for him to make a complete examination and evaluation. Most doctors consider a transient ischemic attack to be a medical emergency requiring prompt evaluation and treatment if stroke is to be prevented.

Other warning symptoms or signs of stroke are less specific. They may include a sudden, unexplained headache, unsteadiness or loss of equilibrium, and drowsiness. These symptoms, too, merit prompt attention.

What is the relationship of hardening of the arteries to stroke?

In hardening of the arteries (or athero- or arteriosclerosis), the arterial passageway gradually becomes smaller, decreasing the supply of blood being circulated through some areas and predisposing the artery to plugging. Several factors are associated with hardening of the arteries. One is blood fats. Studies have shown that excessive cholesterol, a fatlike material found in certain foods as well as in the body, and saturated (animal) fats form plaques (deposits or patches) that build up on the walls of the arteries, narrowing them and preventing adequate blood flow. Since a diet high in cholesterol and saturated fat may speed hardening of the arteries, such a diet may also increase the chances of stroke. Other diseases, such as high blood pressure (sometimes called hypertension) and diabetes, also intensify hardening of the arteries. All of these are known as risk factors in stroke.

How does high blood pressure affect stroke?

Blood pressure itself is simply the amount of force required by the heart to pump blood throughout the body. Normal blood pressure is 120/80 or 120 over 80. The number 120 is the systolic pressure—pressure exerted by the contraction of the heart. The number 80 is the diastolic pressure—pressure remaining in the blood vessels when the heart relaxes. Evaluations above 120/80 do not necessarily indicate high blood pressure, because a moderate increase often occurs as a person grows older. Blood pressure above 140/90, however, usually is considered to mean high blood pressure.

When blood pressure is high, the blood exerts too much force when passing through the arteries, and this excess force may weaken an artery in the brain. If blood pressure remains too high, the weakened artery may rupture, causing a cerebral hemorrhage. High blood pressure is also related to the other types of stroke because it accelerates hardening of the arteries. Therefore, it is probably a major cause of stroke.

What makes high blood pressure so dangerous, too, is that at least 20 million Americans are hypertensive—and most of them don't know it. One reason is the common misconception that if you have high blood pressure, you have symptoms, such as headaches. Actually, most people with high blood pressure have no symptoms—which is why it's called a "silent disease." Any personality type can have high blood pressure. High-strung, excitable people may have lower blood pressure than phlegmatic people who always seem calm. The only way you can tell whether you have high blood pressure is to have your blood pressure checked, and have it checked regularly.

At the same time, some factors may predispose a person to high blood pressure. Since high blood pressure tends to run in families, if a close blood relative has or had it, your chances of having it are greater. If you're overweight, you have more of a tendency toward high blood pressure than if you're slimmer. The high incidence of high blood pressure in Blacks and Orientals may be related to a high salt intake. Thus, a person who uses a lot of salt or eats a lot of salty foods may run an increased risk of high blood pressure. However, this relationship is still not proven.

Are stress, environment, and exercise related to stroke?

Stress may accelerate hardening of the arteries and high blood pressure. For example, the stress of visiting a doctor's office may temporarily raise blood pressure, which is why a person with a high reading may need to have it rechecked several times. Stress or tension due to worries about a job, to family problems, or to the pressure of coping with any of the many problems of modern life is another factor. Temporary increases in blood pressure are normal. When stress is maintained over a long period of time with correspondingly elevated blood pressure, however, the blood pressure may remain permanently high, thus enhancing the possibility of a stroke.

The relationship of environment to stroke is less tangible. Reporting of stroke in different countries isn't too reliable. Still, enough comparisons of stroke rates have been made to relate environment, to a certain extent, to stroke. Colder climates, for example, seem to have higher stroke rates than warmer ones. People living in areas where the water is soft have more strokes than people in hard water areas.

As for exercise, studies have shown that people in seder tary jobs suffer the effects of hardening of the arteries moı than people whose work requires moderate exercise.

Is surgery ever used to avoid stroke?

When TIA warning symptoms are caused by a narrowing of a *neck* artery, preventive surgery may be in order. Although generally performed to prevent a stroke, surgery may sometimes be necessary after a stroke to remove a clot. But no surgery in the world can bring back dead brain tissue. The affected part of the brain, our fantastic three-pound computer, is then "out of order."

You should be aware of the warning symptoms of stroke, just as you are aware of symptoms of heart disease and cancer. Any transient weakness in a limb, any transient visual or speech difficulty, or any of the other symptoms require prompt attention.

Can I have a stroke?

Yes. Anyone can have a stroke, but you are less apt to have a stroke the more of the following factors you have in your favor: If you are a woman of childbearing age, not taking birth control pills, and a nonsmoker; if you are lean, close to average weight for your height and age, according to ideal weight tables; if your blood pressure is within normal bounds; if your blood fats are normal; if you follow a lean diet, avoiding foods rich in cholesterol and saturated fats; if you don't smoke or have given up cigarettes; if you avoid undue stress or emotional tension; and if you exercise regularly. Knowing and acting on stroke warning symptoms, moreover, is a big plus in anyone's favor.

How can strokes be prevented?

You and only you can help strike out stroke. If you learn the following "Ten Commandments" and follow them, you have a head start on stroke prevention:

• Promptly report any warning symptoms of stroke to your physician.

• Have your blood pressure checked regularly. If your blood pressure is high, follow your physician's advice for lowering and controlling it and faithfully take any medication prescribed.

• Follow a healthful diet, avoiding cholesterol-rich and saturated-fat foods for which so many Americans have a passion. You can eat wisely and well—eating lean and thinking lean—by keeping to a diet that relies on vegetables, frui' chicken and turkey, fish, skimmed milk, and skimmed milk cheeses. You can omit or keep to a minimum your bacon-and-egg breakfasts, greasy French fries and hamburgers, fatty and salty "junk foods," and rich milk shakes and ice cream.

• Stop smoking and encourage others to stop. Smoking is one of the hardest addictions to break, but it can be done and must be done. This will pay off in better general health, as well as in stroke prevention.

• Exercise regularly and moderately. Exercise can be

valuable in several ways, such as in helping control weight and working off stress. Occasional intense exercise can be dangerous.

- Decrease your salt intake, keeping in mind that practically all foods have their own natural salt content.
- Have regular checkups to detect, prevent, and adequately treat any illness.
- Drink alcohol only in moderation.
- Watch your weight and lose weight, if necessary.
- Avoid stress, relax, and enjoy life.

What can be done about a stroke?

Despite taking all preventive measures, a person can still have a stroke. Treatment is usually begun by the family physician, who may call in specialists—what has been called the stroke team—for assistance. The neurologist assesses the extent of the brain damage, confirms the diagnosis, and recommends treatment. A neurosurgeon may be called upon to evacuate or remove a clot. The physiatrist, a specialist in rehabilitative medicine, may be consulted to initiate a program of progressive therapy to help restore the stroke victim's physical condition. This program, which is vital to a person's recovery from stroke, entails passive and then active exercises. When there are communication and speech difficulties, a speech therapist will be called in. Other specialists and laboratory assistants will perform blood tests, brain scans, and X-rays that may be of help to the family physician and neurologist.

Above all, the positive attitude and the help of family and friends are vital in motivating the stroke victim toward greater effort. The patient's will to practice rehabilitative exercises until recovery is achieved can spell the difference between success and failure.

For additional information on stroke, write to:

National Institute of Neurological and Communicative Disorders and Stroke
National Institutes of Health
Bethesda, Maryland 20205

Council on Stroke
American Heart Association
7320 Greenville Avenue
Dallas, Texas 75231

The National Easter Seal Society for Crippled Children and Adults
2023 West Ogden Avenue
Chicago, Illinois 60612

Stroke Foundation
898 Park Avenue
New York, New York 10021

The Dwight D. Eisenhower Institute for Stroke Research, Inc.
785 Mamaroneck Avenue
White Plains, New York 10605

Heart Attacks

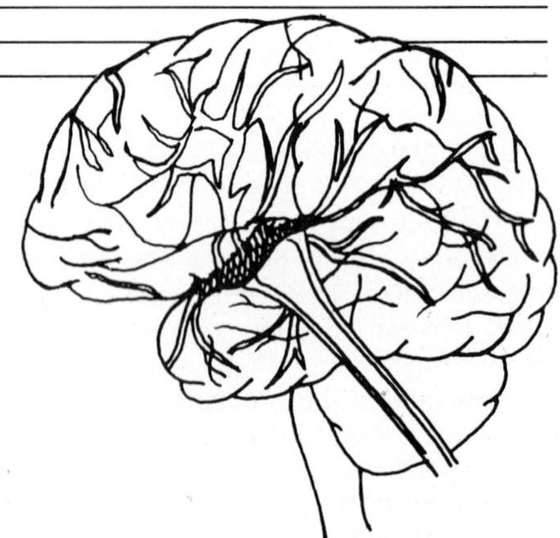

What Causes Heart Attacks?

Arteriosclerosis, which involves both hardening and blocking of the blood vessels, is the major cause of cardiovascular disease and heart attacks.

Arteriosclerosis is a general medical term for a number of diseases of the arteries, including hardening of the arteries. Atherosclerosis is the most common form of arteriosclerosis and it affects primarily the larger arteries of the body. In this condition the inner wall of the artery becomes thickened and irregular with deposits of fatty substances.

Atherosclerosis in any of the vessels of our body develops by a process that is totally silent. At birth our vessels are perfectly smooth and open, but all through our lives fatty deposits or atheromata are slowly developing in the blood vessels. Fortunately, in most of us this develops at a very slow rate and only in certain areas. However, medical evidence shows that more than two-thirds of a coronary artery may be filled with fatty deposits without symptoms. Only when more than two-thirds of the vessel lumen or channel is blocked do we see signs of the occlusion; symptoms may manifest themselves as chest pain called angina pectoris, heart attack, or sudden death.

Arteriosclerosis is responsible for 84 percent of all cardiovascular disease, or using 1975 statistics, for over 850,000 deaths a year. One quarter of these deaths, over 200,000 each year, occur before age 65.

Heart attacks account for nearly two-thirds of all cardiovascular deaths. In 1974 over 665,000 deaths were due to arteriosclerosis of the coronary arteries resulting in heart attack. Another 200,000 deaths were due to strokes caused by arteriosclerosis of the cerebral vessels.

Arteriosclerosis of the coronary arteries, also known as coronary artery disease, is our primary medical problem in terms of mortality, limitation of activity, and social security disability. It also ranks first in number of physician visits and total number of hospital bed days.

How the Heart Works

To understand what happens in a heart attack, we have to think of the heart as a pump. Blood from the body enters the right side of the heart, entering an auricle. From there it enters the right ventricle; it is pumped under relatively low pressure into the lungs where it becomes oxygenated. From the lungs the oxygenated blood goes back to the auricle on the left side of the heart. The left ventricle then pumps the blood under relatively high pressure to the rest of the body, supplying oxygen and nutrients to the tissues.

So, the heart is like a pump, squeezing and forcing blood throughout the body. The most important part of the heart is the muscle, or myocardium. Like all muscles in the body, the myocardium must have oxygen and nutrients in order to do its work. Unfortunately, the myocardium cannot use oxygen and nutrients directly from the blood within the chambers of the heart. Instead, nutrients and oxygen are furnished by blood vessels outside the heart. The two most important vessels are the right and left coronary arteries which begin at the base of the aorta, the large artery that carries blood from the heart to other parts of the body.

When a Heart Attack Occurs

A heart attack happens when these two small coronary vessels are blocked with fatty deposits. If an area of the myocardium is supplied by more than one vessel, the heart muscle may live for a period of time even if one vessel becomes blocked. However, the extent of heart muscle damage occurring with a heart attack depends on which vessel is blocked, whether it is a big or small one, and on the remaining blood supply to that area of the myocardium.

When heart muscle does not get oxygen and nutrients, it dies. The dead heart muscle is surrounded by an area of acute injury and an area of temporary injury or inflammation called an infarction. This injured area causes the heart to lose some of its effectiveness as a pump since there is less muscle to contract and force blood out.

Symptoms

There are many different symptoms of heart attack. Certainly the most common one experienced by most people is chest pain, but even this differs among individuals. Most often the pain is in the midchest; sometimes it radiates to the neck or left shoulder or goes down the left arm. Some describe the pain as vicelike, or constricting, as if a rope were being pulled tightly around the chest. Others describe the feeling as a heavy weight pressing or crushing down on the chest.

Heart attack patients often experience weakness and shortness of breath. A patient acutely ill with a heart attack will appear pale and cold, but may be sweating profusely. Unfortunately, the first sign of disease in the heart and the vessels that supply it could be sudden death. Sudden death is the first sign in about one-quarter of the patients who suffer heart attacks. Also we know that approximately 60 percent of the deaths in patients with chronic heart disease, people who have had one or more heart attacks, occur outside of the hospital.

These deaths occur within two hours of the heart attack, long before most patients can reach or receive effective medical therapy. What does that mean? It tells us that anyone who has a new onset of chest pain or anyone with coronary disease who has sustained pain should seek medical attention as quickly as possible.

What to Do, Where to Go for Help

If you experience any sign of a heart attack, get to a hospital and obtain medical attention as quickly as possible. But what if you or someone in a crowd suddenly collapses? A life-saving technique has been developed to help someone who suffers a heart attack in a shopping center or in the street before an ambulance comes. This new procedure is called cardiopulmonary resuscitation, CPR.

Cardiopulmonary Resuscitation (CPR)

If someone has had a heart attack so severe that heart and breathing has stopped, CPR can keep the person alive until an ambulance and medical treatment is available. CPR is an emergency procedure that is started immediately when cardiac arrest occurs and should only be done by someone thoroughly trained in its use.

CPR involves using a combination of mouth-to-mouth resuscitation and closed chest heart massage to maintain the patient's breathing and circulation. It has been successfully used for some time by doctors and nurses, and it is now recommended that the general public should be trained in its use. More and more people are learning the technique and in some US cities CPR saves almost two hundred lives each year. If you are interested in learning CPR, call your local chapter of the American Heart Association or the American National Red Cross.

Medical Aid

What happens when an ambulance does come, when a paramedic or doctor arrives on the scene? The first task is to try to relax the patient. The anxiety and tension caused by the heart attack produces a vicious cycle as the heart begins to beat more rapidly, and the patient becomes more tense and anxious. Thus, the first effort is to induce relaxation, to calm the patient, and to slow the heart. Doctors handle this primarily by giving an injection of analgesic drugs, usually morphine, which will relieve chest pain, relax the patient, and slow down the heart rate. In addition, oxygen often may be given to keep the heart muscle functioning and to compensate for a deficient blood supply.

Electrocardiograms are used to determine whether a heart attack actually is occurring. By placing sensitive monitors on the chest or arms, the area of heart damage can be located. An electrocardiogram can detect other problems. Is the heart beat regular? Is the heart beat slow? Is the area of heart muscle injury sending out impulses that are causing the heart to beat erratically or ineffectively? Is the heart not beating well at all? Is the heart ventricle beating rapidly and wildly? Is the heart contracting erratically so that the blood is not being pumped very effectively?

Defibrillators

Sometimes after a period of rapid and erratic beating, the heart stops entirely. What happens then? Most ambulances now carry special equipment called defibrillators. The defibrillator allows the paramedic or physician to shock the heart with an electrical impulse which can correct an irregular rhythm or start a heart beating again. Defibrillation is very effective and has saved many, many lives that otherwise would have been lost.

Coronary Care Units

When the ambulance reaches the hospital, the patient is admitted immediately to a coronary care unit where the vital signs (temperature, heart beat, respiration) can be rapidly and effectively monitored.

Blood pressure is measured and blood is drawn for tests that can help diagnose a heart attack as well as rule out other problems like anemia.

In addition, the patient is put on a monitoring system almost immediately, thereby enabling the medical staff to observe and control the heart rate and the blood pressure.

Special Tests

By injecting dye into a vein in the patient's arm, the physician can look at the coronary vessels to determine the extent of the coronary disease. Does this patient have severe three vessel coronary disease, or is just one vessel in trouble? Is the single large vessel that supplies many parts of the heart becoming blocked?

In the coronary care unit, medicines will be given that can relax the patient, relieve pain, or lower the blood pressure, if blood pressure was a factor in provoking the heart attack. Also, there are medicines that can keep the heart beating rhythmically, and slow down or control impulses that may come from dead or dying heart muscle tissue.

Electrical Heart Problems

The heart is normally paced by electrical impulses in certain parts of the heart. If part of the heart's conduction system is injured by disease or heart attack, the heart may stop beating.

Twenty years ago half the attack deaths were from electrical problems in the heart. Today with our ability to monitor electrical impulses, to control them with drugs, to stop and start the heart with defibrillation, and to utilize pacemakers, inhospital electrical causes of death have been virtually eliminated. As a result, the death rate in hospital heart attack patients has been reduced from 35 to 40 percent to about 20 percent. Most of these remaining deaths result from mechanical problems. The heart muscle has been so badly damaged that th heart cannot beat effectively. The result is an insufficient volume of blood pumped out to serve the rest of the body.

Mechanical Heart Problems

Doctors are even making inroads on mechanical problems of the heart. They now have techniques that allow them to measure the amount of heart muscle that has been damaged when a patient sustains a heart attack. Blood tests measure the amount of specific enzymes produced by dying and dead heart muscle and help assess the severity of a heart attack. Physicians can detect and measure specific areas of heart damage and follow the extent of a heart attack by mapping the heart. This is accomplished by placing a special vest with many little electrodes on the patient's chest.

In addition, new techniques allow visualization of the area of heart damage. Certain radioisotopes injected into the patient's vein localize in the heart tissues. Some radioisotopes have an affinity for dead tissue, which allows the doctor to determine the extent of the damaged area. Others collect in healthy heart muscle, thus indicating the boundaries of the injury. The picture produced by this technique looks much like an X-ray of the heart.

The amount of muscle damage occurring during a heart attack is not fixed when the patient enters the coronary care unit; in fact, it is not determined until 24 to 72 hours later. There now are treatments that can decrease the amount of heart muscle damage, such as administering oxygen or lowering the blood pressure. Clinical studies have shown that some antiinflammatory drugs such as hyaluronidase decrease the amount of heart muscle damage. These agents can reduce mechanical failure, which is a second major cause of death.

After a Heart Attack

Rehabilitation for the patient with a heart attack should begin at the time of hospitalization, as the patient enters the coronary care unit. Doctors now realize that many of the symptoms experienced by patients after heart attacks are not due to heart muscle damage but to deconditioning. Laying in a bed for two or three weeks without any activity can make anyone feel weak. Today, patients begin to exercise arm and leg muscles while in the coronary care unit so that on discharge they feel well, their muscles are in shape, and they can return rapidly and progressively to full exercise and activity.

In some patients a heart rhythm abnormality persists because of the area of injury or damage. In these patients pacemakers that can keep the heart beating normally and regularly are implanted on the chest wall.

Coronary Bypass Surgery

Chest pain or angina may persist in some people after a heart attack. Any activity will provoke signs of decreased blood supply, such as pain in the chest or in the left arm. Incapacitating angina can be effectively relieved by bypassing the area of obstruction with a procedure called coronary artery bypass surgery. A large vein called the saphenous vein is removed from the leg. The vein is attached to the aorta well away from the area where coronary vessels originate. The other end of the vein then is connected to a coronary vessel below the obstruction, bypassing the diseased coronary artery. The coronary bypass operation supplies blood to an area of the heart deficient in blood thereby relieving chest pain. Patients who were formerly incapacitated by any activity can be relieved of pain with the bypass procedure.

However, there is no evidence yet that coronary bypass surgery improves the function of the left ventricle or that it makes the heart pump better. In fact, there is some evidence that the bypass surgery may actually decrease efficiency. Clinical investigations are now trying to determine whether bypass surgery improves or impairs heart function and whether it increases a patient's life expectancy.

Coronary bypass surgery now is being done in this country at the rate of 50 to 70 thousand procedures a year at a cost of $12,000 to $18,000 per procedure for a total cost of $1 billion a year. These high figures make it important for us to find out whether we are improving the patient's outlook and prognosis as well as relieving pain.

Heart Transplants

Amazing advances have been made through heart research in the last twenty years. Physicians now have sophisticated resuscitative equipment to treat heart attack victims. Surgeons can stop the heart in order to operate on it and then start it beating again. Doctors can control the rhythm of the heart and improve the well-being of the patient. Heart muscle damage can be decreased and diseased coronary vessels can be bypassed surgically. Surgeons can even transplant irrevocably diseased hearts which have many vessels completely filled with fatty deposits.

Heart transplantation still is an experimental procedure, but in a few large medical centers, the procedure now is remarkably successful. Among patients surviving transplantation, and about 80 percent of the patients do, 60 percent survive for three years and 40 percent for five years. This is remarkable when you consider that patients who are candidates for heart transplantation would not live more than four months without transplanted hearts.

But all of these procedures are expensive and involve patient and family suffering, and none of these new techniques do any good if the patient dies before they can be used. The fact that well over half of our cardiovascular deaths occur outside the hospital and that the first sign of heart disease is sudden death for a quarter of all patients means our attention must focus on an earlier stage of heart disease. The answer is prevention before the problem occurs; if we wait for the first sign of heart attack, we may have waited too long.

Some New Techniques

Cardiovascular physiologists are working on better methods to diagnose heart disease before pain or before any other symptoms occur. For example, using echocardiography, a technique used to chart the oceans, doctors can bounce soundwaves across and through the chest, and can actually see th heart contracting. The thickness of the heart and the heart valves can also be visualized. By monitoring the heart during exercise, doctors can spot potential problems. As exercise causes the heart to work harder, an electrocardiogram can measure the heart's response to the stress.

By injecting a small amount of radioactive material into a vessel in the arm leading to the heart, we can use imaging procedures to see if the heart is contracting normally. In the next ten to fifteen years, new techniques will enable a better view of the coronary arteries themselves and may result in an even better prognosis for the patient.

Prevention

Cardiovascular epidemiologists have given us another clue in the prevention of heart disease. They have defined risk factors, traits, or habits in individuals that suggest increased risk for heart attack long before the heart attack occurs.

Smoking

An important risk factor is smoking. The more a person smokes, the more likely he or she is to sustain a heart attack. Someone who smokes two packs of cigarettes a day is more at risk than a person smoking one pack a day, who is more at risk than the occasional smoker. Certainly all these people are more likely to have a heart attack than a person who does not smoke cigarettes at all.

Blood Pressure

Similarly, high blood pressure is a risk factor for heart attack. Not only does elevated blood pressure make any heart condition worse because the heart must work harder, but high blood pressure accelerates the process of atherosclerosis. If the blood pressure is high, atherosclerosis will occur earlier and develop more rapidly. Just as with smoking, blood pressure is a graded risk; if a person has a normal blood pressure 120/80, which goes up slightly to 150/95— a level not even considered high blood pressure by some physicians—that person is already two and one-half times more likely to have an attack than someone with normal blood pressure.

Cholesterol

High blood cholesterol is a risk factor. The higher the level of cholesterol in the blood, the more likely a subject is to sustain a heart attack. Based on animal studies, it's safe to recommend that if your cholesterol is elevated, try to lower it by dietary changes. Eat lean meat, poultry and fish, vegetable oils and cottage cheese; use foods that are lower in cholesterol and relatively high in unsaturated fats; avoid foods that are high in cholesterol, high in saturated fats, such as milk, butter, cream, eggs, and fatty meats.

Animal studies show that when cholesterol intake in animals is lowered, it not only prevents progression of atherosclerosis, but lessens existent atherosclerosis in the coronary vessel. Although the National Heart, Lung, and Blood Institute doesn't have the evidence in man yet, the Institute is investing about $40 million dollars each year in controlled clinical trials to determine if intervention on factors such as cholesterol will decrease risk.

Diabetes

Another risk factor is diabetes, or high blood sugar. Many of us recognize diabetes as a severe and significant problem and think only about high blood sugars. But the fact is that over 80 percent of patients with both juvenile and adult-onset diabetes die of some form of premature cardiovascular disease, usually heart attack.

Life Style

A sedentary way of life is another factor contributing to heart disease. The less active you are, especially in adult years, the more likely you are to sustain a heart attack. Excess weight is especially interesting because it is not a direct risk factor. Excess weight does not directly affect the heart itself, but it is important because it intensifies other risk factors. Excess weight will make blood pressure, cholesterol, and blood sugar levels higher.

Other Factors

There are other risk factors, such as family history, that we cannot control. If your mother or father or a sibling died of heart problems or a heart attack before age 65, you are at increased risk. Obviously, you cannot preselect a parent or a sibling to control this factor, nor can you control age and sex. Of course, the older you get, the more likely you are to sustain a coronary event. A male is more likely to have a heart attack especially before age 65. So, family history, male sex and age are risk factors that we cannot do anything about. But the other factors—excess weight, high cholesterol, high blood pressure, smoking, and diabetes—we certainly can change. Each factor alone increases the risk of sustaining a heart attack by two to three times. A person with two risk factors is at about three to four times the risk of someone who has none. With three risk factors, your risk increases by some eight- to ten-fold; and so it increases the more risk factors you have. Since there are factors we cannot control, like family history, it makes sense to avoid risks that we can control.

A major question that we face today is whether we can affect heart attack risk by intervening on these risk factors. With some, there is no question. Studies show that if you stop smoking, your risk of heart disease will decrease. If you lower your blood pressure, the risk of stroke, heart failure, and renal failure decreases. But we don't know conclusively about some of the other factors.

What does this mean? There is no doubt that within one year of stopping smoking, the increased risk from smoking will be only 10 percent greater than normal. The rest of the 10 percent increased risk will disappear over the next five to ten years. It has been estimated that if Americans stop smoking, the number of heart attack deaths in this country would be reduced by 150,000 a year! By controlling blood pressure we know we can prevent heart failure and stroke. Just knowing whether your blood pressure is elevated isn't enough. Do something about it. Take prescribed medicines to keep the blood pressure normal, decrease the amount of salt in your diet, and decrease your weight, if necessary.

Exercise

Regular daily exercise and avoidance, when possible, of severe stress can be protective. See your doctor before starting any exercise programs. If you don't exercise now, begin to exercise gradually and regularly until the heart muscle and the other muscles in the body are in relatively good condition. Any exercise such as walking on a regular basis will help prevent heart attack.

The problem with all of this advice is that it may not be what you like to hear. It is difficult to change life styles and to change life-long eating habits. It may be easy to stop smoking, but it is difficult to remain a non-smoker. Today behavioral scientists are working with biomedical scientists to find ways to help people help themselves. They are attempting to develop techniques to help persuade people to seek health-maintaining behavior and to avoid harmful behavior, such as eating habits, and smoking.

Smoking, Tobacco, and Health

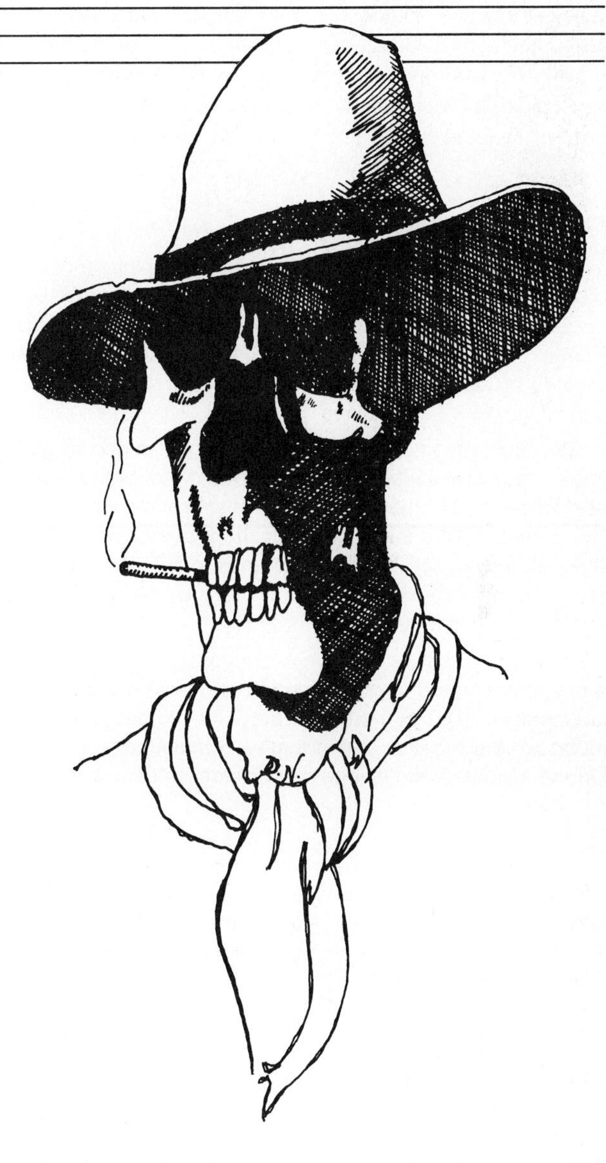

Until the early years of the 20th century, cigarettes were neither a major article of consumption nor an important threat to health. Tobacco was used mainly for chewing and for cigars, pipe tobacco, and snuff. As late as 1915 only about 18 billion cigarettes were consumed annually in this country, as contrasted with more than 600 billion today. Cigarettes in large numbers are thus new in our society, newer than the automobile, the airplane, and the telephone.

The sudden and enormous increase in the use of cigarettes came about for a variety of reasons. Cigarettes are inexpensive, less offensive than other forms of tobacco to many people, and they are the only form of tobacco which has been taken up by large numbers of women. Cigarette smoke is milder than smoke from pipes and cigars, making inhalation easier and thus nicotine absorption into the bloodstream more rapid. Once a person begins smoking cigarettes, addiction in the sense of building up a physiological and psychological dependence can quickly follow. Cigarettes are also profitable to manufacture, which has permitted the cigarette companies over the years to invest immense sums in advertising and promotion.

Scientists became suspicious of cigarettes as a cause of illness and death as early as the 1930's. One reason for their concern was an increase in the incidence of lung cancer. In 1930, less than 3,000 Americans were listed as dying from this disease; by the 1950's this number had grown to 18,000 annually. Estimates put the number of deaths for 1980 at over 100,000.

Since the 1930's, the medical evidence has grown stronger, until cigarette smoking can now be identified as a major cause of death and disability in this country and throughout the world. Cigarettes are linked as a cause of not only lung and other cancers, but heart disease, chronic lung disease, and other diseases as well.

As measured by per capita consumption and the percent of people smoking, cigarette use in the United States reached its peak in the early 1960's. Since then, in the face of the medical evidence, consumption has turned down. What has been called the "epidemic" of cigarette smoking—the chief preventable cause of death in our society—may now be waning.

Who smokes cigarettes

In 1978 about 37 percent of adult men and 31 percent of adult women smoked cigarettes. This is the lowest figure for men since the Government began collecting this information in 1955. Women started smoking later as a group than men. Their smoking increased from 1955 to 1965, but since then, their percentage, too, has declined.

Education, income, and race all play a role in deciding who smokes and who does not. College graduates of both sexes are less likely to smoke than those with less education. Among men the percentage of smokers generally drops as income increases, although for women the opposite tends to be true. Blacks are more apt to be smokers than whites, but on the average they smoke fewer cigarettes.

Among different occupational categories, the highest percentages of male smokers are found either in blue collar jobs or unemployed. The highest percentage of women smokers is found among those in administrative or managerial positions. On the average, men smoke more cigarettes than women.

Teenage smokers

In 1979, about 13 percent of females and about 11 percent of males under 19 were regular cigarette smokers. This is a marked decline from smoking levels in 1974, when the percentages were 15 and 16.

Teenage smoking patterns are similar in many ways to those of adults. There are fewer smokers among adolescents coming from higher socioeconomic backgrounds, and among adolescents taking college preparatory courses in high school.

One of the strongest influences on teenage smoking is the family's smoking habits. Adolescents are more likely to start smoking if one or both of their parents or an older brother or sister smokes. The chances are greater that an adolescent will smoke if one or both parents do not live at home.

In recent years, health education programs presenting the health hazards of smoking have become more common in the nation's schools. These programs, sometimes part of a community-wide antismoking effort, are believed to have helped reduce the percentage of teenage smokers.

Former smokers

One of the interesting things about cigarette smoking is that most people who smoke cigarettes would rather not. About 60 percent of the more than 50 million current adult smokers have tried to stop smoking at one time or other, 27 percent within any given year. Young smokers—those 17 to 24—more frequently reported efforts to stop than did their elders.

A variety of services to help break the habit—counseling, cessation programs, and related efforts—are offered in almost every community through voluntary health agencies, church groups, and private organizations. However, most people who quit smoking do it on their own, without guidance or direction.

Giving up cigarettes is difficult for many people, but for those who succeed the effort pays off: ten years after quitting, their death rates for lung cancer and other smoking related diseases return approximately to those of nonsmokers.

Cigarette smoking and health

The effect of cigarette smoking on the Nation's health is tragic, and staggering in its significance. Although new and further information continues to appear, here is what is already known about these effects:

- Cigarette smoking is clearly the largest preventable cause of illness and premature death in the United States.

- Cigarette smoking is a causal factor for coronary heart disease and arteriosclerotic peripheral vascular disease; cancer of the lung, larynx, oral cavity and esophagus; and chronic bronchitis and emphysema.

- Cigarette smoking is associated with cancer of the urinary bladder and pancreas, and ulcer disease. Maternal cigarette smoking is associated with retarded fetal growth, an increased risk for spontaneous abortion and prenatal death, and slight impairment of growth and development during early childhood.

• Cigarette smoking acts synergistically with oral contraceptives to enhance the probability of coronary and some cerebrovascular disease; with alcohol to increase the risk of cancer of the larynx, oral cavity, and esophagus; with asbestos and some other occupationally encountered substances to increase the likelihood of cancer of the lung; and with other risk factors to enhance cardiovascular risk.

• Involuntary or passive inhalation of cigarette smoke can precipitate or exacerbate symptoms of existing disease states such as asthma and cardiovascular and respiratory diseases. Pneumonia and bronchitis are more common in the first year of life in children whose parents smoke.

• Smoking is the major identifiable cause of fire deaths and injuries as well as contributor to residential accidental injuries and deaths.

Because of cigarette smoking's significant threat to health, virtually every important organization involved with the Nation's health has joined the antismoking campaign. These include the American Cancer Society, the American Heart Association, the American Lung Association, the American Medical Association, and the American Public Health Association. More than 30 of these groups have joined together to form the National Interagency Council on Smoking and Health to coordinate their drive against cigarette smoking.

Outside the United States, many nations have forceful antismoking campaigns. The World Health Organization also has taken a strong position against smoking, calling for a total prohibition, world-wide, of all forms of tobacco promotion.

Death rates for smokers

A major part of the medical evidence establishing cigarette smoking as a cause of death and disease has been derived from a series of seven prospective population studies undertaken in this country and Great Britain. Large numbers of people were enrolled in these studies, information on their smoking habits was obtained, and their life histories were then followed over the ensuing years.

Typical of these studies, and the largest, was one conducted by E. Cuyler Hammond of the American Cancer Society. Volunteers of the Society in 1959 enlisted a total of 1,078,894 adult men and women for this study; collected detailed questionnaires from them on their living styles, habits, and environment; and then, year after year, kept tab on them, obtaining new information from those who were still living and deaths certificates for those who had died.

When data from this and from the other large studies are analyzed, it is found that for every 10 non-smokers who die, there are 17 deaths among cigarette smokers. The differences are most striking for lung cancer and heart disease, but are present in the case of other cancers and other diseases as well. Death rates are related to how many cigarettes are smoked daily, how long a person has smoked, and the tar and nicotine levels of the product which is used. Male smokers of "high" tar cigarettes had nearly twice the death rates of non-smoking males. For women who smoked "high" tar cigarettes the risk was one and a half times as great.

Life expectancy

One of the prospective studies of the 1950's was made by H. F. Dorn, using the life histories of 293,958 U.S. veterans holding government life insurance. An analysis of this monumental study has been made by E. Rogot, showing the effect of cigarette smoking on life expectancy. As might be expected, cigarette smokers can look forward to fewer years of life than nonsmokers.

The effect of smoking is most serious for those who smoke two or more packs a day. Those who begin smoking as adolescents also have expectancies much shorter than those who begin smoking later. Those who smoke pipes and cigars have life expectancies only slightly less than those who do not smoke, but their mortality rates from cancer of the oral cavity, larynx, pharynx, and esophagus are elevated over those of nonsmokers.

Cigarette smoking and disease

Cigarette smoking causes a number of serious illnesses, chief of which are lung cancer, heart disease, and chronic lung disease. Over the years, death rates from lung cancer and chronic lung disease have soared. For heart disease there was a continuous increase until the late 1960's, when death rates began turning down.

Age-adjusted data are used in this section because they make it possible to compare the rates for different years without the bias introduced by the increasing age of the nation's population. In 1950, adjusted death rates for lung cancer for white males stood at about 19 per 100,000. For the next 20 years they rose year after year, reaching 52 per 100,000 by 1975. Since then the increase has continued at a slower rate. For women, death rates did not begin a dramatic rise until after 1960. In the next 17 years, however, they increased by 220 percent. By 1983, the rate for lung cancer is expected to surpass that of breast cancer, currently the chief cause of cancer deaths for women.

Deaths from emphysema and chronic obstructive lung disease have increased proportionately even more than deaths from lung cancer, rising from a rate of 8.2 per 100,000 in 1960 to 31.3 in 1977 for white males, and from a rate of 1.0 to 9.8 for white females. Changes in methods of reporting deaths from these causes, however, may have somewhat overstated this rapid rate of increase.

Smoking and disabilities

For some years, the National Center for Health Statistics has gathered data on cigarette smokers through its Health Interview Survey. This survey has consistently found that smokers are ill more often than nonsmokers, lose more days from work, and are more apt to suffer from chronic conditions which limit activity.

From these surveys it has been calculated that each year an excess of nearly 150 million days in bed are due to the extra amounts of illness experienced by cigarette smokers who also have more than 81 million "excess" days of job absenteeism.

A number of attempts have been made to calculate the economic costs of smoking. One such estimate, made for the year 1976, placed direct health care costs at $8 billion and losses in productivity at $19 billion. Because of inflation and escalating health care costs, current estimates would be much higher.

Cigarette smoking and pregnancy

There is increasing evidence that smoking during pregnancy has a significant and adverse effect upon the well-being of the fetus, the health of the newborn baby, and the baby's future development.

Babies born to women who smoke during pregnancy are on the average 200 grams (7 ounces) lighter than babies born to comparable women who do not smoke. Smoking during pregnancy increases the risk of spontaneous abortion, fetal death, and neonatal death in otherwise normal infants. Children of smoking mothers may have measurable deficiencies in physical growth and in intellectual and emotional development independent of other known risk factors.

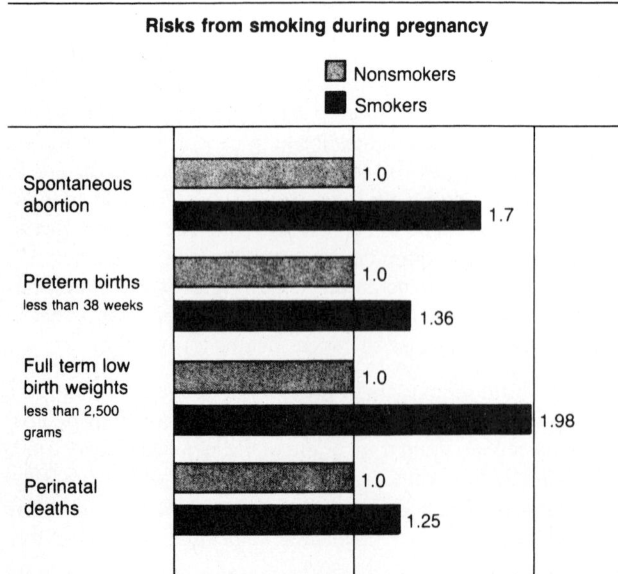

Cigarette smoking and occupational hazards

Scientists today generally agree that workers who smoke have a greater risk of developing occupational respiratory diseases than nonsmoking workers; coal miner's "Black Lung" is one well-known example. This appears to be due to the fact that toxic agents found in the workplace may cause a biological effect additive to that caused by cigarette smoking.

Smoking may also act synergistically with toxic agents found in the workplace to cause a much more profound effect than that anticipated simply from the separate influences of the agent and smoking. This is seen in the case of uranium miners where it has been shown that miners who never smoked had nearly the same rate of respiratory cancer as men in the general population who smoked two or more packs of cigarettes a day. The rates for those uranium miners who were smokers, however, were over six times higher than for the other two groups and about 40 times higher than for other non-smoking white males. One study has shown that for asbestos workers who smoke, the lung cancer risk is eight times that of all other smokers and 92 times the risk of nonsmokers not exposed to asbestos.

There are two other ways in which smoking in the work environment can be unhealthy. Toxic agents in the workplace can contaminate cigarettes and other tobacco products and enter the body orally. Smoking may transform workplace chemicals into more harmful substances. Certain toxic agents in tobacco products or produced by smoking itself may also be present in the work environment, thereby increasing exposure.

The changing cigarette

Cigarettes have changed markedly in the past 25 years. In 1950, when reports linking cigarettes to lung cancer were first appearing, less than one percent of cigarettes were filter tipped. By 1964, at the time of the first Surgeon General's Report, the market share of filter-tipped cigarettes had reached 60 percent. By 1977, that percentage had increased to 90.

The tar and nicotine yields have also changed dramatically. (Tar and nicotine are the particulates in cigarette smoke, as contrasted to gases.) At the same time, the average tar delivery of cigarettes dropped from 37, to 23, to 17 mg.

The decline in tar and nicotine yields has been made possible by changes in cigarette production technology, such as the development of tobacco sheet reconstitution, improvements in cigarette filtration and cigarette paper, and increased use of plant stems and other tobacco portions formerly regarded as waste.

In the past five years, the market share of cigarettes with tar deliveries of 15 mg. or less has increased rapidly and now exceeds 30 percent. Some brands have less than 10 mg., 5 mg., and some even less than 1 mg. Changes in nicotine and tar yields of cigarettes by brand are monitored by the Federal Trade Commission, which publishes the results several times a year.

The FTC plans to monitor carbon monoxide levels in the near future.

In 1966, the Public Health Service found that "the preponderance of scientific evidence strongly suggests that the lower the tar and nicotine content of a cigarette, the less harmful will be the effect." Smokers should understand, however, that in shifting to a less hazardous cigarette, they should be careful not to begin smoking more cigarettes or inhaling more deeply. Most of all, they must realize that even the lowest yield of cigarettes presents health hazards very much higher than would be encountered if they smoked no cigarettes at all. The single most effective way to reduce the hazards associated with smoking is to quit.

Passive smoking

Passive or involuntary smoking occurs when nonsmokers find themselves in a smoke-filled atmosphere—elevators, for example, or restaurants, or automobiles. For most people, passive smoking is a discomfort and nuisance, and for some people—those with lung and heart problems—it can aggravate the symptoms of these diseases.

Now researchers have also shown that for one aspect of pulmonary function healthy nonsmokers who work in a smoky environment show the same amount of abnormality as do smokers who inhale between 1 and 10 cigarettes a day.

More than 30 states and hundreds of local communities now have ordinances restricting smoking in public places, and the number is growing every day. Many restaurants divide their premises into smoking and nonsmoking rooms, a practice practically unheard of a decade ago. Increasingly, employers, including the Federal Government, are setting up regulations which limit smoking in certain work, dining, and recreation areas.

Public attitudes about smoking are also changing. According to a 1978 survey conducted for the Tobacco Institute, "there has been an appreciable rise in the number of people who favor segregation of public smokers to separate sections or facilities." Now even a majority of smokers support such bans in restaurants, theaters, indoor sports arenas, public meeting halls, as well as in airplanes and other forms of public transportation.

Common Ailments: The Mentionables

The Common Cold: What's It All About?

Had you lived in ancient Rome you might have sipped a broth made by soaking *Allium cepa*—an onion—in warm water to relieve the symptoms of the common cold. In Colonial America you might have relied on pennyroyal tea or an herbal concoction made from such unmedicinal sounding plants as sage, hyssop, yarrow, black cohosh, buckthorn, coltsfoot, goldenseal, cubeb berries, or bloodroot. In grandma's time, lemon and honey was a favorite recipe, or in extreme cases, a hot toddy laced with rum—the amount of same determined by the age of the drinker.

Today, if you don't have an old reliable remedy to fall back on, you might take one of literally thousands of drug preparations available without prescription. Some contain ingredients reminiscent of the folk medicine of the past; others are formulated with sophisticated chemical creations. Old or new, simple or sophisticated, many of these remedies will relieve some of the familiar cold symptoms, such as stopped up nose or hacking cough. But not a single one of these products —on which Americans spend an estimated $700 million a year—will prevent, cure, or even shorten the course of the common cold.

So says a panel of non-Government experts called on by the Food and Drug Administration to study the safety, the effectiveness, and the accuracy of claims made on the labels of some 50,000 cold, cough, allergy, bronchodilator, and antiasthmatic drug products. The Panel is one of 17 set up by FDA to examine all nonprescription (over-the-counter) drugs marketed in the United States. The project, mandated by a 1962 Amendment to the Food, Drug, and Cosmetic Act which requires that all drugs be proven effective as well as safe, will eventually lead to the establishment of definitive Federal standards on ingredients and labeling claims for all nonprescription drugs.

The Panel indicated that proper use of nonprescription drugs can be effective in relieving cough, sinus congestion, runny nose, and some of the other symptoms associated with colds, allergies, or asthma. But it made clear that although these products may relieve certain symptoms they will not cure any of these conditions.

One aspect of this class of drugs that concerned the Panel was the relative scarcity of single ingredient products on the market. This is particularly true of cough and cold remedies. The common cold is a self-limiting respiratory infection which lasts from one to two weeks. It usually starts with a sore throat, sneezing, and runny nose. After a few days, the nose becomes stopped up and the eyes become watery. This is followed by lethargy, aches and pains, and sometimes a slight fever. Cough may occur in the later stages. Often these symptoms do not occur at the same time. Nevertheless, almost 90 percent of cough and cold products now available contain a combination of ingredients intended to relieve a number of different symptoms. Only 46 of the cough-cold products examined by the Panel consisted of a single active ingredient.

The Panel said it is "irrational" to take a combination product unless each of the ingredients is necessary to relieve the patient's particular symptoms. Moreover, because of variations in individual reactions to drugs, fixed combinations may not be suitable for some people. Consumers need more choice in selecting the appropriate treatment for their symptoms, the Panel said, and recommended that all products to relieve cough and cold symptoms be available in both combination and single ingredient form.

Another area of concern to the Panel was labeling of cough and cold remedies. It said labeling for these products "tends to be overly complicated, vague, unsupported by scientific evidence, and in some cases is misleading." The Panel called for an end to claims that one product is superior to, stronger than, or contains more active ingredients than another, or is specially formulated. Under its recommendations such words as "cold medicine," "cold formula," or "for the relief of colds" would be banned from drug labels. Such claims suggest the product will cure a cold when the best it can do is relieve specific symptoms, the Panel said.

One of the most distressing symptoms of the common cold is sore throat and many nonprescription drug products claim to provide relief for this condition. The Panel noted, however, that sore throat can be due to serious infection which should not be treated by self-medication. It recommended that labels on cough, cold, and related nonprescription drugs limit their claimed effectiveness to "minor throat irritation" and should advise consumers to seek medical help for serious throat problems.

Timed-release formulations also came under the scrutiny of the Panel, which found advantages and disadvantages in this type of medication. Obviously it is easier to take one pill instead of two or three, especially at night, but variations in the rate at which ingredients dissolve, differences in individual patient reactions, and even technical flaws in the manufacturing process could mean that the medicine could be absorbed erratically or possibly all at one time. Therefore, the Panel recommended that a four-year period be allowed for industry, in cooperation with FDA, to develop suitable tests for the standardization of all nonprescription timed-release cough-cold products and that timed-release claims not be permitted in labeling unless such claims have been documented.

Children represent a substantial portion of the consumers of cough and cold remedies, yet the Panel found that information on how these drugs affect them is "negligible or non-existent." Lacking definitive data, the Panel sought the advice of a group of experts on pediatric drug therapy in developing the following recommendations: the dose for children 6 through 11 should be half the adult dose, and for youngsters 2 through 5 it should be one quarter of the adult dose. Asthma and cough preparations should not be taken by children 2 through 5 in any amount except on the advice of a physician. Any product with an alcoholic content of more than 10 percent is not for children under 6, the Panel noted.

As for infants up to 2 years of age, the Panel said dosage should be determined by a physician and the labels on nonprescription drug products should make this clear. Labels should never carry a recommended dose for these youngsters unless the product has been demonstrated to be safe for them, the Panel said.

In reviewing all cough, cold, allergy, bronchodilator, and antiasthmatic nonprescription drug products the Panel studied some 90 active ingredients. These ingredients were divided into six groups (plus a miscellaneous classification):

- Antitussives, which are cough suppressants.
- Expectorants, which help bring up mucus in the bronchial airways so it can be spit out.
- Bronchodilators, which enlarge the bronchial passages to make it easier for people with asthma to breathe.
- Anticholingerics, which dry up watery secretions in the nose and eyes.
- Nasal decongestants, which open up the nasal passages.
- Antihistamines, a class of drugs used to relieve sneezing and watery

and itchy eyes, usually associated with hay fever and other allergies.

Each ingredient reviewed was placed in one of three categories:

Category I—Generally recognized as safe and effective and not mislabeled.

Category II—Not generally recognized as safe and effective or mislabeled. Such ingredients and labeling claims will be removed from products within six months after FDA issues its final regulations on cough, cold, and related nonprescription drug products.

Category III—Available data insufficient to permit final classification at this time. The Panel recommended that when FDA issues its final regulations ingredients which are placed in this category be permitted to remain on the market for a stipulated length of time if the manufacturer immediately begins tests to satisfy the questions raised by the Panel.

Lucky is the cold victim who has only an annoying tickle in his throat or a stuffed up nose. The Panel found 7 ingredients both safe and effective as cough suppressants and 14 safe and effective as nasal decongestants. It recommended that one of the cough suppressants and four of the nasal decongestants which are now available only in dosage levels that require a prescription be made available in effective dosages that could be sold without a prescription.

Not so fortunate is the person whose cough is "nonproductive" or produces only small amounts of thick phlegm. Not one ingredient was found by the Panel to be both safe and effective as an expectorant. Similarly, the Panel found no ingredient both safe and effective as an anticholinergic to relieve watery secretions of nose and eyes.

Fifteen of the ingredients it studied are not generally recognized as safe and effective for cough and cold symptoms and should be taken off the market, the Panel reported. One of these is chloroform, which FDA already has banned on the basis of evidence that high doses of it can cause cancer in test animals.

A wide array of ingredients—52 all told—were considered by the Panel to be safe enough, but further proof of their effectiveness in relieving coughs and stuffy or runny noses is needed. Scattered throughout the list are names reminiscent of patent medicines and home remedies of the past: cod liver oil, slippery elm, cedar leaf oil, horehound, camphor, menthol, and oil from the koala bear's favorite food, eucalyptus leaves. The Panel recommended that these familiar remedies—as well as the rest of the 52 whose effectiveness it questioned—be permitted to stay on the market for from three to five years if their manufacturers undertake further tests to prove (or disprove) that grandma knew all along what was good for the sniffles.

As for the labeling of cough and cold remedies, the Panel recommended that cough suppressants be permitted to claim that they temporarily relieve coughs due to minor throat irritation, help to quiet the cough reflex, or help you to cough less. But the labels should warn that a cough may be a sign of a serious condition and that a physician should be consulted if it lasts more than one week. The Panel also recommended a warning that cough suppressants should not be used for persistent or chronic coughs such as occur with smoking, asthma, and emphysema. In such cases, coughing is essential to rid the bronchial airways of mucus and other secretions. Cough suppressant labels should not refer to lung or chest conditions, the Panel said, nor should they claim the product works by soothing the bronchial passages.

The Panel said expectorant labels should be permitted to claim that the product helps loosen phlegm or rid passageways of bothersome mucus, but it called for a warning against taking expectorants for persistent chronic cough associated with smoking, asthma, or emphysema, or if there are excessive secretions, except under the advice of a physician.

Labels on anticholinergics could promise temporary relief of watery nasal discharge, or runny nose or watering of the eyes, but such statements as "clears nasal passages" or

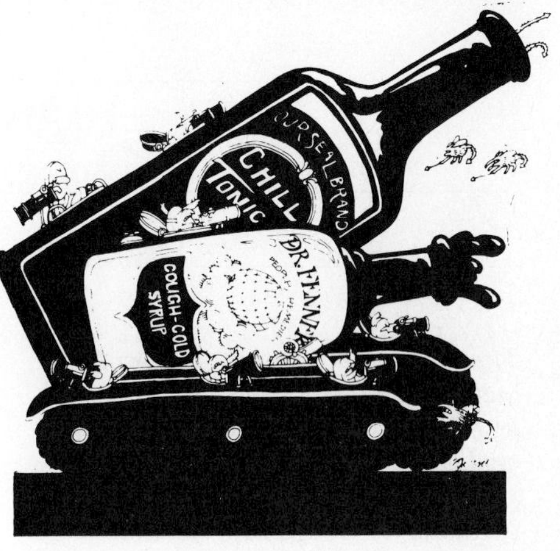

"opens airways" would not be permitted under the Panel's recommendations. Consumers should be warned not to take anticholinergics if they have asthma, glaucoma, or difficulty in urinating, the Panel said.

Topical nasal decongestants, those applied directly in the nose, present a unique problem. These drugs help clear up stuffy noses by constricting enlarged blood vessels in the nasal passage. But if they are used for too long a time or too frequently they can have the opposite effect and actually enlarge, rather than constrict, the blood vessels. Therefore, the Panel recommended that labeling for topical nasal decongestants warn users not to exceed the recommended dosage and not to use the product for more than three days. If symptoms persist, a physician should be consulted.

Oral nasal decongestant labels should warn against use by persons suffering from high blood pressure, heart disease, diabetes, or thyroid disease unless under a physician's supervision, the Panel said. And products that are inhaled should carry the caution statement: "Not for use by mouth."

Approximately six million people in this country suffer from asthma, a disease marked by wheezing, coughing, and shortness of breath. Many of these people use nonprescription drugs called bronchodilators to help them breathe more easily, and the Panel found 12 ingredients safe and effective for this purpose. Five of them are now available only by prescription, and the

Ingredients: What The Panel Said

Cough and Cold Remedies

The Panel found that the following ingredients are generally recognized as safe and effective and are not mislabeled.

Antitussives (cough suppressants)

Codeine
Codeine alkaloid
Codeine phosphate
Codeine sulfate
Dextromethorphan
Dextromethorphan hydrobromide
Diphenhydramine hydrochloride

Expectorants

none

Anticholinergics

none

Nasal Decongestants

Ephedrine
Ephedrine hydrochloride
Ephedrine sulfate
Racephedrine hydrochloride
Naphazoline hydrochloride (topical)
Oxymetazoline hydrochloride (topical)
Phenylephrine hydrochloride (oral/topical)
Phenylpropanolamine bitartrate (oral)
Phenylpropanolamine hydrochloride (oral)
Phenylpropanolamine maleate (oral)
Propylhexedrine (inhalant)
Pseudoephedrine hydrochloride (oral)
Pseudoephedrine sulfate (oral)
Xylometazoline hydrochloride (topical)

The Panel found that the following ingredients are not generally recognized as safe and effective or are mislabeled.

Antitussives

Hydrocodone bitartrate
Oil of turpentine (oral)

Expectorants

Antimony potassium tartrate
Calcium iodide anhydrous
Chloroform
Hydriodic acid syrup
Iodized lime
Ipecac fluidextract
Potassium iodide
Squill
Squill extract
Oil of Turpentine (oral)

Anticholinergics

Atropa belladonna (inhalant)
Datura stramonia (inhalant)

Nasal Decongestants

Mustard oil (topical/inhalant)
Oil of turpentine (oral)

The Panel found that there are insufficient data to classify the following ingredients. It recommended that these ingredients be permitted to remain on the market from three to five years if their manufacturers immediately begin tests to answer the questions raised by the Panel.

Antitussives

Beechwood creosote
Camphor (topical/inhalant)
Caramiphen edisylate
Carbetapentane citrate
Cod liver oil
Elm bark
Ethylmorphine hydrochloride
Eucalyptol/eucalyptus oil (topical/inhalant)
Horehound (horehound fluidextract)
Menthol/peppermint oil (topical/inhalant)
Noscapine (noscapine hydrochloride)
Oil of turpentine (topical/inhalant)
Thymol

Nasal Decongestants

Beechwood creosote
Bornyl acetate (topical)
Camphor (topical/inhalant)
Cedar leaf oil (topical)
1-Desoxyephedrine (inhalant)
Ephedrine (oral)
Ephedrine hydrochloride (oral)
Ephedrine sulfate (oral)
Eucalyptol/eucalyptus oil (topical/inhalant)
Menthol/peppermint oil (topical/inhalant)
Oil of turpentine (topical/inhalant)
Phenylpropanolamine hydrochloride (topical)
Racephedrine hydrochloride (oral)
Thenyldiamine hydrochloride (topical)
Thymol (inhalant)

The Panel found that there are insufficient data to classify the following ingredients. It recommended that these ingredients be permitted to remain on the market from three to five years if their manufacturers immediately begin tests to answer the questions raised by the Panel.

Anticholinergics

Atropine sulfate (oral)
Atropine (d, dl hyoscyamine) (oral)
Scopolamine (l-hyoscine) (oral)

Expectorants

Ammonium chloride
Beechwood creosote
Camphor (topical/inhalant)
Compound tincture of benzoin (inhalant)
Compound white pine syrup
Eucalyptol/eucalyptus oil (topical/inhalant)
Extract white pine compound
Glyceryl guaiacolate
Ipecac syrup
Menthol/peppermint oil (topical/inhalant)
Oil of turpentine (topical/inhalant)
Pine tar
Potassium guaiacol sulfonate
Sodium citrate
Syrup of pine tar
Terpin hydrate
Terpin hydrate elixir
Tincture of benzoin (inhalant)
Tolu
Tolu balsam
Tolu balsam tincture
White pine

Allergy Remedies (Antihistamines)

The Panel found that the following ingredients are generally recognized as safe and effective and are not mislabeled.

Brompheniramine maleate
Chlorpheniramine maleate
Diphenhydramine hydrochloride
Doxylamine succinate
Methapyrilene fumarate
Methapyrilene hydrochloride
Phenindamine tartrate
Pheniramine maleate
Promethazine hydrochloride
Pyrilamine maleate
Thonzylamine hydrochloride

The Panel found that there are insufficient data to classify the following ingredients. It recommended that they be permitted to remain on the market for three years if their manufacturers immediately begin tests to answer the questions raised by the Panel.

Phenyltoloxamine citrate
Thenyldiamine hydrochloride (oral)

Asthma Remedies (bronchodilators)

The Panel found that the following ingredients are generally recognized as safe and effective and are not mislabeled.

Ephedrine
Ephedrine hydrochloride
Ephedrine sulfate
Racephedrine hydrochloride
Epinephrine
Epinephrine bitartrate
Epinephrine hydrochloride (racemic)
Methoxyphenamine hydrochloride
Aminophylline
Theophylline anhydrous
Theophylline calcium salicylate
Theophylline sodium glycinate

The Panel found that the following ingredients are not generally recognized as safe and effective or are mislabeled.

Atropa belladonna (inhalant)
Datura stramonia (inhalant)
Pseudoephedrine hydrochloride
Pseudoephedrine sulfate

The Panel found that there are insufficient data to classify the following ingredient. It recommended that this ingredient be permitted to remain on the market for three years if the manufacturer immediately begins tests to answer the questions raised by the Panel.

Euphorbia pilulifera

Panel proposed that they be changed to over-the-counter status.

Because of variations in the way the body breaks down the two types of drugs most often used as bronchodilators, the Panel said that single ingredient preparations are more effective and safer to use than combination products. It also cautioned that bronchodilators not be used unless a diagnosis of asthma has been made and then only under the supervision of a physician.

Because bronchodilators can have adverse effects on the circulatory and central nervous systems, they should carry labels warning against use by persons suffering from high blood pressure, heart disease, thyroid disease, diabetes, or enlargement of the prostate gland, the Panel said. Labeling also should warn the patient to seek help immediately if symptoms are not relieved in one hour—or in 20 minutes in the case of epinephrine taken by an inhaler. Bronchodilator labels should be permitted to claim that the product is for temporary relief or symptomatic control of bronchial asthma only, the Panel recommended, and there should be no suggestion that it will relieve hay fever or have any effect on the nasal passages.

The relief of hay fever should be left to the antihistamines, the Panel indicated. It found 11 ingredients from this class of drugs safe and effective for relieving the symptoms of allergic rhinitis, or hay fever. Four of these are now available by prescription only, but the Panel recommended that they be approved for over-the-counter sale. Two antihistamines now used in hay fever products require further testing to demonstrate their effectiveness, the Panel said.

Although the antihistamines that are rated safe and effective have a low potential for side effects and toxicity

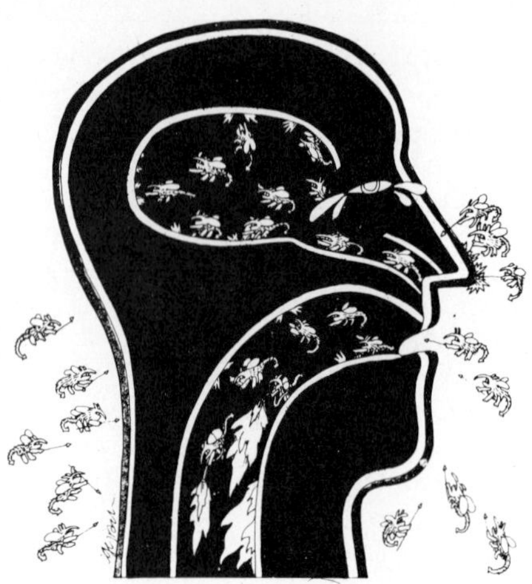

they may cause drowsiness, the Panel pointed out, and it said this fact should be made known on the label. The label also should include a warning against use by people who have asthma, glaucoma, or enlargement of the prostate gland unless under the supervision of a physician.

Acceptable label claims for antihistamines should be that they are for the temporary relief of runny nose, sneezing, itching of the nose or throat, and itchy and watery eyes as may occur in hay fever, but not for the relief of nasal symptoms, such as stopped up nose, nasal stuffiness, or clogged up nose, the Panel said.

Although antihistamines are widely used in the treatment of common cold symptoms, the Panel said there is "little valid evidence" that they are effective for this purpose. Claims that antihistamines are effective for cold symptoms have not been substantiated by appropriate research, the Panel said, but it suggested ways these drugs could be tested for the common cold.

The Panel considered a number of ingredients which are often found in nonprescription cough-cold preparations, but which did not fall within the six main categories under review. These included antihistamines added to some cough-cold products as a sedative or sleep-aid. The Panel questioned the validity of adding an antihistamine to a cough or cold preparation for purposes of sedation and recommended that such combinations be taken off the market. But it said combinations that include an antihistamine "for restful sleep" should be allowed to stay on the market provided testing is undertaken by the manufacturer to establish an effective dose.

The Panel also called for additional testing to prove the effectiveness of caffeine, which is added to some cough-cold products to counteract drowsiness caused by other ingredients, and phenobarbital, which is added to offset central nervous system stimulants.

Label claims that vitamins, when used either alone or in combination with other products, are effective as cold preventives or cures should not be permitted, the Panel said. But the Panel added that manufacturers should be allowed to use vitamin C in cold products for three years if they want to do so in an effort to demonstrate its effectiveness, on the condition that no claims are made about the vitamin C.

The Panel's report, the culmination of three years of study of this vast array of ingredients, is advisory in nature. It was published by FDA in the FEDERAL REGISTER to allow for comments from industry and consumers. After reviewing the report and the comments on it, FDA will issue final standards for acceptable ingredients and labeling claims for cough, cold, and related over-the-counter drug products. As a result, many products may have to be reformulated and labeling and advertising claims may have to be changed, a process which may take place even before the final standards are issued.

Canker Sores and Fever Blisters

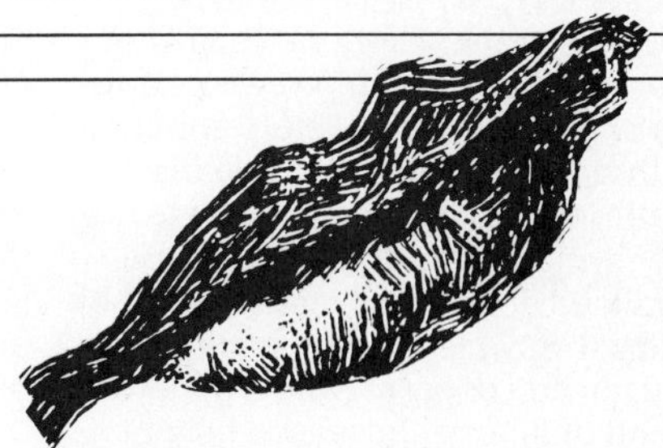

Canker Sores

The medical term for canker sore is aphthous stomatitis or aphthous ulcer.

What are they? Aphthous ulcers are recurring sores that form inside the mouth. They often appear in groups. By and large, canker sores are limited to the movable areas of the lining of the mouth - the inside of the cheeks and lips, the tongue or soft palate. On occasion, they may appear in areas covered with mucous membrane other than the mouth, such as the genital organs.

The ulcer looks like a small punched-out hole. It begins under the surface of the lining of the mouth and works outward through several layers of tissue. The ulcer is round or oval, grayish-white, and has a bright red edge. There may be some swelling in nearby tissue.

The diameter of the sore may vary from about an eighth of an inch to an inch and a quarter, although in early attacks the sores are rarely large. The first incident is usually between ages 10 and 20 years of age, but these ulcers may appear as early as 2 years.

Fever is rare, and there is no association of canker sores with any other disease. Most people feel pain before the ulcer is visible.

Recurrences are variable. Some people do not have more than one or two canker sores a year. Others may experience a continuous series of mouth ulcerations.

Who is susceptible? Women are twice as likely to have canker sores as men. About 90 percent of the time similar oral ulcers are found in other members of the family. The disease is not contagious, however, and it is not limited to any climate or economic condition.

What causes canker sores? The cause is not known. The ulcers tend to appear when the patient has experienced some physical or emotional stress. A study of a group of university students revealed that canker sores were more likely to develop during examination periods than during vacations. They may flare up occasionally with the onset of menstruation.

Anything that affects the lining of the mouth can aggravate canker sores. It may be physical damage such as cuts, bruises, or the scratch of a nut or a stray toothbrush bristle, or it may be a chemical effect. Food allergies may be a factor. Some people avoid chocolates, walnuts, or acid foods such as citrus fruit, tomatoes, and condiments such as vinegar because they seem to trigger the ulcers.

Treatment. If left untreated, canker sores usually heal in 10 to 14 days. In severe cases they may leave scars. Neither vitamins nor special foods help the condition unless a specific deficiency exists. Although physical and emotional stress are serious factors in the intensity and severity of the disease, tranquilizers seem to give little relief.

Fortunately, canker sores can be helped by other treatment. A clinical study done at NIDR has shown that holding a suspension of tetracycline in the mouth for a few minutes and then swallowing it is helpful. The antibiotic reduces healing time, the size of the ulcer, and the pain. Repetition of this treatment several times a day usually relieves pain in 24 hours. It reduces the bacteria sufficiently to allow complete healing in 5 to 7 days. Although the antibiotic promotes healing, the U.S. Food and Drug Administration has warned doctors that administering tetracyclines to pregnant women and young children can cause permanent staining of the teeth. In very severe chronic cases in which ulcers appear elsewhere than in the mouth, topical applications of steriods may be prescribed. Both treatments require a prescription and care of a doctor.

Fever Blisters

Fever blisters or cold sores, recurrent sores on the lips and areas around the mouth, are caused by the herpes simplex virus.

Primary Herpes. The first attack, known as primary herpes, usually occurs in children under 5 years of age. One or more whitish blisters appear in the throat or elsewhere inside the mouth. Most of the time, there are no other symptoms and the blisters go unnoticed. In more severe cases, the child will have fever, which may rise to 101 or 102 degrees, and a general feeling of illness. Increased flow of saliva, bad breath, loss of appetite, and swollen neck glands may also appear as signs and symptoms.

The blisters tend to run together and then collapse, leaving a flat sore. The sore may be red around the edges and is covered with yellowish material.

Since viruses cannot live long outside the body, the infection must come directly from other persons. Herpes simplex is very contagious. The risk of infection is high in such places as nurseries, orphanages, and overcrowded urban areas.

Recurrent labial herpes. Following the initial attack, the individual carries the virus in a latent form and may suffer repeated secondary infections around the nose and lips. These blisters are called cold sores or fever blisters and may appear at intervals from once a month to once a year.

Generally, a blister, surrounded by swelling, appears at the outside edge of the lip, but it may also form at the edge of the nostril. In a day or two the blister breaks and the ulcer becomes covered with a yellow crust. In many people, these blisters form in the same spot, time after time.

Fever blisters often appear when physical resistance is low as a result of illness (particularly upper respiratory infections), fever, or trauma. The blisters also are associated with periods of emotional stress or with overexposure to the sun's ultraviolet rays.

Treatment. Although most viral infections cannot be cured by drugs, the blisters should not be neglected. Local anesthetics can relieve pain, antibiotics can control secondary bacterial infections when they occur, and ointments can soften crusts. Steroid hormone ointments are not recommended because they lessen defenses against infections and may spread the virus. Dye-light therapy and smallpox vaccinations, too, are of questionable value and are potentially harmful. Fortunately, the sores seldom scar and usually heal by themselves in a week or two. Unless the individual is badly malnourished, vitamins do not appear to help.

What Can I Do About My Aching Head?

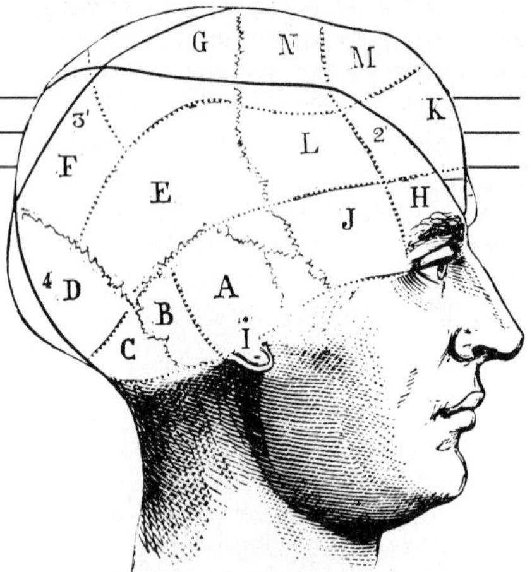

"But what can I do about my headache?"

Why Is Headache Important?

Headache is important because it can be the symptom—perhaps the first warning—of a serious condition which probably could be controlled if detected early. Only your doctor is professionaly trained to find out what your headache symptom points to. If you remove the warning, day after day, with a painkiller, you may pass the point of easy control.

Some of the headaches which are alarm signals for prompt and thorough medical checkup are:

Sudden, severe headache "out of the blue."
Headache associated with fever.
Headache associated with convulsions.
Headache accompanied by confusion or lessening of consciousness.

Headache following a blow on the head.
Headache associated with local pain in the eye, ear, or elsewhere.
Headache beginning in the older person, previously free of headache.
Recurring headache in children.
Headache at any age which interferes with normal living.
Daily or frequent headache.

Learning to handle your headache, like learning to swim, generally requires a teacher. Books and pamphlets help, but expert human direction is invaluable.

For emergency treatment of headache, you are wise to try a prompt fresh-air test. This will get you away from any deadly, odorless, carbon monoxide poisoning from a downdraft in heating equipment or a leaky car exhaust. Or it takes you temporarily out of a crowded, overexciting, tension-creating gathering.

A few first-aid measures may be practiced while waiting for an appointment with your doctor:

Rest, quiet, and fresh air end many common headaches. Lying down and possibly falling asleep may help.

Muscle-contraction (tension) headaches are often handled with massage of the neck muscles, heat from an electric pad, or a shower or warm tub soak, plus any medicine the doctor has prescribed.

Because hunger may be overlooked as a headache source, make a habit of regular meals. If a meal must be postponed for more than an hour, a snack helps you avoid a hunger headache.

An aspirin tablet and a cup of coffee tide some persons over till their date with the doctor. Unless a physician so orders, no more than two aspirin tablets should be taken at one time. **More aspirin at one time, according to present evidence, has little or no effect on pain relief. Too much aspirin may be harmful, even causing headache.**

See your family doctor first

For professional treatment of headache, think first of your family doctor. If he finds it necessary, he will refer you to an appropriate specialist, for example, an internist or a neurologist. Glaucoma, a potentially blinding eye disease, may cause headache. For this reason, all patients with unexplained headache should have a thorough ophthalmologic examination and appropriate treatment if necessary. If your doctor suspects dental trouble as a headache cause, follow his advice about seeing your dentist and having any needed dental work done.

Some hospitals have a special "headache unit" to which your family doctor may refer you for study.

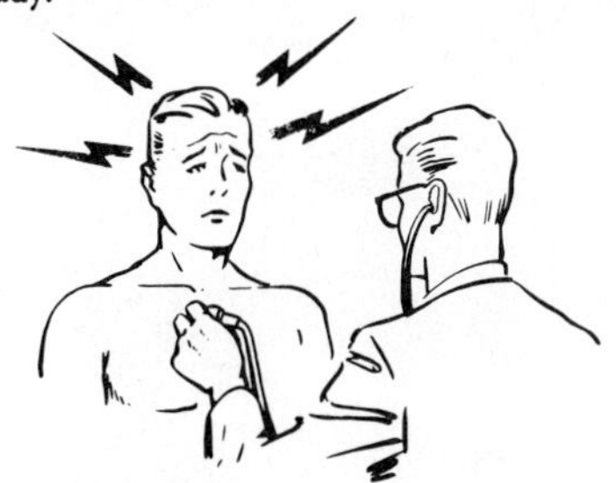

How Do Doctors Classify Headache?

Headache may be classified as acute or chronic. The acute headache occurs suddenly and occasionally, and is an unpleasant part of many illnesses.

Chronic headaches recur more or less frequently, and doctors classify them in various ways, such as:

1. Migraine and other headaches due to blood vessel (vascular) changes.

Headaches associated with blood vessel (vascular) changes include the painful *migraine* or "sick" headache and its variations, such as *cluster headache* which is also called *histamine headache.*

Research proved that a temporary narrowing (vasoconstriction) of the blood vessels in the head marks the early painless stage of migraine. Perhaps 8 to 10 percent of migraine patients experience a warning of the impending headache, such as jagged streaks of light or other "fireworks" of vision, numbness, tingling, and perhaps nausea. Some feel weak, tired, or over-excited.

This warning "aura" allows the individual to lie down in a dark, quiet room, or to take immediately the medicine his doctor has prescribed. These means may ward off the threatening head pain.

The second and painful stage begins in minutes or hours with a severe, throbbing, one-sided or two-sided headache, and distended, throbbing arteries sensitized by certain chemical substances. Distension of arteries by the sun or a hot bath does not cause pain unless sensitization of the arteries also occurs. Medicine to contract dilated arteries may end a migraine attack.

A third stage may follow—the steady headache—which is either part of the original migraine attack, or a complicating muscle-contraction (tension) headache resulting from muscles held stiffly in the neck.

2. The muscle-contraction (tension) headache

Undoubtedly the commonest of chronic headaches is the muscle-contraction headache which comes from stiffly set muscles in the neck. A popular name is "tension headache."

The trigger which sets the person to holding these muscles stiffly is some kind of conflict or stress. It could be an emotional conflict when a person or event is hated or viewed with anxiety.

Or, the trigger could be physical—a cold draft from an air conditioner, eye-muscle fatigue, straining to hear because of partial deafness, or pain anywhere in the body. Muscle-contraction headache can complicate other types of headache.

Muscle-contraction headache comes without warning symptoms or signs. It usually affects both sides of the head, or the back of the head and neck, or the forehead, face, or jaw muscles, or a band around the head. The pain is steady or pressing or "tight" rather than throbbing.

Muscle-contraction headache may occur occasionally or frequently. Such a headache at times disappears quickly, at other times lasts for days or weeks. The pain can be mild, or more severe than some "dangerous" headaches.

3. Headaches associated with various structural changes

A small but important group of recurring headaches are associated with a variety of structural changes. These include headaches due to high blood pressure, virus infection, tumors, brain abscesses, defects and malformations of blood vessels, and certain diseases of the neck and spine, and headache related to the menstrual cycle.

In women with migraine, the attacks may appear just before, during, or after the menses. The exact role that hormones play in menstrual migraine is still to be determined. Research indicates that retention of fluid is not the direct and invariable cause of menstrual headache. Recent evidence suggests that falling levels of estradiol (estrogen) may play a role in menstrual migraine but the role is not completely understood.

Headache in persons with ***high blood pressure*** takes many forms, and can accompany sudden rises of blood pressure. A distinct type of hypertensive headache occurs in the morning upon awakening and eases as the day goes on.

Certain headaches involving structural changes may resemble migraine, adding to the doctor's problem of diagnosis.

4. Other headaches involving special problems

Post-traumatic headaches follow an injury, commonly a fall or an auto accident. Structures on the outside or inside of the head may be damaged. Every person who has been knocked unconscious should have a medical examination. Medical care should be continued as long as headache continues after an accident involving the head.

Headaches sometimes follow the neck strain called "whiplash" or "hyperextension." One expert said. "Bed rest is best, to relieve the neck from the stress of holding up the weight of the head, combined if necessary with pain relievers and muscle relaxants. Next best to bed rest is a 'cervical collar.'

After the initial phase, wet hot packs and range-of-motion exercises and resistance exercise may be prescribed by the physician."

Insomnia: Triumph of Mind Over Mattress

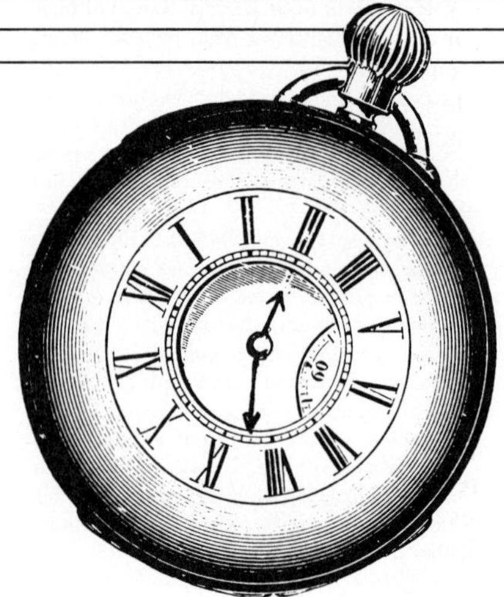

Insomnia is the triumph of mind over mattress, as one joke has it. But for many people insomnia is no laughing matter.

Americans spend approximately $25 million a year on over-the-counter (OTC) sleep aids, and additional millions are spent by the approximately 8.5 million Americans who take prescription sleeping pills. In 1977, about two million of these insomniacs took prescription sleep medications every night for two consecutive months or longer.

But the recent recall of OTC sleep aids containing methapyrilene and a previous FDA warning about the efficacy of OTC sleep aids, coupled with an Institute of Medicine report on prescription sedatives and hypnotics, has brought into question the wisdom of indiscriminate and widespread use of both OTC and prescription sleep medications.

In 1975, FDA's expert panel on sleep aids, daytime sedatives, and stimulants cautioned those with chronic sleep problems to seek medical help. It warned against using sleep aids containing bromides and scopolamine compounds, and found "irrational" the use of passion flower extract and vitamin B_1 (thiamine hydrochloride) in sleep aids. Although most sleep aids containing these ingredients were reformulated after the panel's report, some remain on the market.

More recently, OTC sleep aids containing the antihistamine methapyrilene, a carcinogen, were recalled down to the retail level in June (See FDA CONSUMER, July-August 1979). Manufacturers again reformulated their products, mostly with a chemically similar antihistamine, pyrilamine, which has not yet been tested for carcinogenicity. This action leaves thousands of users of OTC sleep aids wondering if they should continue to take these drugs, see their doctor for a prescription medication, or possibly look for other ways to relieve insomnia.

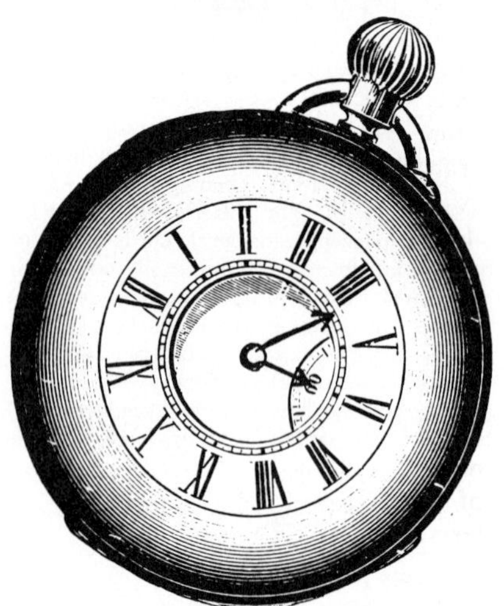

Adding to the insomniac's quandary is the recent study on sedative-hypnotic drugs issued by the National Academy of Science's Institute of Medicine (IOM). IOM conducted the study at the request of the White House Office of Drug Policy and the National Institute on Drug Abuse. Of significance to insomniacs seeking prescription drugs was the IOM report's advice to physicians to restrict use of sedative-hypnotic drugs to short-term treatment of insomnia. IOM found little evidence that sedative hypnotics in general continue to be effective when used nightly over long periods. Indeed, sleep laboratory research on sleeping pills shows that practically all lose their sleep promoting effectiveness after 3 to 14 days of continuous use.

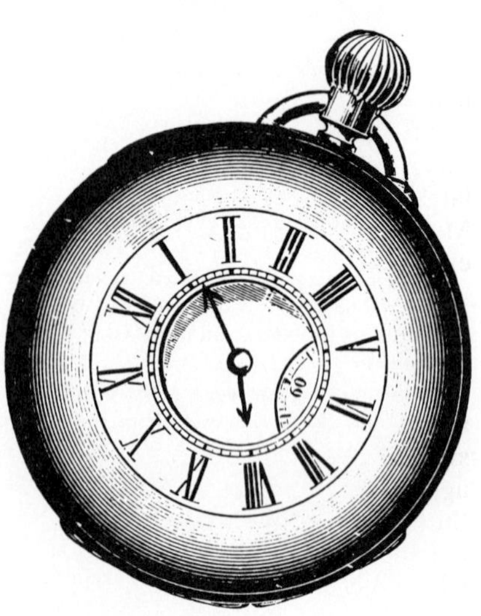

In addition to the time limitations on effectiveness, studies show that many of the prescription drugs interfere with various stages of sleep. The barbiturates suppress REM (Rapid Eye Movement) sleep during which persons dream. In the last several years, this knowledge, together with the association of barbiturates and drug abuse, has been responsible for a shift away from prescribing barbiturates in favor of the benzodiazepines, most notably Dalmane. However, there is now evidence that the benzodiazepines suppress sleep stages 3 and 4.

To better understand the significance of such suppression, we can look at an explanation of the various stages of sleep.

In their book, INSOMNIA (Doubleday, N.Y., 1969), Gay Gaer Luce and Julius Segal describe what happens when a person falls asleep. At the threshold of sleep, body temperature goes down and what are known as "alpha rhythm" brain waves occur. At this point, after the alpha state is reached, many people experience a sudden jerking awake. This is technically known as the "Myclonic Jerk" and signals neural changes resulting from a sudden burst of activity in the brain. Typically, the sleeper jerks half awake, then quickly enters stage 1 of sleep. Muscles relax and the pulse slows. Sleepers awakened at this point often feel that they have not been asleep.

If unawakened, the sleeper now enters stage 2. At this time if an EEG (electroencephalograph) were being made the tracings would show a burst of activity as the brain waves grow larger. The sleeper's eyes roll from side to side. If the eyes open, they do not see. At this point, although asleep about 10 minutes, a person if awakened might wonder if he or she had been sleeping or might believe no sleep had occurred.

After about 30 minutes of sleep, stage 3 is reached. Brain waves are large and slow, rather like mountains. Muscles are relaxed and breathing even.

The sleeper then enters stage 4, or "delta" sleep. This is the deepest sleep of all and lasts longer in the first part of the night than toward morning. Initially, after about 20 minutes of delta sleep, the sleeper ascends near waking again, but does not awaken. Instead, the sleeper goes into REM sleep, so named for the rapid eye movements which occur during this phase. The sleeper dreams during 85 percent of REM. The heartbeats are irregular and blood pressure fluctuates; the brain waves resemble those of a waking person. The first REM period lasts about 10 minutes, and then the cycle begins again with the sleeper entering sleep stage 2. This cycle repeats itself about once every 90 minutes. Toward morning there is less delta sleep and more REM.

The orders of the sleep cycle and each of its stages seem to be biologically essential. Studies of people deprived of REM show that they become hostile, irritable, and anxious. Those deprived of delta sleep seem to become depressed and apathetic. Both the REM- and the delta-deprived make up the missed stages as soon as possible when allowed to return to normal sleep.

Given this knowledge, it is understandable that medical authorities are questioning the use, especially over extended periods, of sleeping pills that may suppress these important phases of sleep.

What, then, do you do if you don't want to take pills but you can't get a good night's sleep? Just such a question was recently addressed in the JOURNAL OF THE AMERICAN MEDICAL ASSOCIATION (JAMA, Nov. 17, 1978, Vol. 240, No. 21). In an article entitled "What to Use Instead of Sleeping Pills," Thomas J. Coates, Ph.D., and Carl E. Thoresen, Ph.D., point out that the insomniac should be given a thorough physical examination to make sure that the insomnia is not related to liver, kidney, or heart disease, a metabolism problem, or some other physical ailment. With these problems ruled out, the authors then suggest that physicians advise insomniac patients to look to their eating, drinking, exercise, and relaxation habits to see if these might be preventing good sleep.

In another article along the same lines in Harvard University's MEDICAL FORUM (Vol. IV No. 7, May 1979), Dr. Quentin R. Regestein, director of the Sleep Clinic at Peter Bent Brigham Hospital, Boston, observes that most insomnia cases are related to lifestyle problems such as irregular times of going to bed and arising, night work, daytime naps, completely sedentary daytime routine, overuse of caffeine or other stimulants, and chronic abuse of tranquilizers, sleeping pills, or alcohol.

Luce and Segal point out that there are a number of types of insomnia and a variety of reasons a person may be having sleeping problems.

A major problem for many is not inabiiity to sleep but fear they will not sleep. The Greeks had a word for it: *agrypniaphobia*, fear of not being able to sleep. Then there are people who dwell on their sleeplessness, constantly pointing to it as the insurmountable problem in their lives, as a way of avoiding confrontation with more threatening problems.

Others believe mistakenly that they have insomnia. These persons may actually be getting adequate sleep for their needs, but because they have not had a full 8 hours of sleep, believe they have a problem. In fact, 8 hours may be too much sleep for some people and not enough for others. There is no statistical evidence that everyone needs 8 hours of sleep a night. Average amounts of habitual sleep can vary from 5 to 10 hours a night. There are even a few persons who habitually get as little as 2 or 3 hours sleep a night and awake feeling refreshed.

There is a type of insomnia in which persons believe they have not been asleep when they actually were. This occurs, Luce and Segal theorize, because periods of light sleeping and wakefulness are often fused and the insomniac believes he or she has not slept at all. In addition, some persons have more difficulty judging time at night than in daytime and therefore are likely to overestimate wakeful hours.

Another type of insomnia occurs when something upsetting or exciting **happens in a person's life. This type disappears by itself when the crisis is over.**

Then there is pathological insomnia which may be a sign of emotional illness. For example, early morning awakening is often a sign of depression.

If an insomniac's problem does not seem to fall into any of these areas, then he or she should look to environment and habits.

Irregular times of going to bed and awaking may make sleeping more difficult because the body gets used to sleep at certain times. There is the lark and owl syndrome—the larks being those who are at their best when they go to sleep and arise early, and the owls those who excel when they go to bed and get up at later hours. This variation is apparently linked to individual biological rhythms and possibly heredity, and can vary greatly from one individual to another. Therefore, insomniacs might do well to experiment with different times of going to sleep and arising, to see if they can get a better synchronization with their natural body rhythms

Another factor that can affect sleep is age. People require less sleep as they grow older, and this becomes increasingly evident after age 55.

There's sexism in tossing and turning. Several studies indicate that women have more trouble with insomnia than men. The question arises whether this is because, as with other physical or psychological complaints, women tend to seek help more often than men or whether there is an actual biological difference. It is known that women can be more easily roused from sleep than men and that, at an earlier age, they start requiring less sleep than men. In addition, there may be a hormonal factor, the sleepiness of early pregnancy due to progesterone release and the insomnia of pre-menstrual tension being two examples.

Besides these factors, there are environmental variables, such as diet and exercise, which are more amenable to change.

Interestingly, that old folk remedy for sleeplessness, a glass of warm milk, had some scientific basis. In a study, one of the amino acids found in milk was given in large doses to volunteers and was found to have a sedative effect. In another experiment, when persons were deprived of two other amino acids that occur in high protein foods, there was a drop in the amount of REM sleep. Therefore, a good rule of thumb might be to have a high protein dinner and a glass of milk before bedtime.

On the other hand, insomniacs would be wise to avoid beverages containing caffeine, such as coffee, tea, and colas, because they act as stimulants in most people. Smokers should note that nicotine is also a stimulant and that many ex-smokers have reported improved sleep after quitting.

Alcohol, in that old standby the nightcap, may not always work to induce sleep because it, too, can be a stimulant. In addition, some alcoholics report that their problem began with bedtime drinking. There also is evidence showing that at some dosage levels alcohol reduces REM sleep.

Exercise—the right kind at the right time—can be a sleep aid. Exercise during the daytime, especially if followed on a routine basis, has a beneficial effect on sleep. However, exercise at night may make sleeping a bit more difficult, especially if you are not used to it. Similarly, mental stimulation before bedtime can make it harder to fall asleep.

Controlling the environmental factors will often alleviate or completely eliminate sleep problems. Those for whom this approach is insufficient may want to try some of the alternatives to medication alluded to in the JAMA and MEDICAL FORUM articles and also discussed by Luce and Segal.

One solution is referral by a physician to a sleep clinic. Some sleep clinics are set up as part of hospitals. Others are connected with privately owned sleep labs and are thus more research oriented. Some sleep clinics accept people on an in-patient basis only; others accept both in- and out-patients. The program in most sleep clinics includes a thorough physical exam and psychological testing preceding several nights of EEG studies during which the insomniac is monitored to determine what abnormalities exist in his sleep pattern. A list of sleep clinics is available from Peter Bent Brigham Hospital Sleep Clinic, 721 Huntington Avenue, Boston, Mass. 02115, or Dr. William Dement, Association of Sleep Disorders Centers, Stanford University School of Medicine, Stanford, Calif. 94305.

Biofeedback, which came into wide use in the late 1960's as a way of reducing tension, has also been used to relieve insomnia. Although medical experts differ on the extent of its effectiveness for various problems, laboratory tests have shown that people can learn to control, at least partially, body functions—such as blood pressure and heart rate—that are not usually subject to conscious control.

In BIOFEEDBACK: TURNING ON THE POWER OF YOUR MIND (Lippincott, Phila., 1972), Marvin Karlin and Lewis M. Andrews describe a biofeedback training program for insomniacs. In this program, people overcome sleep difficulties by first learning to relax their forehead muscle through feedback from an EMG (electromyograph) that emits a rising tone when the forehead muscle contracts and a falling tone when it relaxes.

After learning to control the forehead muscle, the subjects then learn, through similar EEG feedback, how to produce the alpha brain waves that precede sleep.

Although some insomniacs have found relief through biofeedback techniques, their acceptance is by no means universal, and some experts, such as Beata Jencks, Ph.D., in YOUR BODY: BIOFEEDBACK AT ITS BEST (Nelson Hall, 1977), suggest that the body itself, through exercises and relaxation techniques, can be taught to act as its own biofeedback mechanism.

Certainly a number of relaxation techniques have been successful in helping people attain more beneficial sleep. Simply tensing and relaxing each muscle in the body can make a person more receptive to sleep. Similar methods are included in programs of Hatha Yoga and some forms of meditation.

Hypnosis, in the hands of a qualified professional who gives a posthypnotic suggestion that the subject will sleep and feel rested, can also be a solution to insomnia. Another, similar method, is self-hypnosis. With both these methods, however, one should be certain that there is not a deep psychological problem underlying the insomnia—a problem that may resurface in another perhaps more destructive manner. For those whose insomnia is rooted in emotional problems, psychotherapy may be the best answer.

Whether or not one of these alternatives appeals to you, one thing seems fairly certain: there is a growing body of medical opinion, including the IOM report and the FDA panel recommendations, which sees sleeping pills as, at best, a temporary solution to insomnia. The informed consumer, with expert medical advice, will explore the alternatives to drugs to find an effective, safe, long lasting solution to sleep difficulties.

Diabetes: An Overview

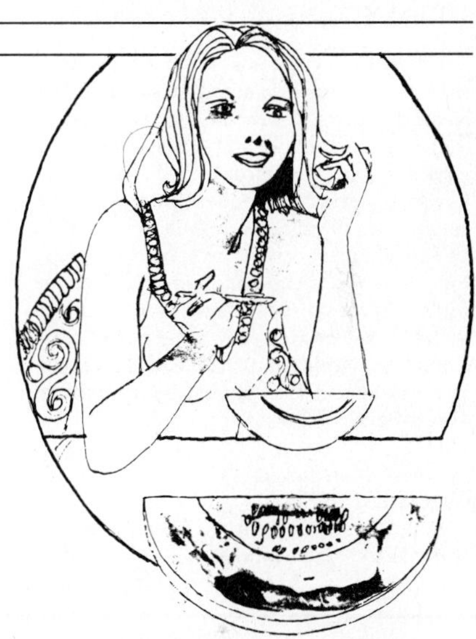

THE NATURE OF THE DISEASE

Diabetes—also known as diabetes mellitus or sugar diabetes—is a disease in which the body is unable to convert certain foods into the heat and energy necessary for normal activity. Normally, the sugars and starches (carbohydrates) in the food we eat are processed by our digestive juices into a form of sugar called glucose which circulates in our blood. This glucose or blood sugar is the fuel with which our body functions. It is burned as needed for energy or stored for later use. Insulin, a hormone produced by the pancreas, is one of the major regulators of the use of our fuel supply. When the right amount of insulin is present at the right time, the right amount of glucose is burned or released for use by the body.

In the diabetic individual, there is an impairment of insulin activity. Either the body doesn't produce enough insulin, or the available insulin is somehow blocked or inactivated by other substances within the body and insulin is prevented from performing its primary function. Because of this impairment, glucose is not properly utilized by the body and excessive glucose accumulates in the blood and tissues and overflows into the urine. Too much glucose in the blood and glucose in the urine are signs of diabetes.

TWO FORMS OF DIABETES—JUVENILE AND ADULT ONSET

There are two main forms of diabetes, which differ from each other in several ways. The more serious of the two is the juvenile-type diabetes, in which there is a total or substantial lack of insulin and daily injections of the hormone are necessary for survival. Before the discovery of insulin a half century ago and its subsequent production from the pancreas of animals, juvenile diabetics did not live more than a year or two after the onset of the disease. As its name implies, juvenile diabetes usually begins in the early years, from infancy to young adulthood. Virtually all juvenile diabetics are insulin-dependent.

In adult onset diabetes, which most often manifests itself in middle-age, insulin is usually present, but it is either insufficient in quantity or it is hindered in some manner from performing at normal efficiency. The adult form of the condition is much more common, accounting for 85 to 90 percent of all cases. Most individuals with adult onset diabetes do not require insulin treatment and can maintain their blood sugar at relatively normal levels by controlling their weight and adhering to a prescribed diet.

WHO IS SUSCEPTIBLE TO DIABETES?

In general, women are more susceptible than men. The disease tends to occur most frequently in certain "high-risk" groups—close relatives of individuals who have diabetes, people who are overweight, or over forty, or women who have given birth to large infants (weighing over 10 pounds).

WHAT CAUSES DIABETES?

The basic cause of the loss of insulin production or activity in diabetes is not known. While there appears to be a strong hereditary factor in diabetes, leading to the belief that it has a tendency to "run in families," not all cases fall in this category. Consequently, other possible causes are continually being explored—previous severe virus infections, environmental factors, some form of autoimmunity. Thus far there is no conclusive evidence linking diabetes to these possible causes. A fact that does seem clear, however, is that obesity worsens and may even precipitate diabetes.

THE SYMPTOMS OF DIABETES

The early symptoms of diabetes stem from the increased amount of sugar in the blood and urine. Since the kidneys excrete excessive amounts of water along with the excess sugar, the uncontrolled diabetic is likely to urinate frequently and to be constantly thirsty. Because the sugar in the blood is not being converted to energy, he will be weak, tired and hungry. Because of the calories lost in the urine he will lose weight, no matter how much he eats. Common symptoms that can be easily recognized and that should be brought to the prompt attention of a physician include:

- Excessive urination
- Increased thirst
- Rapid loss of weight with increased appetite and food intake.
- General weakness, drowsiness and fatigue.
- Visual disturbances, such as blurring.
- Slow healing of cuts and bruises.
- Skin disorders, such as boils, infections and intense itching, especially around the genital areas.

Some diabetics, especially those with the milder adult onset form, may experience none of these symptoms, or the symptoms may be so vague—that "run down" feeling—that they go unrecognized. The only way to detect this so-called "hidden" diabetes is to have a regular checkup at your doctor's office or at the local health department.

HOW DIABETES IS DETECTED

Even when there are no symptoms, a doctor can detect the possibility of diabetes by testing small samples of the urine and blood for sugar. In such cases, a more complicated diagnostic procedure, the Glucose Tolerance Test, is administered. In this test the level of glucose in the blood is measured before and at timed intervals after drinking a prepared glucose drink.

Today, an increasing number of communities and industries are offering diabetes screening programs, in which large numbers of people are tested and referred to their own physicians if the tests indicate the possibility of diabetes.

THE TREATMENT OF DIABETES

Since no two cases of diabetes are exactly alike, treatment must be prescribed on an individual basis. The doctor and patient are mainly concerned with diet, exercise, and insulin when needed. Some form of exercise and dietary regulation are necessary in every case of diabetes. In juvenile diabetes, insulin must be taken regularly to replenish the patient's own supply.

Diet. Years ago, the diet of the diabetic was rigid and unappealing. Today, it may be varied and is much more satisfying. For the most part, the patient can eat the same foods as the rest of the family (meat, fish, eggs, bread, dairy and cereal products, vegetables, fruits within reason and fats), cutting down only on sugars, and sugar-rich foods such as pastry, soft drinks and other sweets. The doctor, however, must decide on the appropriate diet to meet his patient's special needs.

Diets are usually written in precise terms—an ounce of meat, a slice of bread, a cup of milk—but with the help of "Exchange Lists," menus can be endlessly varied. For the overweight patient, some form of weight reducing diet is essential, for it will greatly improve the abnormality of sugar metabolism.

Physical Activity. Exercise in the form of work and play is also important if you have diabetes. A normal amount of regular exercise increases the ability of the body to use food. Here again, the doctor must decide what is best for each patient, balancing diet and medication with the level of activity.

Some of our star athletes have insulin-dependent diabetes. With proper care, young diabetics can engage in sports and other vigorous activities and should be encouraged to do so, for this is important to their emotional as well as physical development.

Insulin. Insulin, a hormone, which is prepared from extract of pancreas of cattle and hogs, must be taken by injection as the digestive juices in the stomach would destroy it if taken by mouth.

In recent years, new and improved forms of insulin have been developed. These are of a higher purity than the earlier forms. Measurement of prescribed doses is now simpler, reducing the chances of error. Substances that cause allergies in some patients have been removed and the incidence of hypersensitive reactions, such as skin rash and pitting of the skin, has been diminished.

All juvenile and some adult diabetics must take insulin in order to use carbohydrates in a comparatively normal manner. In order to gain his freedom and independence, the juvenile diabetic must, as soon as possible, assume full responsibility for his own care. For the rest of his life he will have to take insulin injections daily, give himself the shots at precise times in precise doses, and balance the dosage with his food intake and physical activity. Several times a day, as an indirect check on his blood sugar level, he will have to perform urine tests. The responsible performance of these activities will permit the juvenile diabetic to participate in a productive life.

Infants, the very young and the disabled who cannot perform these tasks need the assistance of an individual who is trained in the procedure.

Oral Drugs. Since 1957, chemical compounds, taken by mouth, have been available for the treatment of adult-onset diabetes.

While these drugs have been widely used, a recent ten-year study of their effects in combating diabetes, conducted at 12 leading medical centers, has raised doubts as to their value in controlling diabetes and its complications and, in fact, about their safety. It was the consensus of the study groups, supported by an international group of experts in biostatistics, that use of the oral anti-diabetic drugs in diabetic patients is attended by a greater risk of death from coronary heart disease than is use of diet plus insulin or diet alone and thus, they should be used only in selected cases: in those patients with maturity-onset diabetes in whom the disorder cannot be controlled by diet alone or by diet plus insulin.

INSULIN SHOCK AND DIABETIC COMA

Insulin shock due to hypoglycemia (too little sugar in the blood) may result when the diet-exercise-insulin balance is disrupted, by not eating enough, engaging in too strenuous exercise, or by taking too much insulin. Symptoms include: tremor, hunger, sweating, headache, nausea, blurred vision and eventually, if not promptly treated, loss of consciousness. Prompt relief can usually be attained with candy,

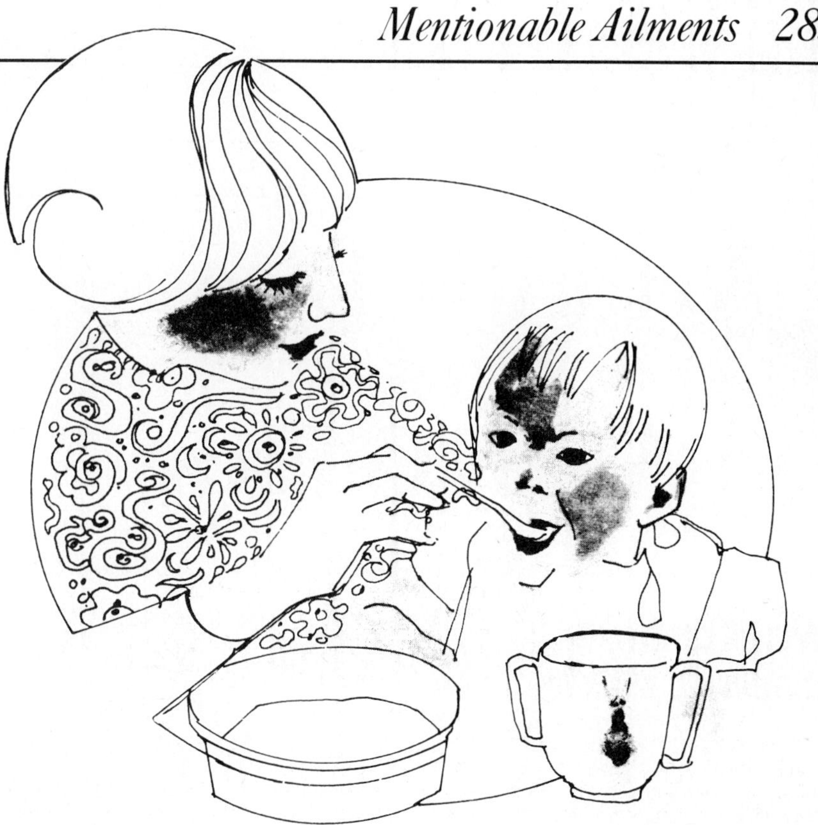

orange juice or some other sugary food or beverage, but, in all cases, symptoms should be reported to your doctor.

Diabetic coma accompanied by hyperglycemia (too much sugar in the blood) can occur when a patient fails to take sufficient insulin or follow his meal plan. Other contributory causes are infection and illness. In this condition, which is the opposite of insulin shock, fat is burned to supply energy and this produces an increasingly acid condition of the blood and other body fluids (acidosis) due to the accumulation of so-called ketone substances, including acetone. Usual symptoms are nausea, drowsiness, extreme thirst, headache, blurred vision, abdominal pains and rapid breathing. Acetone can be detected by the patient in the routine urine tests and should be immediately reported to the doctor, for if it progresses it can lead to loss of consciousness and coma.

As diabetics are more susceptible to infections than other individuals, even minor wounds should receive careful attention. Serious infections should be promptly reported to the physician, as they are frequently a precipitating factor in acidosis and diabetic coma.

THE COMPLICATIONS OF DIABETES

Diabetes is a complex, multi-faceted disorder that affects the entire body, and it involves more than an impaired production or activity of insulin. Despite satisfactory control of blood sugar levels through diet and the administration of insulin, in many cases the long-term complications of diabetes develop, primarily those affecting blood vessels, nerves, kidneys, and the eyes. Both juvenile and adult onset diabetics are susceptible to these complications; in general, however, juvenile diabetics are more severely affected.

Although present-day methods of treatment have improved, complications usually occur at some time in the course of the disease. While treatment of the complications has improved in recent years, finding the cause and methods for the prevention of complications are goals constantly being pursued.

IMPACT OF JUVENILE DIABETES ON THE FAMILY

When diabetes strikes a youngster, every member of the family is affected. Because childhood diabetes presents such complex diverse problems, most families with a diabetic youngster can profit from professional counseling. Fortunately, today, many medical institutions have diabetes clinics or centers where patients and their parents can receive help and support in adjusting to the disease, so that the child can participate actively in life.

In a growing number of such centers across the country, young diabetics and their parents are trained in every aspect of proper management of the patient's particular condition. Doctors, nurses, aides, social workers and family counselors deal with the physical, social and emotional problems involved in each age group and in each patient's situation, temperament and life style. Social and recreational activities conducted by these centers include: summer camps for young diabetics; periodic meetings of patient and parent groups to discuss the wide range of problems that are associated with the disease, such as the interactions of the child with his companions and teachers at school, his attitudes relating to dating and to the possibility of marriage and a family, and his possible uncertainties regarding choice of a career.

Your doctor or county medical society can refer you to these centers. Take advantage of them, for they can be of inestimable value for all diabetics, adult as well as juvenile, in meeting the medical, personal and family problems associated with the disease. With their help, combined with continuing medical supervision by the doctor, the diabetic will best be able to make the necessary adjustments to his disease and to function in every way as well as possible.

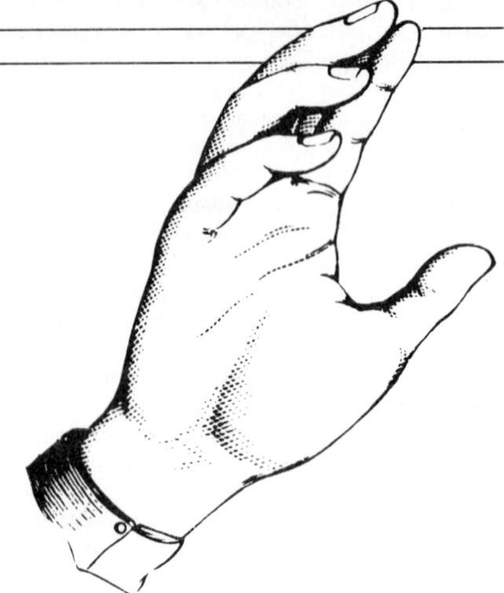

Arthritis: Disease of Many Guises

What are we coping with?

Arthritis is man's oldest known chronic illness. The skeleton of the ancient platycarpus, a large swimming reptile that lived 100 million years ago, shows changes characteristic of arthritis. Bones of the Java Ape Man and the mummies of Egypt show signs of arthritic damage. The ancient Greeks and Romans are known to have been victims of this disease, which throughout the ages has tormented mankind.

Arthritis refers to the types of rheumatic disease which attack the joints. Other types, such as those that involve the muscles, tendons, ligaments, or bursae, are referred to as rheumatism. The effects of rheumatic disease may vary from a slight pain, stiffness or swelling to crippling and total disability.

The word *arthritis* means inflammation of a joint. But arthritis as we now understand it often involves much more than just aches and pains around a joint. In fact, inflamed joints may be only one manifestation of the more than 90 different diseases that can be considered arthritis.

The three most common of these diseases are rheumatoid arthritis, osteoarthritis and gout. Each is a distinct disease with different causes and different prospects for recovery, requiring different methods of treatment.

Rheumatoid arthritis is the most crippling of the rheumatic diseases. It affects three times as many women as men and generally starts between the ages of 25 and 50.

Rheumatoid arthritis usually affects many joints, most commonly the small joints of the hands. Inflammation and thickening of the lining and tissue around the joints may cause destruction of the bones, deformity, and eventually, disability. There may be wide variation, however, from person to person—in some cases, the disease may be mild, while in others it can be crippling.

The cause of rheumatoid arthritis is unknown. There are two leading theories held by many scientists, which have led to a series of aggressive and productive investigations in recent years, but neither has been definitely proved. Much of the research supported by the National Institute of Arthritis, Metabolism, and Digestive Diseases involves these theories of *infection* and *autoimmunity*.

The infection theory holds that rheumatoid arthritis may be due, directly or indirectly, to microorganisms, such as viruses or mycoplasma. According to the autoimmunity theory, the immune processes, or defense mechanisms of the body, may become disrupted and produce abnormal antibodies that are directed against the body's own tissues rather than against invasion of the body by foreign material, as is normally the case.

Abnormal proteins of an antibody-like nature, known as the "rheumatoid factor," have been found in the blood of rheumatoid arthritis patients. This factor seems to be strongly involved in the immunological mechanism of the disease.

Evidence from a series of studies indicates that joint inflammation may be associated with a process by which rheumatoid factor is taken from the surrounding joint fluid by leukocytes (scavenging white blood cells). The ingestion of this material by the leukocytes, some scientists believe, results in the release of certain tissue-eroding enzymes from tiny sacs in the cells (lysosomes). The enzymes previously contained in those sacs now gain access to the joint cartilage and chemically destroy it.

The antibody-like rheumatoid factor has been shown to appear in patients and laboratory animals with unrelated chronic infections and to disappear when these infections are cured, thus tending to link the infection theory to the autoimmunity theory. An even closer link has been suggested in the possibility that an infection may set the stage for a later disruption of the immune process in which abnormal antibodies are produced against the body's own tissues.

Emotional stress has also been investigated as a possible instigator of rheumatoid arthritis. This factor has been exonerated as a cause, but stress can perhaps hasten the onset of its symptoms and can clearly aggravate the disease once it is established. Hereditary factors, as manifested by certain unusual blood proteins are now being actively investigated as possible indicators of individuals more susceptible than others to various kinds of arthritis.

Symptoms and Signs of Rheumatoid Arthritis

The first signs of rheumatoid arthritis usually are fatigue, muscular stiffness, and loss of appetite and weight. Frequently, patients have cold, sweaty hands and feet. Painful swelling may begin at one or more joints; nodules, from the size of a pea to a walnut, may appear under the skin. Gradually, joint motion is lost and deformities of the joints occur. The disease can affect many internal organs and is sometimes accompanied by fever.

Accurate diagnosis of rheumatoid arthritis can be made only by a qualified physician after a careful physical examination and a variety of tests and, frequently, X-rays. The physician will then recommend a comprehensive treatment plan that is geared to the individual patient. This plan may include 1) rest, 2) physical therapy, such as heat and corrective exercises, 3) any one of a number of drugs to control pain and inflammation, and 4) in selected cases, surgery. The physician may also recommend a well-balanced diet, correction of posture, and avoidance of cold and dampness. The doctor's choice of treatment depends largely on the distribution and severity of the disease.

Although it is not possible today to cure rheumatoid arthritis, it is possible for patients to cope successfully with their affliction with the help of their physicians and other specialists. The prime objective of

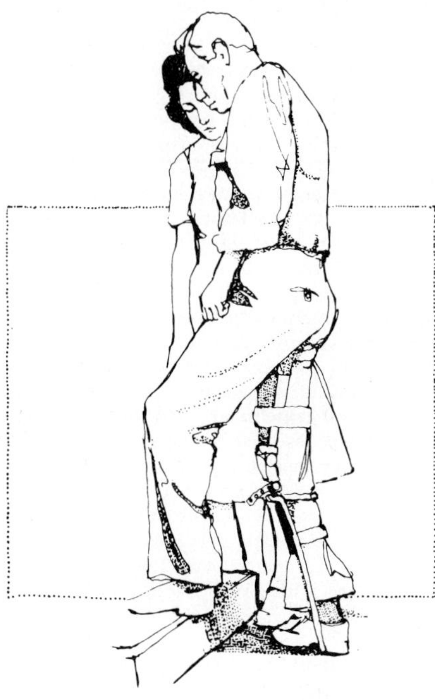

treatment is prevention of joint destruction. The likelihood of complete remission of the disease makes it important that all efforts be made to prevent destruction during the active stage. Past damage may not be reversible.

Control of Rheumatoid Arthritis

Since rheumatoid arthritis is usually chronic and may last a lifetime, physicians try to avoid use of toxic drugs as far as possible. The patient is started on large doses of aspirin, which is the most reliable and least toxic of all anti-arthritic drugs. It is the one that is most likely to provide sustained control of symptoms at the lowest risk of undesirable side-effects.

When conservative drugs prove ineffective in certain cases, physicians have a variety of anti-inflammatory and immuno-suppressive agents, such as gold compounds, phenylbutazone, adrenocortical steroids and others, which can be prescribed. Although these

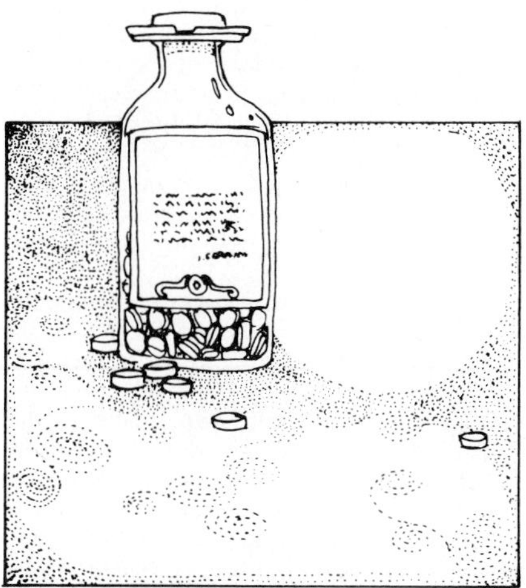

often provide immediate and dramatic improvement, they carry the hazard of possible side-effects, and are used mostly in special situations and for limited periods, under close medical supervision.

Of the new drugs that are constantly being tested, one of the most promising groups is the antimetabolites or anti-cancer drugs, which are known to block cellular mechanisms of antibody production. These have been used in several autoimmune diseases, with greatest success in the blood-destroying leukemias, and offer hope for an effective form of therapy in rheumatoid arthritis, as well as in other diseases involving abnormal immunological processes.

If rheumatoid arthritis is diagnosed early, and if prompt, individualized treatment is instituted as soon after diagnosis as possible, there is evidence that severe crippling now can be prevented in at least seven out of ten cases. Research supported by the National Institute of Arthritis, Metabolism, and Digestive Diseases includes study of the occurrence, frequency and distribution of arthritis in the continuing search for its causes, as well as evaluation and demonstration of new and better therapeutic techniques.

Osteoarthritis

Osteoarthritis seems to result from a combination of aging, irritation of the joints, and normal wear and tear. It is far more common than rheumatoid arthritis, but, as a rule, it is less damaging. Older people are its most frequent victims. Chronic irritation of the joints is the main contributing factor. This may result from overweight, poor posture, injury, or strain from one's occupation or recreation, or a combination of these factors.

The disease is characterized by degeneration of joint cartilage which lines the outside of bones where they move against each other. This cartilage becomes soft and wears unevenly. In some areas, it may wear away completely, exposing the underlying bone and damaging it. Disability most often results from disease in the weight-bearing joints—the knees, hips and spine.

The common symptoms are pain and stiffness. Pain is usually experienced when certain joints are used, especially finger joints and those that bear the body's weight. Enlargement of the fingers at the last joint often occurs. Such enlargements are common and are called Heberden's nodes. Although

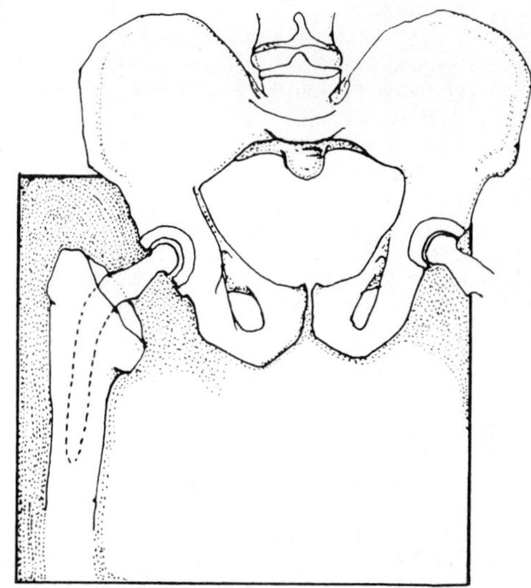

permanent, enlargements of this type seldom lead to disability.

The same general methods of treatment and care that are used for rheumatoid arthritis are equally effective in the treatment of osteoarthritis. Surgical correction of deformed weight-bearing joints, especially hips, has been effective in helping many osteoarthritic patients to walk again without pain.

Other forms of arthritis and rheumatism

Juvenile rheumatoid arthritis is similar in many ways to adult rheumatoid arthritis, but there are also marked differences. Juvenile rheumatoid arthritis affects primarily those under the age of 16 years. Its complications can be quite variable. It causes growth disturbances and results in high fever and skin rash more frequently than is the case among older patients. There are also characteristic accompanying disorders in other body tissues and organs. Some 30 percent of patients develop severe crippling. Often there is absence of rheumatoid factor in the blood. Because of these distinctions, arthritis in children is looked upon as a separate disease, or group of diseases. In the majority of cases, it can be controlled with proper treatment.

Psoriatic arthritis affects about ten percent of people with psoriasis, a common skin disease. This arthritis closely resembles the rheumatoid type, and it is treated in a similar manner, with special attention to the skin disorder.

Systemic lupus erythematosus is an uncommon disease of connective tissue which produces changes in the structure and functions of the skin, joints, and internal organs. It is found most often in people between the ages of 20 and 40 years, and affects women more frequently than men. There is no specific and complete treatment for this disease, of which the cause is not known, so supportive treatment must be tailored to fit each specific case.

Ankylosing spondylitis is also known as rheumatoid spondylitis and as Marie-Strumpell disease. It is a systemic disorder which affects mostly males in late adolescence or young adulthood. It is characterized by back pain, stiffness, and loss of spinal mobility due to involvement of spinal joints. The disease is treated with pain-relieving and anti-inflammatory drugs; and exercise, posture training and orthopedic correction are important forms of therapy.

Reiter's syndrome is a combination of urethritis (inflammation of the urethra), arthritis, and conjunctivitis (inflammation of the delicate membrane that lines the eyelids). It occurs most commonly in young male adults, and usually lasts only a matter of weeks or months.

Bursitis is inflammation of a bursa, a small sac containing fluid, which is usually situated between a tendon and the bone over which the tendon glides. "Tennis elbow" and "housemaid's knee" are examples of bursitis. The condition may be relieved through application of heat, resting the part involved, and with aspirin. In severe cases, anti-inflammatory agents may be injected directly into the painful area.

Fibrositis is the most common rheumatic condition that does not affect the joints directly. It involves pain, stiffness or soreness of fibrous tissue, especially in the coverings of the muscles. Attacks may follow an injury, repeated muscular strain, prolonged mental tension or depression. Fibrositis within the muscles is sometimes called myositis. Lumbago is fibrositis in the lumbar region. The condition may disappear spontaneously or as a result of treatment. It is not a destructive, progressive disease and not a crippler.

Gout

Gout is the easiest form of arthritis to detect and treat and the best understood. It most commonly affects the joints of the feet, particularly the big toe, although other joints are frequently involved. Nearly all cases of gout occur in men.

In gout, too much of a certain body chemical, uric acid, is deposited in the tissues. Crystals of uric acid form in the joints causing inflammation and severe pain. The excess of uric acid may result either from overproduction within the body or from decreased urinary excretion of it.

Attacks of gout may follow minor injury, excessive eating or drinking, overexercise, or

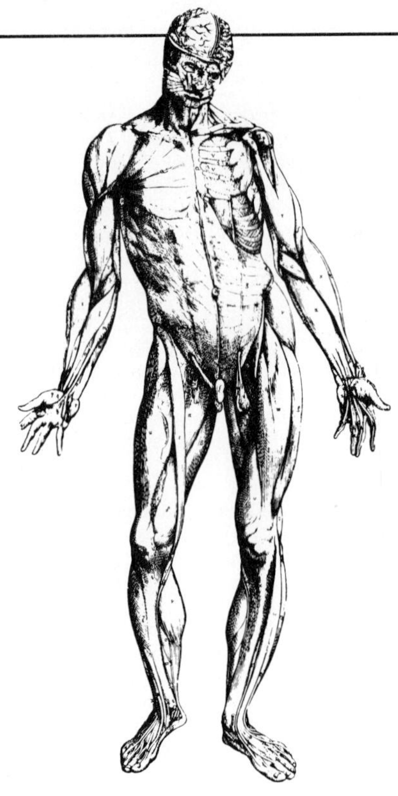

surgery. Often, attacks, very sudden in onset, occur for no apparent reason, and may last for days or weeks, during which the patient suffers acute pain and tenderness in his affected joints. Between attacks he may be free of symptoms. Many years after the onset, chronic arthritis may set in. Gouty kidney disease and consequent high blood pressure can develop if the condition is not detected and treated in its early stages.

Gout responds more satisfactorily to treatment and is more effectively controlled than any other type of arthritis. Drugs are used successfully to reduce the excessive amount of uric acid in the blood and tissue. These medications can diminish the frequency of recurrent acute attacks of painful gout, although they have no effect in reducing the inflammation and pain when attacks do occur. Other drugs, however, can be employed to prevent or control these acute flare-ups.

Victims of gouty arthritis now can be maintained with reasonable comfort, and if their disease is diagnosed early and treated properly, it will neither cripple them nor seriously interfere with their daily life or general health.

Scientists believe that research currently being conducted in clinical centers and laboratories throughout the world may result in identification of other basic defects which underlie gout. Such a finding could lead to even more effective methods of treatment, and, perhaps, to an ultimate cure for this ancient disease.

You can sit in an abandoned radium mine, hang a Vryllium tube on your lapel, bury yourself up to the neck in horse manure, swill Dr. Fenby's Formula X, or take a dose of "Chuei-Fong-Tou-Geu-Wan," but you will not be able to cure your arthritis.

It is a distressing fact of life that although there are drugs to relieve the pain and reduce the inflammation of arthritis—plain aspirin being one of the most effective—there is no cure for this painful and oftentimes crippling disease. Yet many arthritis sufferers turn to quack devices and "miracle" cures, such as those listed above. They do no good and in some cases can do considerable harm. According to CONSUMER REPORTS (June 1979), for every dollar spent on arthritis research $25 is spent on useless nostrums, unapproved devices, unnecessary food supplements, and diet books. The total annual tab is estimated to be $950 million. In 1966, the Arthritis Foundation had put that figure at $310 million. Obviously arthritis quackery is big business and growing every year.

The various forms of arthritis have different causes, symptoms, and types of treatment. Medication, rest, heat, special exercises, and surgery are all used to relieve the symptoms of these diseases. But what's best for individual patients depends on an accurate diagnosis of the type of arthritis they have. Treatment programs also have to be tailored to fit the individual because the disease varies from patient to patient, and patients themselves vary in the way they react to different therapies.

Medical quacks don't take such factors into consideration when they peddle their wares. Arthritis, rheumatism, gout—it's all the same to them. One drug or one device cures all. Unfortunately, arthritis quackery persists even in this age of technological enlightenment. In part, that's because of a quirk of the disease called spontaneous remission. Arthritis has a way of coming and going unpredictably. The pain and swelling can simply disappear for days, weeks, or even months. Victims who experience such a remission are easily convinced that whatever they were taking or doing brought relief.

The Food and Drug Administration has long been concerned about fraudulent drugs and devices and has, over the years, taken legal action to get many of them off the market.

One of the earliest quack gadgets to make its appearance in this country was "Perkins Tractors," two pointed rods about 3 inches long—one gold-colored, the other silver. A number of conditions, especially gout, pleurisy, rheumatism, violent insanity, "inflammatory tumors," and yellow fever, resulted from a surcharge of an electric fluid in the body, inventor Elisha Perkins claimed. This electricity could be released through drawing the tractors over the affected area. Perkins and his "tractors" were the biggest thing going—in 1796.

The 20th century arthritis victim has been lured by an astounding variety of quack devices, ranging from the simple copper or magnetic bracelet to complex "electronic" mechanisms, such as the Palorator device seized by FDA in 1954. It had two electromagnetic coils that vibrated a couple of knobs on the front of a box. The Gonsertron, billed as "A New Concept in the Field of Electrotherapy," was a cabinet filled with various electrical components connected to a chair and, not coincidentally, to the house current. Another was the Magnetron, a 6,000-volt transformer hooked up to a homemade condenser; the claim was that it provided an adequate and effective treatment for diabetes, tumors, varicose veins, and rheumatoid arthritis. Other devices, such as Diapulse Electro Magnetic Energy Generators and Solarama Microthermal Panels are still turning up despite FDA efforts to get them out of circulation.

Things that vibrate—chairs and mattresses—also have been "hot" items in the arthritis quack's bag of tricks. The vibrators may produce interesting sensations but they certainly are not harmless since the vibrations could further aggravate already inflammed joints. So too could the Slim-Twist Exerciser, two pieces of wood connected by a ball bearing swivel joint. Stand on the top piece, pretend to dance the "Twist," and you can lose weight, cure heart and vascular problems, or relieve arthritis, asthma, and diabetes, the promoters claimed.

One of the most dangerous quack gadgets was the Detoxacolon, a pressurized enema device. Promoter Roy W. DeWelles claimed all ailments known to man, including cancer, asthma, arthritis, colitis, epilepsy, and high and low blood pressure, were caused by toxins in the colon that could be eliminated through irrigation with water and oxygen. What he didn't tell patients was that this treatment could spread infection and possibly perforate the colon wall. FDA seized Detoxacolon machines on four occasions. Despite these actions and the efforts of the California State Department of Health to put him out of business, DeWelles managed to stay out of jail for 20 years. His first conviction came in 1964 on a charge of mail fraud.

Another popular item of arthritis quackery has been uranium. Not only have patients sat in abandoned mines to soak up the "curative" powers of this dangerous ore, but they have been hoodwinked into buying mittens, gloves, mattresses, and pads of assorted sizes supposedly filled with radioactive material. Crushed rock with less radiation than a watch dial emits is what they receive.

Even more dangerous is Leifcort, a powerful drug making a comeback as an unapproved arthritis treatment. Leifcort is a hormone compound developed and promoted nearly 20 years ago by a Dr. Robert Leifmann, who fled to Canada because he was wanted by U.S. marshals for selling a baldness cure. Leifmann prescribed his compound in Montreal until 1968 when the Canadian Food and Drug Directorate raided his clinic. Charged with marketing an unapproved drug and with other violations, Leifmann continued treating his own patients while various appeals were pending. He died in 1972.

FDA became concerned about Leifcort after the death of an American woman who went to Canada and came back with a year's supply of the drug on the strength of a glowing report in a popular magazine. The Agency issued press information alerting the public to the dangers of this drug.

Apparently, the warning bears repeating, since a number of Leifmann's colleagues are back in business in the United States operating as the Arthritis Medical Offices and the Arthritis Medical Center. Leifcort, renamed variously "Hormone Balance Treatment," "Balanced Hormone Treatment," "Holistic Balance Treatment," and "Rheumatril," is being sold in clinics often set up in hotel rooms. Arthritis victims visiting these clinics are given a cursory physical examination and a 6-month supply of the drug for $640. What they take home for continued self-treatment is a combination of prednisone, estrogen, and testosterone—all hormones.

Promoters of the drug claim their product is perfectly legal since the components are all approved drugs. That may be, says FDA, but the combination has not been approved and, furthermore, it poses a real danger to health. Prednisone, which is very similar to cortisone, is used in arthritis treatment, but only in small amounts and under close medical supervision. Patients who go to the Arthritis Medical Center clinics may get immediate relief, but the danger lies in taking high doses for long periods. This misuse of the combination can lead to thinning of bones, lowered resistance to infection, high blood pressure, cataracts, glaucoma, and peptic ulcers. In addition, patients who are also taking cortisone may not realize they are getting a double dose of a powerful hormone.

FDA is investigating the activities of the Arthritis Medical Center. Outside of the Agency's jurisdiction are other dispensers of the Leifmann formula in Santo Domingo in the Dominican Republic, and in Mexicali and Juarez, Mexico.

The British, it seems, have encountered a slightly different version of the hormone-arthritis treatment. According to a number of letters to the BRITISH MEDICAL JOURNAL unsuspecting patients have ordered drugs from Hong Kong with such exotic names as Chuei-Fong-Tou-Geu-Wan (meaning "chase the wind through the bones") and Tsai-Tsao-Wan. Like the Americans taking Leifcort, these British patients may get immediate relief from pain but also get the kind of adverse reaction that comes from overdoses of corticosteroids.

Snake venom made the news last year as an arthritis treatment after CBS's "Sixty Minutes" featured the work of Dr. Ben Sheppard, a Florida practitioner, who had been giving a combination of cobra and krait venom to victims of multiple sclerosis and rheumatoid arthritis. FDA's Bureau of Biologics had held a public workshop in November 1979 on Sheppard's snake venom treatment. Scientific experts at the workshop felt Dr. Sheppard's experiences did not prove that his product, incidentally called PROven, was effective and suggested that further laboratory testing in animals might be helpful. Dr. Sheppard died early this year, but the snake venom treatment is being offered by a number of other doctors in Florida.

While no one would consider aspirin a form of quackery, a number of medical writers have labeled the "glorification" of the more expensive forms of aspirin a kind of medical misrepresentation. Special arthritis strength formulas are nothing more than plain aspirin with small amounts of caffeine or antacid added. The tablet may be bigger than an ordinary aspirin, but so is the price.

A few years ago, a panel of non-Government experts evaluating aspirin and other pain relievers for FDA said that terms such as "arthritis strength" or "arthritis pain formula" should not be included in the labels or advertising of aspirin products. Ads suggesting arthritis is a minor disease or that alleviation of pain with "extra strength aspirin" will control the disease could delay proper diagnosis and treatment, the group said.

Arthritis is not a minor disease, but its pain can be relieved and its crippling effects can be prevented in many cases by prompt and proper treatment. Victims of the disease should be wary of products that offer "special" or "secret" formulas, that promise quick or easy cures, and that are promoted by case histories and testimonials. Such products should be shunned or left capped—there are no genies in those bottles, and the products can do more harm than good.

Therapies For Arthritis Victims

Current therapy for arthritis depends on the type of disease being treated, its severity, and the response of the patient. Here are some forms of treatments currently being used for the major types of arthritis.

Rheumatoid Arthritis

Medication: Anti-inflammatory Drugs:

Aspirin—must be taken in large doses, regularly, day after day.

Nonsteroidal anti-inflammatory drugs, such as fenoprofen, ibuprofen, indomethacin, naprozen, sulindac, tolectin.

Phenylbutazone—reduces inflammation but can have

serious side effects and use must be closely supervised by a physician.

Corticosteroids (cortisone)—can give dramatic reduction in pain but can cause serious side effects; therefore are being prescribed less often by specialists. Direct injection into joints provides temporary relief.

Other Drugs:

Gold Salts—used for about 50 years. Takes time to determine correct dosage. Effective for many patients, but not all.

Penicillamine—reserved for patients with severe rheumatoid arthritis who do not respond well to other therapy.

Antimalarials—derivatives of quinine. May be helpful in limited dosage over long periods of time.

Rest and Exercise:

Rest, usually in bed, helps decrease inflammation, but can lead to temporary stiffening of diseased joints; individual joints are sometimes rested in removable lightweight splints.

Exercise—special "quiet" exercises, done daily, put joints gently through their full range of motion.

Heat:

Relaxing and soothing, helps joints move better with less pain; various forms are used: hot baths, hydrotherapy, hot packs, heat lamps, paraffin wax applications.

Surgery:

"Frozen" joints can be made movable by plastic surgery, useless joints can be made stable by fusion, and artificial joints can replace those diseased by arthritis.

Osteoarthritis

Medication:

Aspirin

Phenylbutazone

Indomethacin

Pain relievers such as codeine

Cortisone—not used orally for osteoarthritis, but may be injected in joints for temporary relief.

Physical Therapy:

May be the most valuable treatment for the patient. Objective is to restore maximum degree of physical function by helping patient make the best use of remaining abilities.

Exercises are aimed at making sure affected joints are moved through their full range of motion. Some are performed by patient alone, others are done with assistance of a physical therapist or other trained person.

Heat:

May include a hot bath first thing in the morning or warm packs, heated wax, heat lamp treatments.

Surgery:

Can be very effective in preventing some deformities, in relieving pain, and improving overall function. Progress is being made in perfecting artificial joints, especially for total hip replacement.

Splints, crutches, braces:

Used to rest joints or reduce pressures on them. Orthopedic collar may be used to limit motion of vertebrae of the neck.

Gout

Medication:

Colchicine—extremely powerful, can cause side effects.

Phenylbutazone

Oxyphenbutazone

Indomethacin

Probenecid—helps body discharge more uric acid

Allopurinol—reduces body's production of uric acid

Arthritis and Your Diet

Diet has nothing to do with causing or curing arthritis, say experts at the National Institute of Arthritis, Metabolism, and Digestive Diseases and at the Arthritis Foundation. People with arthritis should, of course, watch their weight since extra pounds can mean an extra burden on weight-bearing joints, and those with gout should avoid overindulgence in alcohol and stay away from liver, sweetbreads, and kidneys. Nevertheless, "special" arthritis diets abound.

Everything from cod liver oil, alfalfa, pokeberries, and blackstrap molasses to a mixture of honey, vinegar, iodine, and kelp have been sold for arthritis diets. At one time "immune milk" was a big item. This supposedly came from cows injected with streptococcus and staphylococcus vaccines. Seawater was highly promoted in the early 1960's by a physician who claimed to have rejuvenated his 97-year-old father with this treatment. Serious complications were reported in cardiac and rheumatic patients who were swept up by what then FDA Commissioner George Larrick called a "nation-wide seawater swindle." FDA moved in Texas, California, Indiana, Ohio, Pennsylvania, and Michigan to seize about 2,000 bottles of seawater packaged by a Florida laboratory.

Diet cookbooks for arthritics have appeared on the scene as have special biological health regimens. One book, THERE IS A CURE FOR ARTHRITIS, recommends a treatment that includes elimination of all drugs, therapeutic fasting, enemas two or three times a day, and a diet heavy in fresh fruits, raw vegetables, herb teas, and other so-called natural or whole grain foods. Recently, two professors at Rutgers University theorized that arthritis is caused by eating vegetables classed as "nightshades." This includes tomatoes, white potatoes, green pepper, and eggplant. Honey and the sting of the honey maker also have been recommended treatments, but not by experts in rheumatology. Such treatments have not been studied scientifically. An off-beat diet might not do too much injury, but an unapproved drug could. "Groff's Arthra Tone," "Ar-Thry-Go Tablets," "Ring's Golden Herb Tonic," and "Elmore's R'heumative Goutaline" were some of the drugs seized by FDA in the 1950's and 1960's because of false and misleading claims. Dr. Fenby's Formula X is a more recent entry in the field. Postal authorities charged its manufacturer with false advertising in 1979. Many of these "cures" were combinations of herbs, aspirin, and alcohol.

Not so innocuous was the Tri-Wonda Treatment, a three-part concoction consisting of one bottle of dilute hydrochloric and dilute nitric acid with traces of tartaric and acetic acid; a second bottle containing cream of tartar, senna, sulfur, and phenophthalein, a laxative; and a third bottle containing a 44 percent alcohol solution of fluid extract of Jamaica dogwood, thiamine hydrochloride, and wild cherry flavoring. It took 7 years for FDA to get Tri-Wonda off the market, because of legal maneuvering by the manufacturer.

Arthritis, Medical Treatment and Mental Health

In the management of arthritis, the physician must consider the whole person. He must treat not only the pain and stiffness in the patient's joints but the anxieties in his mind, taking fully into account his character, background and personal problems. He may suggest a change of jobs or household routine or some other measure to alleviate a stressful situation.

No factor is more important in the treatment and rehabilitation of the arthritis patient than maintenance of psychological balance under the stressful conditions imposed by the disease. Complex emotional and vocational problems resulting from chronic disability often require the attention of psychologists, social workers and vocational specialists. In the overall management of arthritis, these specialists must work in close cooperation with each other and with the doctors, surgeons, therapists, relatives of the patient and others involved, if best results are to be achieved.

In most cases, your own physician can best prescribe treatment. If you suffer pain, stiffness or swelling in a joint, see a physician. Do not try self-treatment. You should also be aware that not all physicians are expert rheumatologists; if things are not going well in the treatment of your disease, your physician may wish to ask for consultation with a doctor who specializes in the rheumatic diseases.

You may also wish to contact the Arthritis Foundation, a non-profit voluntary agency with chapters throughout the country, which supports research, promotes public education and expands community services to arthritis patients and their families. The Arthritis Foundation chapter may assist you in locating a qualified rheumatologist, a physician who specializes in treating rheumatic disorders. The American Rheumatism Association is the professional arm of the Foundation and guides its medical and scientific programs.

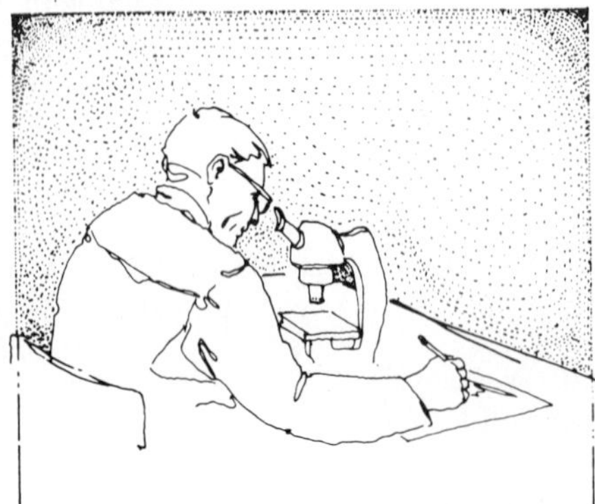

Research in Arthritis

The National Institute of Arthritis, Metabolism, and Digestive Diseases (NIAMDD), a component of the Federal Government's National Institutes of Health, Bethesda, Maryland, is the focal point of an intensive, multifaceted program of research and support of research in arthritis and related disorders. This program is two-fold: it conducts laboratory and clinical research in Bethesda, and supports financially through grants many different research projects directly related to arthritis at various nongovernmental institutions across the country. Current clinical research concerns the processes of arthritis inflammation and tissue destruction and the immunologic mechanisms which may be related. These studies are fundamental to understanding and treatment of arthritis. Other studies are concerned with perfection of such procedures as total hip or knee replacement. These research efforts are continually adding to a valuable fund of basic knowledge and to improving the control of rheumatic diseases.

Common Ailments: The Unmentionables

Anorectal Disease a.k.a. Hemorrhoids

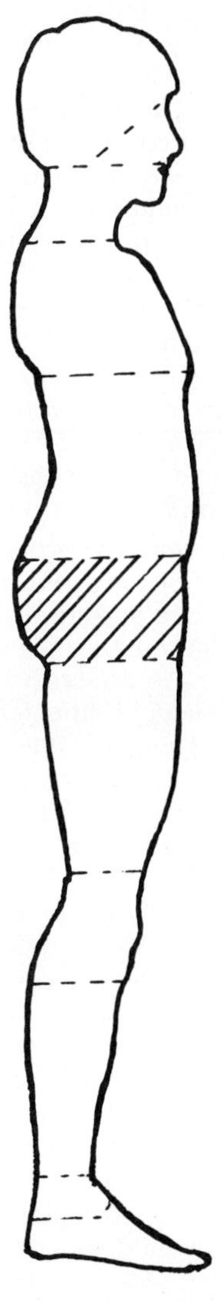

It all started when our ancestors came down out of the trees and began walking on two legs. Standing upright may have been a forward step in evolution, but it also has led to one of the more uncomfortable scourges of the human race—hemorrhoids.

For the many who suffer from this condition, and other disorders of the lower end of the intestinal tract, relief of some of the symptoms is available in nonprescription drugs, according to a panel of non-Government experts. The group identified 24 ingredients that are safe and effective in providing relief. However, they warned that consumers should not use these products for more than 7 days at a time, and that medical advice should be sought if symptoms persist.

At the start of its review, the panel decided that "hemorrhoidal" was too restrictive a term when OTC preparations for "hemorrhoidal disease" were considered. They opted instead for "anorectal" disease or disorders because this more accurately describes the area of the anatomy involved. (Anorectal involves the anus and rectum.) No one knows exactly what causes diseases of the anorectal area, the panel said.

Erect posture, eating more refined foods, and drinking fewer liquids, plus an over concern with "irregularity" and the subsequent overuse of laxatives are believed to play a part. The reason so little is known, according to the panel, is that there has been no concerted effort to study this problem. The panel noted that its review represented the first expenditure of Federal funds related to the study of anorectal disorders.

Despite the universality of anorectal disease—and no human is immune—society's attitude toward the subject is one of secrecy, reticence, shyness, and embarrassment, the panel noted in its report, published in the May 27 issue of the FEDERAL REGISTER. Indeed, the entire subject is often the butt of jokes. Thus inhibited, the average person, as well as some physicians, feel it is not proper to talk about anorectal function or disease. The sufferer finds it difficult to get information and help and, as a result, turns to OTC products even when he should be seeing a physician. Social and medical shyness also were blamed by the panel for the lack of research interest in anorectal disease.

The panel grouped the anorectal ingredients under review into nine categories according to their pharmacological activity. A 10th category included miscellaneous ingredients that didn't fall into the other classifications. Ingredients were judged according to their safety and effectiveness for external use—that is, on the skin around and just inside the anus—or for use within the lower rectum.

Twenty-four of the ingredients in six categories were found by the panel to be safe and effective for their claimed use (see chart). They include:

- *local anesthetics* to relieve pain, irritation, itching, or burning
- *vasoconstrictors* to reduce swelling
- *protectants* to provide a coating over inflamed tissues and relieve itching
- *counterirritants* to detract from the sensation of pain
- *astringents* to relieve irritation and burning
- *keratolytics* to relieve itching

Twenty-six ingredients in these categories were deemed not safe and effective by the panel, which recommended they be taken off the market. Additional tests would be required for 26 other ingredients if they are to continue to be marketed for their respective claims. Guidelines set up by the panel call for ingredients to be tested in the area of the human anatomy where they will be used and in the final form the product will take, i.e., as cream, gel, foam, or suppository.

None of the anorectal ingredients was considered safe and effective as a *wound-healing agent*. No studies have yet conclusively correlated the use of such agents with relief of anorectal symptoms, the panel said. However, the group did identify six ingredients for which such claims might be made if they pass tests of effectiveness.

The panel said claims of *antiseptic* properties in ingredients used in the intrarectal area are scientifically unsound because of the high number of microorganisms normally in the anorectal area. The group recommended that six of the submitted ingredients be banned as antiseptics, and called for additional testing of a seventh ingredient to establish its safety and effectiveness as an external antiseptic.

The panel said there is no place in OTC anorectal products for *anticholinergics*, substances that prevent transmission of nerve impulses, and called for a ban of two such ingredients. Finally the panel said the five miscellaneous ingredients should be taken off the market because there is no information on which to judge their safety and effectiveness.

Labeling of anorectal products should reflect the intended use, rather than the pharmacological activity of the active ingredients, the panel said. Acceptable labeling claims would include such phrases as: "for the temporary relief of itching associated with hemorrhoids and other anorectal disorders," "for the temporary relief of symptoms associated with hemorrhoids and other anorectal disorders," "for the temporary relief of itching."

The panel emphasized that personal hygiene is essential for the product to do its job. Thus, under "directions for use," the group recommended the following: "When practical, wash the anorectal area with mild soap and warm water and rinse off all soap before application of this product."

Under general "warnings" the panel recommended that users be advised not to use the product for more than 7 days, and to consult a physician if symptoms do not improve, if itching persists longer than 7 days, or if bleeding develops. For products containing perfume, label warnings should advise users to seek medical help if redness, burning, itching, swelling, pain, or other symptoms develop.

Hemorrhoids frequently develop during pregnancy, but no studies on the use of anorectal products in pregnant women were found by the panel. The group was concerned that ingredients used intrarectally might be absorbed into the mother's system through the rectal mucosa and thus harm the infant. For this reason, the panel called for the following statement on all products intended for intrarectal use, except protectants: "The safety of this product has not been established for use by pregnant women or by nursing mothers."

With the exception of protectants and astringents, anorectal products should carry a warning against use in children under 12 unless under a doctor's supervision, because hemorrhoids in children may be due to a serious underlying cause requiring diagnosis and treatment by a doctor. Labels on vasoconstrictors should warn against use by anyone who has heart disease, high blood pressure, hyperthyroidism, diabetes, difficulty in urination, or who is taking tranquilizers or "nerve pills," according to the panel.

What is inappropriate or misleading, according to the panel, are label claims that the products are for the treatment of anorectal conditions. OTC products are primarily for the relief of symptoms and not the treatment of disease, the panel said. Similarly, labels should not suggest that use of the product will bring about a permanent change in the condition. Thus, labels on vasoconstrictors cannot claim the product will "shrink hemorrhoids" or "shrink hemorrhoidal tissue." The most the product will do is temporarily reduce swelling, the panel pointed out.

Also taboo are words or phrases describing conditions that are not easily diagnosed by the consumer, such as "anal eczema" or "psoriasis." Labeling that leads the consumer to believe one product is superior to another because of such phrases as "contains no narcotic, anesthetic, or habit forming ingredients" would be banned by the panel, as would wording that suggests the product is "recommended by doctors" or is "doctor tested."

In addition to its recommendations regarding OTC anorectal products, the expert panel called for a study program on the history and management of anorectal diseases; a reevaluation of drugs that have been abandoned but that might be of value; formation of a committee of appropriate professional groups to develop and define acceptable anorectal terminology; formation of research groups to carry out long-range projects on anorectal disease with Federal funding; and a greater emphasis on the anorectal area of diseases of the anorectum in medical schools.

The expert panel is one of 17 such groups assisting FDA in a monumental review of the ingredients in all over-the-counter (OTC) drugs. Their report was published by FDA in the FEDERAL REGISTER to allow the public to comment on the panel's recommendations. Following a review of these comments, and its own evaluation of the report, the Agency will put into final form a monograph establishing the ingredients and labeling for this class of drugs. The panel's findings and recommendations do not necessarily reflect FDA's position.

Classification Of Anorectal Ingredients

External Use—(E) Intrarectal Use—(I)

Classification: Safe and Effective

Local Anesthetics	Protectants	Counterirritants	Antiseptics
Benzocaine in polyethylene glycol ointment (E)	Aluminum hydrochloride gel (E,I)	Menthol in aqueous solution (E)	None
Pramoxine hydrochloride (jelly and cream formulation) (E)	Calamine (E,I)		
	Cocoa butter (E,I)		**Keratolytics**
	Cod liver oil (E,I)	**Astringents**	Alcloxa (E)
	Glycerin in aqueous solution (E)	Calamine (E,I)	Resorcinol (E)
Vasoconstrictors	Kaolin (E,I)	Witchhazel water (Hamamelis water) (E)	
Ephedrine sulfate (E,I)	Lanolin (E,I)	Zinc oxide (E,I)	**Anti-cholinergics**
Epinephrine hydrochloride (E)	Mineral oil (E,I)		None
Phenylephrine hydrochloride (E,I)'	Shark liver oil (E,I)		
	Starch (E,I)	**Wound-healing Agents**	**Miscellaneous**
	White petrolatum (E,I)	None	None
	Wood alcohols (E,I)		
	Zinc oxide (E,I)		

Classification: Not Safe and Effective

Local Anesthetics	Protectants	Astringents	Antiseptics
Diperodon (E)	Bismuth subnitrate (E,I)	Tannic acid (E,I)	Boric acid (E,I)
Phenacaine hydrochloride (E,I)			Boroglycerin (E,I)
Vasoconstrictors	**Counterirritants**	**Wound-healing Agents**	Hydrastis (E,I)
Epinephrine hydrochloride (I)	Camphor (E,I)	None	Phenol (E,I)
Epinephrine undecylenate (I)	Hydrastis (E,I)	**Miscellaneous**	Resorcinol (I)
Keratolytics	Menthol (I)	Collinsonia extract (E,I)	Sodium salicylic acid phenolate (E,I)
Precipitated sulfur (I)	Turpentine oil rectified (E,I)	*E. coli* vaccines (E,I)	
Resorcinol (I)	**Anti-cholinergics**	Lappa extract (E,I)	
Sublimed sulfur (I)	Atropine (E,I)	Leptandra extract (E,I)	
	Belladonna extract (E,I)	Mullein (E,I)	

Classification: Data Insufficient For Classification (further testing required)

Local Anesthetics	Vasoconstrictors	Astringents	Keratolytics
Benzocaine in polyethylene glycol ointment (I)	Epinephrine (E,I)	None	Precipitated sulfur (E)
Benzyl alcohol (E,I)	Epinephrine undecylenate (E)	**Wound-healing Agents**	Sublimed sulfur (E)
Dibucaine (E,I)	Phenylephrine hydrochloride suppositories (I)	Cod liver oil (E,I)	**Anti-cholinergics**
Dibucaine hydrochloride (E,I)	**Protectants**	Live yeast cell derivative (E,I)	None
Diperodon (I)	Bismuth oxide (E,I)	Peruvian balsam (E,I)	**Miscellaneous**
Dyclonine hydrochloride (E,I)	Bismuth subcarbonate (E,I)	Shark liver oil (E,I)	None
Lidocaine (E,I)	Bismuth subgallate (E,I)	Vitamin A (E,I)	
Pramoxine hydrochloride in cream formulation (I)	**Counterirritants**	Vitamin D (E,I)	
Pramoxine hydrochloride jelly formulation (I)	Juniper tar (E,I)	**Antiseptics**	
Tetracaine (E,I)		Resorcinol (E)	
Tetracaine hydrochloride (E,I)			

Zits or Acne Vulgaris

ZITS . . . Those yucky blackheads, pimples, and sores your mother more politely calls acne and your doctor more graphically terms "*acne vulgaris*." At the first sign of a telltale spot on your chin you fear the worst, your looks will be ruined, nobody will go out with you, and you'll be on the fringes of society for the rest of your life.

If it makes you feel any better, this is one time when you definitely are not alone. Some 80 percent of the population develops acne to some extent during adolescence—that awkward time when you're older than a child, but younger than an adult. Acne may persist beyond the age of 25, particularly in women.

Acne is not something to make jokes about. It is a real disease of the skin that can last a long time and often can lead to severe scarring. And it can have a great effect on the life of the person suffering from it.

Technically, acne is a disease of the pilosebaceous unit in the skin.

The pilosebaceous unit is made up of a hair follicle (A) and a sebaceous gland (B), which are connected to the surface of the skin by a duct (C) through which the hair passes. ("Pilo" comes from the Latin word *pilus*, meaning hair.) The sebaceous gland produces sebum, a mixture of fats and waxes which travels through the duct and spreads over the surface of the skin to help keep the skin and hair moist.

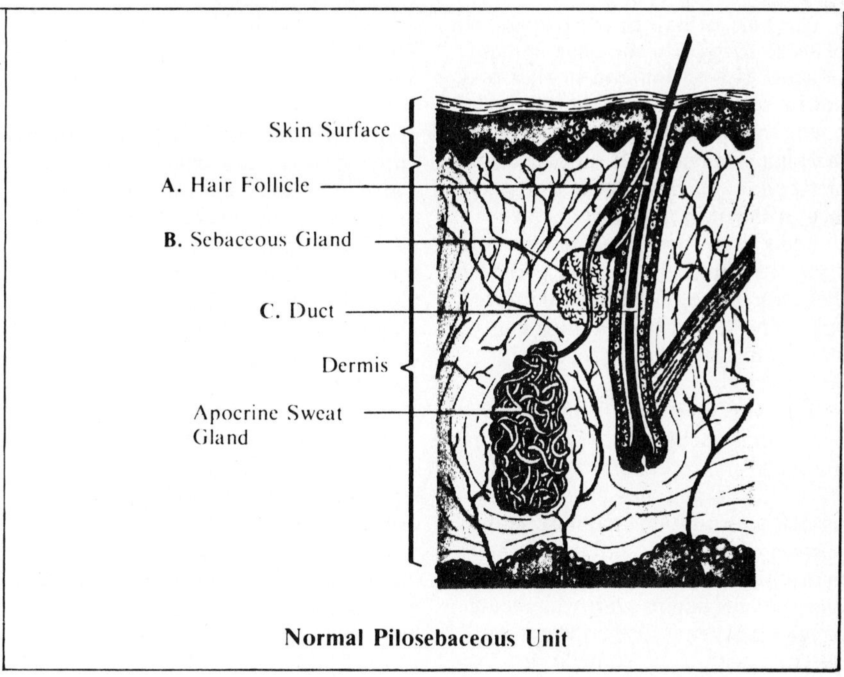

Normal Pilosebaceous Unit

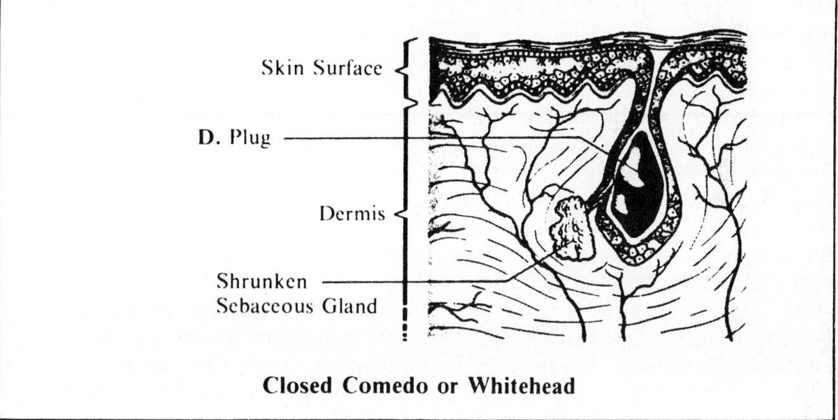

Closed Comedo or Whitehead

Acne develops when the sebaceous glands and the lining of the duct begins to work overtime. The glands produce more sebum, making the skin more oily. Normally the lining of the duct sheds cells which are carried to the surface of the skin by the sebum. When acne develops, these cells stick together to form a thick layer that blocks the duct. More cells and more sebum pile up behind this layer and form a plug called a comedo (D).

If the plug stays below the surface of the skin it is called a "closed" comedo or whitehead. If the plug enlarges and pops out of the duct it is called an "open" comedo. An open comedo (plural: comedones) is known as a blackhead because the tip is dark. This is not dirt and it won't wash away. The discoloration is due to a buildup of melanin, the dark pigment in your skin.

The kind of hair in the hair follicle plays some part in the development of acne. If it is thin and small it may not be capable of keeping the duct open. Instead, it becomes trapped in the plug. Heavier hair on the scalp or face may push the plug to the surface of the skin and thus keep the comedo from forming. Pilosebaceous units are found all over the body, but there are more of them on the face, upper chest, and back, which explains why acne usually occurs in these places.

If all you've got are some whiteheads and blackheads you have what is called "noninflammatory" acne. But if the comedones become inflamed and pimples, papules, and pustules develop, you have "inflammatory" acne. Inflammatory acne almost always begins with whiteheads, never blackheads. When excessive pressure within the comedo produces leakage into the surrounding tissue, disfiguring cysts and abcesses can form.

What makes the sebaceous glands become more active and thus causes acne to develop is not completely understood. However, it is known that acne almost always starts when the body begins to mature—at about age 11 for girls and 13 for boys. At this time boys' bodies begin to produce male hormones, called androgens, that stimulate the activity of the sebaceous gland. Girls also produce these hormones, but not as many of them. Acne tends to be more severe among boys than girls. There does seem to be a connection between a girl's menstrual cycle and the appearance of acne, perhaps the result of changes in hormone levels. Some scientists have suggested that acne may run in families, but no research has been done to prove or disprove this theory.

No germ or virus is known to cause acne, although bacteria that are normally on the skin do contribute to the development of inflammatory acne by causing the breakdown of skin fats into irritating chemicals.

Bodily changes are not the only factors in the development of acne. The disease can get its start, or certainly can be aggravated, in a number of other ways. For instance, you may find those nasty pimples forming under a tight head band or bra strap. Turtleneck shirts or sweaters that rub on the neck can make it difficult to treat acne in those areas. If you're in the habit of resting your chin on your hand, you may find acne starting up along the edge of your jaw. Using certain cosmetics, pomades (greasy hair dressing), abrasive soaps, and cleansers also can lead to acne.

Acne also can result from using some drugs, such as hormones, epileptic drugs, and antituberculosis drugs. Acne-like skin eruptions can develop from exposure to excessive humidity, industrial oils and grease, and chemicals such as the PCB's that have been in the news lately. Birth control pills seem to work in both directions. They cause acne in some women and help clear it up in others. In fact, The Pill is sometimes used to treat acne in girls and women.

One thing is fairly certain. Chocolate, nuts, cola drinks, and "fast foods" haven't a thing to do with acne. Neither does long hair, unless it is particularly oily.

What can you do about acne? First off, it is important to understand that there is no "magic bullet" that will dispose of acne once and for all. Acne can't be cured or prevented. There are things you can do and medicines you can use that will reduce your symptoms and prevent ugly scarring, but they all take time. Time, indeed, may be the best healer in some cases of mild acne that clears up as the individual suffering from it grows up.

Acne has been with us a long time. Here, for instance, is the treatment suggested by one Marcellus of Bordeaux in 350 A.D.: "Watch a falling star, then instantly while the star is still shooting from the sky, wipe the pimples with a cloth or anything that comes to hand. Just as the star falls from the sky, so the pimples will fall from your body, only you must be very careful not to wipe them with your bare hand or the pimples will be transferred to it."

On the other hand, your chances of improvement will be better if you follow a few simple rules. Don't use facial creams or moisturizers since they may block those pilosebaceous ducts. Don't wear tight-fitting garments such as head bands and turtleneck sweaters or shirts. You will want to clean your skin when it feels oily, but don't scrub it. This can only make the acne worse because it further irritates the skin. The idea is to make the skin dry. If the skin feels tight, cut down on the number of times you wash.

Ultraviolet light from sunlamps and old Sol himself helps clear up milder forms of acne. However, you should stay out of the sun if you are taking certain drugs, including some acne drugs.

While it may be tempting to pick at pimples and squeeze your blackheads the cardinal rule is—DON'T. You can cause injury to the skin and the underlying tissues. There are medical instruments called comedo extractors that are used to remove blackheads. Some doctors suggest that their patients use such an instrument themselves. Other doctors would rather remove blackheads in their office or clinic.

There are a number of medicines you can get without a doctor's prescription to treat mild acne. Sulfur, resorcinol, salicylic acid, and benzoyl peroxide are some of the ingredients found in these drug products. They are called "peeling agents" because they cause a mild irritation and a peeling of the top layer of the skin. This helps keep the pilosebaceous ducts open and get rid of the comedones.

Preparations containing benzoyl peroxide are usually applied at night after the skin has been thoroughly cleaned. Benzoyl peroxide is irritating so you should be careful not to get any on your eyelids, lips, or neck.

Don't decide to improve your suntan while you're using benzoyl peroxide since the ultraviolet rays will increase the irritation to your skin. Some people won't be able to use this medicine at all because it produces a sensitivity reaction.

If you have more than a few pimples and blackheads, you should see a dermatologist—a doctor who specializes in the treatment of skin conditions. He or she will know best how to treat your particular type of acne. One drug that might be prescribed is retinoic acid, also called "vitamin A acid" or "tretinoin." Be sure to follow the doctor's orders to the letter if this drug is prescribed for you. It can cause excessive skin irritation. Other medication should be used with caution if you are using retinoic acid. And, what is most important, you should stay out of the sun and avoid using a sunlamp no matter how pale and pasty you think you look.

When retinoic acid first came on the market in 1971 the manufacturer knew that it would make patients more sensitive to sunlight. In recent years, studies on laboratory animals have shown that the combination of retinoic acid and sunlight can increase the chance that you might get skin cancer later in life.

Some antibiotics also are used to treat and to prevent the development of pustules, papules, and cysts. They are not used to treat whiteheads or blackheads. Tetracycline is the antibiotic most often used. Because it is used over lengthy periods the daily oral dose is usually low. Once in a while a girl who is on tetracycline will develop an infection called candidal vaginitis. Other side effects that sometimes develop are irritation of the gastrointestinal system and sensitivity to light. Women who are pregnant should never take tetracyclines since these drugs will affect the developing teeth of their babies. Anytime you take tetracycline, whether for acne or some other infection, it is important to remember that this drug should never be washed down with a glass of milk or taken along with any dairy product. The milk interferes with the effectiveness of the drug. Take this medicine 1 hour before or 2 hours after meals.

There also is a topical form of tetracycline, that is, one that is applied directly to the skin. Don't be surprised if this drug makes your skin yellow. The color washes off. You may find yourself the hit of the disco dance if your doctor prescribes topical tetracycline. The drug will make treated areas of your skin fluoresce under ultraviolet light.

Sulfones and corticosteroids sometimes are used to treat very bad cases of acne.

An investigational drug that may ultimately be approved for treating very severe cases of acne is a synthetic member of the vitamin A family known as "13-cis-retinoic acid." Researchers at the Federal Government's National Cancer Institute have been testing this drug as a possible cancer preventive. They used it to treat 14 people with acne who had not been helped by any other medicines. The results were dramatic. However, numerous side effects were observed. This drug is still being tested and it is not known at this time when it might be available for the general public.

Even though some of the drugs used for acne are related to vitamin A, doctors warn that you should not try to treat yourself with large amounts of vitamin A that you can buy in drugstores or health food stores. Such self treatment could lead to serious side effects, including damage to your liver.

In very bad cases of acne the dermatologist may use surgery to drain large pustules or abcesses. Another form of surgery, called cryosurgery, involves use of liquid nitrogen or solid carbon dioxide to reduce inflamed areas of the skin. ("Cryo" means cold, and both liquid nitrogen and solid carbon dioxide are very cold.) Dermabrasion—a technique that is like sandpapering the skin—sometimes is used to remove scars left by old acne, but it is not used on new inflamed acne sores.

Although it is unlikely that a quick cure for acne is on the way, the prospects that treatments will improve are good, according to a recent report to Congress. The report is called "Analysis of Research Needs and Priorities in Dermatology" and was prepared by the leading dermatologists in this country. These prospects depend on getting financial support for basic research on such subjects as why the lining of the hair follicle behaves the way it does, how the hormones control the sebaceous glands, and on the relationship between the skin bacteria and acne. More information is needed on the natural history of the disease and the role of skin type, menstrual cycle, dietary factors (including trace metals), and stress, according to the report. And there should be more work done to develop drugs that can be applied directly to the skin.

Cellulite: Hard to Budge Pudge

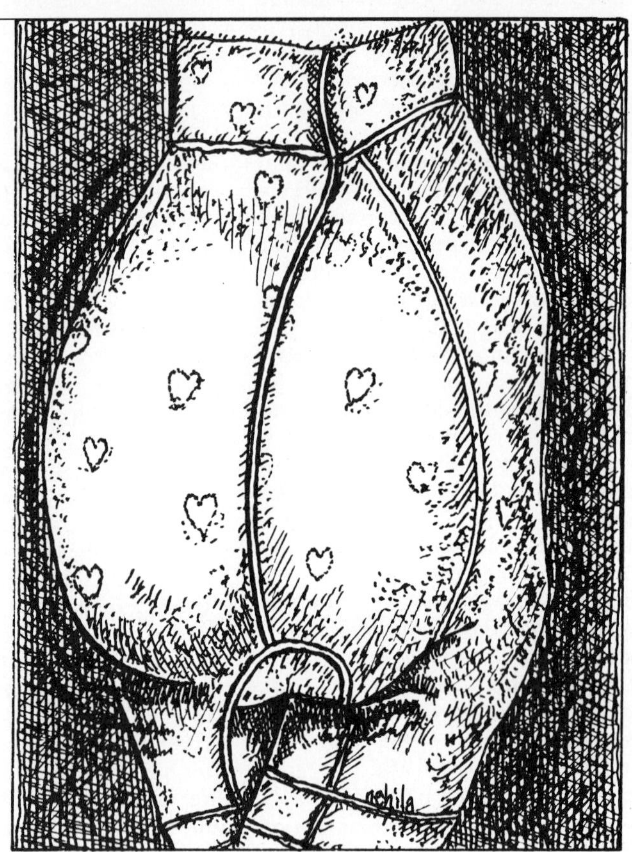

Best described as that waffly looking fat found on women's hips and thighs, cellulite is the subject of many advertisements. Supposedly it's unusual fat that can be removed only in unusual ways. But just as a rose is a rose is a rose, so fat is fat is fat.

"You don't have to be overweight to have cellulite," warns the advertisement. "Try the cellulite pinch test. No matter how thin you are, those ugly bumps just won't go away."

So thousands of women pinch the backs of their legs, watch the skin dimple and pucker until it resembles orange peel, and send away for the cream or pill or sponge that works like magic to take the "cellulite" away.

"Cellulite" (pronounced cell-u-leet) is a term coined in European salons and spas to describe those deposits of fat on women's thighs and buttocks that seem to stubbornly resist diet and exercise. It is alleged to be a special type of "fat-gone-wrong," a combination of fat, water, and toxic wastes that should have been eliminated from the body but wasn't. Cellulite theorists claim that cellulite afflicts nearly eight out of ten women, while most men aren't affected because of their different hormones and physical makeup. Because cellulite isn't "ordinary" fat, these self-styled experts claim, only extraordinary treatments will be effective.

Although the word "cellulite" was popular in European health spas back in the early 1900's, it didn't become well known in the United States until publication in 1973 of a book titled CELLULITE: THOSE LUMPS, BUMPS AND BULGES YOU COULDN'T LOSE BEFORE. The author was a Frenchwoman, Nicole Ronsard, owner of a beauty salon in New York City specializing in skin and body care, including cellulite treatment. Her book sold more than 200,000 hardcover copies, and several books on cellulite by other authors quickly followed. Articles debating the pros and cons of treatment for cellulite appeared in many popular women's magazines, particularly in the mid-1970's, and numerous beauty salons featuring "European-styled" cellulite treatments opened up around the country.

Advertisements for mail-order products to banish cellulite still appear in such publications as COSMOPOLITAN. Among products promoted as sure-fire cellulite remedies are "loofah" sponges, cactus fiber washcloths, horsehair mitts, creams that "dissolve" cellulite, vitamin-mineral supplements with herbs, exercise books, liquids to be used in the bath, massagers, rubberized pants, brushes, rollers, and toning lotions. The costs can mount quickly, especially for a complete cellulite "program," such as a $10 bottle of vitamin-mineral tablets and a $15 jar of cream.

Although these mail-order items can easily ruin a $20 bill, their cost pales in comparison with beauty salon treatments for cellulite. For instance, one skin and body care center in Chevy Chase, Md., offers 10 appointments for $250 to $280, and a New York establishment provides 12 treatments for $475. Visitors to such salons may find themselves hooked up to electrical muscle stimulators, vibrating machines, whirlpool baths, inflatable hip-high pressurized boots, tubes that shoot streams of warm air, and other marvelous gadgets. Some salons offer "hormone" or "enzyme" injections, thermal treatments with warm wax or heating pads, or vitamin-mineral supplements. Massage is particularly popular, and customers are generally given diet and exercise plans. However, even with the $200 to $500 investment they require, the salons offer no guarantees.

Before walking into one of these salons or sending money for a mail-order cellulite remedy, consumers should consider this: There is no medical evidence that these remedies work. In fact, it is difficult to find scientific evidence that cellulite even exists. None of three medical dictionaries published since 1974 (Dorland's, Steadman's, and Gould's) lists cellulite. Although the American Medical Association (AMA) has taken no position, a brief statement in the June 21, 1976, issue of AMA's journal (JAMA) says flatly: "There is no medical condition known or described as cellulite in this country."

A position paper from the Medical Society of the County of New York agrees with AMA and also says: "It is our opinion that . . . books [on cellulite] exploit women through a gimmick . . . . The truth is that fat is fat, and wherever it may be located in the body, it maintains its common characteristics."

Nevertheless, the promoters of cellulite claim that this type of fat is not the ordinary kind and is harder to dislodge. They say the connective tissues holding fat cells just underneath the skin's surface become saturated with water and waste products that aren't properly eliminated by the liver, kidneys, and other organs. These connective tissues harden and combine with fat and water to form pockets of a gel-like substance—cellulite—that bulges out to produce the characteristic orange peel appearance on the skin. Nicole Ronsard's book proposes a six-point program to rid the body of toxic wastes, hence cellulite, involving diet, elimination, breathing, exercise, massage, and relaxation.

Plausible as it may sound, the cellulite theory simply does not agree with medical knowledge. "There is absolutely no medical evidence that the connective tissue or the fat cells are subjected to toxins in response to the inability of the liver or other organs to function properly," said the New York County Medical Society in its position paper. "To present cellulite as a disorder of the liver and, by confused association, of the kidneys, intestine and skin, is a distortion of science and shows total ignorance of pathophysiology."

Vincent F. Cordaro, M.D., an FDA medical officer who has worked with the U.S. Postal Service on a number of false representation cases involving cellulite-removal products, pointed out that no evidence exists to indicate that wastes or toxins are held in any one part of the body. He pointed out that retention of body wastes is associated with serious health problems, such as kidney or intestinal diseases. "A person who retained wastes and toxins would be very ill and could die if not treated," he said. "The whole concept is irrational and unscientific."

If cellulite were really different from other fat, some chemical or structural variation should be evident. However, this is not the case, according to Neil Solomon, M.D., former secretary of Maryland's Department of Health and Mental Hygiene and author of a nationally syndicated newspaper column on health. He conducted a double-blind study with 100 people at Johns Hopkins University and City Hospital in Baltimore, in an attempt to determine if cellulite is different from common fat. Needle biopsies were taken from people with dimply, lumpy, fatty tissue resembling what the promoters call cellulite, as well as from people without cellulite. Pathologists were then asked to compare the samples. There was no difference—they all looked like ordinary fat cells.

So if it's just plain fat, why does cellulite look so bumpy?

Certain cells in the body have the capacity to store enormous amounts of fat, and about half of the body's fat is deposited in these cells immediately beneath the skin. Strands of fibrous tissue connect the skin to deeper tissue layers, and also separate the fat cell compartments. When the fat cells increase in size, this apparently causes the compartments of fat to bulge and produce a waffled appearance of the skin.

In his book ENERGETICS: YOUR KEY TO WEIGHT CONTROL, Dr. Grant Gwinup, director of research on obesity and related disorders at the University of California at Irvine, says: "Fat under the skin has a characteristic appearance which makes its identification an easy matter. It produces a waffled appearance which is similar to the pattern of irregularities on the surface of an orange and becomes more apparent when the skin fold is compressed lightly between the fingers." He also points out that most Americans carry substantially more fat than is good for them.

If there is any excess fat, it has to be stored somewhere. Several factors influence this, with sex and heredity two of the most important. Men tend to deposit fat in the abdomen, while in women, the breasts, hips, buttocks, and thighs are the choice spots.

Individuals vary in their patterns of fat distribution, and offspring are likely to follow the same pattern as their parents. A good example of this was reported by two German physicians in the JOURNAL OF DERMATOLOGIC SURGERY AND ONCOLOGY (March 1978). They were able to study the course of so-called cellulite in combination with obesity in four generations: an 8-year-old girl, her 33-year-old mother, 59-year-old grandmother, and 79-year-old great grandmother. The 8-year-old's buttocks had a waffled appearance when pinched—this was designated the "mattress phenomenon"—and in each older generation this characteristic became more pronounced and highly visible without pinching.

The mattress phenomenon was defined as a "compression and bulging of the upper fat cell chamber system that causes the overlying skin to protrude."

The German researchers found certain characteristics in women's skin and underlying tissue that they suggested would explain why women exhibit the phenomenon and men generally don't. For one thing, the connective tissue beneath women's skin creates large, round fat cell chambers, while in men the fat cell chambers are divided into small, polygonal units that don't readily bulge when filled. In addition, certain outer layers of skin in women—the epidermis and corium—are thinner than men's and more likely to reveal any bulging of fat cells underneath. These layers become even thinner and less elastic with age.

It is important to avoid being overweight from childhood on, the research team advised. "Where there is no obesity there is no so-called cellulite. We make this statement without qualification."

Since obesity—excess fat—is seen as the major culprit in forming cellulite it is not surprising that the suggested treatment for it is to lose weight. "The only effective measure, from our studies, is weight loss by means of low-calorie diets and exercises," the German researchers reported. There was one qualification, however: For the weight loss therapy to be effective, it should be done when the skin is still elastic enough to spring back when the volume of fat is reduced (that is, before 35–40 years of age).

The same remedy for cellulite was recommended by Solomon, who now runs a private practice specializing in weight control at Baltimore. "The treatment is the same in all cases—diet and exercise," he said. He emphasized that in his studies of weight loss in overweight people with significant dimpling of the skin on their thighs and buttocks, "those who lost weight lost some of the dimpling."

Unfortunately, dieting and exercising aren't easy solutions and many people are lured by unproven remedies. They are destined to be disappointed. For example, enzyme injections have been shown in European double-blind studies to be no more effective than a placebo (an inert, nonactive substance). A recent study conducted by Solomon at his Baltimore clinic, using diet, exercise, and vitamin-mineral injections similar to a formula popular in France, showed "absolutely no difference" between patients who received the formula and those who received injections of a placebo.

Another sure disappointment are the tablets claiming to use "all-natural" ingredients to remove cellulite bulges. These usually consist of a few vitamins, minerals, and herbs with possible diuretic properties, which may cause a temporary loss of water that makes the body appear slimmer. As soon as any liquid is consumed, the effect is reversed. Furthermore, no diuretic should be used without advice from a physician.

Mail-order creams and lotions that are claimed to be capable of dissolving cellulite contain essentially the same type of ingredients as common lubricating lotions: water, emollients, emulsifying agents, preservatives, colors, and fragrances. An interesting addition to some creams is capsicum, or hot pepper, which can act as a local irritant and cause the skin to redden and tingle. This sensation may help convince the purchaser that the product is more than an ordinary lotion, even when no proof of any cellulite-dissolving effect is offered.

In the past few years, the U.S. Postal Service has filed complaints against more than a dozen promoters of cellulite treatments for obtaining money through the mails by false representation. Most signed consent agreements promising to cease representing that their products could cause weight loss and control cellulite. In addition, money sent by prospective purchasers was returned.

The Food and Drug Administration works with the Postal Service in false representation cases by reviewing the products and advertisements in question and providing advisory opinions about whether the product will perform as claimed.

On another front, FDA routinely obtains imports of cellulite-reducing devices. In recent years the Agency has also caused the seizure and destruction of a number of weight-control and "body-altering" products, including two cellulite treatment devices that had been imported prior to the restriction and were in use in New York City and Helena, Mont. The Italian-made machines, which had been leased to salons specializing in cellulite treatment, combined a heating pad, electrical muscle stimulator, and iontopheresis device (normally used in skin care). On the machines' labeling and literature were claims that the device could reduce and reproportion the body, help destroy thick fat deposits, improve circulation, and provide benefits to the muscles equivalent to 9 hours of exercise. A U.S. district court found the devices were misbranded because of false and misleading claims and inadequate directions for use, including failure to bear adequate warnings against unsafe use.

Obesity experts agree that no equipment, exercise, or treatment can remove fat exclusively from a single area of the body. Ironically, some studies have shown that spot exercises can sometimes make the exercised limbs look bulkier instead of slimmer. In one study at UC Irvine, Gwinup compared the arm circumference and fat pad (fat measurement using special calipers) on the arms of tennis players to determine if their more active arm carried less fat. Not only did the fat pad measure exactly the same on both arms, but the arm used more often by the players had a larger circumference because the muscles were bigger.

In another study, Gwinup measured the fat pad and circumference of the thighs of a group of slightly obese girls, then required them to exercise only one leg in a gym for 13 weeks. At the end of that period he remeasured the fat pad and found no difference between the exercised and non-exercised legs. However, the exercised legs were larger in circumference because the size of the muscles had increased.

This is not intended to discourage exercising to help lose weight. Exercise uses up energy, and if the body does not obtain enough energy from food, it will eventually turn to its own fat deposits. Exercise can also improve appearance by tightening and strengthening the muscles—for example, it can be easier to hold in your stomach when the muscles are in good shape. However, most obesity experts agree with Gwinup: "There's no such thing as spot reducing. The only way to get rid of fat on your thighs is to get rid of it all over your body."

Obviously, there are no easy answers. Dieting and exercise require much discipline and the appeal of effortless slenderizing promised through other means is understandable. Unfortunately scientific and medical evidence doesn't support the fantasies these remedies offer.

It's enough to make you wish for the days when round, well-fed figures were being glorified by the Flemish painter Peter Paul Rubens. His voluptuous models were the ideal of womanhood back in the early 1600's. You can be sure *they* didn't worry about cellulite.

Not for Women Only: Varicose Veins

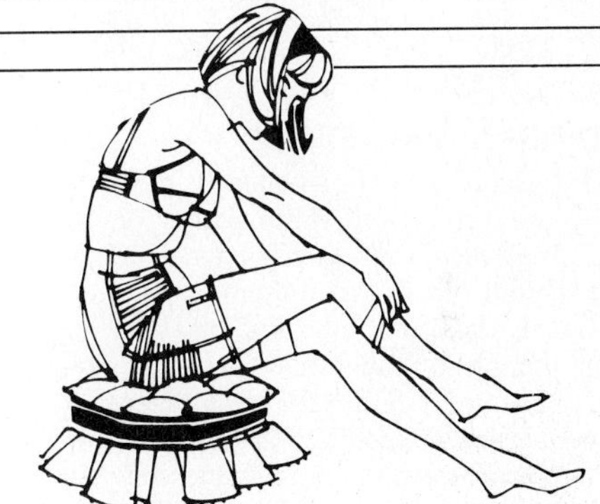

WHAT ARE VARICOSE VEINS?

The word, "varicose," means "swollen." Thus, varicose veins, which doctors may call "varicosities," are swollen, enlarged veins. They are found most frequently on the inner side and back of the calf and on the inner side of the thigh. Bluish in color, they are visible through the skin when close to its surface—and look something like a map's drawing of a river and the streams that flow into it.

The superficial veins, those lying just under the skin, are most commonly affected. The deep veins, which run inside the muscles of the leg and thigh, are seldom seriously afflicted with varicosities because they are surrounded and supported by the muscles.

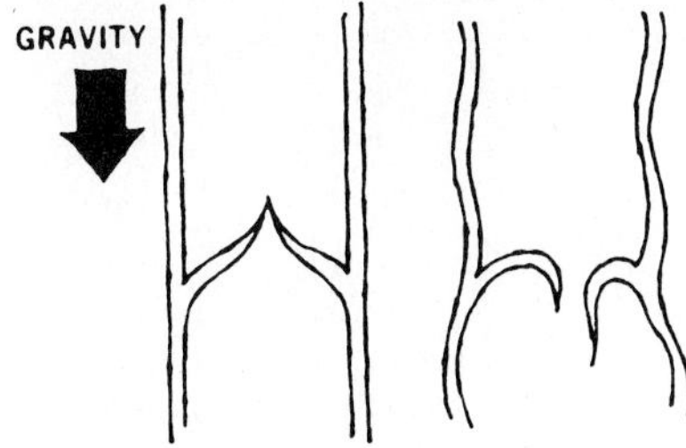

WHAT CAUSES VARICOSE VEINS?

Veins contain valves which permit the blood to flow only in the direction of the heart. One of the main causes of varicose veins seems to be valves that leak, allowing blood to flow backward into the vessel rather than continuing on its way to the heart.

This increases blood pressure in the section of the vein below the faulty valve. Veins are low-pressure vessels. Their walls are thinner and have less muscle in them than do the walls of arteries. When continually subjected to abnormally high pressures, the veins become stretched and swollen. The result is the condition which we know as "varicose veins."

Inherited weakness in the structure of the veins greatly increases the individual's susceptibility to varicose veins. Other contributing factors are diseases, such as phlebitis—an inflammation of the veins, which weakens or damages the walls and valves of the veins.

Abdominal pressure, from the stomach muscles—such as that caused by heavy lifting, coughing, and straining—may also contribute to the development of varicose veins.

Obesity and increasing age are other factors in causing varicose veins. Obesity's useless, fat weight may play a role in overworking the veins. With increasing age there is a loss of tone of the skin and tissues which surround the veins and help to support them.

WHO HAS VARICOSE VEINS?

Varicose veins are widespread throughout the population and affect almost all ages. However, they are most common in people over forty, affecting one out of every two women and one out of every four men in this age group.

Occupation may be a factor in acquiring varicose veins. Persons in occupations that require a great deal of standing, such as elevator operators, beauticians, dentists, and salespeople, seem more prone to varicose veins than people with sit-down jobs. To illustrate this point: it has been found that pressure in the leg veins is increased 5 times when a person stands erect from lying down.

But people in jobs requiring sitting in one place for long periods of time also have a problem. These people should walk around or elevate their feet from time to time to prevent excessive pooling of blood in the veins of the lower leg.

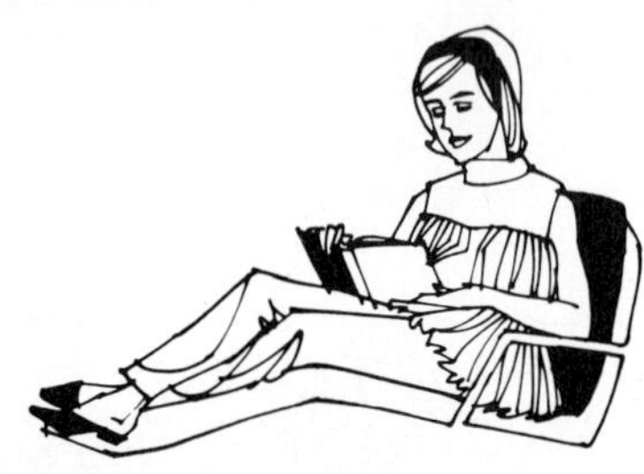

WOMEN IN PARTICULAR

Pregnant women frequently develop varicose veins, sometimes rather early in pregnancy, but more often during later months. The main factors contributing to their development are:

- increased abdominal pressure resulting from the enlarging uterus
- increased bloodflow to and from the lower abdominal and pelvic areas

Both factors act indirectly to hinder return flow from the leg veins, thus increasing blood pressure in these blood vessels.

Unless severe, varicose veins of pregnancy frequently improve substantially without treatment, after delivery.

One of the main kinds of varicose veins, the smaller "spidery type," appears most frequently among women, particularly among women of middle age and those past the menopause.

Among women, a contributing cause of varicose veins is the use of tight garters, girdles, and other clothing which tends to obstruct the veins' bloodflow and thus to increase pressure on the veins. By eliminating or reducing the use of these constricting items from the wardrobe, women can themselves do much to prevent varicose veins or to reduce their severity.

Girdles are made primarily for the standing woman and tend to press down and tightly constrict the big veins of the leg when she sits down. Those with varicose veins, or with a tendency toward them, should not wear girdles, especially if they are going to sit for a long time, as on a long trip by plane, automobile, or train.

SYMPTOMS

Most victims of varicose veins have a combination of many symptoms. Among these symptoms are changes in the appearance of the leg; increased tendency to fatigue of the leg muscles; a sensation of fullness and congestion; soreness in the region of the veins after standing for a long period of time; muscular cramps, particularly at night; and itching and burning sensations in the region of varicose veins.

DIAGNOSING VARICOSE VEINS

In medical terms, there are several kinds of varicose veins. Some can be helped by surgery, some by injection therapy, and some by other simpler measures. An examination is necessary for the doctor to determine the best treatment.

All who have, or suspect they may have, varicose veins should have a complete physical examination. This is important because the presence or absence of other possible diseases is significant for the physician in considering diagnosis and treatment.

Although the doctor, by inspecting and manipulating areas of the leg, can usually establish their presence, various other tests have been developed to aid in diagnosing varicose veins. One of these procedures is called venography. In this test, a radiopaque substance is injected into the veins. Then the blood flow and the working of the valves in the vessels are checked by means of X-rays.

TREATMENT

Conservative Therapy. In mild cases of varicose veins it may be possible to relieve much of the discomfort and to prevent the veins from becoming worse by wearing support hosiery. This hosiery helps to provide additional support to offset excessive blood pressure within the veins. Support hosiery, available in stockings for women and socks for men, should be carefully fitted on the basis of precise leg measurements. With the improved stretch yarns now available, it is possible to make this hosiery attractive and at the same time functional in giving needed support to the legs.

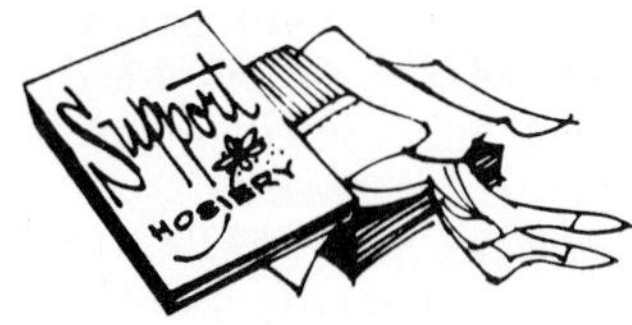

The person with mild varicose veins should also get adequate periods of rest with his feet and legs elevated. He should try to avoid prolonged periods of standing. But, if this is unavoidable because of occupation or other factors, elastic bandages may provide better support than can usually be obtained with support hosiery.

"Bicycling" exercises while lying on the back, swimming, and walking are recommended forms of exercise for persons with mild varicose veins.

Injection. Varicose veins can be injected with a sclerosing (hardening) solution to block off the part of the vein that is swollen. The blood normally carried by that vessel is re-routed through other veins. For a time after injection, the injected vein may be swollen and tender, but this subsides within a few hours or days. Thereafter, the injected section usually withers and gradually disappears over a period of weeks to months. This process may be hastened by removing some of the coagulated blood from the blocked section through a small incision.

Injection is probably best reserved for the treatment of the small varicose veins lying very near the surface of the skin.

Injection treatment has some drawbacks, however. Permanent results cannot be guaranteed, numerous injections may be necessary, and elastic pressure bandages have to be worn for the duration of treatment.

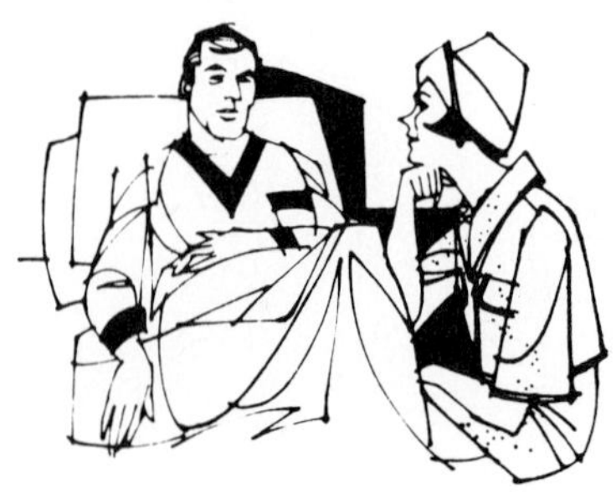

Surgery. Surgery for tying off or removing the vein is quicker and the results are more likely to be permanent. If the patient is otherwise in good health, the surgical risk is slight. However, surgery does require a hospital stay and is relatively expensive.

To the question of how well a victim can get along without the veins that are being injected, tied off, or removed, the answer is: far better than he can get along with them. Varicose veins are inefficient in carrying out their function of returning blood "uphill" to the heart. In fact, in a severely affected vein, blood flow may be in the opposite direction. Thus, blocking or removing that vein actually improves the overall performance of the system of veins.

The physician is the only one who can determine the best course of treatment. After the examination, he will take into account such factors as the patient's general state of health, weight, reaction to drugs, and high or low blood pressure. Then he can suggest the best specific therapy indicated for the individual case. The fact that one has varicose veins does not always have to mean discomfort. Even the worst case is usually responsive to treatment.

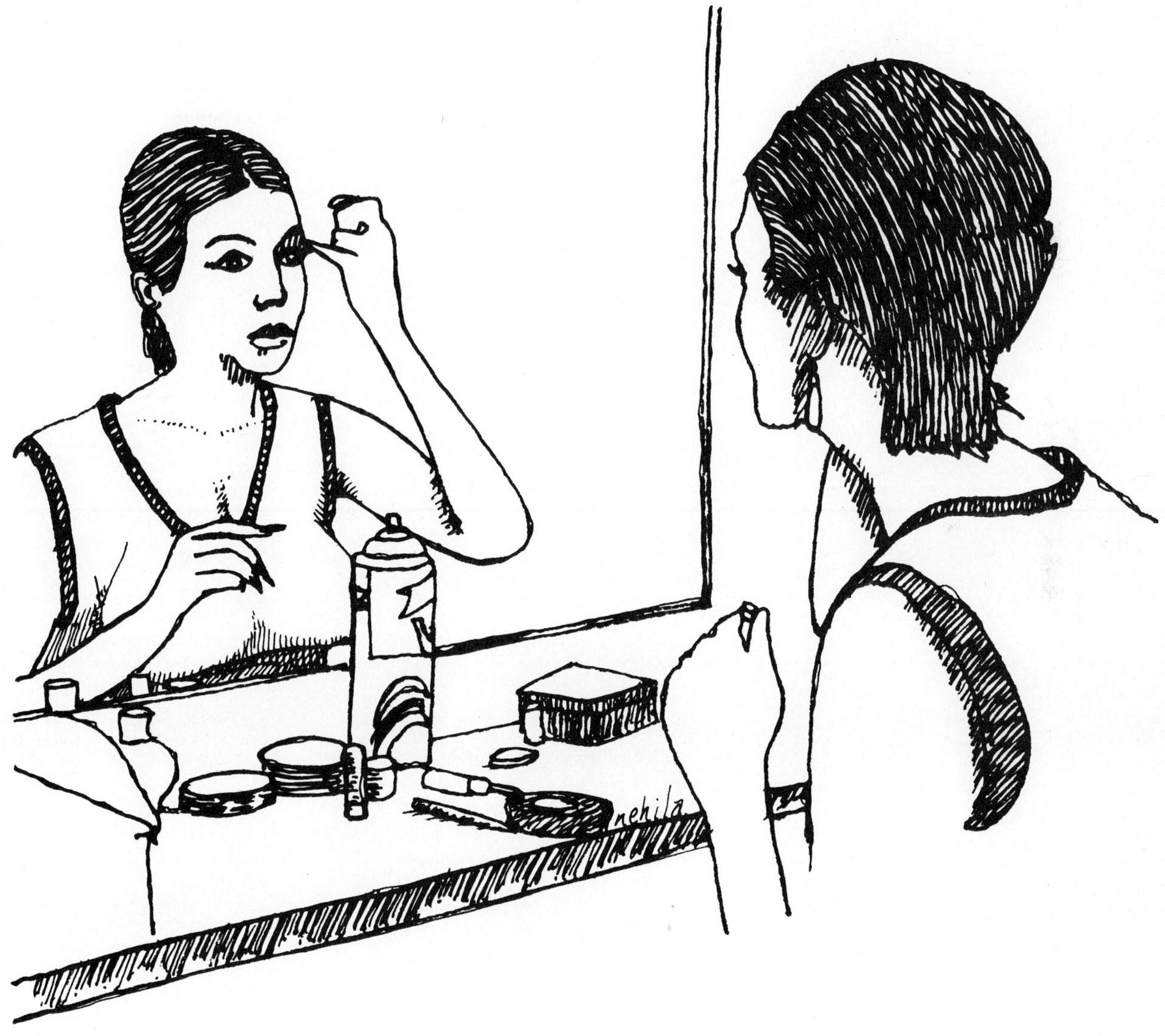

Fitness Programs

Adult Physical Fitness: A Program for Women and Men

INTRODUCTION

If you have decided that it is time to get in shape, you have a rewarding adventure ahead.

The two programs in this book—one for women, one for men—are designed to help you condition yourself and achieve physical fitness on a sound, progressive basis.

Each incorporates principles which, research has shown, can help you increase your strength, stamina and flexibility; look, feel and work better; enjoy life more zestfully, and—very probably—enjoy it longer.

Like millions of adult Americans who today recognize the desirability of physical fitness and would earnestly like to achieve it, you probably have wondered what to do, how to begin, how far to go—and, not least of all, whether you can spare the time, whether fitness is something that can be achieved by busy people with little time to spare.

The programs are designed so that:

You will know exactly how and where to begin—and what to do every step of the way.

You will begin easily—without strain or upset—no matter how long since you engaged in vigorous physical activity.

You will make steady progress toward a level of fitness that you will be able to determine is most suitable for you—and that you will be able to maintain.

You will have the satisfaction of being able to measure your progress as you proceed.

You will be able to proceed at home—without special equipment—and at a convenient time.

And the time required will not be excessive.

Physical fitness can be achieved at any age. You do not achieve it overnight. It does take effort. But the resulting feelings of well-being, renewed strength and vitality are well worth the effort—and you can start on your way right now.

SPECIFIC FACTS YOU'LL WANT TO KNOW ABOUT PHYSICAL FITNESS

What it is

In a technical sense, physical fitness can be viewed as a measure of the body's strength, stamina and flexibility. In more meaningful personal terms, it is a reflection of your ability to work with vigor and pleasure, without undue fatigue, with energy left for enjoying hobbies and recreational activities, and for meeting unforeseen emergencies. It relates to how you look and how you feel—and, because the body is not a compartment separate from the mind, it relates to how you feel mentally as well as physically.

Physical fitness is many-faceted. Basic to it are proper nutrition, adequate rest and relaxation, good health practices, and good medical and dental care.

But these are not enough. An essential element is physical activity—exercise for a body that needs it.

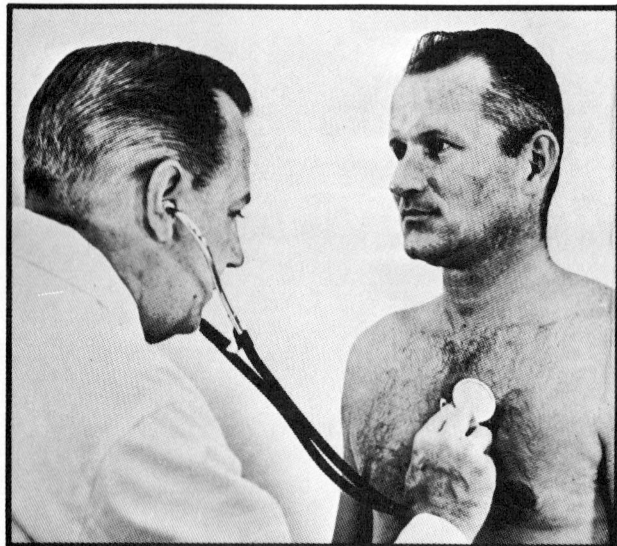

Why exercise?

Wherever there is muscle there is need of movement.

The human body contains more than 600 muscles; overall, it is more than half muscle.

Muscles make possible every overt motion. They also push food along the digestive tract, suck air into the lungs, tighten blood vessels to raise blood pressure when you need more pressure to meet an emergency. The heart itself is a muscular pump.

Technological advances have changed our way of living, have made strenuous physical exertion largely unnecessary. The word "chore" has virtually gone out of use.

But the needs of the human body have not changed. Muscles are meant to be used. When they are not used, or not used enough, they deteriorate. If we are habitually inactive—if we succumb to the philosophy of easy living—we must then pay the price in decreased efficiency.

Research support for regular physical activity as an essential for healthful and vigorous living is increasing constantly.

That we are, to a great degree, what our muscles make us—weak or strong, vigorous or lethargic—is a growing conviction among medical men.

Offering strong support for this conviction is the following observation by a former president of the American Medical Association: "It begins to appear that exercise is the master conditioner for the healthy and the major therapy for the ill."

A 1962 survey of a cross section of physicians—nearly 4,000—showed that almost all now believe strongly that positive health benefits, both physical and mental, accompany physical fitness resulting from regular, moderate exercise. It also revealed that the great majority have come to favor the inclusion of tests of physical fitness in periodic health examinations—and are convinced that physical fitness programs, which have been largely aimed at children, are even more necessary for adults.

Some specific benefits

An obvious effect of regular exercise is the firming of flabby muscles.

In addition, research indicates that exercise produces beneficial changes in the functioning of internal organs—especially the heart, lungs and circulatory system. The heart beat becomes stronger and steadier, breathing becomes deeper and circulation improves.

Research lists these benefits experienced by people who, after a prolonged period of sedentary living, undertake a systematic conditioning program:

- Increased strength, endurance and coordination
- Increased joint flexibility
- Reduction of minor aches, pains, stiffness and soreness
- Correction of remediable postural defects
- Improvement in general appearance
- Increased efficiency with reduced expenditure of energy in performing both physical and mental tasks
- Improved ability to relax and to voluntarily reduce tension
- Reduction of chronic fatigue

Exercise and chronic fatigue

Ranking today as one of the most frequently voiced of all complaints, chronic tiredness can stem from illness. But in many people, investigators report, it is the result of gradual deterioration of the body for lack of enough vigorous physical activity.

Continual inactivity produces muscular atrophy and the individual soon becomes under-muscled for his weight. The result: he lacks the strength and endurance to do his daily work easily and efficiently.

One important end result of the increased muscular strength and general endurance provided by exercise is an increase in the body's capacity for carrying on normal daily activities, a pushing back of fatigue limits.

Valid research indicates that a fit person uses less energy for any given movement or effort than a flabby or weak person.

Exercise and the heart

An old-fashioned idea—that exercise may be bad for the heart—has been shown to be without scientific foundation. Not only that—it has been proven that appropriate exercise strengthens the heart.

A noted heart specialist recently commented: "The best insurance against coronary (heart) disease is exercise—lots of it."

Backing up this conviction is a growing body of evidence. It includes findings of lower cholesterol values in active people, faster clearing of fats from the blood after meals—and sharply reduced heart attack rates.

A recent study covering 120,000 American railroad employees revealed the heart attack incidence among sedentary office workers to be almost twice that of men working in the yards. Other studies—in the United States, England and elsewhere—also show a higher rate of heart attacks among the sedentary than among the physically active.

Additionally, the studies indicate that, when a heart attack does occur, the physically active person is more likely to recover. One possible reason: there is evidence that exercise may promote development of supplementary blood vessels which can take over the burden of nourishing the heart muscle when a coronary artery is blocked in a heart attack.

Exercise and aging

There is strong authoritative support for the concept that regular exercise can help prevent degenerative disease and slow down the physical deterioration that accompanies aging.

The evidence is conclusive: individuals who consistently engage in proper physical activity have better job performance records, fewer degenerative diseases, and probably a longer life expectancy than the population at large. By delaying the aging process, proper exercise also prolongs your active years.

A special note about weight

A common misconception is that exercise does not aid in weight control. This is not the case. Research shows:

That fat piles up in most people by only a few calories a day;

That an excess of only 100 calories a day can produce a 10-pound gain in a year—and that the extra calories could be burned up by a 15- to 20-minute daily walk;

That obese people almost invariably tend to be much less active than those of normal weight;

That individual weight, moreover, is a factor in energy expenditure. If you are overweight, you will burn up more calories in performing exercise than a person of normal weight.

According to studies by the Harvard School of Public Health, one-half hour of proper exercise each day can keep off or take off as much as 26 pounds a year.

Inactivity is the most important factor explaining the frequency of "creeping" overweight in modern Western society. And the consensus now among medical and health authorities is that the most effective way to take off weight and keep it off is through a program which combines proper exercise and reasonable diet.

If you need to lose weight, do so under the direction of your physician. Don't lose more than two pounds per week without his knowledge and consent. Determine to reduce gradually and consistently. Determine to develop proper eating habits. A change in diet—perhaps a change as slight as taking a little less sugar or none in beverages—may be all that is necessary to bring your weight down and keep it down, especially if coupled with the essential exercise regimen.

If you're handicapped

Where there is impairment or illness, any and all exercise should be medically prescribed and regulated.

Today, physicians are using exercise as an aid in combatting many chronic problems, including arthritis, asthma, diabetes and emphysema. A common type of low back pain has been traced to weakened back muscles, and exercise has been used both to produce relief and to help prevent recurrences.

If you have a handicap, your doctor may find that some or many of the exercises given in this manual—perhaps with modifications—could be of value to you.

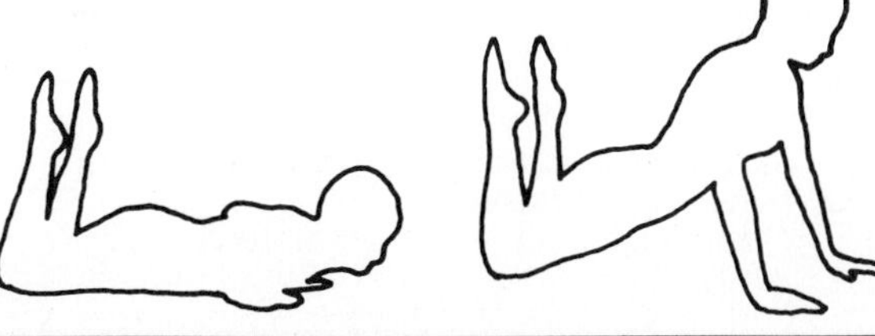

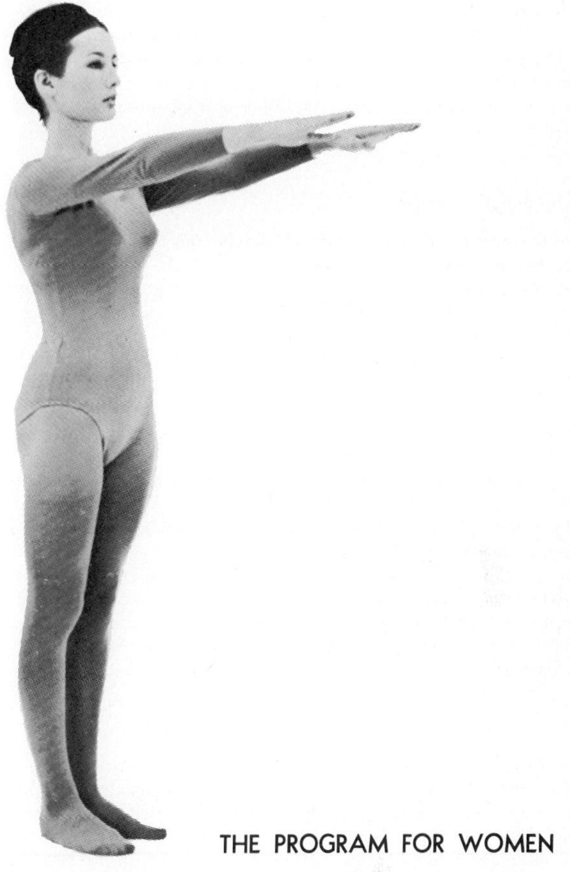

THE PROGRAM FOR WOMEN

Before you begin

A medical examination at least once a year is generally advisable for every adult. It's an excellent idea to get such an examination now before beginning your conditioning program.

Very probably your physician will be able to recommend that you proceed without restriction. If he should find any physical problem, he can take steps to correct it—and may have suggestions for modifying the program to make it more suitable for you.

Once you have had an examination, you can proceed confidently.

A reassuring word about muscles

As you make use of the program in the following pages, you need have no fear of becoming heavily, unattractively muscled. On the contrary:

With disuse or little use, muscles tend to become less elastic, weaker, softer. They lose tone.

The exercises you will be working with are designed to firm your muscles, restore their tone, increase their strength and flexibility. Your appearance will improve as certain muscles—in the abdomen and back, for example—become able to provide better support. As others—in the arms, legs—become more responsive, every move you make is likely to be easier and more graceful.

About the program

It assumes that you have not been engaging recently in consistent, vigorous, all-round physical activity—even though, in housework or other daily routines, you have put some muscles to extensive use.

It starts with an orientation or "get-set" series of exercises that will allow you to bring all major muscles into use easily and painlessly.

There are then five graded levels.

As you move from one to the next, you will be building toward a practical and satisfying level of fitness.

By building gradually, progressively, you will be building soundly.

What the exercises are for

There are three general types—warmup exercises, conditioning exercises and circulatory activities.

The warmup exercises stretch and limber up the muscles and speed up the action of the heart and lungs, thus preparing the body for greater exertion and reducing the possibility of unnecessary strain.

The conditioning exercises are systematically planned to tone up abdominal, back, leg, arm and other major muscles.

The circulatory activities produce contractions of large muscle groups for relatively longer periods than the conditioning exercises—to stimulate and strengthen the circulatory and respiratory systems.

The plan calls for doing 10 mild exercises during the orientation period and, thereafter, the warmup exercises and the seven conditioning exercises listed for each level. The first six exercises of the orientation program are used as warmup exercises throughout the graded levels.

When it comes to the circulatory activities, you choose one each workout. Alternately running and walking . . . skipping rope . . . running in place. All are effective. You can choose running and walking on a pleasant day, one of the others for use indoors when the weather is inclement. You can switch about for variety.

How you progress

A sound physical conditioning program should take into account your individual tolerance—your ability to execute a series of activities without undue discomfort or fatigue. It should provide for developing your tolerance by increasing the work load so you gradually become able to achieve more and more with less and less fatigue and with increasingly rapid recovery.

As you move from level to level, some exercises will be modified so they call for increased effort.

Others will remain the same but you will build more strength and stamina by increasing the number of repetitions.

You will be increasing your fitness another way as well.

At level 1, your objective will be to gradually reduce, from workout to workout, the "breathing spells" between exercises until you can do the seven conditioning exercises without resting. You will proceed in the same fashion with the more difficult exercises and increased repetitions at succeeding levels.

You will find the program designed—the progression carefully planned—to make this feasible. You will be able to proceed at your own pace, competing with yourself rather than with anyone else—and this is of great importance for sound conditioning.

Note: Gradually speeding up, from workout to workout, the rate at which you do each exercise will provide greater stimulation for the circulatory and respiratory systems and also help to keep your workouts short. However, the seven conditioning exercises should not be a race against time. Perform each exercise correctly to insure maximum benefit.

Choosing your goal

There is no need to pick the level to which you want to go—now.

Many women will be able to advance through the first three levels. While the fourth is challenging, some women will be able to achieve it. The fifth is one which only extremely vigorous, well-conditioned women will reach.

The level of fitness you can reach depends upon your age, your body's built-in potential capacity and previous conditioning. It also depends upon your state of mind; as you know, when you want to do something and believe you can, it is much easier to do than otherwise.

While there will be no dramatic overnight changes, gradually over the next weeks and months, as you progress through the first levels, you will begin to notice a new spring in your step, a new ease with which you accomplish your ordinary daily activities. You will find yourself with more energy left at the end of the working day and a new zest for recreation in the evening. Quite likely, you will be sleeping more soundly than you have slept for many years and waking more refreshed in the morning.

After completing the early levels, you may come to realize that you can—and want to—go further. Go as far as you can.

The important point is that, no matter what level you choose, you will greatly improve your physical fitness and you will be able to maintain the improvement and continue to enjoy the benefits.

When and how often to work out

To be most beneficial, exercise should become part of your daily routine—as much so as bathing, dressing.

Five workouts a week are called for throughout the program.

You can choose any time that's convenient. Preferably, it should be the same time every day—but it doesn't matter whether it's upon arising, at some point during the morning or afternoon, or in the evening.

How long at each level

Your objective at each level will be to reach the point where you can do all the exercises called for, for the number of times indicated, without resting between exercises.

But, start slowly.

It cannot be emphasized enough that by moving forward gradually you will be moving forward solidly, avoiding sudden strains and excesses that could make you ache and hold you back for several days.

If you find yourself at first unable to complete any exercises—to do continuously all the repetitions called for—stop when you encounter difficulty. Rest briefly, then take up where you left off and complete the count. If you have difficulty at first, there will be less and less with succeeding workouts.

Stay at each level for at least three weeks. If you have not passed the prove-out test at the end of that time, continue at the same level until you do. The prove-out test calls for performing—in three consecutive workouts—the seven conditioning exercises without resting and satisfactorily fulfilling the requirement for one circulatory activity.

A measure of your progress

You will, of course, be able to observe the increase in your strength and stamina from week to week in many ways—including the increasing facility with which you do the exercises at a given level.

In addition, there is a 2-minute step test you can use to measure and keep a running record of the improvement in your circulatory efficiency, one of the most important of all aspects of fitness.

The immediate response of the cardiovascular system to exercise differs markedly between well-conditioned individuals and others. The test measures the response in terms of pulse rate taken shortly after a series of steps up and down onto a bench or chair.

Although it does not take long, it is necessarily vigorous. Stop if you become overly fatigued while taking it. You should not try it until you have completed the orientation period.

The test

Use any sturdy bench or chair 15–17 inches in height.

Count 1—Place right foot on bench.

Count 2—Bring left foot alongside of right and stand erect.

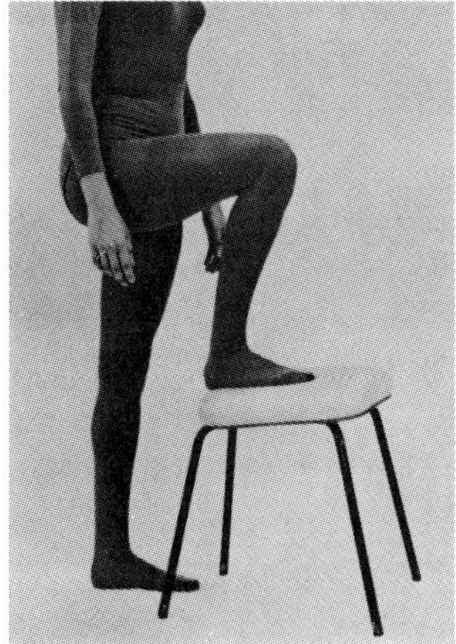

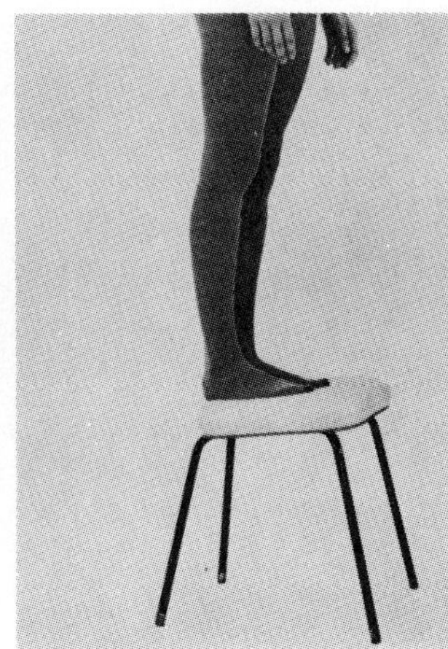

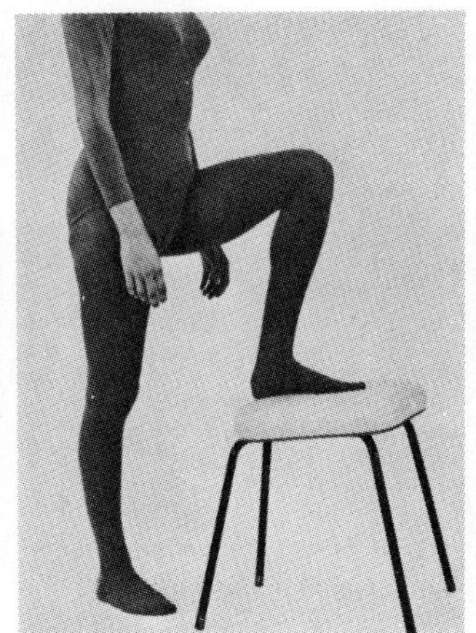

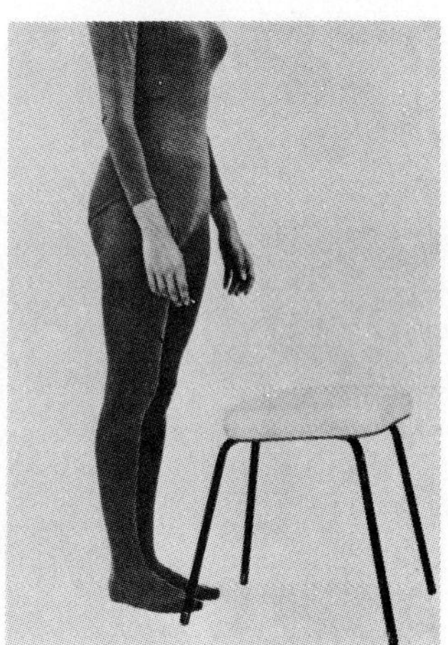

Count 3—Lower right foot to floor.
Count 4—Lower left foot to floor.

REPEAT the 4-count movement 30 times a minute for two minutes.

THEN sit down on bench or chair for two minutes.

FOLLOWING the 2-minute rest, take your pulse for 30 seconds. Double the count to get the per-minute rate. (You can find the pulse by applying middle and index finger of one hand firmly to the inside of the wrist of the other hand, on the thumb side.)

Record your score for future comparisons. In succeeding tests—about once every two weeks—you probably will find your pulse rate becoming lower as your physical condition improves.

Three important points:

1. For best results, do not engage in physical activity for at least 10 minutes before taking the test. Take it at about the same time of day and always use the same bench or chair.

2. Remember that pulse rates vary among individuals. This is an individual test. What is important is not a comparison of your pulse rate with that of anybody else—but rather a record of how your own rate is reduced as your fitness increases.

3. As you progress, the rate at which your pulse is lowered should gradually level off. This is an indication that you are approaching peak fitness.

Your progress records

Charts are provided for the orientation program and for each of the five levels.

They list the exercises to be done and the goal for each exercise in terms of number of repetitions, distance, etc.

They also provide space in which to record your progress—(1) in completing the recommended 15 workouts at each level, (2) in accomplishing the three prove-out workouts before moving on to a succeeding level, and (3) in the results as you take the step test from time to time.

A sample chart and progress record for one of the five levels is shown below.

You do the warmup exercises and the conditioning exercises along with one circulatory activity for each workout.

Check off each workout as you complete it. The last three numbers are for the prove-out workouts, in which the seven conditioning exercises should be done without resting. Check them off as you accomplish them.

You are now ready to proceed to the next level.

As you take the step test—at about 2-week intervals—enter your pulse rate.

When you move on to the next level, transfer the last pulse rate from the preceding level. Enter it in the margin to the left of the new progress record and circle it so it will be convenient for continuing reference.

SAMPLE	GOAL
Warmup Exercises	**Exercises 1–6 of Orientation program**
Conditioning Exercises	**Uninterrupted repetitions**
1. Bend and stretch	10
2. Sprinter	6
3. Sitting stretch	15
4. Knee pushup	12
5. Situp (fingers laced)	10
6. Leg raiser	10 each leg
7. Flutter kick	30
Circulatory activity (choose one each workout)	
Jog-walk (jog 50, walk 50)	½ mile
Rope (skip 30 secs.; rest 60 secs.)	3 series
Run in place (run 100, hop 25 – 2 cycles)	3 minutes
Water activities—See recommendations in Section IV.	

Your progress record	1	2	3	4	5	6	7	8	9	10	11	12	13 14 15 Prove-out workouts
Step test (pulse)													

Getting set—orientation workouts

With the series of mild exercises listed in the chart on the next page and illustrated and described on the next two pages, you can get yourself ready—without severe aches or pains—for the progressive conditioning program.

Plan to spend a minimum of one week for preliminary conditioning. Don't hesitate to spend two weeks or three if necessary for you to limber up enough to accomplish all the exercises easily and without undue fatigue.

The Exercises

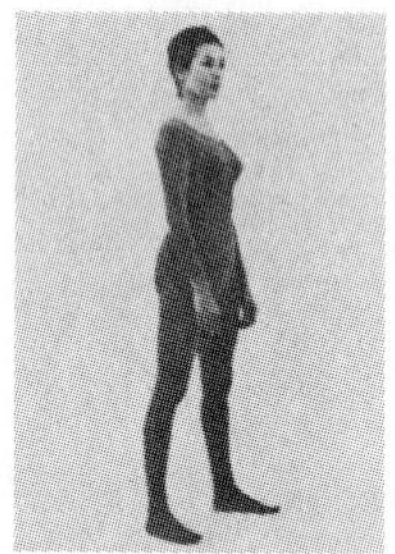
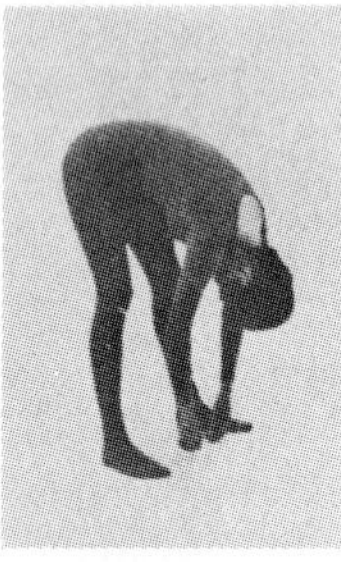

1. BEND AND STRETCH

Starting position: Stand erect, feet shoulder-width apart.
Action: Count 1. Bend trunk forward and down, flexing knees. Stretch gently in attempt to touch fingers to toes or floor. Count 2. Return to starting position.
Note: Do slowly, stretch and relax at intervals rather than in rhythm.

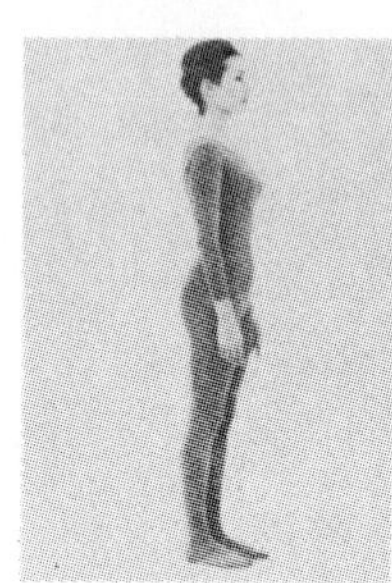
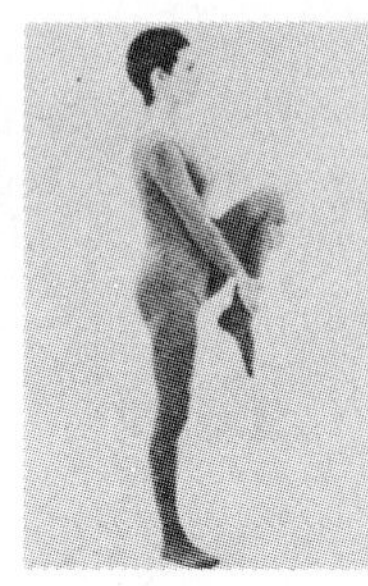

2. KNEE LIFT

Starting position: Stand erect, feet together, arms at sides.
Action: Count 1. Raise left knee as high as possible, grasping leg with hands and pulling knee against body while keeping back straight. Count 2. Lower to starting position. Counts 3 and 4. Repeat with right knee.

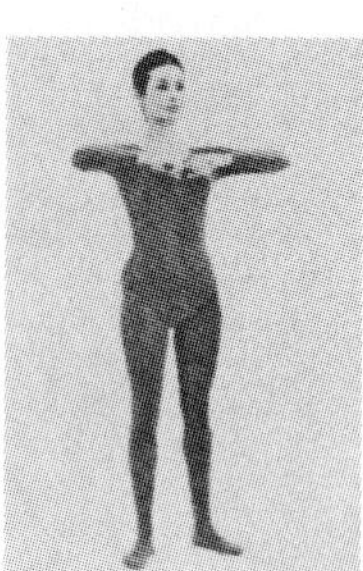
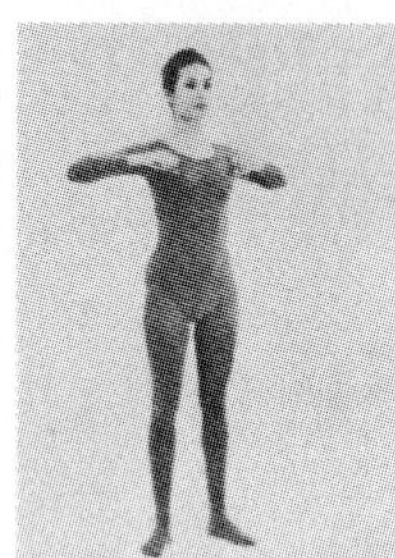

3. WING STRETCHER

Starting position: Stand erect, elbows at shoulder height, fists clenched in front of chest.
Action: Count 1. Thrust elbows backward vigorously without arching back. Keep head erect, elbows at shoulder height. Count 2. Return to starting position.

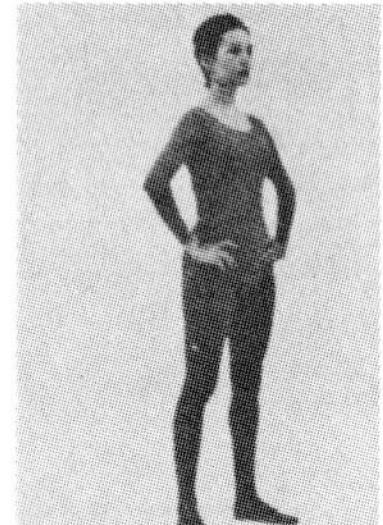
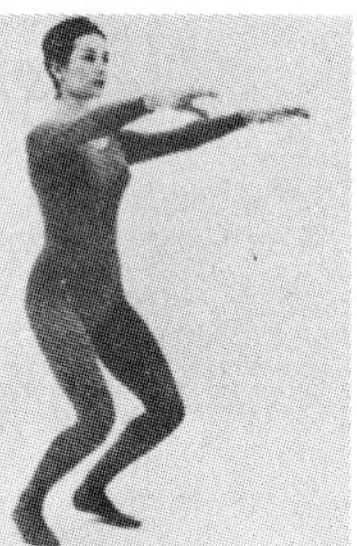

4. HALF KNEE BEND

Starting position: Stand erect, hands on hips.
Action: Count 1. Bend knees halfway while extending arms forward, palms down. Count 2. Return to starting position.

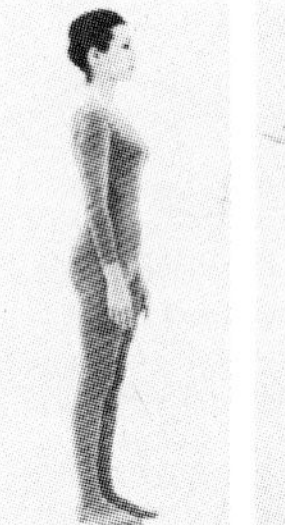
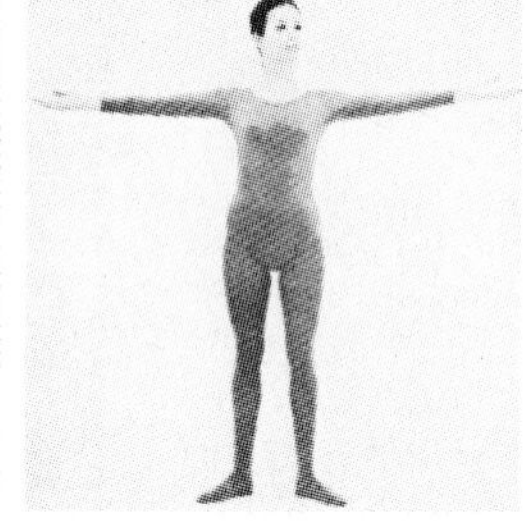

5. ARM CIRCLES

Starting position: Stand erect, arms extended sideward at shoulder height, palms up.
Action: Describe small circles backward with hands. Keep head erect. Do 15 backward circles. Reverse, turn palms down and do 15 small circles forward.

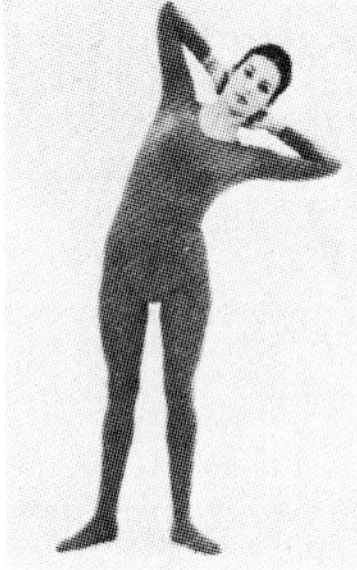
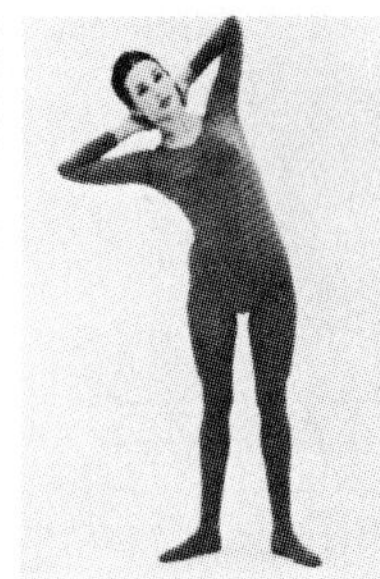

6. BODY BENDER

Starting position: Stand, feet shoulder-width apart, hands behind neck, fingers interlaced.
Action: Count 1. Bend trunk sideward to left as far as possible, keeping hands behind neck. Count 2. Return to starting position. Counts 3 and 4. Repeat to the right.

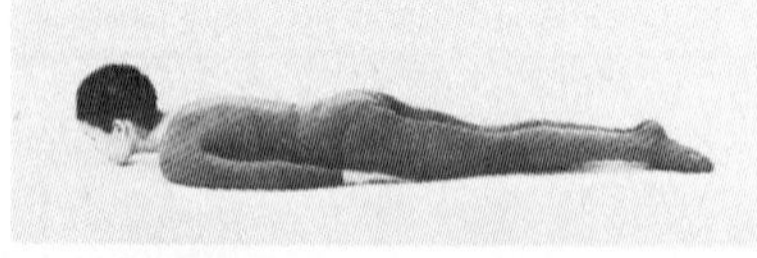
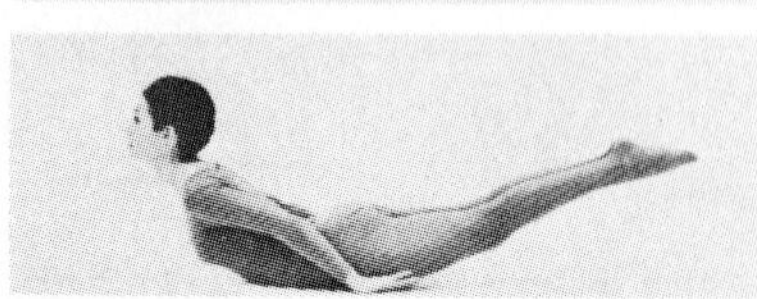

7. PRONE ARCH

Starting position: Lie face down, hands tucked under thighs.
Action: Count 1. Raise head, shoulders and legs from floor. Count 2. Return to starting position.

ORIENTATION PROGRAM

Conditioning exercises	GOAL Repetitions
*1. Bend and stretch	10
*2. Knee lift	10 left, 10 right
*3. Wing stretcher	20
*4. Half knee bend	10
*5. Arm circles	15 each way
*6. Body bender	10 left, 10 right
7. Prone arch	10
8. Knee pushup	6
9. Head and shoulder curl	5
10. Ankle stretch	15
Circulatory activity (choose one each workout)	
Walking	½ mile
Rope (skip 15 sec.; rest 60 sec.)	3 series

*The first six exercises of the orientation program will be used as warmup exercises throughout the graded levels.
Step Test Record—After completing the orientation program, take the 2-minute step test
Record your pulse rate here: _____. This will be the base rate with which you can make comparisons in the future.

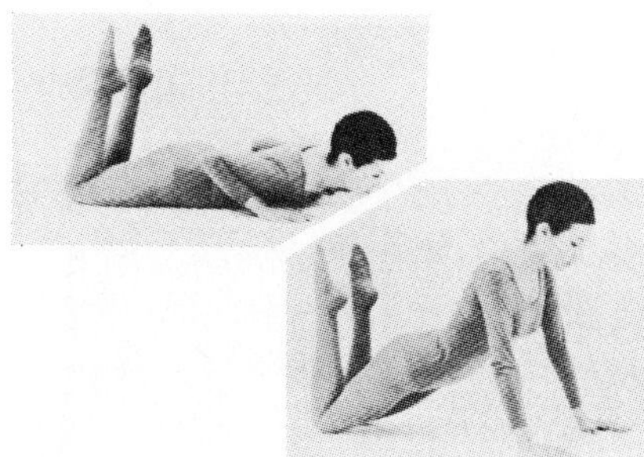

8. KNEE PUSHUP

Starting position: Lie on floor, face down, legs together, knees bent with feet raised off floor, hands on floor under shoulders, palms down.
Action: Count 1. Push upper body off floor until arms are fully extended and body is in straight line from head to knees. Count 2. Return to starting position.

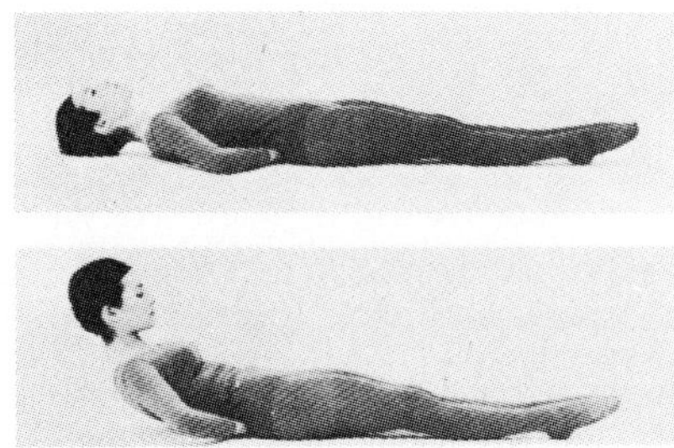

9. HEAD AND SHOULDER CURL

Starting position: Lie on back, hands tucked under small of back, palms down.
Action: Count 1. Tighten abdominal muscles, lift head and pull shoulders and elbows off floor. Hold for four seconds. Count 2. Return to starting position.

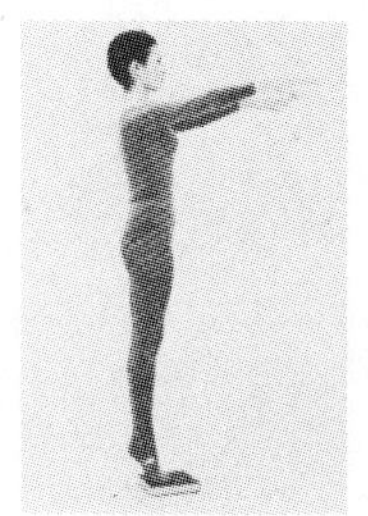

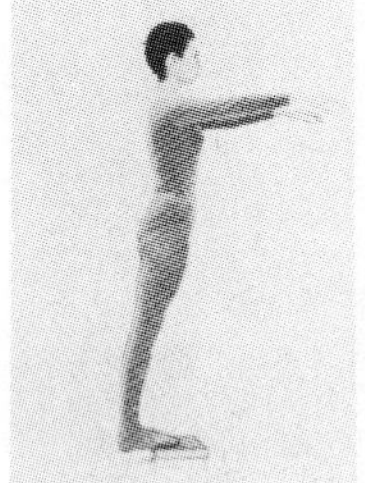

10. ANKLE STRETCH

Starting position: Stand on a stair, large book, or block of wood, with weight on balls of feet and heels raised.
Action: Count 1. Lower heels. Count 2. Raise heels.

CIRCULATORY ACTIVITIES

WALKING—Step off at a lively pace, swing arms and breathe deeply. *ROPE*—Any form of skipping or jumping is acceptable. Gradually increase the tempo as your skill and condition improve.

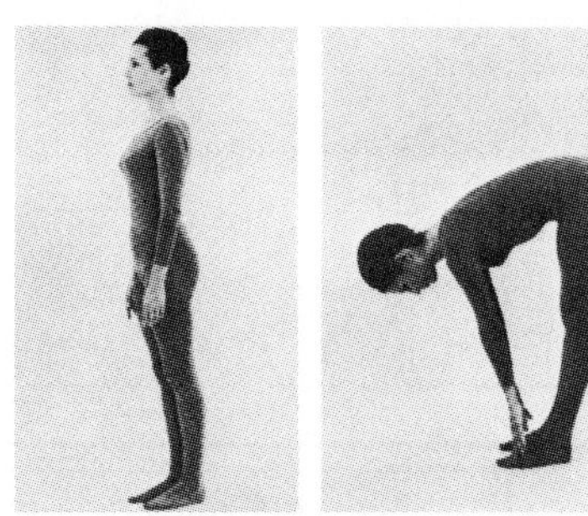

1. TOE TOUCH

Starting Position: Stand at attention.
Action: Count 1. Bend trunk forward and down, keeping knees straight, touching fingers to ankles. Count 2. Bounce and touch fingers to top of feet. Count 3. Bounce and touch fingers to toes. Count 4. Return to starting position.

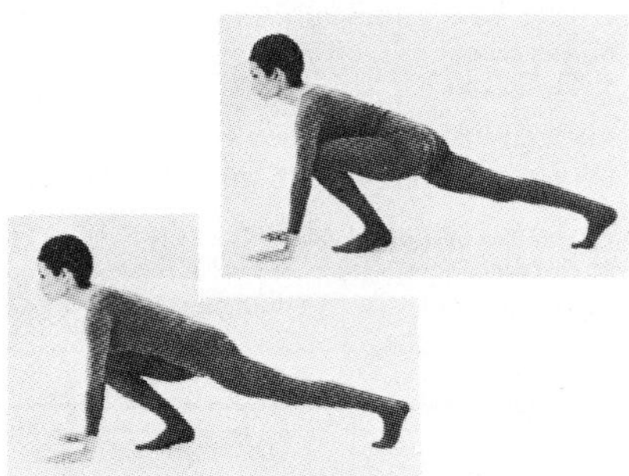

2. SPRINTER

Starting position: Squat, hands on floor, fingers pointed forward, left leg fully extended to rear.
Action: Count 1. Reverse position of feet in bouncing movement, bringing left foot to hands, extending right leg backward—all in one motion. Count 2. Reverse feet again, returning to starting position.

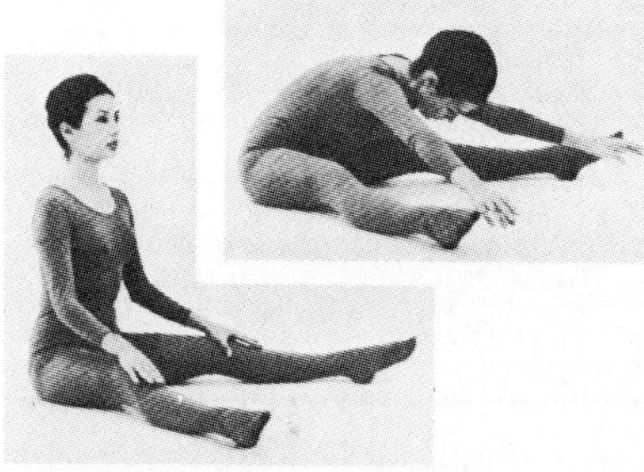

3. SITTING STRETCH

Starting position: Sit, legs spread apart, hands on knees.
Action: Count 1. Bend forward at waist, extending arms as far forward as possible. Count 2. Return to starting position.

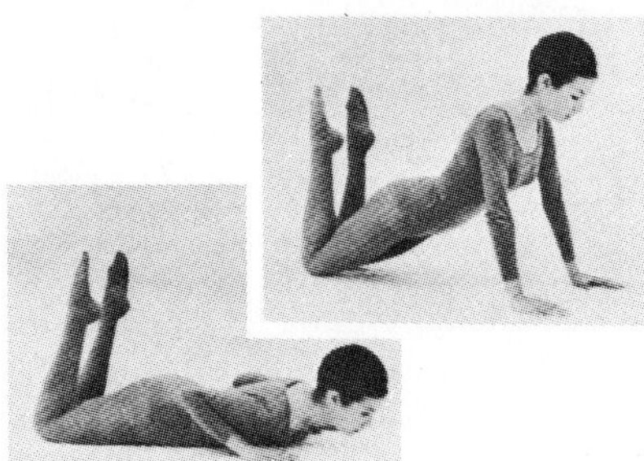

4. KNEE PUSHUP

Starting position: Lie on floor, face down, legs together, knees bent with feet raised off floor, hands on floor under shoulders, palms down.
Action: Count 1. Push upper body off floor until arms are fully extended and body is in straight line from head to knees. Count 2. Return to starting position.

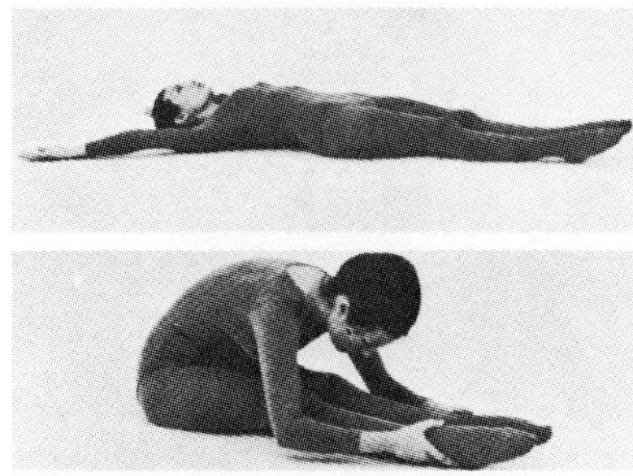

5. SITUP (ARMS EXTENDED)

Starting position: Lie on back, legs straight and together, arms extended beyond head.
Action: Count 1. Bring arms forward over head, roll up to sitting position, sliding hands along legs, grasping ankles. Count 2. Roll back to starting position.

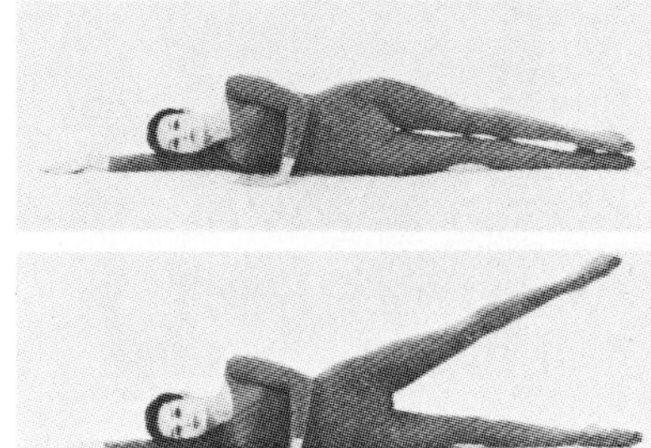

6. LEG RAISER

Starting position: Right side of body on floor, head resting on right arm.
Action: Lift left leg about 24″ off floor, then lower it. Do required number of repetitions. Repeat on other side.

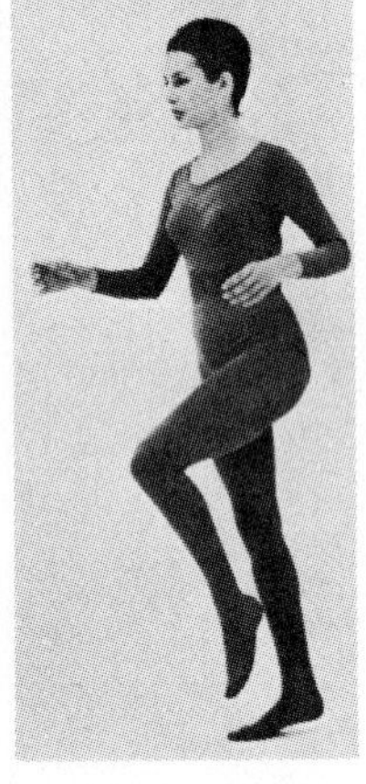

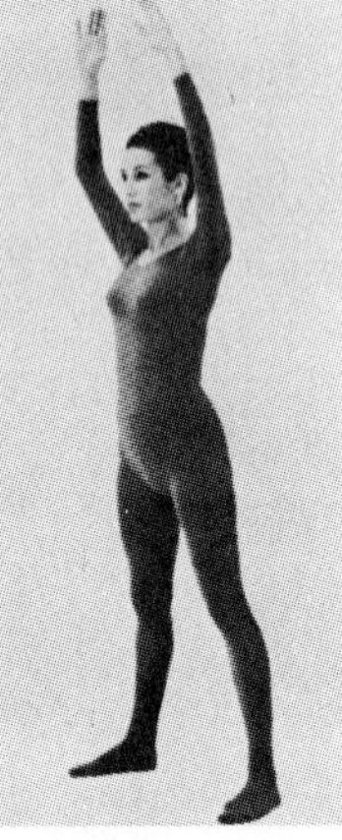

CIRCULATORY ACTIVITIES

WALKING—Maintain a pace of 120 steps per minute for a distance of ½ mile. Swing arms and breathe deeply.
ROPE—Skip or jump rope continuously using any form for 30 seconds and then rest 60 seconds. Repeat 2 times.
RUN IN PLACE—Raise each foot at least 4″ off the floor and jog in place. Count 1 each time left foot touches floor. Complete number of running steps called for in chart, then do specified number of straddle hops. Complete 2 cycles of alternate running and hopping for time specified on chart.
STRADDLE HOP—*Starting position:* At attention.
Action: Count 1. Swing arms sideward and upward, touching hands above head (arms straight) while simultaneously moving feet sideward and apart in a single jumping motion. Count 2. Spring back to starting position. Two counts in one hop.

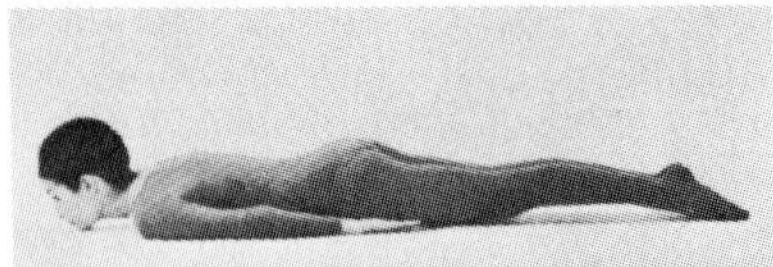

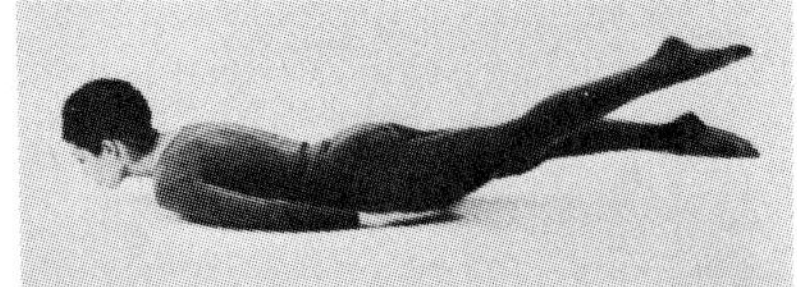

7. FLUTTER KICK

Starting position: Lie face down, hands tucked under thighs.
Action: Arch the back, bringing chest and head up, then flutter kick continuously, moving the legs 8″–10″ apart. Kick from hips with knees slightly bent. Count each kick as one.

WOMEN: LEVEL ONE ★ GOAL

Warmup Exercises	**Exercises 1–6 of Orientation program**
Conditioning Exercises	**Uninterrupted repetitions**
1. Toe touch	5
2. Sprinter	8
3. Sitting stretch	10
4. Knee pushup	8
5. Situp (arms extended)	5
6. Leg raiser	5 each leg
7. Flutter kick	20
Circulatory activity (choose one each workout)	
Walking (120 steps a minute)	½ mile
Rope (skip 30 secs.; rest 60 secs.)	2 series
Run in place (run 50; straddle hop 10 – 2 cycles)	2 minutes
Water activities—See recommendations in Section IV.	

Your progress record	1	2	3	4	5	6	7	8	9	10	11	12	13	14	15
Step test (pulse)													Prove-out workouts		

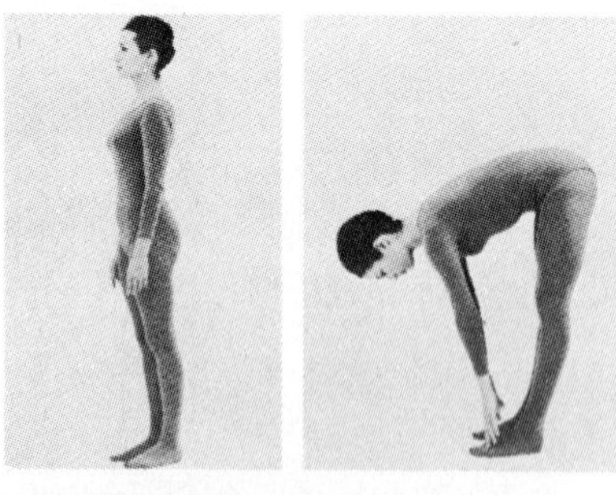

1. TOE TOUCH

Starting position: Stand at attention.
Action: Count 1. Bend trunk forward and down, keeping knees straight, touching fingers to ankles. Count 2. Bounce and touch fingers to top of feet. Count 3. Bounce and touch fingers to toes. Count 4. Return to starting position.

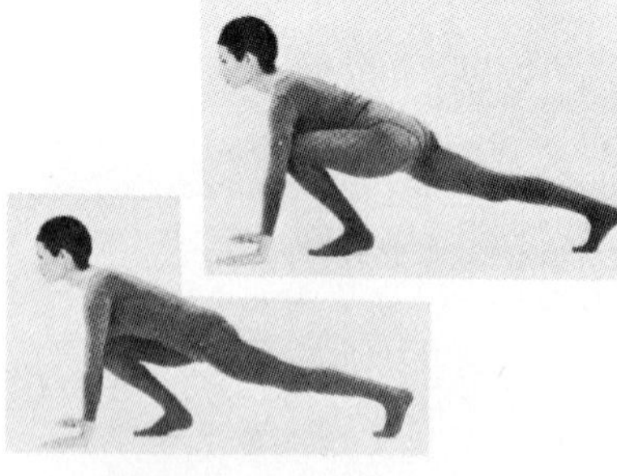

2. SPRINTER

Starting position: Squat, hands on floor, fingers pointed forward, left leg fully extended to rear.
Action: Count 1. Reverse position of feet in bouncing movement, bringing left foot to hands, extending right leg backward—all in one motion. Count 2. Reverse feet again, returning to starting position.

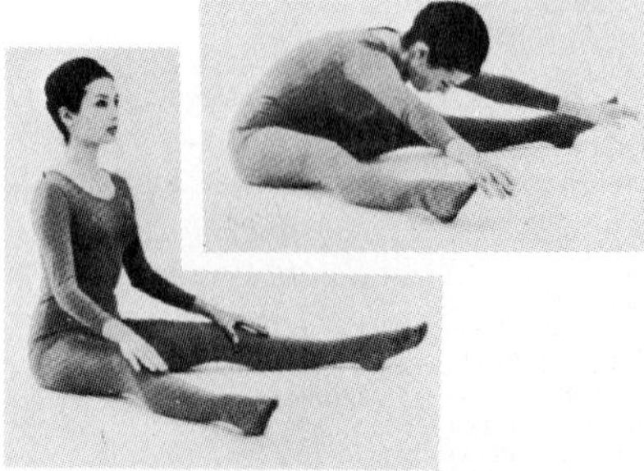

3. SITTING STRETCH

Starting position: Sit, legs spread apart, hands on knees.
Action: Count 1. Bend forward at waist, extending arms as far forward as possible. Count 2. Return to starting position.

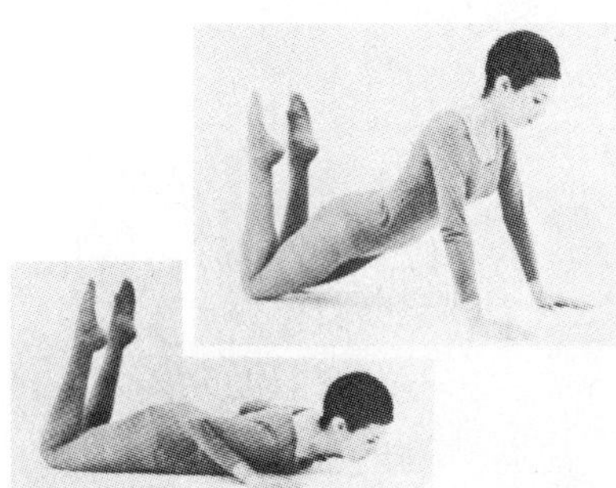

4. KNEE PUSHUP

Starting position: Lie on floor, face down, legs together, knees bent with feet raised off floor, hands on floor under shoulders, palms down. *Action:* Count 1. Push upper body off floor until arms are fully extended and body is in straight line from head to knees. Count 2. Return to starting position.

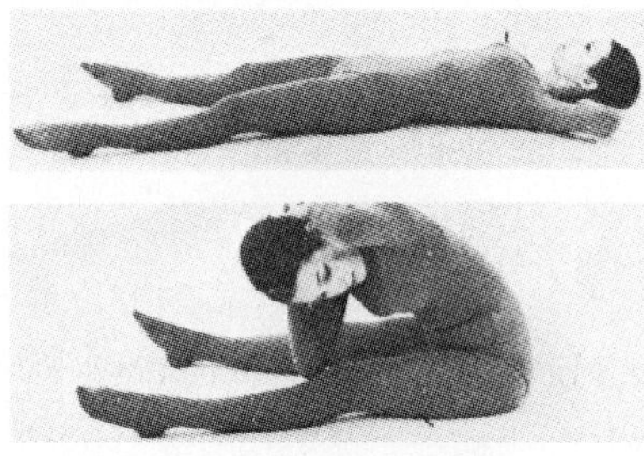

5. SITUP (FINGERS LACED)

Starting position: Lie on back, legs straight and feet spread approximately 1′ apart. Fingers laced behind neck. *Action:* Count 1. Curl up to sitting position and turn trunk to left. Touch right elbow to left knee. Count 2. Return to starting position. Count 3. Curl up to sitting position and turn trunk to right. Touch left elbow to right knee. Count 4. Return to starting position. Score one situp each time you return to starting position. Knees may be bent as necessary.

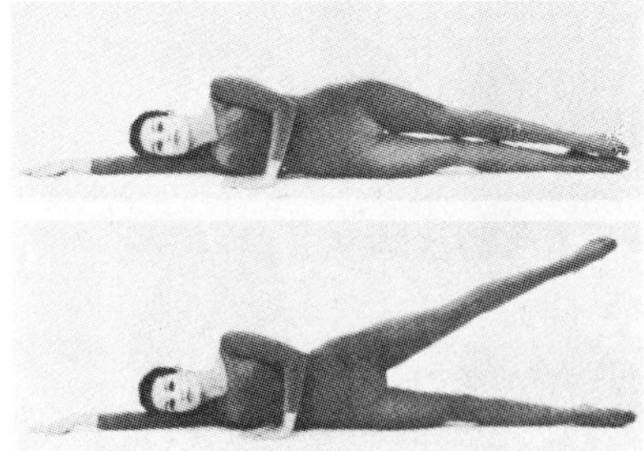

6. LEG RAISER

Starting position: Right side of body on floor, head resting on right arm. *Action:* Lift left leg about 24″ off floor, then lower it. Do required number of repetitions. Repeat on other side.

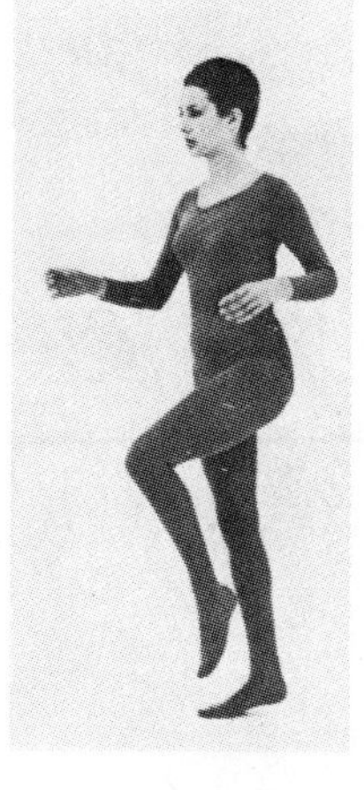

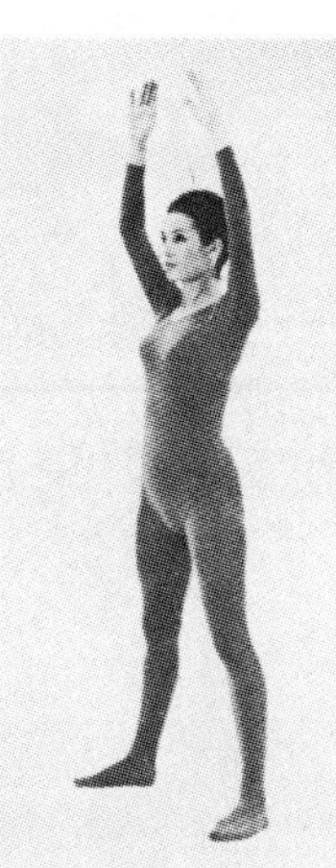

CIRCULATORY ACTIVITIES

JOG-WALK—Jog and walk alternately for number of paces indicated on chart for distance specified.
ROPE—Skip or jump rope continuously using any form for 30 seconds and then rest 60 seconds. Repeat 3 times.
RUN IN PLACE—Raise each foot at least 4″ off floor and jog in place. Count 1 each time left foot touches floor. Complete number of running steps called for in chart, then do specified number of straddle hops. Complete 2 cycles of alternate running and hopping for time specified on chart.
STRADDLE HOP—Starting position: At attention.
Action: Count 1. Swing arms sideward and upward, touching hands above head (arms straight) while simultaneously moving feet sideward and apart in a single jumping motion. Count 2. Spring back to starting position. Two counts in one hop.

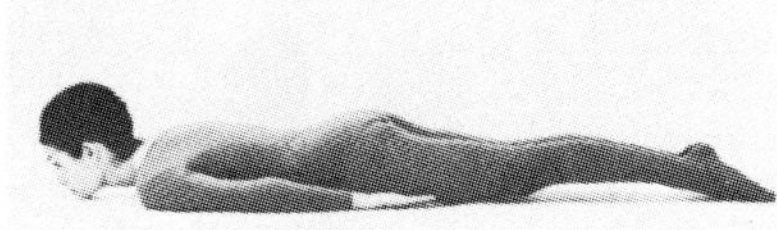

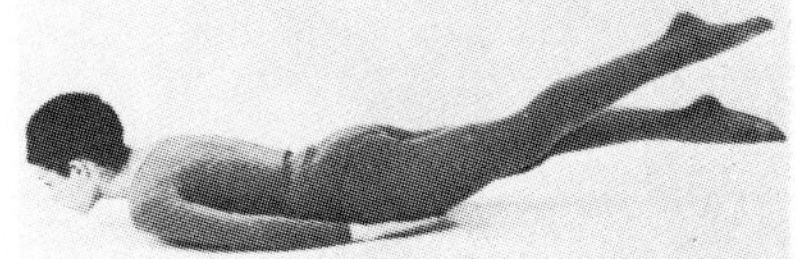

7. FLUTTER KICK

Starting position: Lie face down, hands tucked under thighs. *Action:* Arch the back, bringing chest and head up, then flutter kick continuously, moving the legs 8″–10″ apart. Kick from hips with knees slightly bent. Count each kick as one.

WOMEN: LEVEL TWO ☆☆ — GOAL

Warmup Exercises	Exercises 1–6 of Orientation program
Conditioning Exercises	**Uninterrupted repetitions**
1. Toe touch	10
2. Sprinter	12
3. Sitting stretch	15
4. Knee pushup	12
5. Situp (fingers laced)	10
6. Leg raiser	10 each leg
7. Flutter kick	30
Circulatory activity (choose one each workout)	
Jog-walk (jog 50, walk 50)	½ mile
Rope (skip 30 secs.; rest 60 secs.)	3 series
Run in place (run 80, hop 15 – 2 cycles)	3 minutes

Water Activities—See recommendations in Section IV.

Your progress record	1	2	3	4	5	6	7	8	9	10	11	12	13	14	15
Step test (pulse)													Prove-out workouts		

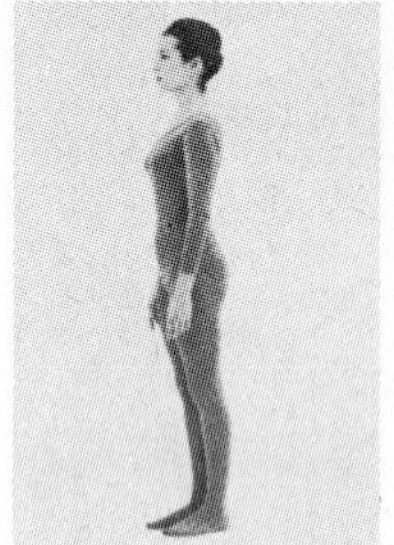
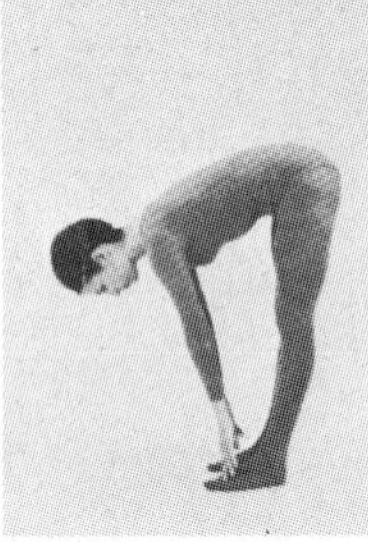

1. TOE TOUCH

Starting position: Stand at attention.
Action: Count 1. Bend trunk forward and down, keeping knees straight, touching fingers to ankles. Count 2. Bounce and touch fingers to top of feet. Count 3. Bounce and touch fingers to toes. Count 4. Return to starting position.

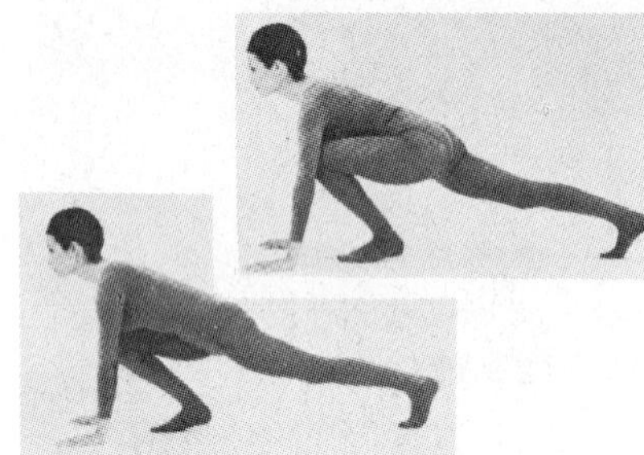

2. SPRINTER

Starting position: Squat, hands on floor, fingers pointed forward, left leg fully extended to rear.
Action: Count 1. Reverse position of feet in bouncing movement, bringing left foot to hands, extending right leg backward—all in one motion. Count 2. Reverse feet again, returning to starting position.

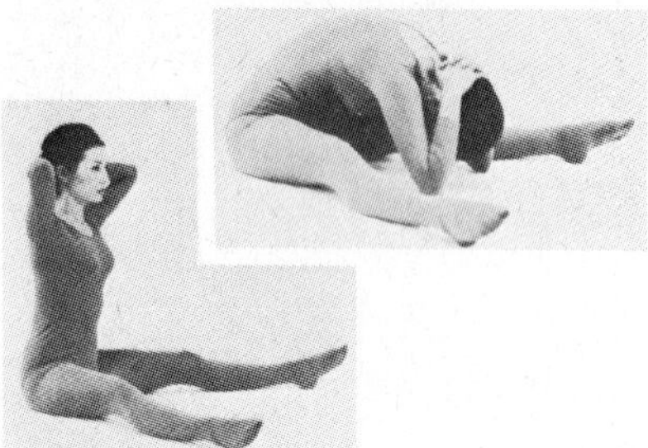

3. SITTING STRETCH (FINGERS LACED)

Starting position: Sit, legs spread apart, fingers laced behind neck.
Action: Count 1. Bend forward at waist, reaching elbows as close to floor as possible. Count 2. Return to starting position.

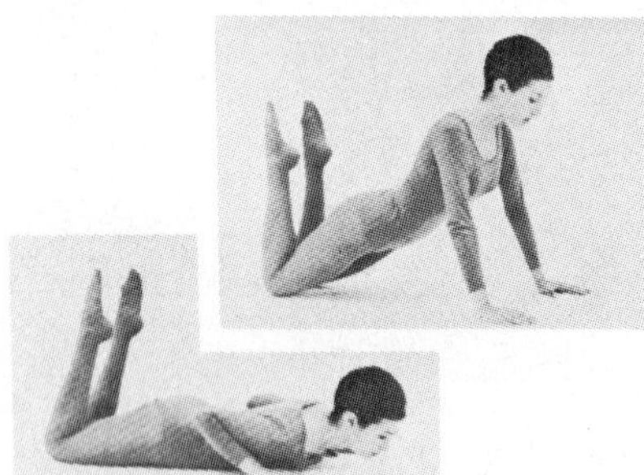

4. KNEE PUSHUP

Starting position: Lie on floor, face down, legs together, knees bent with feet raised off floor, hands on floor under shoulders, palms down.
Action: Count 1. Push upper body off floor until arms are fully flexed and body in straight line from head to knees. Count 2. Return to starting position.

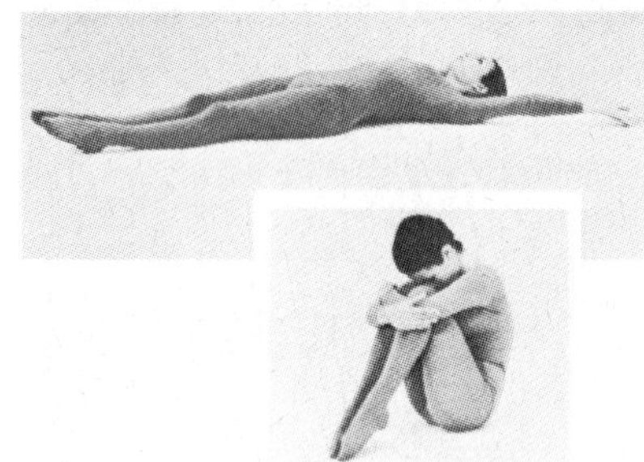

5. SITUP (ARMS EXTENDED, KNEES UP)

Starting position: Lie on back, legs straight, arms extended overhead.
Action: Count 1. Sit up, reaching forward with arms encircling knees while pulling them tightly to chest. Count 2. Return to starting position. Do this exercise rhythmically, without breaks in the movement.

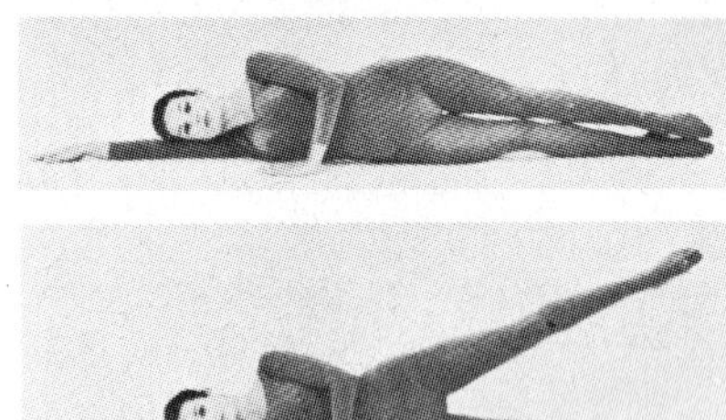

6. LEG RAISER

Starting position: Right side of body on floor, head resting on right arm.
Action: Lift left leg about 24″ off floor, then lower it. Do required number of repetitions. Repeat on other side.

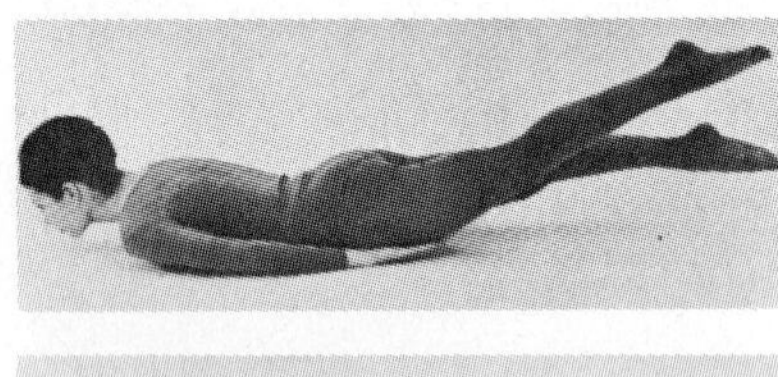
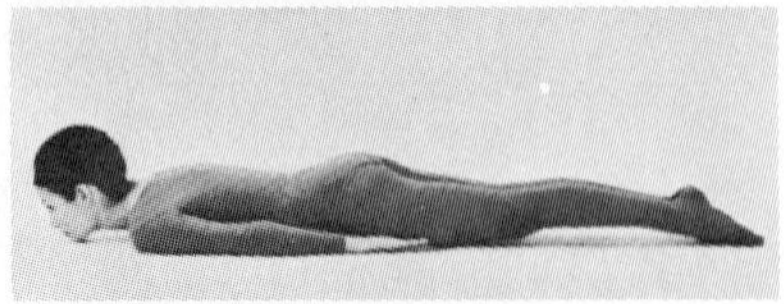

7. FLUTTER KICK

Starting position: Lie face down, hands tucked under thighs.
Action: Arch the back, bringing chest and head up. Then flutter kick continuously, moving the legs 8″–10″ apart. Kick from hips with knees slightly bent. Count each kick as one.

CIRCULATORY ACTIVITIES

JOG-WALK—Jog and walk alternately for number of paces indicated on chart for distance specified.
ROPE—Skip or jump rope continuously using any form for 45 seconds and then rest 30 seconds. Repeat 3 times.
RUN IN PLACE—Raise each foot at least 4″ off floor and jog in place. Count 1 each time left foot touches floor. Complete number of running steps called for in chart, then do specified number of straddle hops. Complete 2 cycles of alternate running and hopping for time specified on chart.
STRADDLE HOP—Starting position: At attention.
Action: Count 1. Swing arms sideward and upward, touching hands above head (arms straight) while simultaneously moving feet sideward and apart in a single jumping motion. Count 2. Spring back to starting position. Two counts in one hop.

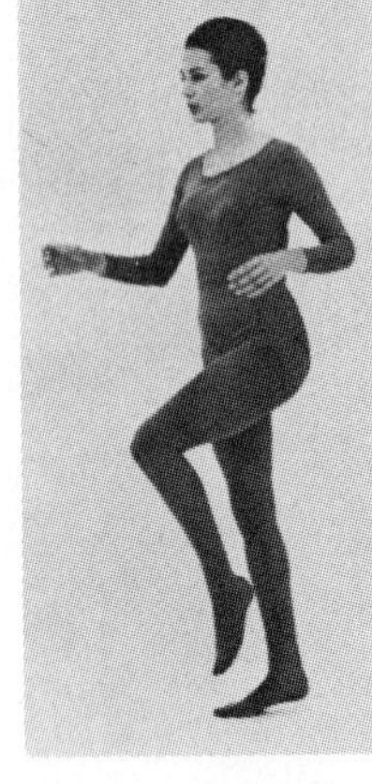
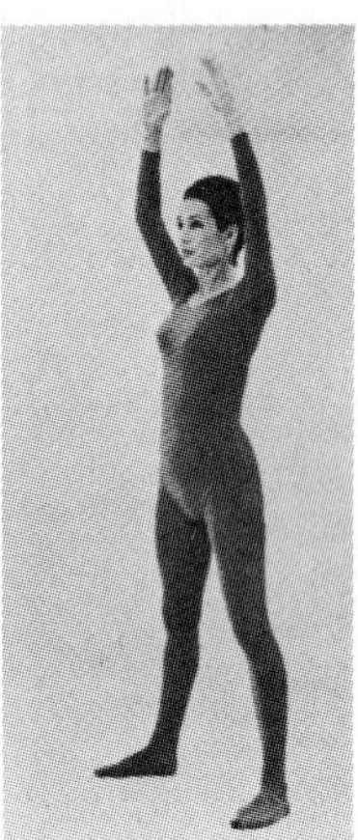

WOMEN: LEVEL THREE ☆☆☆ — GOAL

Warmup Exercises	Exercises 1–6 of Orientation program
Conditioning Exercises	**Uninterrupted repetitions**
1. Toe touch	20
2. Sprinter	16
3. Sitting stretch (fingers laced)	15
4. Knee pushup	20
5. Situp (arms extended, knees up)	15
6. Leg raiser	16 each leg
7. Flutter kick	40
Circulatory activity (choose one each workout)	
Jog-wc (jog 50, walk 50)	¾ mile
Rope (skip 45 secs.; rest 30 secs.)	3 series
Run in place (run 110, hop 20 – 2 cycles)	4 minutes
Water activities—See recommendations in Section IV.	

Your progress record	1	2	3	4	5	6	7	8	9	10	11	12	13	14	15
Step test (pulse)													Prove-out workouts		

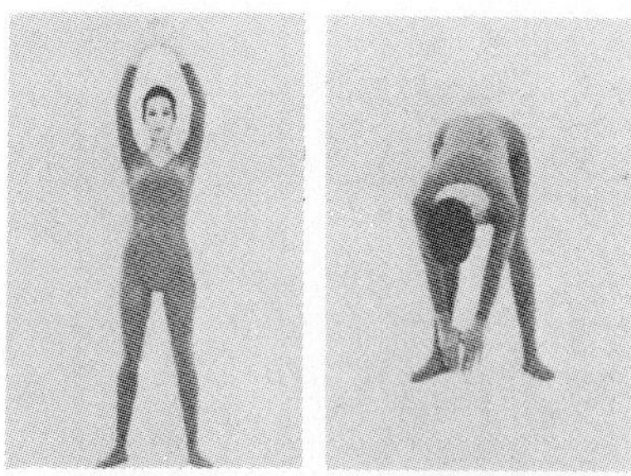

1. TOE TOUCH (TWIST AND BEND)

Starting position: Stand, feet shoulder-width apart, arms extended overhead, thumbs interlocked.
Action: Count 1. Twist trunk to right and touch floor inside right foot with fingers of both hands. Count 2. Touch floor outside toes of right foot. Count 3. Touch floor outside heel of right foot. Count 4. Return to starting position, sweeping trunk and arms upward in a wide arc. On the next four counts, repeat action to left side.

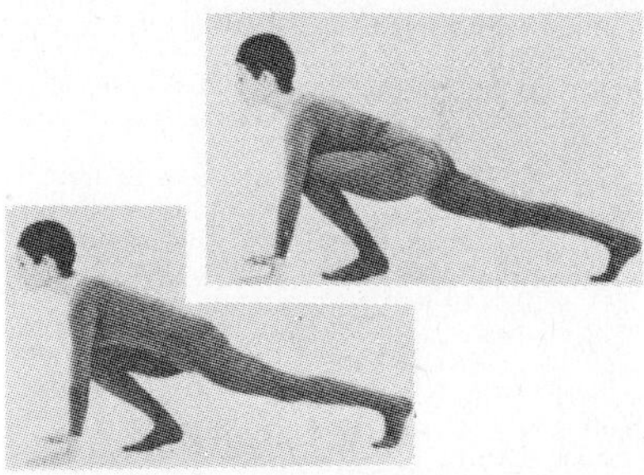

2. SPRINTER

Starting position: Squat, hands on floor, fingers pointed forward, left leg fully extended to rear.
Action: Count 1. Reverse position of feet in bouncing movement, bringing left foot to hands, extending right leg backward—all in one motion. Count 2. Reverse feet again, returning to starting position.

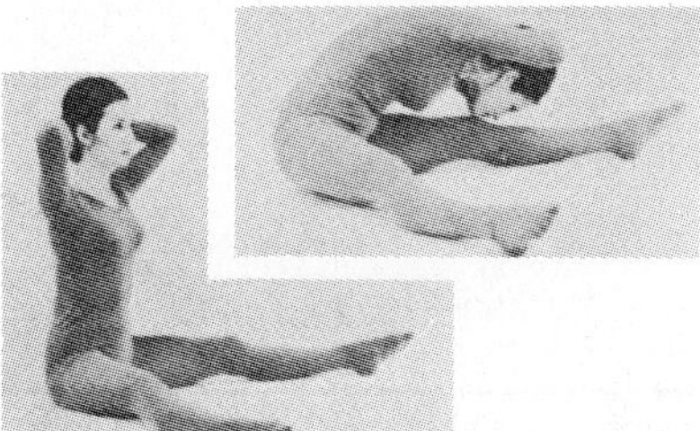

3. SITTING STRETCH (ALTERNATE)

Starting position: Sit, legs spread apart, fingers laced behind neck, elbows back.
Action: Count 1. Bend forward to left, touching forehead to left knee. Count 2. Return to starting position. Counts 3 and 4. Repeat to right. Score one repetition each time you return to starting position. Knees may be bent if necessary.

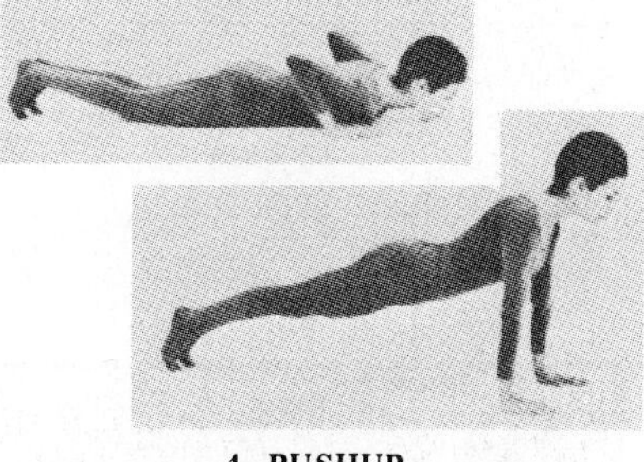

4. PUSHUP

Starting position: Lie on floor, face down, legs together, hands on floor under shoulders with fingers pointing straight ahead.
Action: Count 1. Push body off floor by extending arms so that weight rests on hands and toes. Count 2. Lower the body until chest touches floor.
Note: Body should be kept straight, buttocks should not be raised, abdomen should not sag.

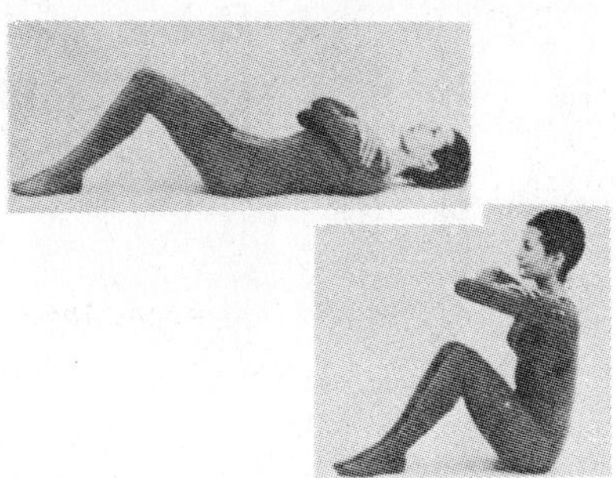

5. SITUP (ARMS CROSSED, KNEES BENT)

Starting position: Lie on back, arms crossed on chest, hands grasping opposite shoulders, knees bent to right angle, feet flat on floor.
Action: Count 1. Curl up to sitting position. Count 2. Return to starting position.

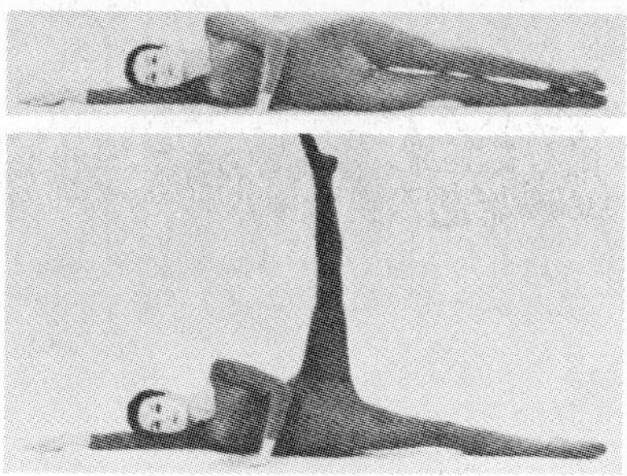

6. LEG RAISER (WHIP)

Starting position: Right side of body on floor, right arm supporting head.
Action: Whip left leg up and down rapidly lifting as high as possible off the floor. Count each whip as one. Reverse position and whip right leg up and down.

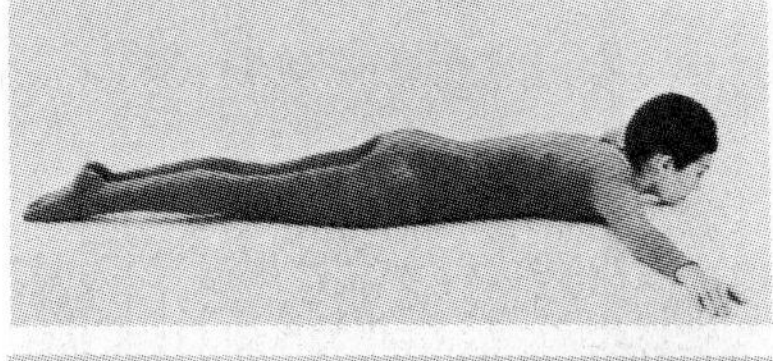

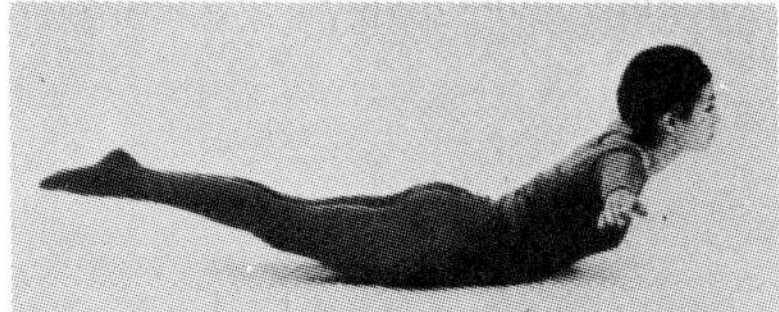

7. PRONE ARCH (ARMS EXTENDED)

Starting position: Lie face down, legs straight and together, arms extended to sides at shoulder level.
Action: Count 1. Arch the back, bringing arms, chest and head up, and raising legs as high as possible. Count 2. Return to starting position.

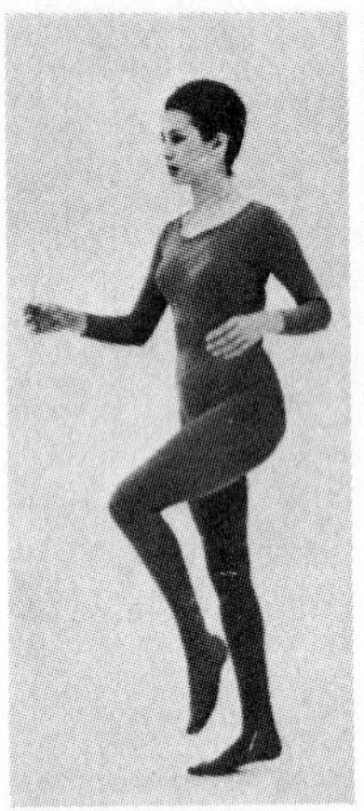
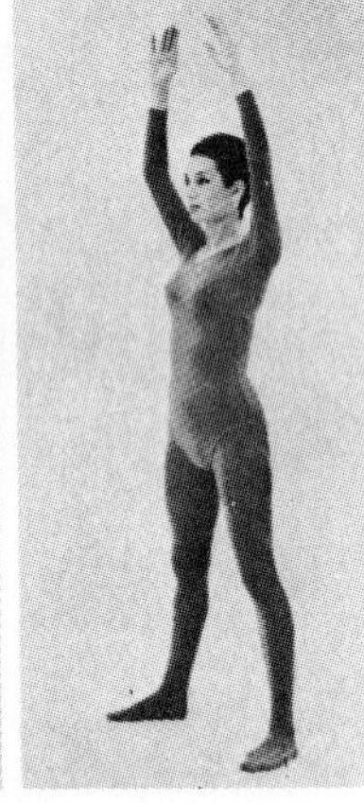

CIRCULATORY ACTIVITIES

JOG-WALK—Jog and walk alternately for number of paces indicated on chart for distance specified.
ROPE—Skip or jump rope continuously using any form for 60 seconds and then rest 30 seconds. Repeat 3 times.
RUN IN PLACE—Raise each foot at least 4" off floor and jog in place. Count 1 each time left foot touches floor. Complete number of running steps called for in chart, then do specified number of straddle hops. Complete 2 cycles of alternate running and hopping for time specified on chart.
STRADDLE HOP—*Starting position:* At attention.
Action: Count 1. Swing arms sideward and upward, touching hands above head (arms straight) while simultaneously moving feet sideward and apart in a single jumping motion. Count 2. Spring back to starting position. Two counts in one hop.

WOMEN: LEVEL FOUR ☆☆☆☆ GOAL

Warmup Exercises	Exercises 1–6 of Orientation program
Conditioning Exercises	**Uninterrupted repetitions**
1. Toe touch (twist and bend)	15 each side
2. Sprinter	20
3. Sitting stretch (alternate)	20
4. Pushup	8
5. Situp (arms crossed, knees bent)	20
6. Leg raiser (whip)	10 each leg
7. Prone arch (arms extended)	15
Circulatory activity (choose one each workout)	
Jog-walk (jog 100; walk 50)	1 mile
Rope (skip 60 secs.; rest 30 secs.)	3 series
Run in place (run 145, hop 25 – 2 cycles)	5 minutes
Water activities—See recommendations in Section IV.	

Your progress record	1	2	3	4	5	6	7	8	9	10	11	12	13	14	15
Step test (pulse)													Prove-out workouts		

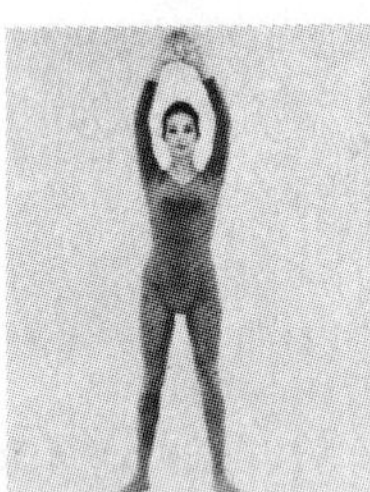
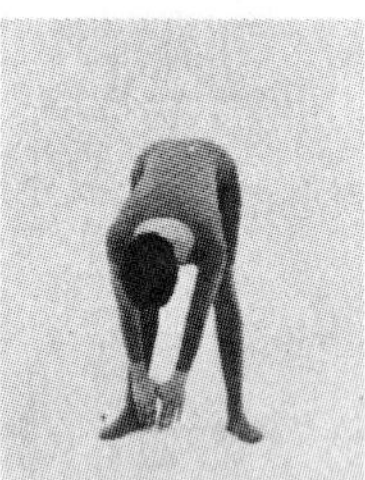

1. TOE TOUCH (TWIST AND BEND)

Starting position: Stand, feet shoulder-width apart, arms extended overhead, thumbs interlocked.
Action: Count 1. Twist trunk to right and touch floor inside right foot with fingers of both hands. Count 2. Touch floor outside toes of right foot. Count 3. Touch floor outside heel of right foot. Count 4. Return to starting position, sweeping trunk and arms upward in a wide arc. On the next four counts, repeat action to left side.

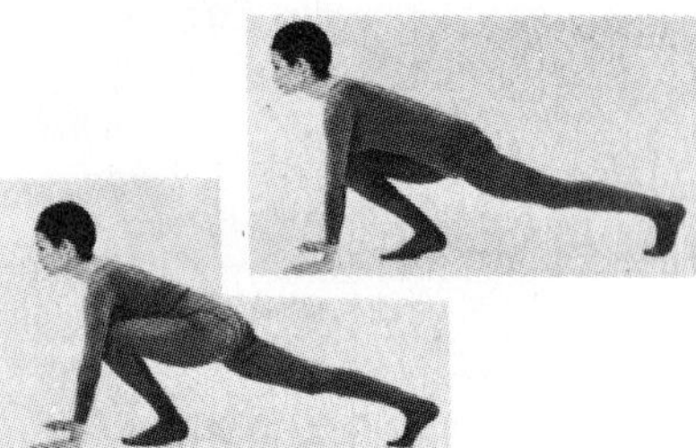

2. SPRINTER

Starting position: Squat, hands on floor, fingers pointed forward, left leg fully extended to rear.
Action: Count 1. Reverse position of feet in bouncing movement, bringing left foot to hands and extending right leg backward—all in one motion. Count 2. Reverse feet again, returning to starting position.

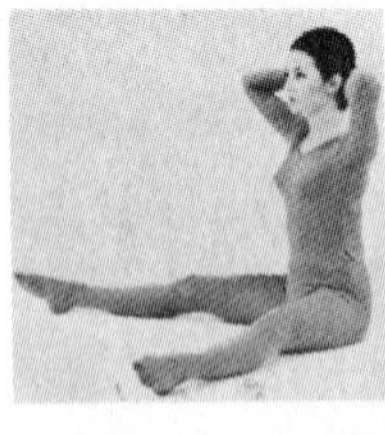
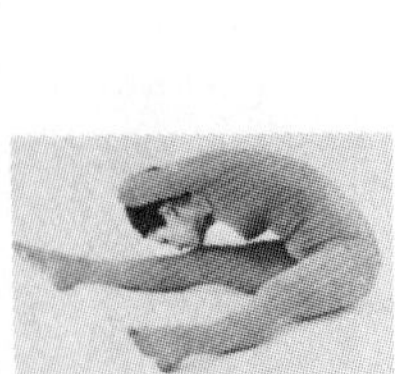

3. SITTING STRETCH (ALTERNATE)

Starting position: Sit, legs spread apart, fingers behind neck, elbows back.
Action: Count 1. Bend forward to left, touching forehead to left knee. Count 2. Return to starting position. Counts 3 and 4. Repeat to right. Score one repetition each time you return to starting position. Knees may be bent if necessary.

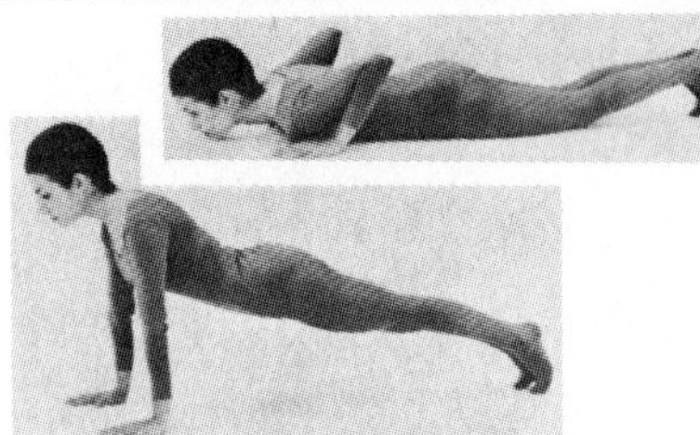

4. PUSHUP

Starting position: Lie on floor, face down, legs together, hands on floor under shoulders with fingers pointing straight ahead.
Action: Count 1. Push body off floor by extending arms so that weight rests on hands and toes. Count 2. Lower the body until chest touches floor.
Note: Body should be kept straight, buttocks should not be raised, abdomen should not sag.

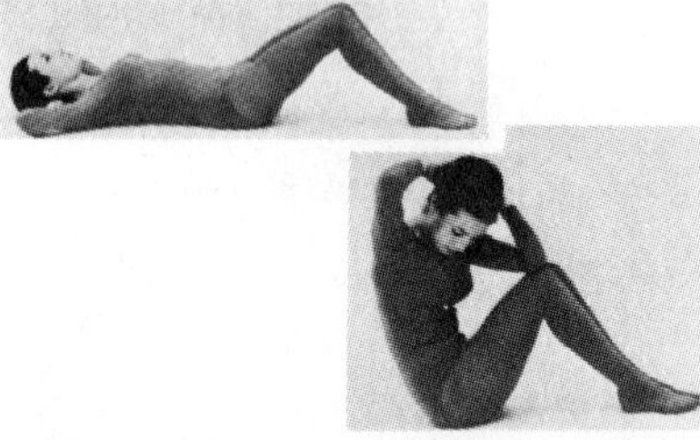

5. SITUP (FINGERS LACED, KNEES BENT)

Starting position: Lie on back, fingers laced behind neck, knees bent, feet flat on floor.
Action: Count 1. Sit up, turn trunk to right, touch left elbow to right knee. Count 2. Return to starting position. Count 3. Sit up, turn trunk to left, touch right elbow to left knee. Count 4. Return to starting position. Score one each time you return to starting position.

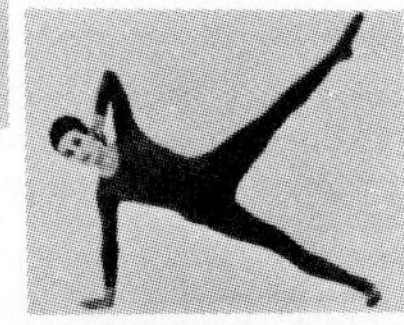

6. LEG RAISER (ON EXTENDED ARM)

Starting position: Body rigidly supported by extended right arm and foot. Left arm is held behind head.
Action: Count 1. Raise left leg high. Count 2. Return to starting position slowly. Repeat on other side. Do required number of repetitions.

WOMEN: LEVEL FIVE ☆☆☆☆☆ — GOAL

Warmup Exercises	**Exercises 1–6 of Orientation program**
Conditioning Exercises	**Uninterrupted repetitions**
1. Toe touch (twist and bend)	25 each side
2. Sprinter	24
3. Sitting stretch (alternate)	26
4. Pushup	15
5. Situp (fingers laced, knees bent)	25
6. Leg raiser (on extended arm)	10 each side
7. Prone arch (fingers laced)	25
Circulatory activity (choose one each workout)	
Jog-run	1 mile
Rope (skip 2 mins.; rest 45 secs.)	2 series
Run in place (run 180, hop 30 – 2 cycles)	6 minutes
Water Activities—See recommendations in Section IV	

Your progress record	1	2	3	4	5	6	7	8	9	10	11	12	13	14	15
Step test (pulse)													Prove-out workouts		

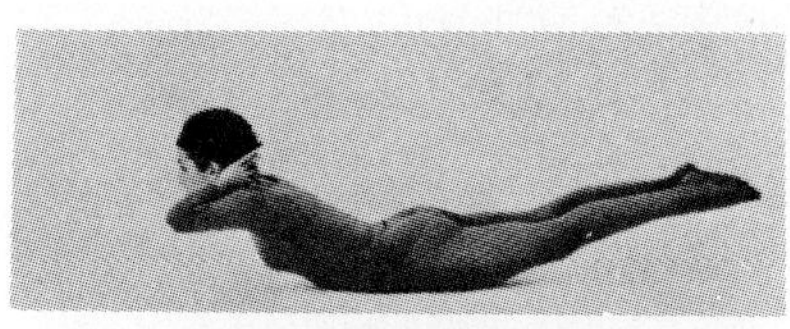

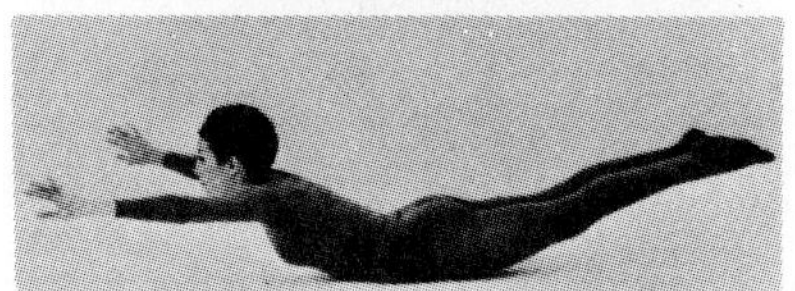

7. PRONE ARCH (FINGERS LACED)

Starting position: Lie face down, fingers laced behind neck.
Action: Count 1. Arch back, legs and chest off floor. Count 2. Extend arms fully forward. Count 3. Return hands to behind neck. Count 4. Flatten body to floor.

CIRCULATORY ACTIVITIES

JOG-RUN—Jog and run alternately for distance specified on chart.
ROPE—Skip or jump rope continuously using any form for 2 minutes and then rest 45 seconds. Repeat 2 times.
RUN IN PLACE—Raise each foot at least 4″ off floor and jog in place. Count 1 each time left foot touches floor. Complete number of running steps called for in chart, then do specified number of straddle hops. Complete 2 cycles of alternate running and hopping in time specified on the chart.
STRADDLE HOP—*Starting position:* At attention.
Action: Count 1. Swing arms sideward and upward, touching hands above head (arms straight) while simultaneously moving feet sideward and apart in a single jumping motion. Count 2. Spring back to starting position. Two counts in one hop.

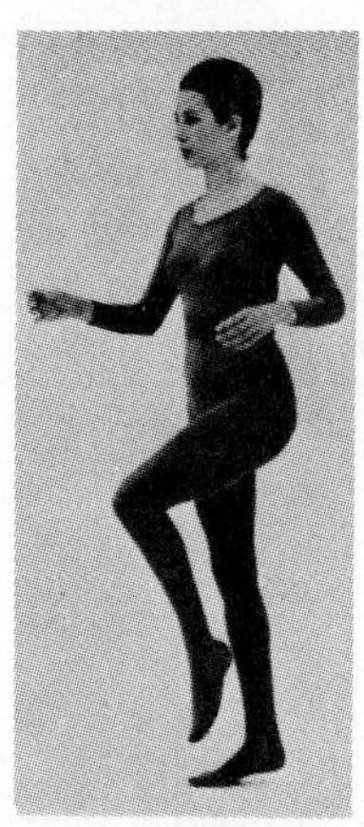

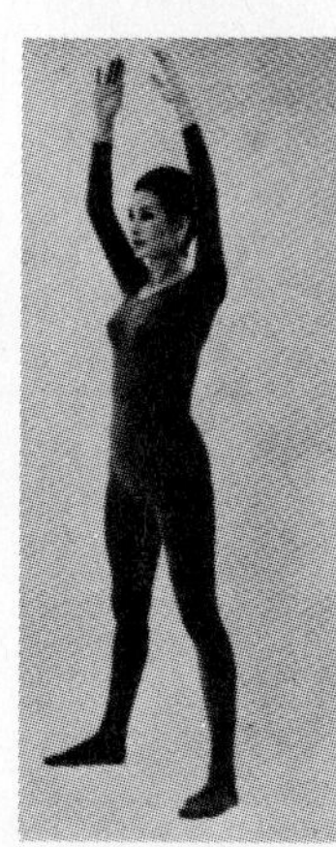

Staying fit

Once you have reached the level of conditioning you have chosen for yourself, you will wish to maintain your fitness.

To do so, continue the workouts at that level.

While it has been found possible to maintain fitness with three workouts a week, ideally, exercise should be a daily habit. If you can, by all means continue your workouts on a five-times-a-week basis.

If at any point—either after reaching your goal or in the process of doing so—your workouts are interrupted because of illness or other reason for more than a week, it will be best to begin again at a lower level. If you have had a serious illness or surgery, proceed under your physician's guidance.

SEPTEMBER

SUNDAY	MONDAY	TUESDAY	WEDNESDAY	THURSDAY	FRIDAY	SATURDAY
1	2	3	4	5	6	7
8	9	10	11	12	13	14
15	16	17	18	19	20	21
22	23	24	25	26	27	28
29	30		September			

Broadening your program

The exercises and activities you have engaged in are basic—designed to take you soundly and progressively up the ladder to physical fitness without need for special equipment or facilities.

There are many other activities and forms of exercise which, if you wish, you may use to supplement the basic program.

They include a variety of sports; water exercises you can use if you have access to a pool; and isometrics—sometimes called exercises without movement—which take little time (6–8 seconds each). One isometric—the abdominal—is particularly valuable for many women; it helps strengthen muscles that can act like a girdle to maintain a trim waistline.

You'll find suggestions, too, for improving posture—and also for taking advantage of many daily opportunities for sound physical activity.

THE PROGRAM FOR MEN

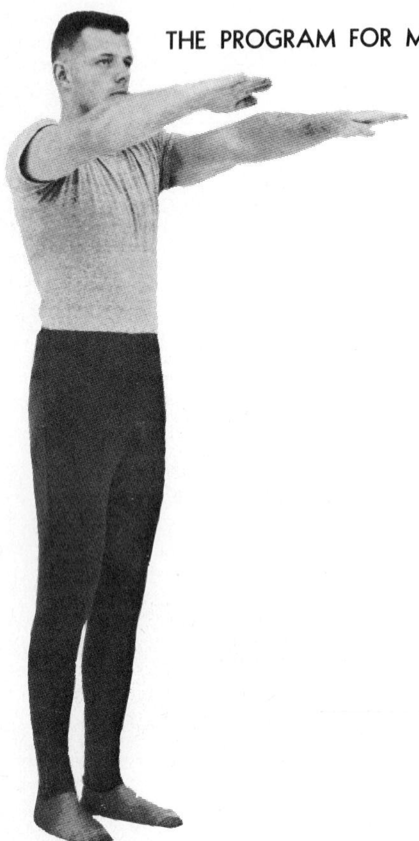

Before you begin

A medical checkup at least once a year is generally advisable for every man. It's an excellent idea to have such an examination now before beginning your conditioning program.

Very probably, you'll get an unlimited go-ahead. If there should be a health problem, your doctor can take steps to correct it and may have suggestions, too, for modifying the program to make it more suitable and effective for you.

With an examination under your belt, you can proceed confidently.

About the program

It assumes you have not—recently and consistently—been exposed to vigorous, all-round physical activity . . . which could be true even if you play golf once or twice a week or engage in some other sport; no one sport provides for balanced development of all parts of the body.

The plan starts with an orientation—"get-set"—series of mild exercises to limber up all major muscle groups and help assure a painless transition.

There are then five graded levels.

As you move up from one to the next, you will be building toward a practical and satisfactory level of fitness.

By building gradually—progressively—you will be building soundly.

What the exercises are for

There are three general types—warmup exercises, conditioning exercises and circulatory activities.

The warmup exercises stretch and limber up the muscles and speed up the action of the heart and lungs, thus preparing the body for greater exertion and reducing the possibility of unnecessary strain.

The conditioning exercises are systematically planned to tone up abdominal, back, leg, arm and other major muscles.

The circulatory activities produce contractions of large muscle groups for relatively longer periods than the conditioning exercises—to stimulate and strengthen the circulatory and respiratory systems.

The plan calls for doing 10 mild exercises during the orientation period and, thereafter, the warmup exercises and the seven conditioning exercises listed for each level. The first six exercises of the orientation program are used as warmup exercises throughout the graded levels.

When it comes to the circulatory activities, you select one each workout. Alternately running and walking . . . skipping rope . . . running in place. All are effective. You can switch about for variety.

How you progress

Right now, you have limited tolerance for exercise, can do just so much without discomfort and fatigue.

A sound conditioning program should gradually stretch your tolerance. It should give unused or little-used muscles moderate tasks at first, then make the tasks increasingly more demanding so you become able to achieve more and more with less and less fatigue and with increasingly rapid recovery.

As you move from level to level, some exercises will be modified so they call for more effort. Others will remain the same but you will build strength and stamina by increasing the number of repetitions.

You will be increasing your fitness another way as well.

At level 1, your objective will be to gradually reduce, from workout to workout, the "breathing spells" between exercises until you can do the seven conditioning exercises without resting. You will proceed in the same fashion with the more difficult exercises and increased repetitions at succeeding levels.

You will find the program designed—the progression carefully planned—to make this feasible. You will be able to proceed at your own pace, competing with yourself rather than with anyone else—and this is of great importance for sound conditioning.

Note: Gradually speeding up, from workout to workout, the rate at which you do each exercise will provide greater stimulation for the circulatory and respiratory systems and also help to keep your workouts short. However, the seven conditioning exercises should not be a race against time. Perform each exercise completely to insure maximum benefit.

What should your goal be?

There is no need to decide that now.

Many men will be able to complete the first three levels. Some will go on to level 4, which is challenging. The fifth is one which only extremely vigorous, well-conditioned men will reach.

Not everybody is physically constituted to play par golf or run a mile in under four minutes. Other factors in determining what your peak level will be is your body's built-in capacity, your age and previous conditioning.

But another factor can be very important.

As you know, it's much easier to accomplish something when you wish to accomplish it, believe you can, and enjoy the process.

Chances are, after several months of workouts, you will find it hard to believe you could do so little at the beginning.

As your physical tolerance for exercise increases, your psychological tolerance also will stretch—especially as you enjoy such results of your increasing fitness as trimmer appearance, growing energy for daily activities, more zest for play and a marked sense of well-being.

As you progress, you may realize that you can—and want to—go a long way. Go as far as you can.

The important point *is* that no matter what level you choose—three, four, or five—you will have gone far, achieved great improvement—*and you will be able to maintain that improvement.*

When and how often to work out

To be most beneficial, exercise should become part of your regular daily routine—as much as bathing, shaving, dressing.

Five workouts a week are called for throughout the program.

You can choose any time that is convenient. Preferably, it should be the same time every day—but it does not matter whether it's first thing in the morning, before dinner in the evening, just before retiring, any other time.

How long at each level

The time can vary between individuals. It may vary, too, for you from one level to another.

Your objective, as already noted, will be to reach a point at each level at which you can do all the exercises called for, for the number of times indicated, without resting.

But start slowly. There is no rush. You are building for a lifetime of physical fitness and by avoiding rush you will avoid sudden strains and excesses that could make you ache and hold you back.

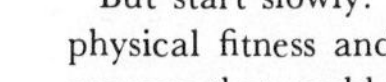

If you find yourself unable at first to complete any exercise—to do, continuously, all the repetitions called for—stop when you encounter difficulty. Rest briefly, then take up where you left off and complete the count. If you have difficulty at first, you will have less and less in succeeding workouts.

Stay at each level for at least three weeks. If you have not passed the prove-out test at the end of that time, continue at the same level until you do. The prove-out test calls for performing—on three consecutive days—the seven conditioning exercises without resting and satisfactorily fulfilling the requirement for one circulatory activity.

A measure of your progress

You will, of course, be able to observe the increase in your strength and stamina from week to week in many ways—including the increasing facility with which you do the exercises at a given level.

In addition, there is a 2-minute step test you can use to measure and keep a running record of the improvement in your circulatory efficiency, one of the most important of all aspects of fitness.

The immediate response of the cardiovascular system to exercise differs markedly between well-conditioned individuals and others. The test measures the response in terms of pulse rate taken shortly after a series of steps up and down onto a bench or chair.

Although it does not take long, it is necessarily vigorous. Stop if you become overly fatigued while taking it. You should not try it until you have completed the orientation period.

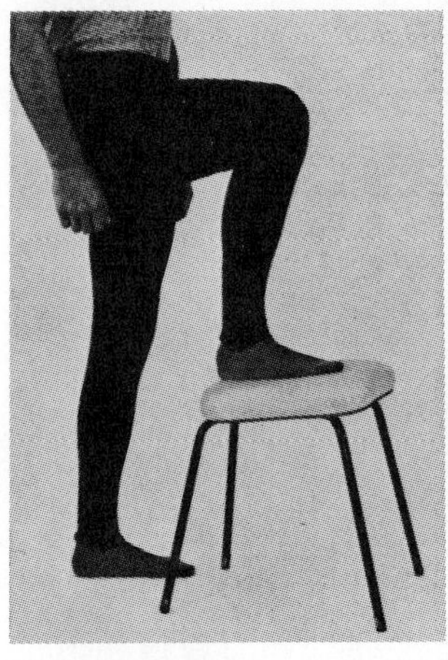

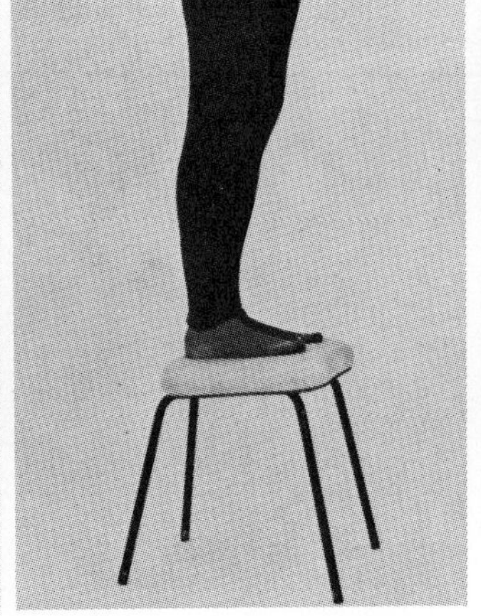

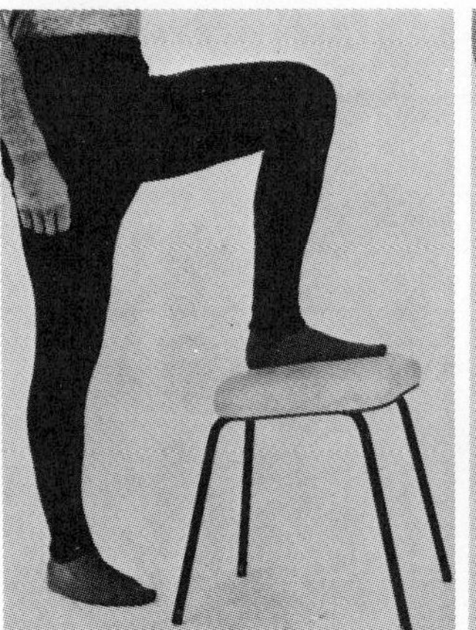

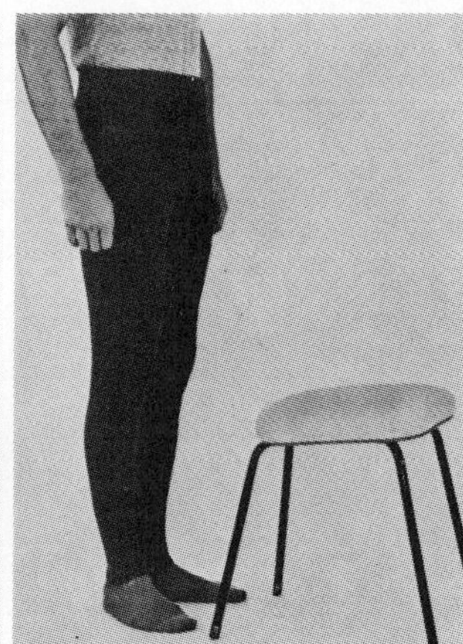

The test

Use any sturdy bench or chair 15–17 inches in height.

Count 1—Place right foot on bench.

Count 2—Bring left foot alongside of right and stand erect.

Count 3—Lower right foot to floor.

Count 4—Lower left foot to floor.

Repeat the 4-count movement 30 times a minute for two minutes.

THEN sit down on bench or chair for two minutes.

FOLLOWING the 2-minute rest, take your pulse for 30 seconds. Double the count to get the per-minute rate. (You can find the pulse by applying middle and index fingers of one hand firmly to the inside of the wrist of the other hand, on the thumb side.)

Record your score for future comparisons. In succeeding tests—about once every two weeks—you probably will find your pulse rate becoming lower as your physical condition improves.

Three important points:

1. For best results, do not engage in physical activity for at least 10 minutes before taking the test. Take it at about the same time of day and always use the same bench or chair.

2. Remember that pulse rates vary among individuals. This is an individual test. What is important is not a comparison of your pulse rate with that of anybody else—but rather a record of how your own rate is reduced as your fitness increases.

3. As you progress, the rate at which your pulse is lowered should gradually level off. This is an indication that you are approaching peak fitness.

Your progress records

Charts are provided for the orientation program and for each of the five levels.

They list the exercises to be done and the goal for each exercise in terms of of number of repetitions, distance, etc.

They also provide space in which to record your progress—(1) in completing the recommended 15 workouts at each level, (2) in accomplishing the three prove-out workouts before moving on to a succeeding level, and (3) in the results as you take the step test from time to time.

A sample chart and progress record for one of the five levels is shown below.

You do the warmup exercises and the conditioning exercises along with one circulatory activity for each workout.

Check off each workout as you complete it. The last three numbers are for the prove-out workouts, in which the seven conditioning exercises should be done without resting. Check them off as you accomplish them.

You are now ready to proceed to the next level.

As you take the step test—at about 2-week intervals—enter your pulse rate.

When you move on to the next level, transfer the last pulse rate from the preceeding level. Enter it in the margin to the left of the new progress record and circle it so it will be convenient for continuing reference.

SAMPLE	GOAL
Warmup Exercises	**Exercises 1–6 of Orientation program**
Conditioning Exercises	**Uninterrupted repetitions**
1. Toe touch	20
2. Sprinter	16
3. Sitting stretch	18
4. Pushup	10
5. Situp (fingers laced)	15
6. Leg raiser	16 each leg
7. Flutter kick	40
Circulatory activity (choose one each workout)	
Jog-walk (jog 100, walk 100)	1 mile
Rope (skip 60 secs.; rest 60 secs.)	3 series
Run in place (run 95, hop 15 – 2 cycles)	3 minutes
Water activities—See recommendations in Section IV.	

Your progress record	1	2	3	4	5	6	7	8	9	10	11	12	13 14 15 Prove-out workouts
Step test (pulse)													

Getting set—orientation workouts

With the series of preliminary exercises listed in the chart at the bottom of the next page and illustrated and described on the next two pages, you can get yourself ready—without severe aches or pains—for the progressive conditioning program.

Even if these preliminary exercises should seem easy—and they are deliberately meant to be mild—plan to spend a minimum of one week with them. Do not hesitate to spend two weeks or even three if necessary for you to limber up enough so you can accomplish all the exercises easily and without undue fatigue.

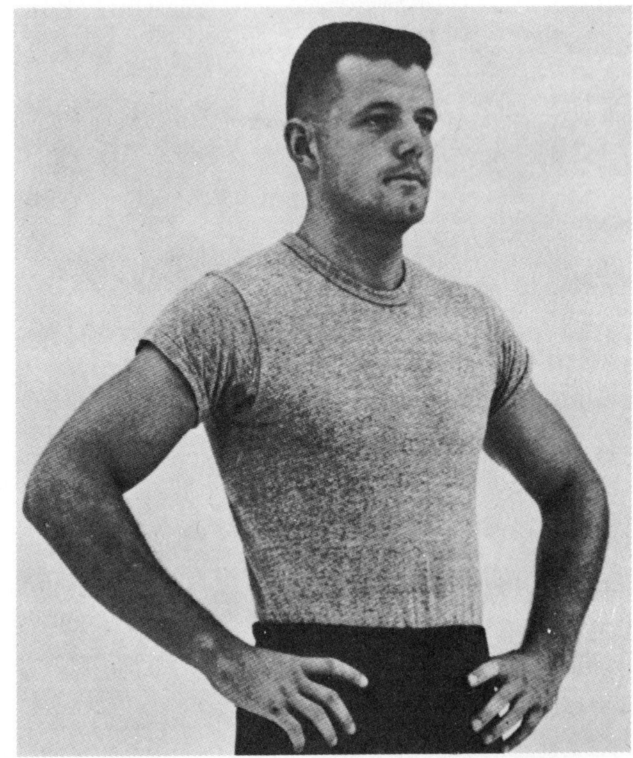

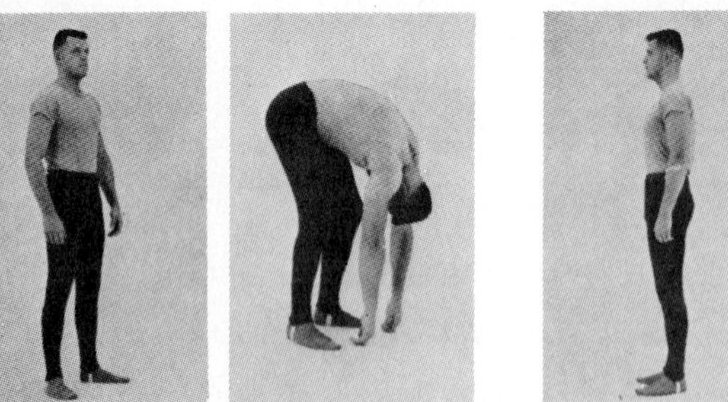

1. BEND AND STRETCH

Starting position: Stand erect, feet shoulder-width apart.
Action: Count 1. Bend trunk forward and down, flexing knees. Stretch gently in attempt to touch fingers to toes or floor. Count 2. Return to starting position.
Note: Do slowly, stretch and relax at intervals rather than in rythm.

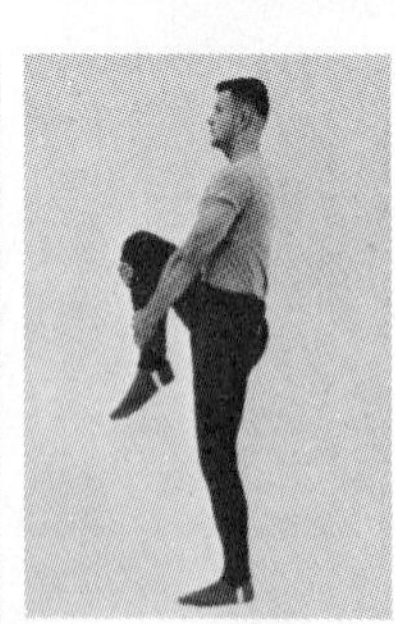

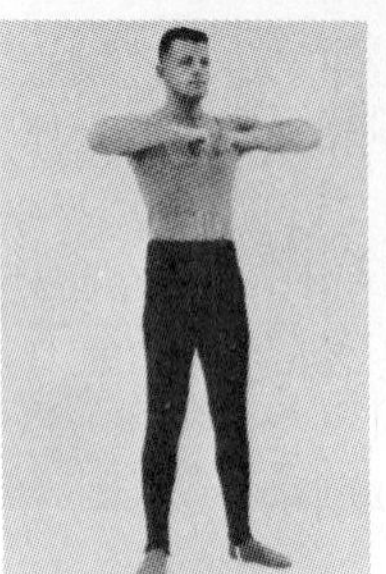

2. KNEE LIFT

Starting position: Stand erect, feet together, arms at sides.
Action: Count 1. Raise left knee as high as possible, grasping leg with hands and pulling knee against body while keeping back straight. Count 2. Lower to starting position. Counts 3 and 4. Repeat with right knee.

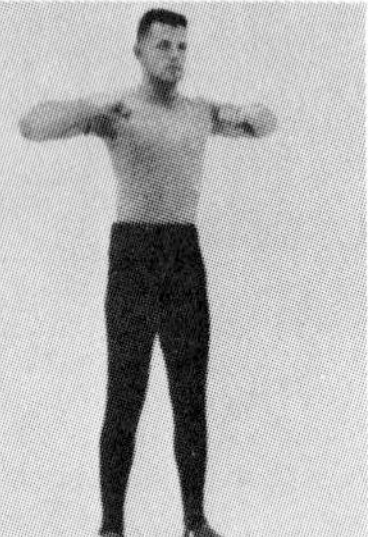

3. WING STRETCHER

Starting position: Stand erect, elbows at shoulder height, fists clenched in front of chest.
Action: Count 1. Thrust elbows backward vigorously without arching back. Keep head erect, elbows at shoulder height. Count 2. Return to starting position.

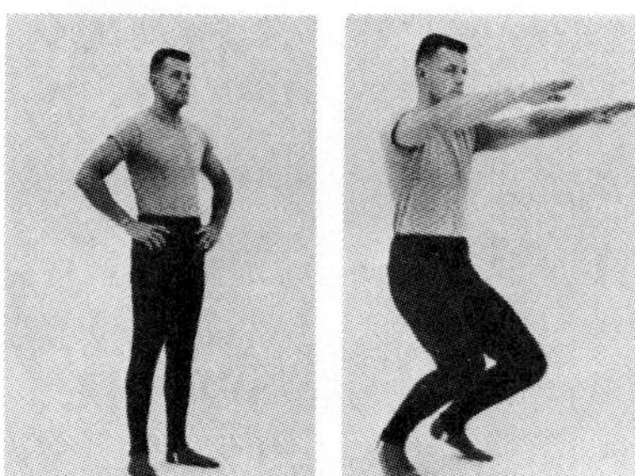

4. HALF KNEE BEND

Starting position: Stand erect, hands on hips. *Action:* Count 1. Bend knees halfway while extending arms forward, palms down. Count 2. Return to starting position.

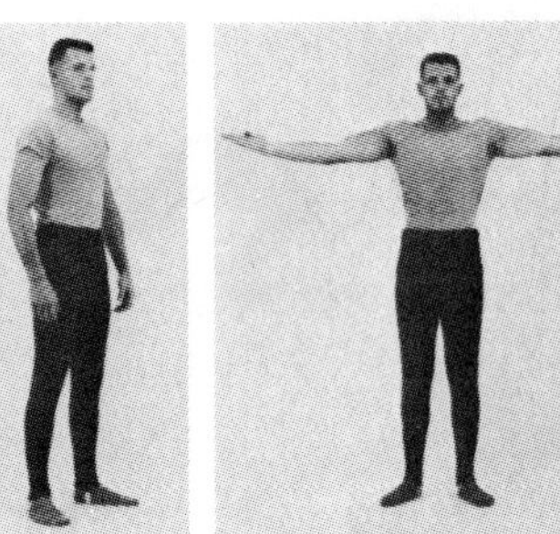

5. ARM CIRCLES

Starting position: Stand erect, arms extended sideward at shoulder height, palms up. *Action:* Describe small circles backward with hands. Keep head erect. Do 15 backward circles. Reverse, turn palms down and do 15 small circles forward.

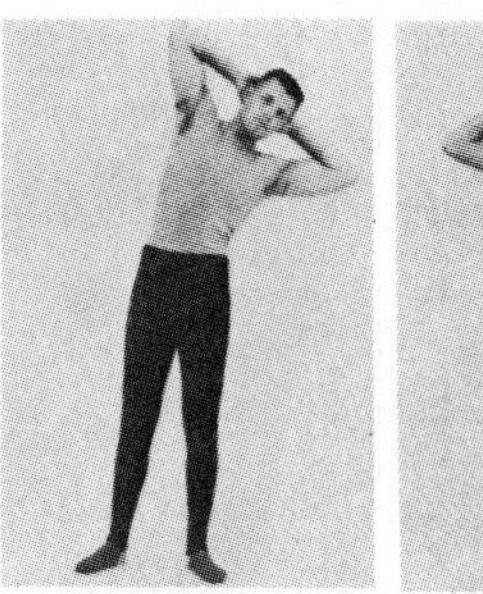

6. BODY BENDER

Starting position: Stand, feet shoulder-width apart hands behind neck, fingers interlaced. *Action:* Count 1. Bend trunk sideward to left as far as possible, keeping hands behind neck. Count 2. Return to starting position. Counts 3 and 4. Repeat to the right.

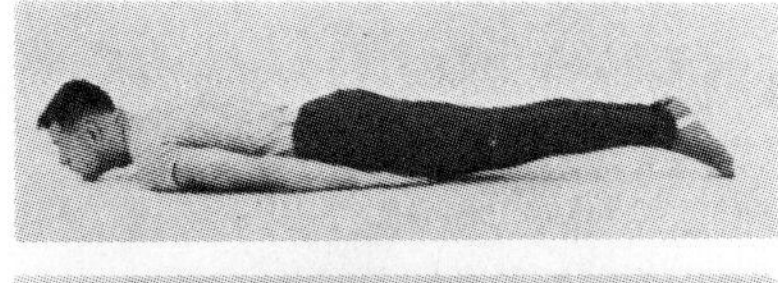

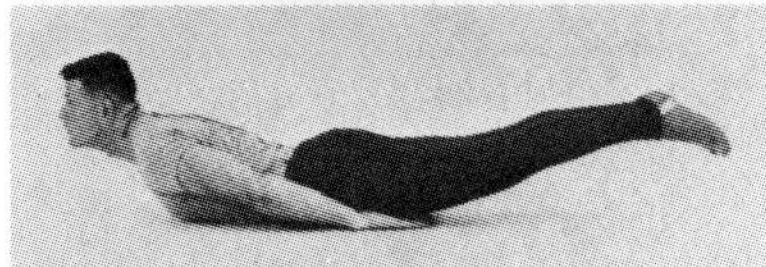

7. PRONE ARCH

Starting position: Lie face down, hands tucked under thighs. *Action:* Count 1. Raise head, shoulders, and legs from floor. Count 2. Return to starting position.

ORIENTATION PROGRAM — GOAL

Conditioning Exercises	Repetitions
*1. Bend and stretch	10
*2. Knee lift	10 left, 10 right
*3. Wing stretcher	20
*4. Half knee bend	10
*5. Arm circles	15 each way
*6. Body bender	10 left, 10 right
7. Prone arch	10
8. Knee pushup	6
9. Head and shoulder curl	5
10. Ankle stretch	15

Circulatory activity (choose one each workout)	
Walking	½ mile
Rope (skip 15 secs.; rest 60 secs.)	3 series

*The first six exercises of the Orientation program will be used as warmup exercises throughout the graded levels. *Step Test Record*—After completing the orientation program, take the 2-minute step test (as described on pp. 38–39). Record your pulse rate here: _____ This will be the base rate with which you can make comparisons in the future.

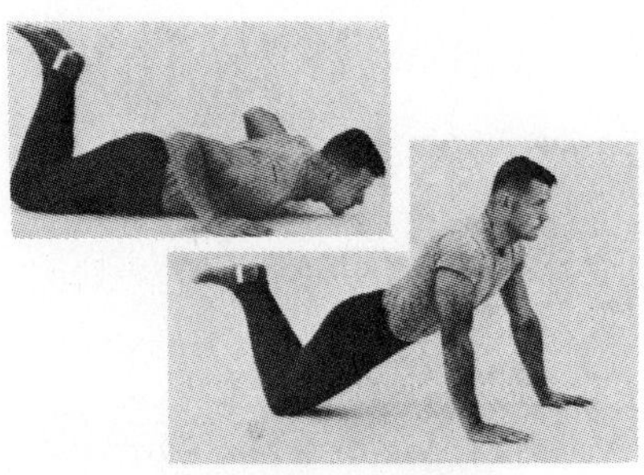

8. KNEE PUSHUP

Starting position: Lie on floor, face down, legs together, knees bent with feet raised off floor, hands on floor under shoulders, palms down. *Action:* Count 1. Push upper body off floor until arms are fully extended and body is in straight line from head to knees. Count 2. Return to starting position.

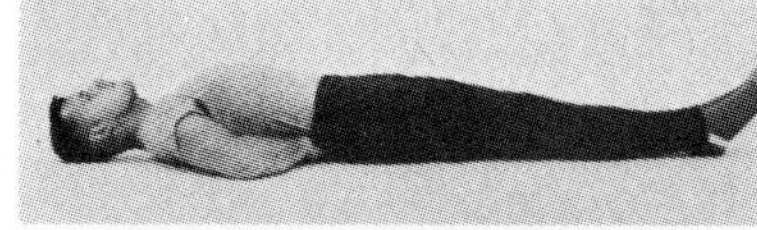

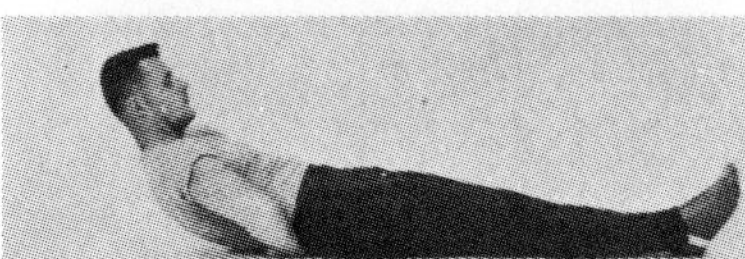

9. HEAD AND SHOULDER CURL

Starting position: Lie on back, hands tucked under small of back, palms down. *Action:* Count 1. Tighten abdominal muscles, lift head and pull shoulders and elbows up off floor. Hold for four seconds. Count 2. Return to starting position.

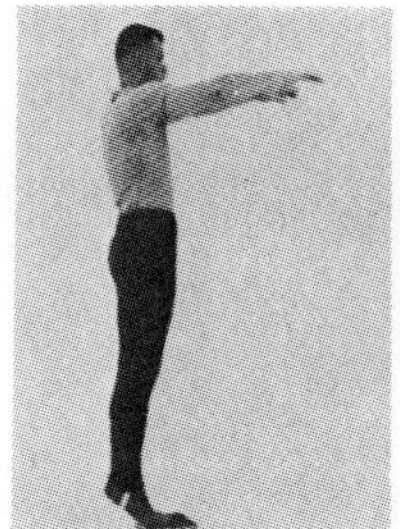

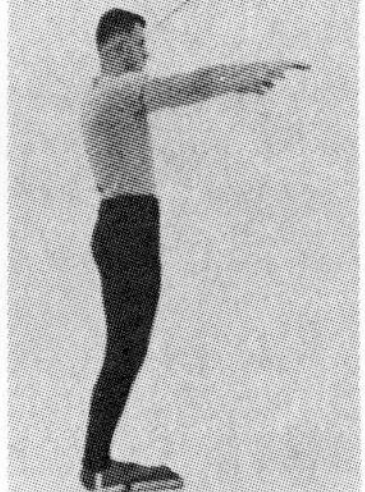

10. ANKLE STRETCH

Starting position: Stand on a stair, large book or block of wood, with weight on balls of feet and heels raised. *Action:* Count 1. Lower heels. Count 2. Raise heels.

CIRCULATORY ACTIVITIES

WALKING—Step off at a lively pace, swing arms and breathe deeply. *ROPE*—Any form of skipping or jumping is acceptable. Gradually increase the tempo as your skill and condition improve.

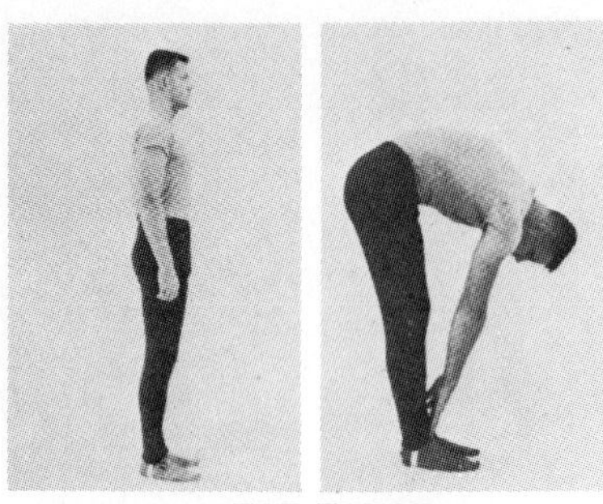

1. TOE TOUCH

Starting position: Stand at attention.
Action: Count 1. Bend trunk forward and down keeping knees straight, touching fingers to ankles. Count 2. Bounce and touch fingers to top of feet. Count 3. Bounce and touch fingers to toes. Count 4. Return to starting position.

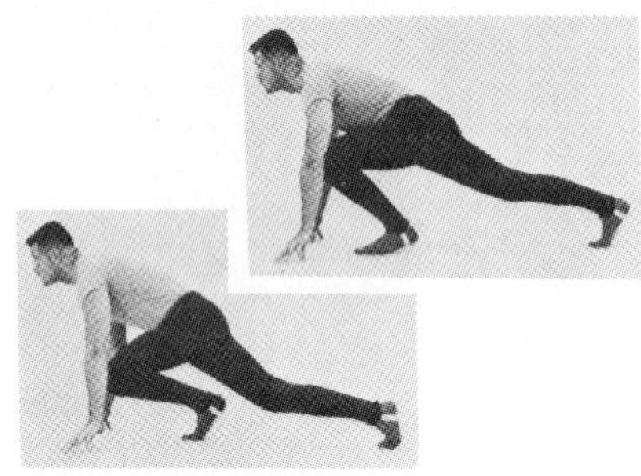

2. SPRINTER

Starting position: Squat, hands on floor, fingers pointed forward, left leg fully extended to rear.
Action: Count 1. Reverse position of feet in bouncing movement, bringing left foot to hands and extending right leg backward—all in one motion. Count 2. Reverse feet again, returning to starting position.

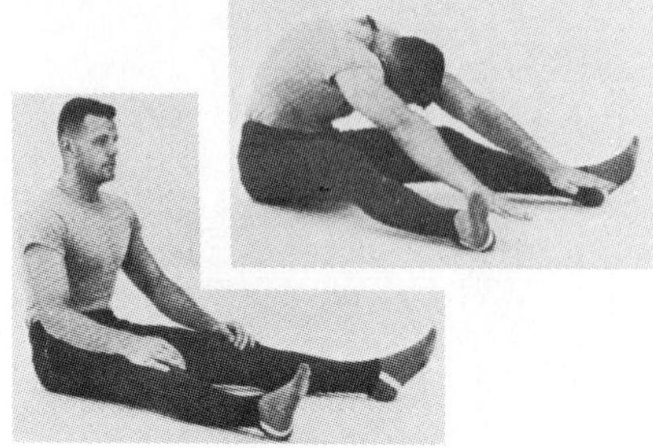

3. SITTING STRETCH

Starting position: Sit, legs spread apart, hands on knees.
Action: Count 1. Bend forward at waist, extending arms as far forward as possible. Count 2. Return to starting position.

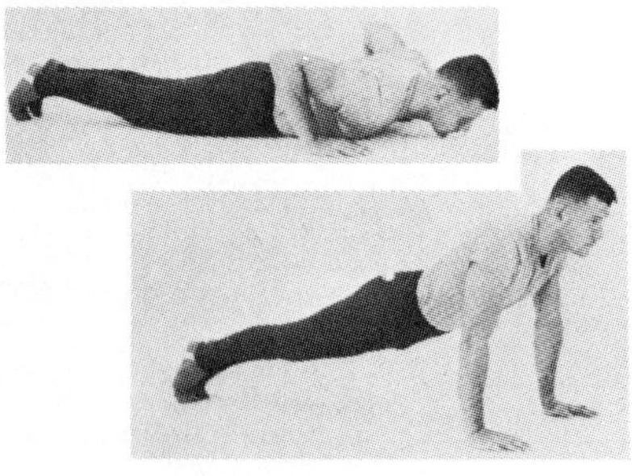

4. PUSHUP

Starting position: Lie on floor, face down, legs together, hands on floor under shoulders with fingers pointing straight ahead.
Action: Count 1. Push body off floor by extending arms, so that weight rests on hands and toes. Count 2. Lower the body until chest touches floor.
Note: Body should be kept straight, buttocks should not be raised, abdomen should not sag.

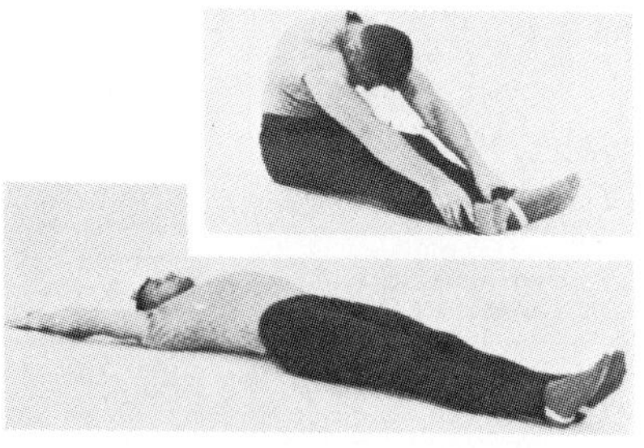

5. SITUP (ARMS EXTENDED)

Starting position: Lie on back, legs straight and together, arms extended beyond head.
Action: Count 1. Bring arms forward over head, roll up to sitting position, sliding hands along legs, grasping ankles. Count 2. Roll back to starting position.

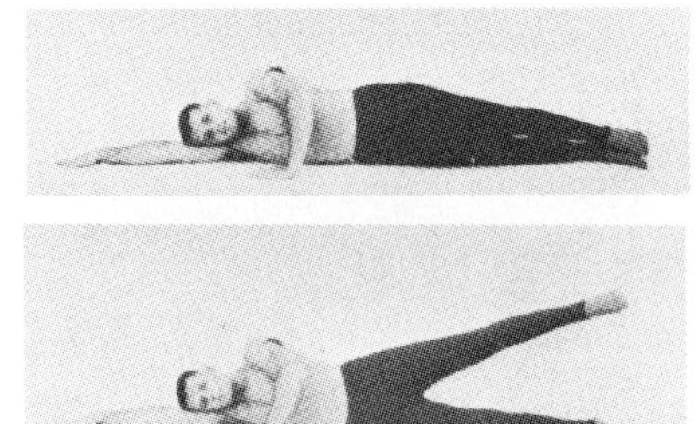

6. LEG RAISER

Starting position: Right side of body on floor, head resting on right arm.
Action: Lift left leg about 24″ off floor, then lower it. Do required number of repetitions. Repeat on other side.

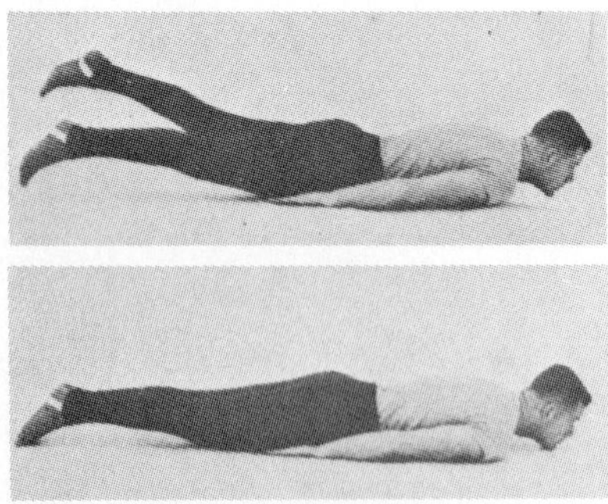

7. FLUTTER KICK

Starting position: Lie face down, hands tucked under thighs.
Action: Arch the back, bringing chest and head up, then flutter kick continuously, moving the legs 8″–10″ apart. Kick from hips with knees slightly bent. Count each kick as one.

CIRCULATORY ACTIVITIES

WALKING—Maintain a pace of 120 steps per minute for a distance of 1 mile. Swing arms and breathe deeply.
ROPE—Skip or jump rope continuously using any form for 30 seconds and then rest 30 seconds. Repeat 2 times.
RUN IN PLACE—Raise each foot at least 4″ off floor and jog in place. Count 1 each time left foot touches floor. Complete the number of running steps called for in chart, then do specified number of straddle hops. Complete 2 cycles of alternate running and hopping for time specified on chart.
STRADDLE HOP—*Starting position:* At attention.
Action: Count 1. Swing arms sideward and upward, touching hands above head (arms straight) while simultaneously moving feet sideward and apart in a single jumping motion. Count 2. Spring back to starting position. Two counts in one hop.

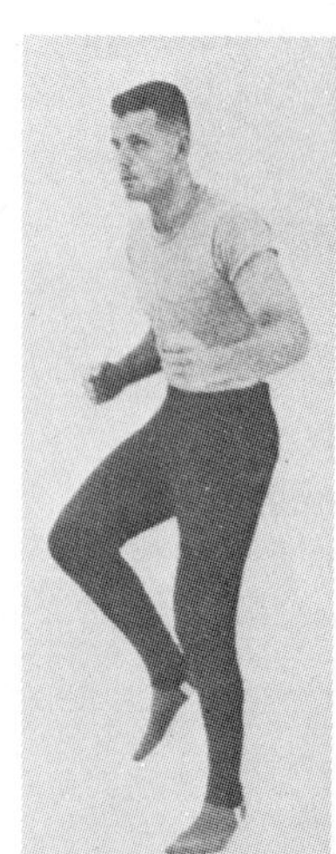

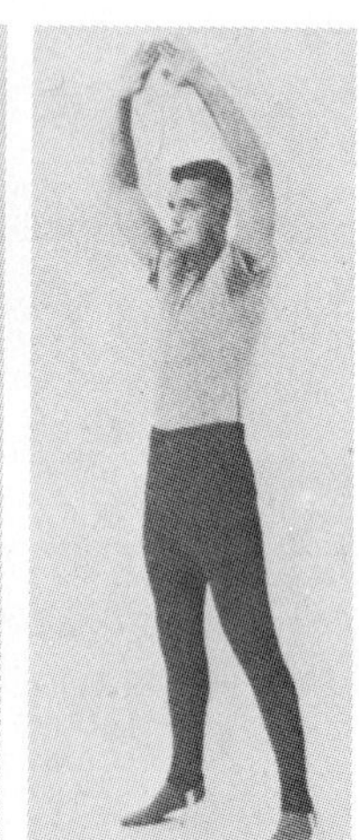

MEN: LEVEL ONE ★ GOAL

Warmup Exercises	**Exercises 1–6 of Orientation program**
Conditioning Exercises	**Uninterrupted repetitions**
1. Toe touch	10
2. Sprinter	12
3. Sitting stretch	12
4. Pushup	4
5. Situp (arms extended)	5
6. Leg raiser	12 each leg
7. Flutter kick	30
Circulatory activity (choose one each workout)	
Walking (120 steps a minute)	1 mile
Rope (skip 30 secs.; rest 30 secs.)	2 series
Run in place (run 60, hop 10 – 2 cycles)	2 minutes

Water activities —See recommendations in Section IV.

Your progress record	1	2	3	4	5	6	7	8	9	10	11	12	13	14	15
Step test (pulse)													Prove-out workouts		

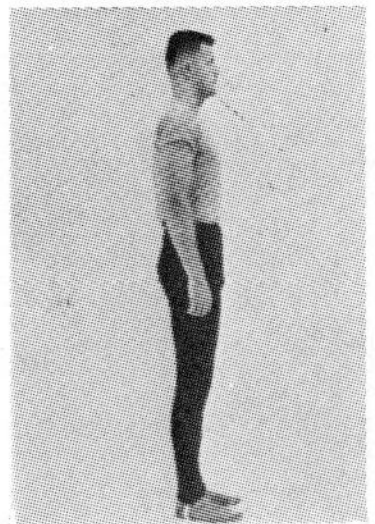
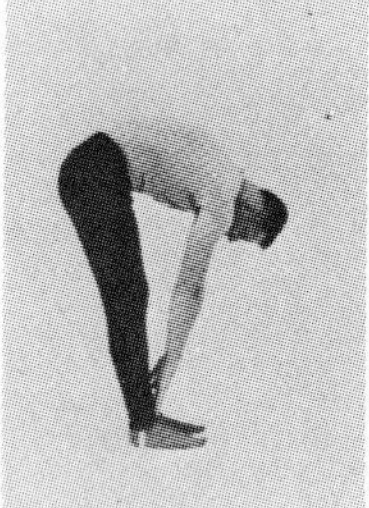

1. TOE TOUCH

Starting position: Stand at attention.
Action: Count 1. Bend trunk forward and down keeping knees straight, touching fingers to ankles. Count 2. Bounce and touch fingers to top of feet. Count 3. Bounce and touch fingers to toes. Count 4. Return to starting position.

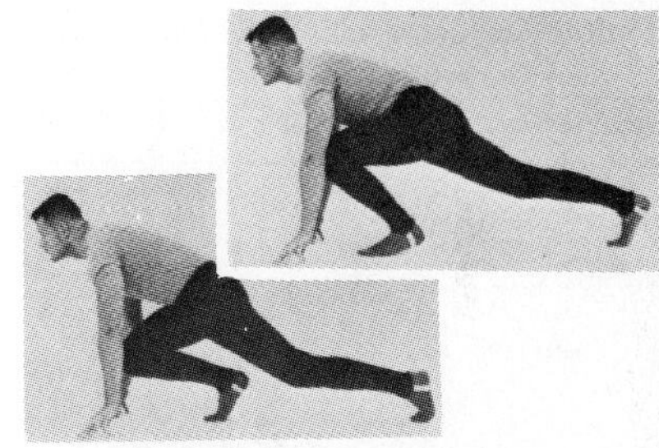

2. SPRINTER

Starting position: Squat, hands on floor, fingers pointed forward, left leg fully extended to rear.
Action: Count 1. Reverse position of feet in bouncing movement, bringing left foot to hands and extending right leg backward—all in one motion. Count 2. Reverse feet again, returning to starting position.

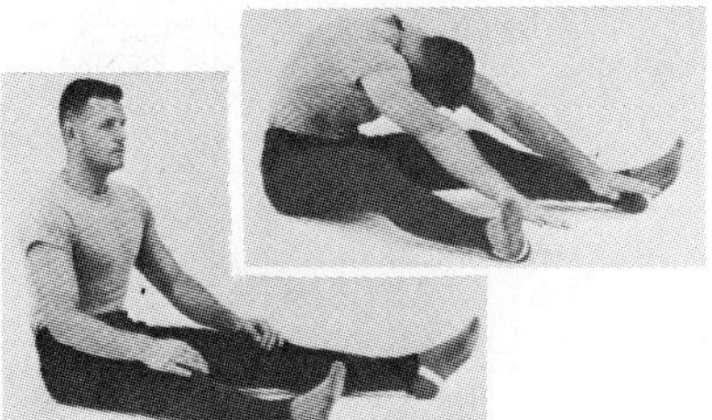

3. SITTING STRETCH

Starting position: Sit, legs spread apart, hands on knees.
Action: Count 1. Bend forward at waist, extending arms as far forward as possible. Count 2. Return to starting position.

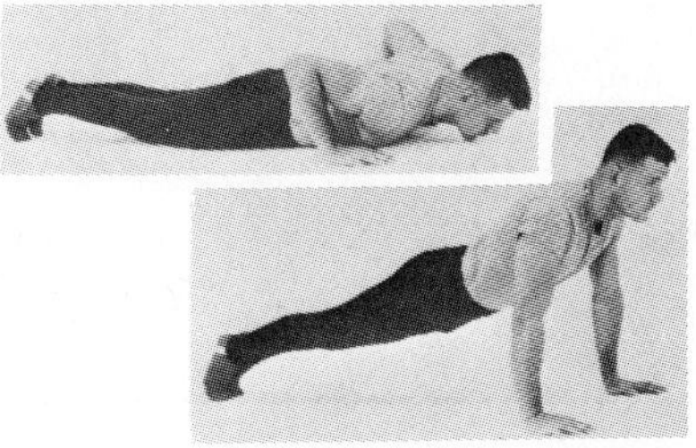

4. PUSHUP

Starting position: Lie on floor, face down, legs together, hands on floor under shoulders with fingers pointing straight ahead.
Action: Count 1. Push body off floor by extending arms, so that weight rests on hands and toes. Count 2. Lower the body until chest touches floor.
Note: Body should be kept straight, buttocks should not be raised, abdomen should not sag

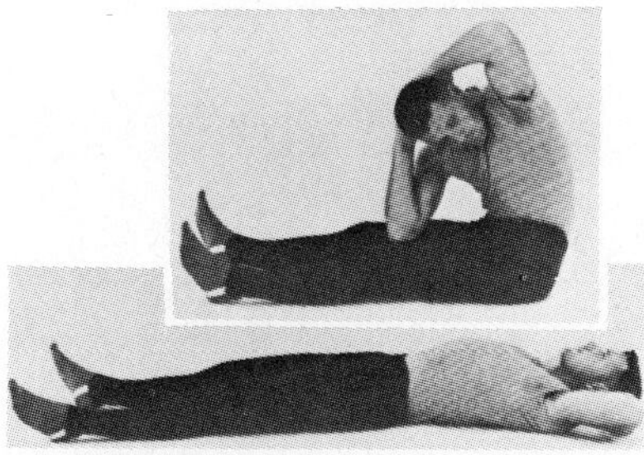

5. SITUP (FINGERS LACED)

Starting position: Lie on back, legs straight and feet spread approximately 1′ apart. Fingers laced behind neck.
Action: Count 1. Curl up to sitting position and turn trunk to left. Touch the right elbow to left knee. Count 2. Return to starting position. Count 3. Curl up to sitting position and turn trunk to right. Touch left elbow to right knee. Count 4. Return to starting position. Score one situp each time you return to starting position. Knees may be bent as necessary.

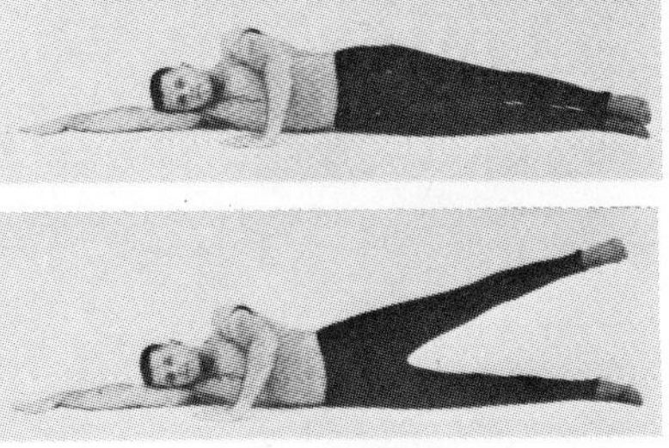

6. LEG RAISER

Starting position: Right side of body on floor, head resting on right arm.
Action: Lift left leg about 24″ off floor, then lower it. Do required number of repetitions. Repeat on other side.

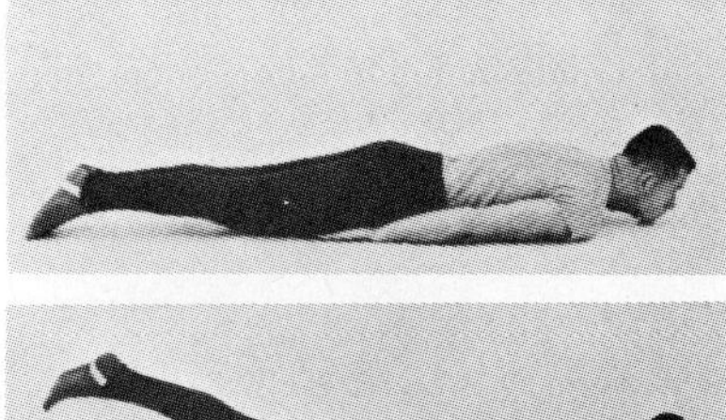
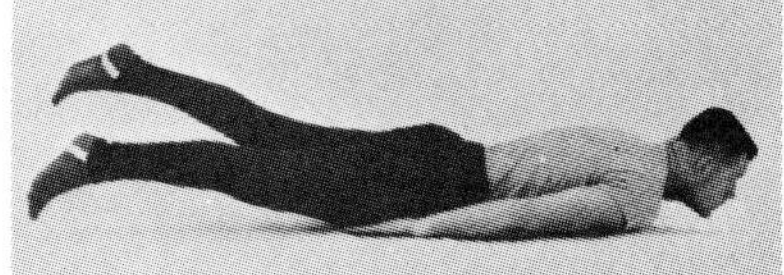

7. FLUTTER KICK

Starting position: Lie face down, hands tucked under thighs.
Action: Arch the back, bringing chest and head up, then flutter kick continuously, moving the legs 8″–10″ apart. Kick from hips with knees slightly bent. Count each kick as one.

MEN: LEVEL TWO ☆☆

GOAL

Warmup Exercises	Exercises 1–6 of Orientation program
Conditioning Exercises	**Uninterrupted repetition**
1. Toe touch	20
2. Sprinter	16
3. Sitting stretch	18
4. Pushup	10
5. Situp (fingers laced)	20
6. Leg raiser	16 each leg
7. Flutter kick	40
Circulatory activity (choose one each workout)	
Jog-walk (jog 100; walk 100)	1 mile
Rope (skip 1 min.; rest 1 min.)	3 series
Run in place (run 95, hop 15 – 2 cycles)	3 minutes

Water activities—See recommendations in Section IV.

Your progress record	1	2	3	4	5	6	7	8	9	10	11	12	13	14	15
Step test (pulse)													Prove-out workouts		

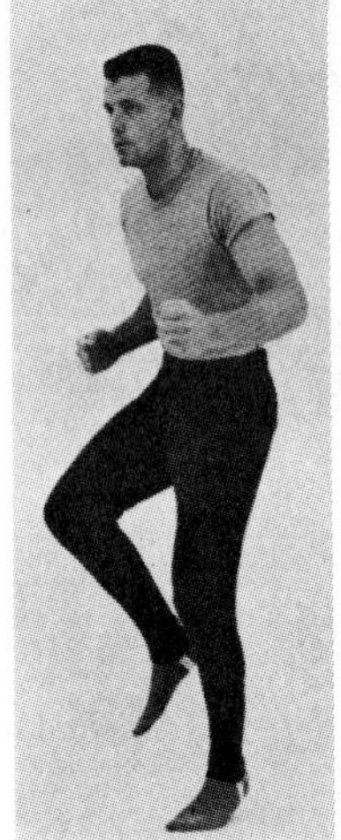
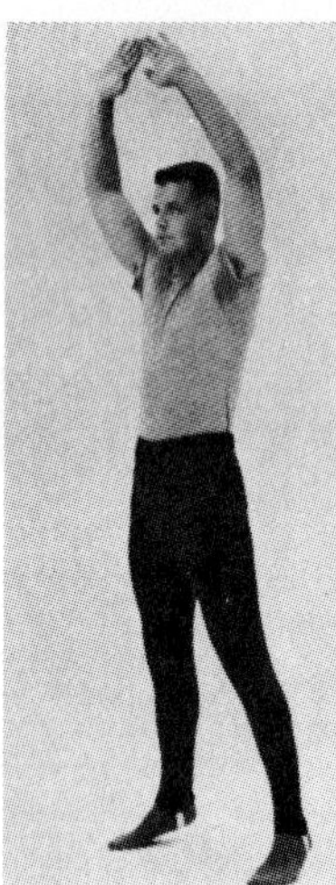

CIRCULATORY ACTIVITIES

JOG-WALK—Jog and walk alternately for number of paces indicated on chart for distance specified.
ROPE—Skip or jump rope continuously using any form for 60 seconds and then rest 60 seconds. Repeat 3 times.
RUN IN PLACE—Raise each foot at least 4'' off floor and jog in place. Count 1 each time left foot touches floor. Complete the number of running steps called for in chart, then do specified number of straddle hops. Complete 2 cycles of alternate running and hopping for time specified on chart.
STRADDLE HOP—Starting position: At attention.
Action: Count 1. Swing arms sideward and upward, touching hands above head (arms straight) while simultaneously moving feet sideward and apart in a single jumping motion. Count 2. Spring back to starting position. Two counts in one hop.

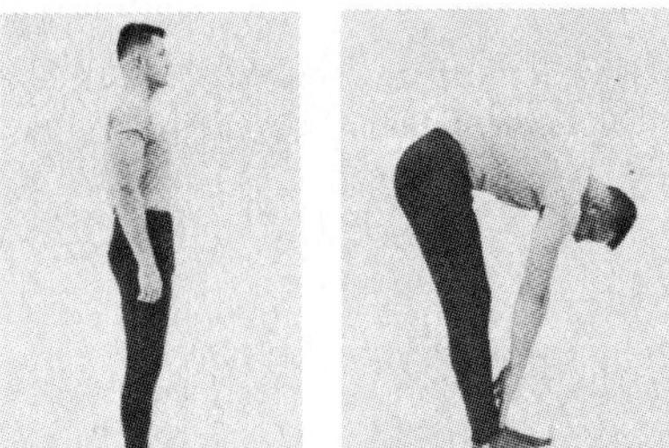

1. TOE TOUCH

Starting position: Stand at attention.
Action: Count 1. Bend trunk forward and down keeping knees straight, touching fingers to ankles. Count 2. Bounce and touch fingers to top of feet. Count 3. Bounce and touch fingers to toes. Count 4. Return to starting position.

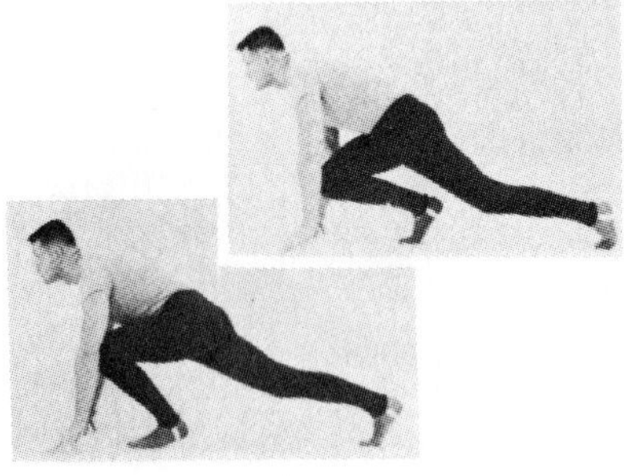

2. SPRINTER

Starting position: Squat, hands on floor, fingers pointed forward, left leg fully extended to rear.
Action: Count 1. Reverse position of feet in bouncing movement, bringing left foot to hands, extending right leg backward—all in one motion. Count 2. Reverse feet again, returning to starting position.

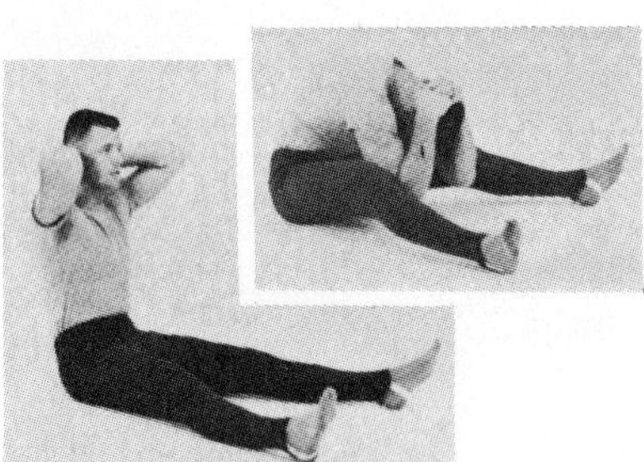

3. SITTING STRETCH (FINGERS LACED)

Starting position: Sit, legs spread apart, fingers laced behind neck, elbows back.
Action: Count 1. Bend forward at waist, reaching elbows as close to floor as possible. Count 2. Return to starting position.

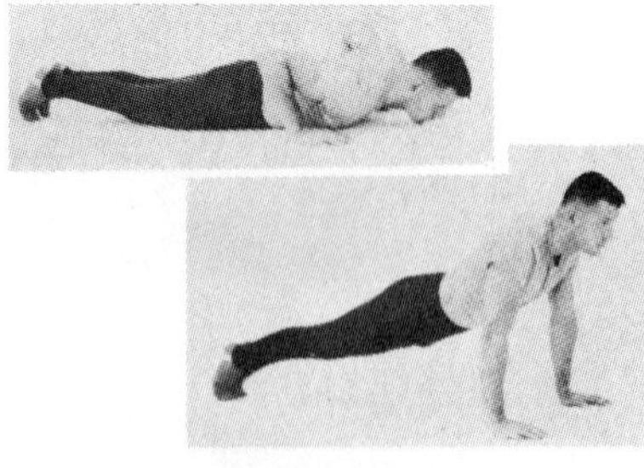

4. PUSHUP

Starting position: Lie on floor, face down, legs together, hands on floor under shoulders with fingers pointing straight ahead.
Action: Count 1. Push body off floor by extending arms, so that weight rests on hands and toes. Count 2. Lower the body until chest touches floor.
Note: Body should be kept straight, buttocks should not be raised, abdomen should not sag.

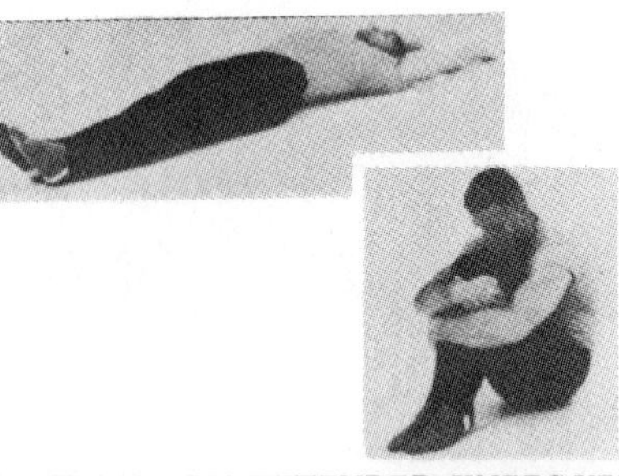

5. SITUP (ARMS EXTENDED, KNEES UP)

Starting position: Lie on back, legs straight, arms extended overhead.
Action: Count 1. Sit up, reaching forward with arms encircling knees while pulling them tightly to chest. Count 2. Return to starting position. Do this exercise rhythmically, without breaks in the movement.

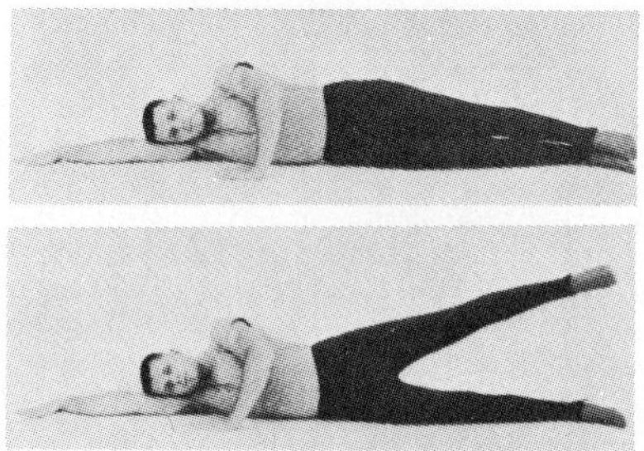

6. LEG RAISER

Starting position: Right side of body on floor, head resting on right arm.
Action: Lift left leg about 24″ off floor then lower it. Do required number of repetitions. Repeat on other side.

MEN: LEVEL THREE ☆☆☆ GOAL

Warmup Exercises	Exercises 1–6 of Orientation program
Conditioning Exercises	**Uninterrupted repetition**
1. Toe touch	30
2. Sprinter	20
3. Sitting stretch (fingers laced)	18
4. Pushup	20
5. Situp (arms extended, knees up)	30
6. Leg raiser	20 each leg
7. Flutter kick	50
Circulatory activity (choose one each workout)	
Jog-walk (jog 200; walk 100)	1½ miles
Rope (skip 1 min.; rest 1 min.)	5 series
Run in place (run 135, hop 20 – 2 cycles)	4 minutes
Water activity—See recommendations in Section IV.	

Your progress record	1	2	3	4	5	6	7	8	9	10	11	12	13	14	15
Step test (pulse)													Prove-out workouts		

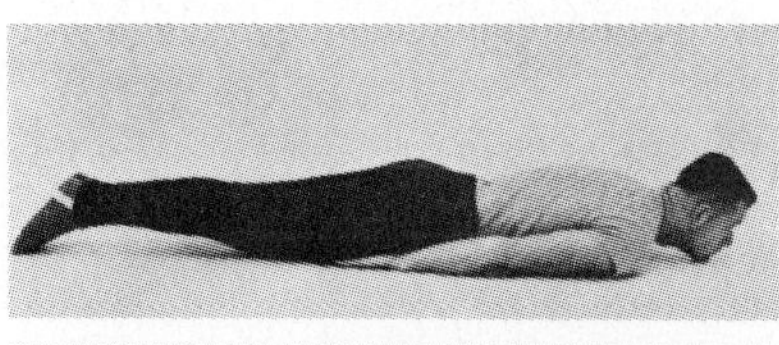

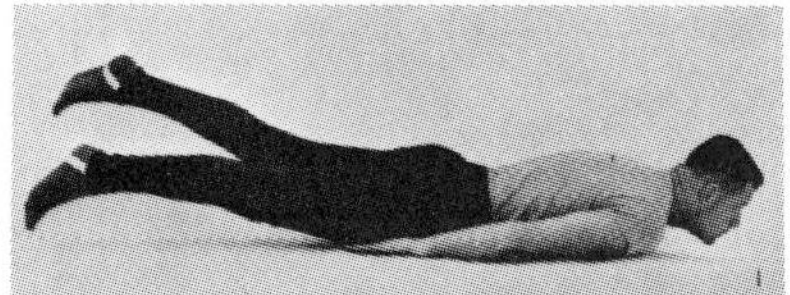

7. FLUTTER KICK

Starting position: Lie face down, hands tucked under thighs.
Action: Arch the back, bringing chest and head up, then flutter kick continuously, moving the legs 8″–10″ apart. Kick from hips with knees slightly bent. Count each kick as one.

CIRCULATORY ACTIVITIES

JOG-WALK—Jog and walk alternately for number of paces indicated on chart for distance specified.
ROPE—Skip or jump rope continuously using any form for 60 seconds and then rest 60 seconds. Repeat 5 times.
RUN IN PLACE—Raise each foot at least 4″ off floor and jog in place. Count 1 each time left foot touches floor. Complete number of running steps called for in chart, then do specified number of straddle hops. Complete 2 cycles of alternate running and hopping for time specified on chart.
STRADDLE HOP—*Starting position:* At attention.
Action: Count 1. Swing arms sideward and upward, touching hands above head (arms straight) while simultaneously moving feet sideward and apart in a single jumping motion. Count 2. Spring back to starting position. Two counts in one hop.

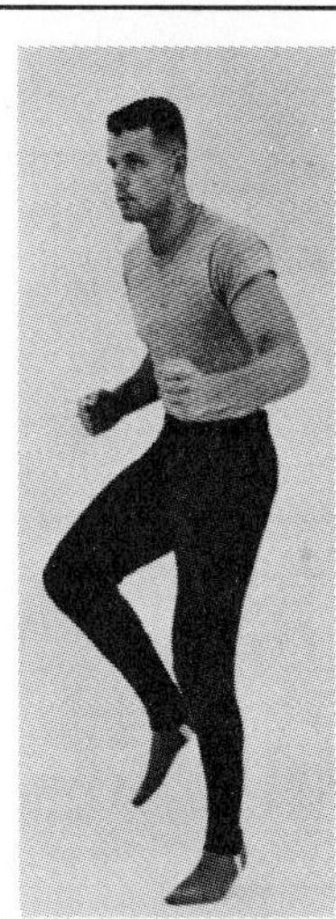

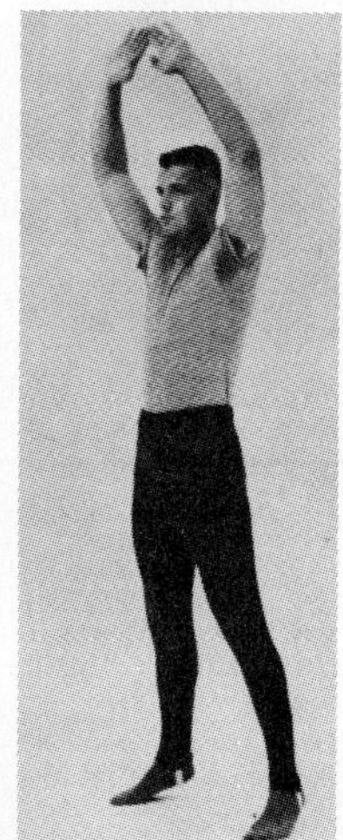

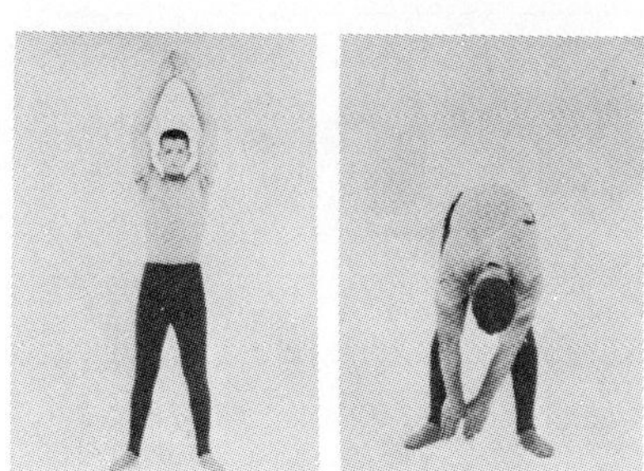

1. TOE TOUCH (TWIST AND BEND)

Starting position: Stand, feet shoulder-width apart, arms extended overhead, thumbs interlocked.
Action: Count 1. Twist trunk to right and touch floor inside right foot with fingers of both hands. Count 2. Touch floor outside toes of right foot. Count 3. Touch floor outside heel of right foot. Count 4. Return to starting position, sweeping trunk and arms upward in a wide arc. On the next four counts, repeat action to left side.

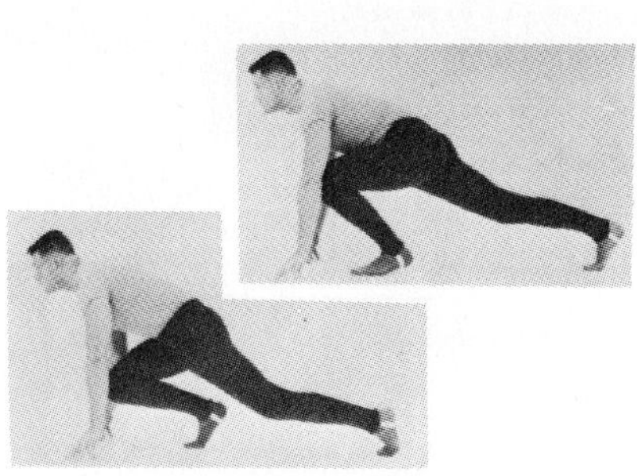

2. SPRINTER

Starting position: Squat, hands on floor, fingers pointed forward, left leg fully extended to rear.
Action: Count 1. Reverse position of feet in bouncing movement, bringing left foot to hands, extending right leg backward—all in one motion. Count 2. Reverse feet again, returning to starting position.

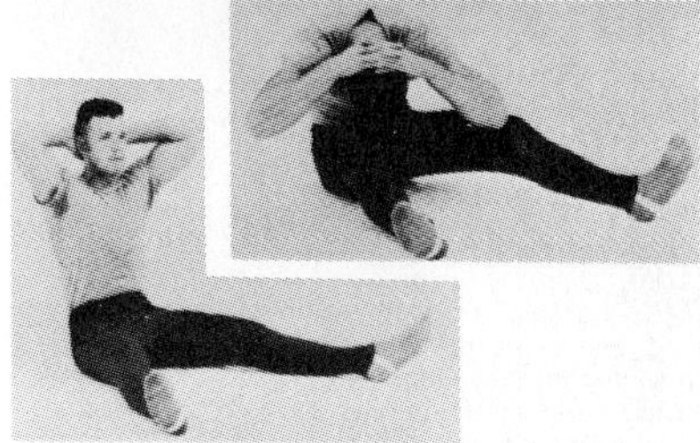

3. SITTING STRETCH (ALTERNATE)

Starting position: Sit, legs spread apart, fingers laced behind neck, elbows back.
Action: Count 1. Bend forward to left, touching forehead to left knee. Count 2. Return to starting position. Counts 3 and 4. Repeat to right. Score one repetition each time you return to starting position. Knees may be bent if necessary.

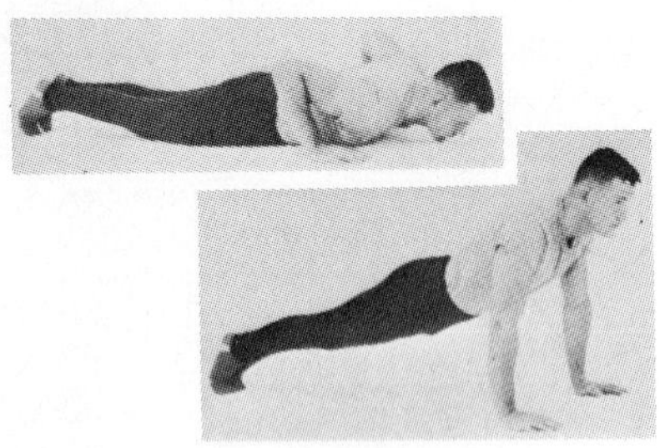

4. PUSHUP

Starting position: Lie on floor, face down, legs together, hands on floor under shoulders with fingers pointing straight ahead.
Action: Count 1. Push body off floor by extending arms, so that weight rests on hands and toes. Count 2. Lower the body until chest touches floor.
Note: Body should be kept straight, buttocks should not be raised, abdomen should not sag.

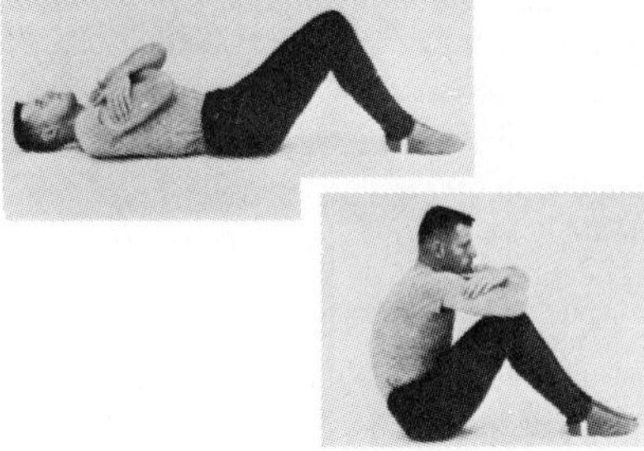

5. SITUP (ARMS CROSSED, KNEES BENT)

Starting position: Lie on back, arms crossed on chest, hands grasping opposite shoulders, knees bent to right angle, feet flat on floor.
Action: Count 1. Curl up to sitting position. Count 2. Return to starting position.

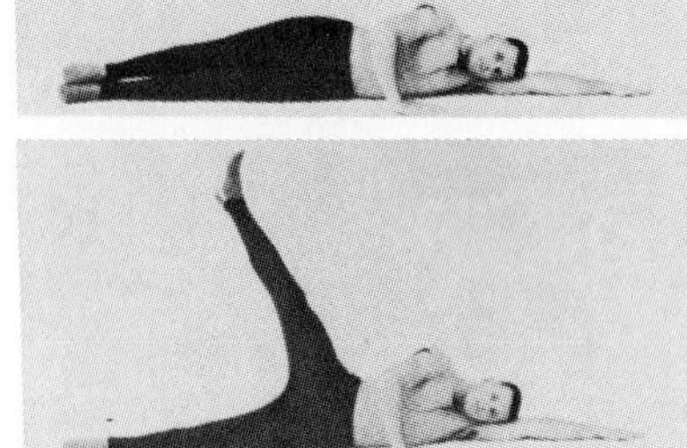

6. LEG RAISER (WHIP)

Starting position: Right side of body on floor, right arm supporting head.
Action: Whip left leg up and down rapidly, lifting as high as possible off the floor. Count each whip as one. Reverse position and whip right leg up and down.

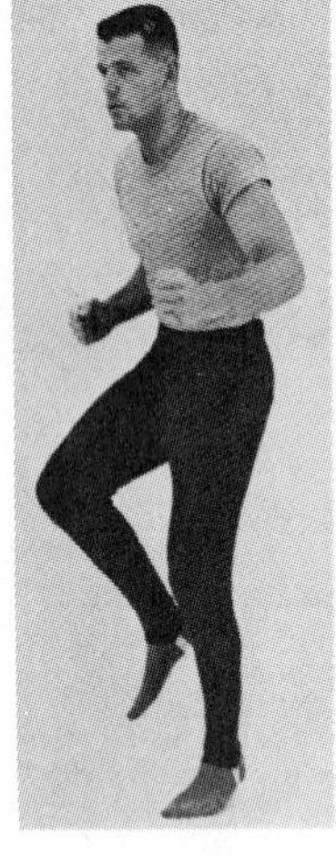

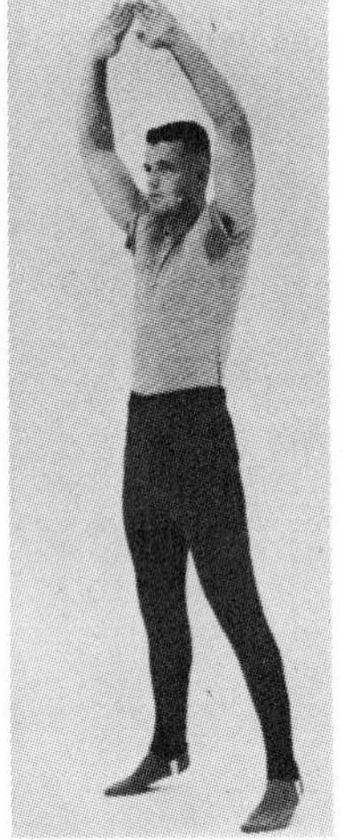

CIRCULATORY ACTIVITIES

JOG—Jog continuously for 1 mile.
ROPE—Skip or jump rope continuously using any form for 90 seconds and then rest for 30 seconds. Repeat 3 times.
RUN IN PLACE—Raise each foot at least 4″ off floor and jog in place. Count 1 each time left foot touches floor. Complete number of running steps called for in chart, then do specified number of straddle hops. Complete 2 cycles of alternate running and hopping in time specified on chart.
STRADDLE HOP—*Starting position:* At attention.
Action: Count 1. Swing arms sideward and upward, touching hands above head (arms straight) while simultaneously moving feet sideward and apart in a single jumping motion. Count 2. Spring back to starting position. Two counts in one hop.

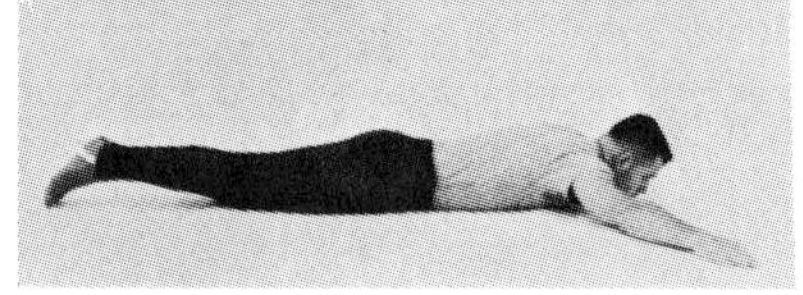

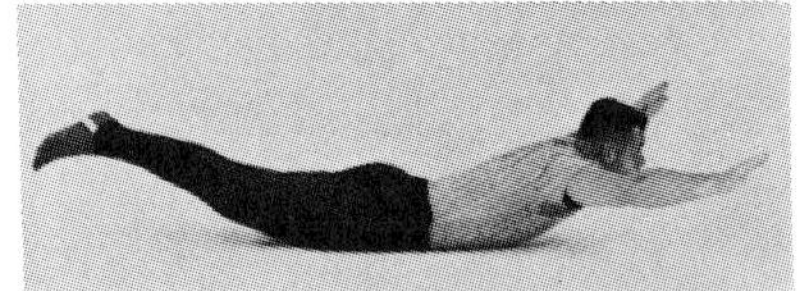

7. PRONE ARCH (ARMS EXTENDED)

Starting position: Lie face down, legs straight and together, arms extended to sides at shoulder level.
Action: Count 1. Arch the back, bringing arms chest and head up, and raising legs as high a possible. Count 2. Return to starting position

MEN: LEVEL FOUR ☆☆☆☆ GOAL

Warmup Exercises	**Exercises 1–6 of Orientation program**
Conditioning Exercises	**Uninterrupted repetitions**
1. Toe touch (twist and bend)	20 each side
2. Sprinter	28
3. Sitting stretch (alternate)	24
4. Pushup	30
5. Situp (arms crossed, knees bent)	30
6. Leg raiser (whip)	20 each leg
7. Prone arch (arms extended)	20
Circulatory activity (choose one each workout)	
Jog	1 mile
Rope (skip 90 secs.; rest 30 secs.)	3 series
Run in place (run 180; hop 25 – 2 cycles)	5 minutes
Water activities—See recommendations in Section IV.	

Your progress record	1	2	3	4	5	6	7	8	9	10	11	12	13	14	15
Step test (pulse)													Prove-out workouts		

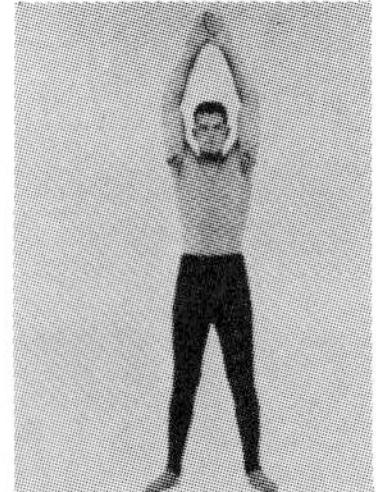
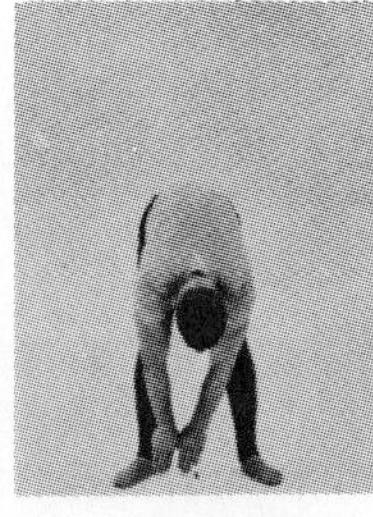

1. TOE TOUCH (TWIST AND BEND)

Starting position: Stand, feet shoulder-width apart, arms extended over head, thumbs interlocked.
Action: Count 1. Twist trunk to right and touch floor inside right foot with fingers of both hands. Count 2. Touch floor outside toes of right foot. Count 3. Touch floor outside heel of right foot. Count 4. Return to starting position, sweeping trunk and arms upward in a wide arc. On the next four counts, repeat action to left side.

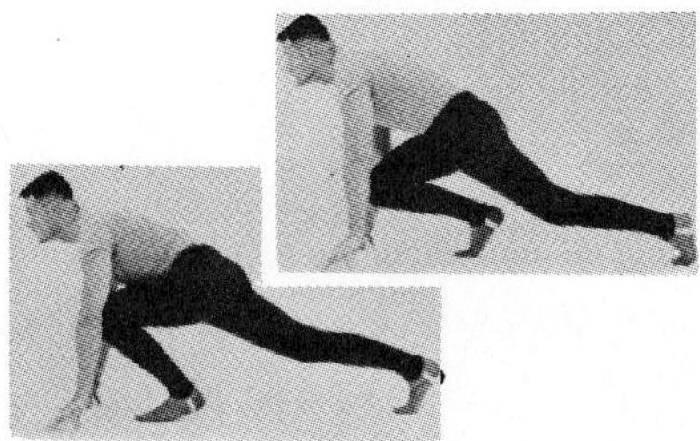

2. SPRINTER

Starting position: Squat, hands on floor, fingers pointed forward, left leg fully extended to rear.
Action: Count 1. Reverse position of feet in bouncing movement, bringing left foot to hands and extending right leg backward—all in one motion. Count 2. Reverse feet again, returning to starting position.

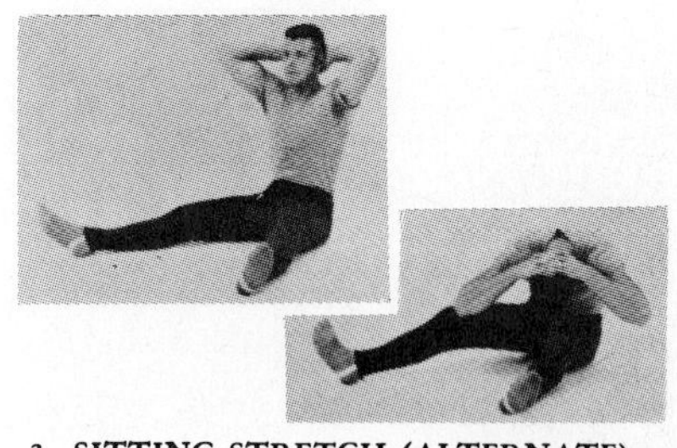

3. SITTING STRETCH (ALTERNATE)

Starting position: Sit, legs spread apart, fingers laced behind neck, elbows back.
Action: Count 1. Bend forward to left, touching forehead to left knee. Count 2. Return to starting position. Counts 3 and 4. Repeat to right. Score one repetition each time you return to starting position. Knees may be bent if necessary.

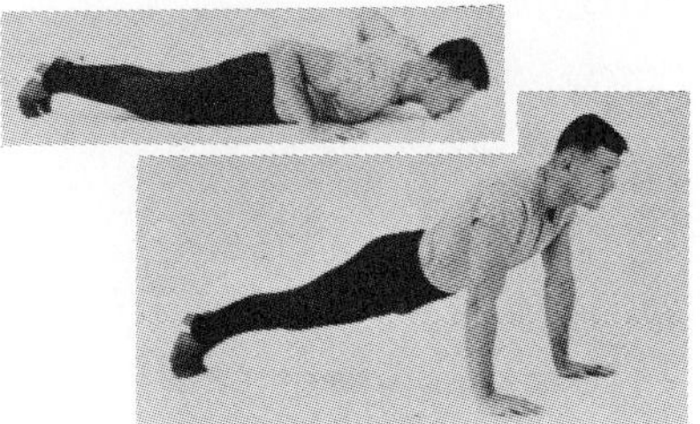

4. PUSHUP

Starting position: Lie on floor, face down, legs together, hands on floor under shoulders with fingers pointing straight ahead.
Action: Count 1. Push body off floor by extending arms so that weight rests on hands and toes. Count 2. Lower body until chest touches floor.
Note: Body should be kept straight, buttocks should not be raised, abdomen should not sag.

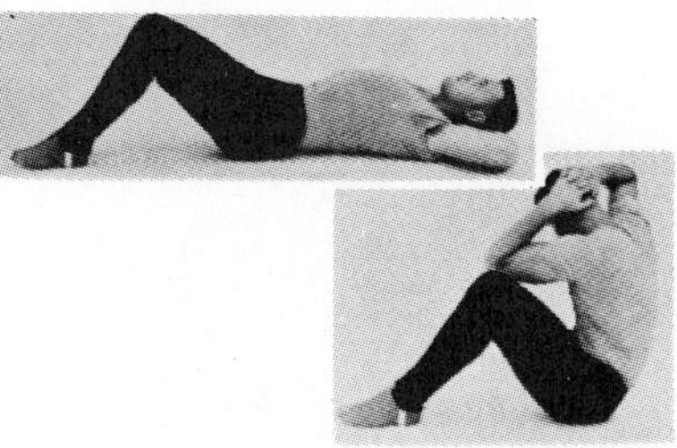

5. SITUP (FINGERS LACED, KNEES BENT)

Starting position: Lie on back, fingers laced behind neck, knees bent, feet flat on floor.
Action: Count 1. Sit up, turn trunk to right, touch left elbow to right knee. Count 2. Return to starting position. Count 3. Sit up, turn trunk to left, touch right elbow to left knee. Count 4. Return to starting position. Score one each time you return to starting position.

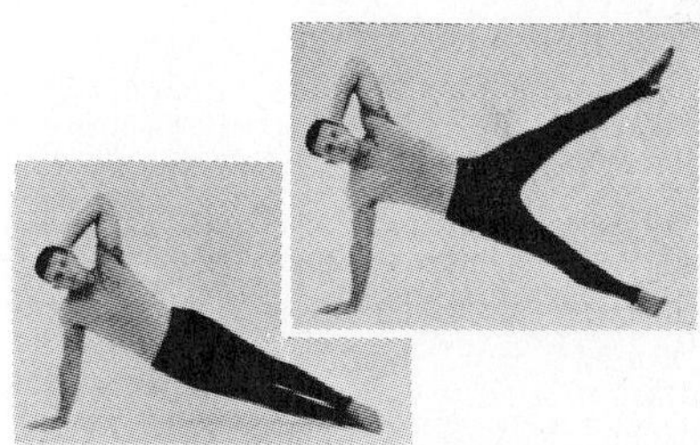

6. LEG RAISER (ON EXTENDED ARM)

Starting position: Body rigidly supported by extended right arm and foot. Left arm is held behind head.
Action: Count 1. Raise left leg high. Count 2. Return to starting position slowly. Do required number of repetitions. Repeat on other side.

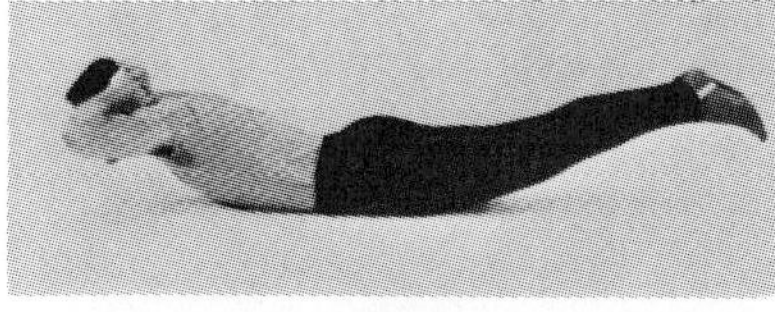
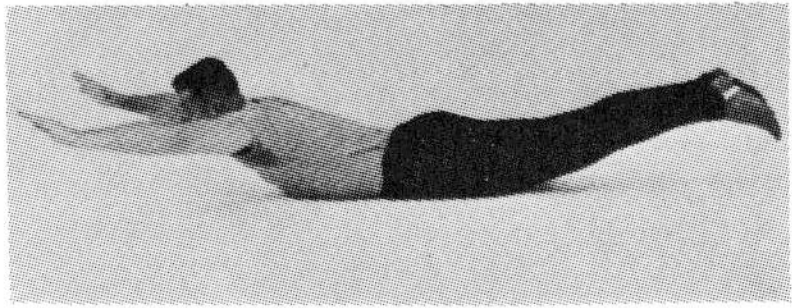

7. PRONE ARCH (FINGERS LACED)

Starting position: Lie face down, fingers laced behind neck.
Action: Count 1. Arch back, legs, and chest off floor. Count 2. Extend arms forward. Count 3. Return hands to behind neck. Count 4. Flatten body to floor.

MEN: LEVEL FIVE ☆☆☆☆☆ GOAL

Warmup Exercises	**Exercises 1–6 of Orientation program**
Conditioning Exercises	**Uninterrupted repetitions**
1. Toe touch (twist and bend)	30 each side
2. Sprinter	36
3. Sitting stretch (alternate)	30
4. Pushup	50
5. Situp (fingers laced, knees bent)	40
6. Leg raiser (on extended arm)	20 each side
7. Prone arch (fingers laced)	30
Circulatory activity (choose one each workout)	
Jog-run	3 miles
Rope (skip 2 mins.; rest 30 secs.)	3 series
Run in place (run 216, hop 30 – 2 cycles)	6 minutes
Water activities—See recommendations in Section IV	

Your progress record	1	2	3	4	5	6	7	8	9	10	11	12	13	14	15
Step test (pulse)													Prove-out workouts		

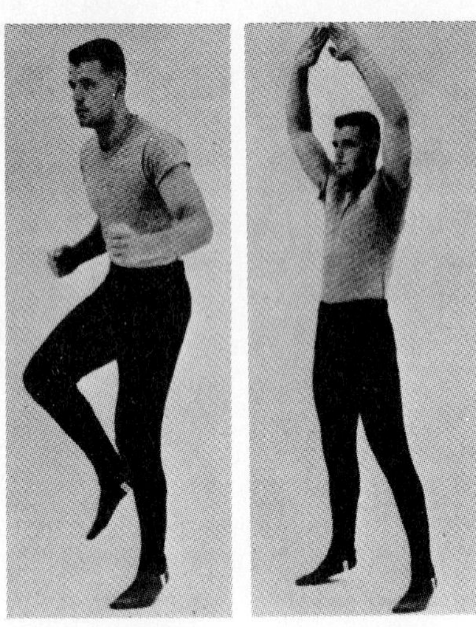

CIRCULATORY ACTIVITIES

JOG-RUN—Alternately jog and run the specified distance. Attempt to increase the proportion of time spent running in each succeeding workout.
ROPE—Skip or jump rope continuously using any form for 2 minutes and then rest 30 seconds, Repeat 3 times.
RUN IN PLACE—Raise each foot at least 4" off floor and jog in place. Count 1 each time left foot touches floor. Complete number of running steps called for in chart, then do specified number of straddle hops. Complete 2 cycles of alternate running and hopping for time specified on the chart.
STRADDLE HOP—*Starting position:* At attention.
Action: Count 1. Swing arms sideward and upward, touching hands above head (arms straight) while simultaneously moving feet sideward and apart in a single jumping motion. Count 2. Spring back to starting position. Two counts in one hop.

Staying fit

After you reach the level of conditioning you have decided is most suitable for you, you can keep yourself fit by continuing the workouts for that level.

While it has been found possible to maintain fitness with three workouts a week, ideally, exercise should be a daily habit. If you can, by all means continue your workouts on a five-times-a-week basis.

If at any point—either after reaching your goal or in the process of doing so—your workouts are interrupted because of illness or other reason for more than a week, it will be best to begin again at a lower level. If you have had a serious illness or surgery, proceed under your physician's guidance.

Broadening your program

The exercises and activities you have engaged in are basic—designed to take you up the ladder of fitness without need for special equipment or facilities.

There are many other activities which, if you wish, you may use to supplement the basic program. They include:

Isometrics—"exercises without movement"—that require no equipment, can be done quickly (6–8 seconds each), and add to muscular strength.

Water exercises you can use if you have access to a pool.

Sports that help maintain or increase fitness.

You will find a discussion of these—and a guide to their use—in the next section.

Also in that section are suggestions for taking advantage of many daily opportunities for sound physical activity—and pertinent tips on good posture.

BROADENING YOUR PROGRAM FOR FITNESS

Daily opportunities for adding to fitness

Isometrics—"exercise without movement"

Water activities

Weight training

Sports

Fitness and posture—improving each with the other

DAILY OPPORTUNITIES FOR ADDING TO FITNESS

There are many—and, by taking advantage of them, you can speed your progress to—and more easily maintain—your top level of fitness.

Here are some examples:

Stairs—versus elevator or escalator: At least now and then, choose the stairs. And bound up them—take two at a time as often as possible.

Breaks—along with, or instead of, those midmorning and midafternoon time-outs for coffee, take exercise breaks. No need to get into a sweat. Do a conditioning exercise or two if convenient. If you lack privacy, do some of the inconspicuous isometric exercises.

Pull-ins—suck in your abdomen now and then, hold it taut for a few seconds.

Up for a stretch—if you must work in a static, sitting position, get up occasionally, stand erect, stretch a bit, move around.

Rub away—after a shower or bath, towel yourself vigorously. That's exercise, too—stimulating for muscles as well as skin.

Walk—every chance you get.

Walking deserves special emphasis

Walking is actually one of the best all-round physical activities. The massaging action the leg muscles exert on the veins as you walk improves the flow of blood back to the heart; when you walk you're improving not only your leg muscles but also the pumping action they provide. Walking costs nothing; there are many possible daily opportunities for it, and it can be enjoyable. Develop a brisk step, breathe deeply, swing your arms.

Allow extra time to get to the train, to the store, to meetings, other places you have to go so you can go, at least now and then, by footpower.

Whenever you feel tense and nervous, try a walk—the brisker and longer, the better; but even a brief one will help discharge tension. Use a before-bed walk as an aid to sleep; it can be a big help in overcoming insomnia.

On an occasional weekend, plan walking as a family enterprise. Set a goal; take a walking tour to a park, other scenic spot, or some place of historical interest.

Whenever possible adult men and women should join physical fitness groups conducted under professional supervision. Such classes are available at local clubs, churches, schools, colleges, community recreation centers, and at the Y's and other voluntary agencies.

ISOMETRICS

Isometric contraction exercises take very little time, require no special equipment. They're excellent muscle strengtheners and, as such, valuable supplements.

The idea of isometrics is to work out a muscle by pushing or pulling against an immovable object such as a wall . . . or by pitting it against the opposition of another muscle.

The basis is the "overload" principle of exercise physiology—which holds that a muscle required to perform work beyond the usual intensity will grow in strength. And research has been indicating that one hard, 6- to 8-second isometric contraction per workout can, over a period of six months, produce a significant strength increase in a muscle.

The exercises illustrated and described in the following pages cover major large muscle groups of the body.

They can be performed almost anywhere and at almost any time.

There is no set order for doing them—nor do all have to be completed at one time. You can, if you like, do one or two in the morning, others at various times during the day whenever you have half a minute or even less to spare.

For each contraction, maintain tension *no more than eight seconds*. Do little breathing during a contraction; breathe deeply between contractions.

And start easily. Do *not* apply maximum effort in the beginning.

For the first three or four weeks, you should exert only about one-half what you think is your maximum force.

Use the first three or four seconds to build up to this degree of force—and the remaining four or five seconds to hold it.

For the next two weeks, gradually increase force to more nearly approach maximum. After about six weeks, it will be safe to exert maximum effort.

Pain indicates you're applying too much force; reduce the amount immediately. If pain continues to accompany any exercise, discontinue using that exercise for a week or two. Then try it again with about 50 percent of maximum effort and, if no pain occurs, you can go on to gradually build up toward maximum.

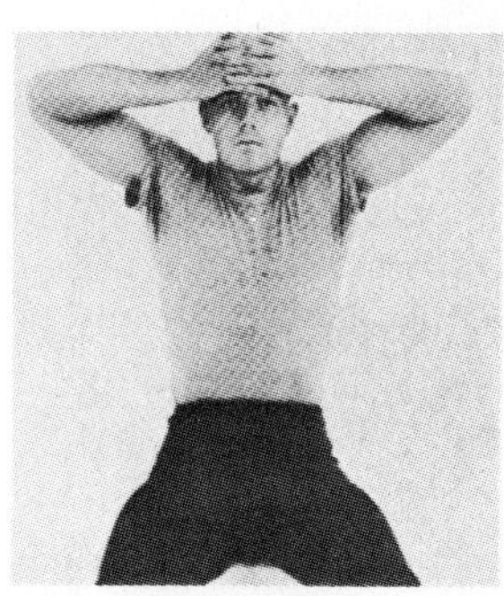

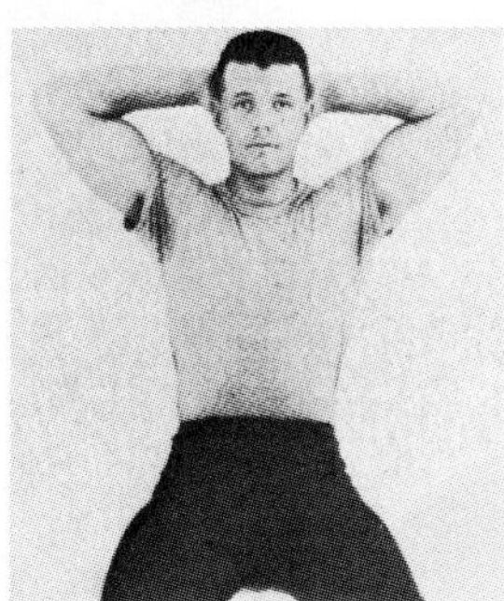

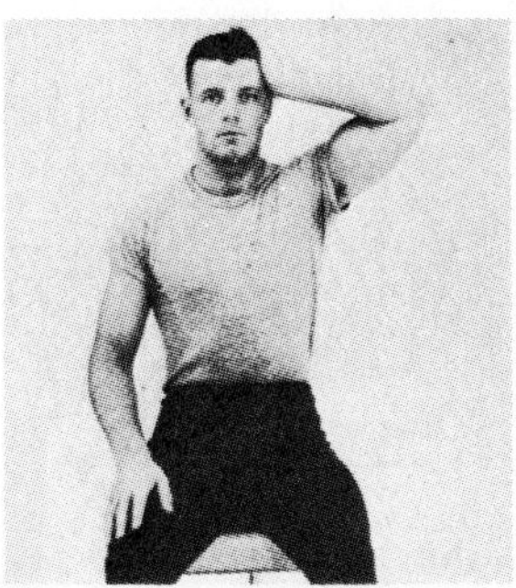

NECK

Starting position: Sit or stand, with interlaced fingers of hands on forehead.
Action: Forcibly exert a forward push of head while resisting equally hard with hands.
Starting position: Sit or stand, with interlaced fingers of hands behind head.
Action: Push head backward while exerting a forward pull with hands.
Starting position: Sit or stand, with palm of left hand on left side of head.
Action: Push with left hand while resisting with head and neck. Reverse using right hand on right side of head.

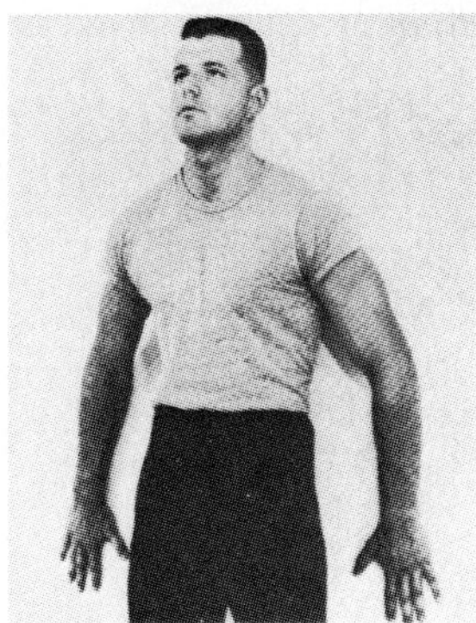

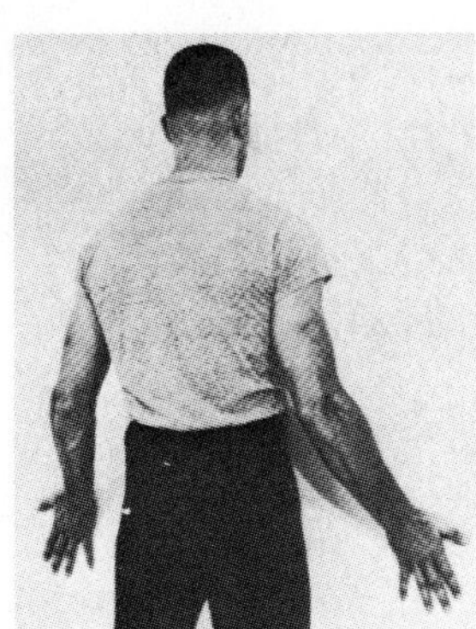

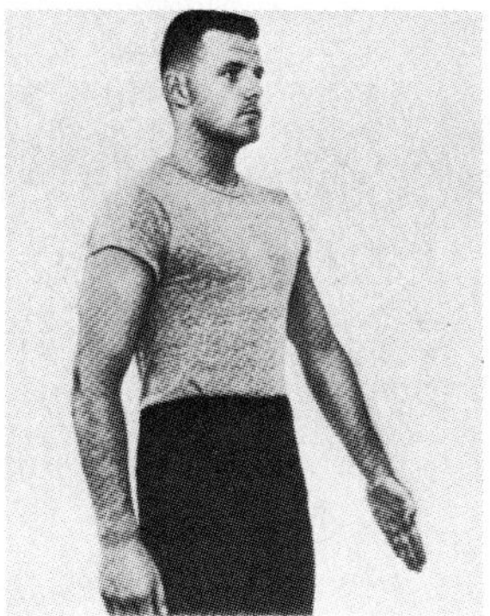

UPPER BODY

Starting position: Stand, back to wall, hands at sides, palms toward wall.
Action: Press hands backward against wall, keeping arms straight.
Starting position: Stand, facing wall, hands at sides, palms toward wall.
Action: Press hands forward against wall, keeping arms straight.
Starting position: Stand in doorway or with side against wall, arms at sides, palms toward legs.
Action: Press hand(s) outward against wall or doorframe, keeping arms straight.

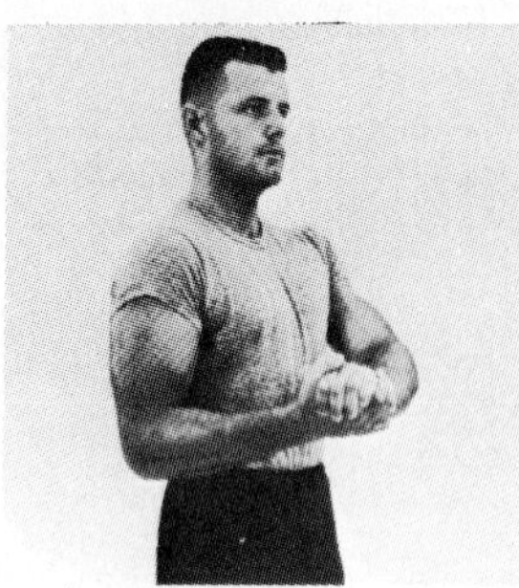

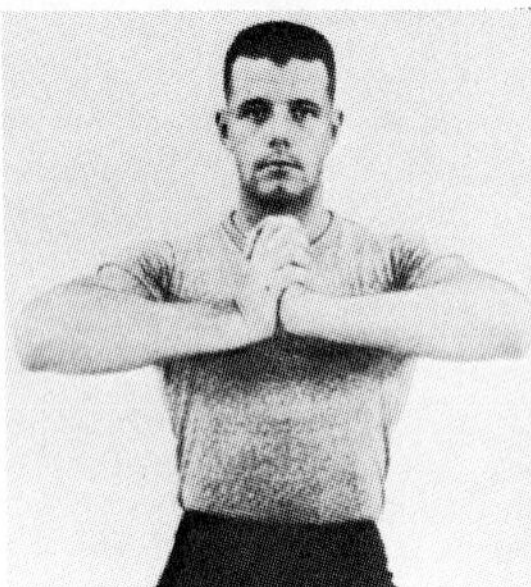

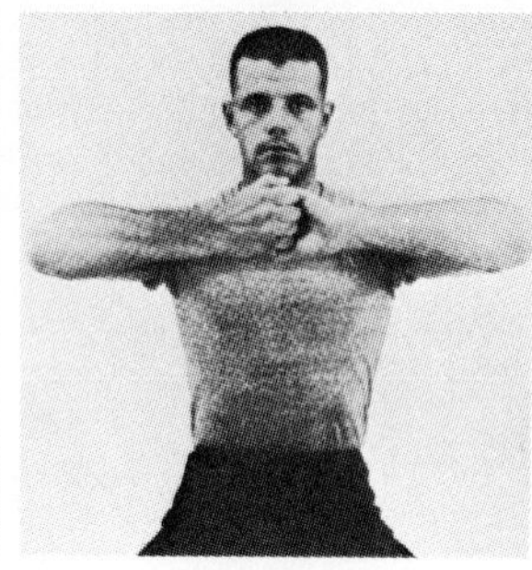

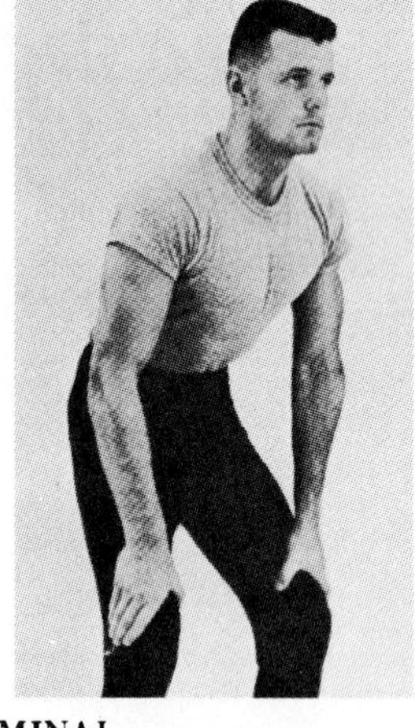

ARMS

Starting position: Stand with feet slightly apart. Flex right elbow, close to body, palm up. Place left hand over right.
Action: Forcibly attempt to curl right arm upward, while giving equally strong resistance with the left hand. Repeat with left arm.

ARMS AND CHEST

Starting position: Stand with feet comfortably spaced, knees slightly bent. Clasp hands, palms together, close to chest.
Action: Press hands together and hold.
Starting position: Stand with feet slightly apart, knees slightly bent. Grip fingers, arms close to chest.
Action: Pull hard and hold.

ABDOMINAL

Starting position: Stand, knees slightly flexed, hands resting on knees.
Action: Contract abdominal muscles.

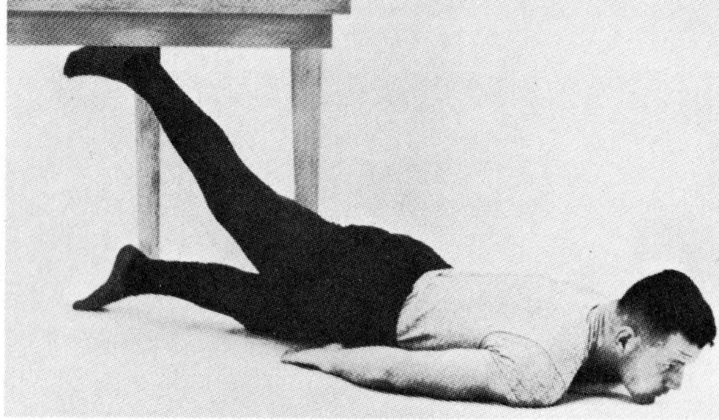

LOWER BACK, BUTTOCKS AND BACKS OF THIGHS

Starting position: Lie face down, arms at sides, palms up, legs placed under bed or other heavy object.
Action: With both hips flat on floor, raise one leg, keeping knee straight so that heel pushes hard against the resistance above. Repeat with opposite leg.

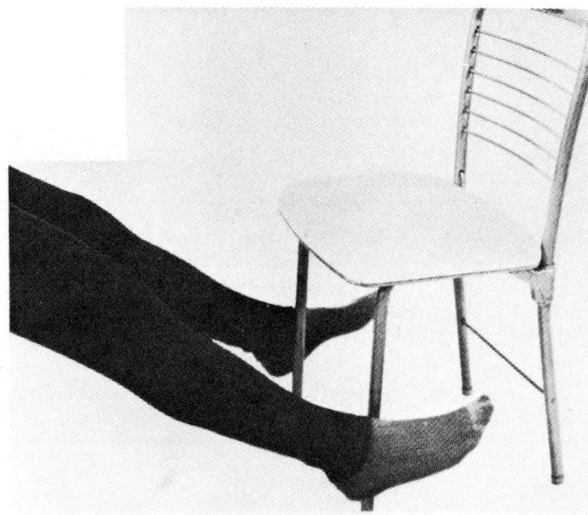

INNER AND OUTER THIGHS

Starting position: Sit, legs extended with each ankle pressed against the outside of sturdy chair legs.
Action: Keep legs straight and pull toward one another firmly. For outer thigh muscles, place ankles inside chair legs and exert pressure outward.

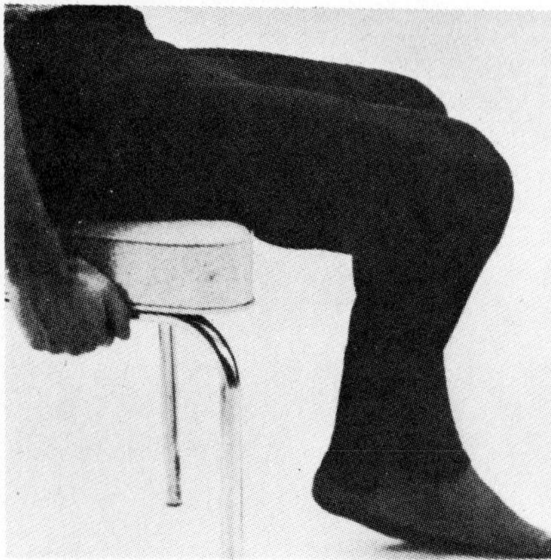

LEGS

Starting position: Sit in chair with left ankle crossed over right, feet resting on floor, legs bent at 90 degree angle.
Action: Forcibly attempt to straighten right leg while resisting with the left. Repeat with opposite leg.

WEIGHT TRAINING

Weight training also is an excellent method of developing muscular strength—and muscular endurance. Where equipment is available, it may be used as a supplement to the seven conditioning exercises.

Because of the great variety of weight training exercises, there will be no attempt to describe them here. Both barbells and weighted dumbbells—complete with instructions—are available at most sporting goods stores. A good rule to follow in deciding the maximum weight you should lift is to select a weight you can lift six times without strain.

SPORTS

Soccer, basketball, handball, squash, ice hockey and other sports that require sustained effort can be valuable aids to building circulatory endurance.

But if you have been sedentary, it's important to pace yourself carefully in such sports, and it may even be advisable to avoid them until you are well along in your physical conditioning program. That doesn't mean you should avoid all sports.

There are many excellent conditioning and circulatory activities in which the amount of exertion is easily controlled and in which you can progress at your own rate. Bicycling is one example. Others include hiking, skating, tennis, running, cross-country skiing, rowing, canoeing, water skiing and skindiving.

You can engage in these sports at any point in the program, if you start slowly. Games should be played with full speed and vigor only when your conditioning permits doing so without undue fatigue.

On days when you get a good workout in sports you can skip part or all of your exercise program. Use your own judgment.

If you have engaged in a sport which exercises the legs and stimulates the heart and lungs—such as skating—you could skip the circulatory activity for that day, but you still should do some of the conditioning and stretching exercises for the upper body. On the other hand, weight-lifting is an excellent conditioning activity, but it should be supplemented with running or one of the other circulatory exercises.

Whatever your favorite sport, you will find your enjoyment enhanced by improved fitness. Every weekend athlete should invest in frequent workouts.

POSTURE

There is a relationship between good posture and physical fitness—one helps the other.

Good posture acts to avoid cramping of internal organs, permits better circulation, prevents undue tensing of some muscles and undue lengthening of others. It thus contributes to fitness.

In turn, physical conditioning, by developing muscle tone, helps to make good posture more readily maintainable—and will help, too, if you have any bad postural habits you need to break.

For good posture, the centers of gravity of many body parts—feet, legs, hips, trunk, shoulders and head—must be in a vertical line. As viewed from the side when you are standing, the line should run through ear lobe, tip of shoulder, middle of hips, just back of kneecap, just in front of outer ankle bone.

Proper posture positions are:

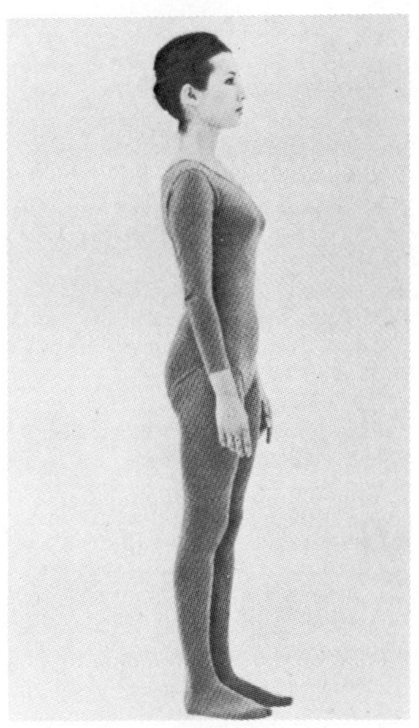

STANDING

1. Feet parallel, about 6″ apart. 2. Head high, as if balancing a book. 3. Chest out. 4. Stomach and hips firm. 5. Abdomen and back as flat as possible. 6. Knees very lightly flexed—not stiffly locked. 7. Weight evenly distributed on both feet—most of it on balls of feet.

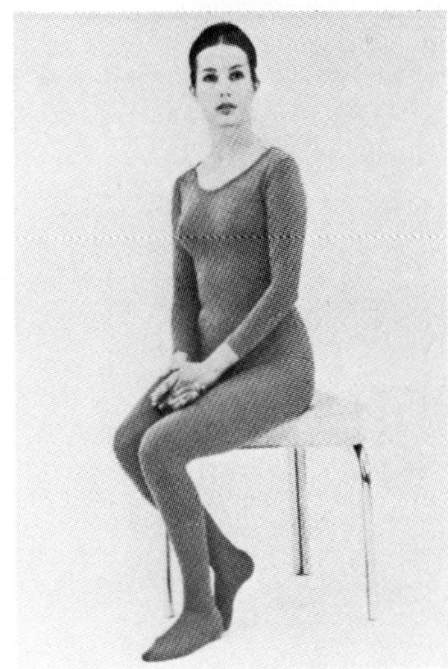

SITTING

1. Sit tall and back, with hips touching the back of the chair, feet flat on floor. 2. Chest out, back of neck nearly in line with upper back. 3. When writing, lean forward from the hips so you keep head and shoulders in line.

The position of the hips is one reliable indicator of posture. They should rest squarely upon the legs without tilting forward or backward.

Flabby abdominal muscles and excess weight—particularly in the abdominal region—are frequent causes of poor posture. Weak abdominal muscles permit the internal organs to drop. The results: the abdomen protrudes, the pelvis tilts forward and the curve of the lower back is accentuated. Lower back pains may occur.

The obese person's "paunch" upsets his center of gravity. As it pulls him forward he compensates by leaning backward, bending his knees slightly and increasing the curve of his back.

This produces the characteristic "old man's stance."

Excessive use of high-heeled shoes can produce the same effect in women—even young women. Additionally, the muscles in the calves and the backs of the thighs are shortened, so that it may be uncomfortable to go barefoot or wear low heels.

Forward head, or "poked neck," is another common posture fault. When the head is out of line, some other part of the body compensates and also moves out of line.

Get the "feel" of proper posture positions. Practice them until they become habitual.

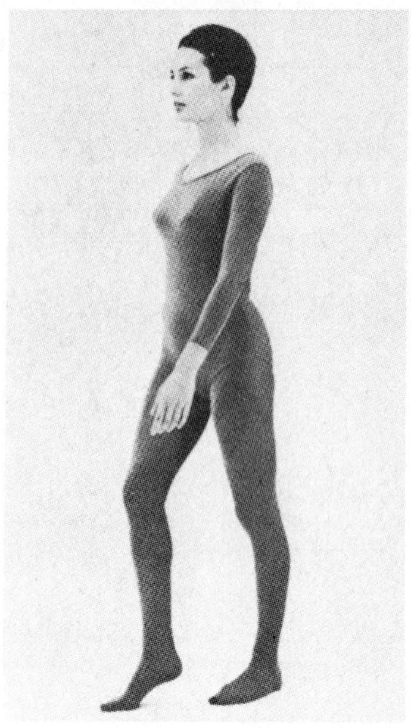

WALKING

1. Knees and ankles limber, toes pointed straight ahead. 2. Head and chest high. 3. Swing legs directly forward from hip joints. 4. Push feet off the ground—don't shuffle. 5. Swing shoulders and arms freely and easily.

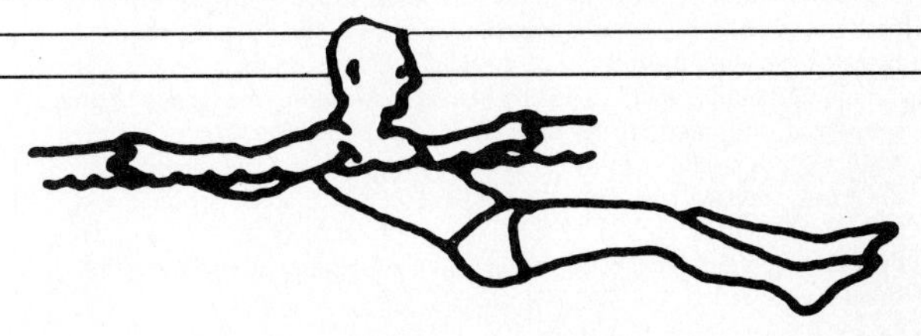

Aqua Dynamics

PHYSICAL CONDITIONING THROUGH WATER EXERCISES

Swimming—A Priority Physical Fitness Activity

Swimming is recognized as America's most popular active sport. It is an activity that may be used for recreation on one day; physical conditioning on the next; and survival on another. It is one of the best physical activities for people of all ages and for many persons who are handicapped. Vigorous water activities can make a major contribution to the flexibility, strength, and circulatory endurance of individuals. With the body submerged in water, blood circulation automatically increases to some extent; pressure of water on the body also helps promote deeper ventilation of the lungs; and with well-planned activity, both circulation and ventilation increase still more.

Increased flexibility work is performed more easily in water because of the lessening of gravitational pull. A person immersed to the neck in water experiences an apparent loss of 90% of his weight. This means that the feet and legs of a woman weighing 130 lbs. immersed in water only has to support a weight of 13 lbs. Thus, individuals and especially older people with painful joints or weak leg muscles will usually find it possible and comfortable to move in the water. It is much easier to do leg straddle or stride stretches in water than on the floor. Too, many individuals could do leg "bobbing" or jogging in the water who could never do so on land.

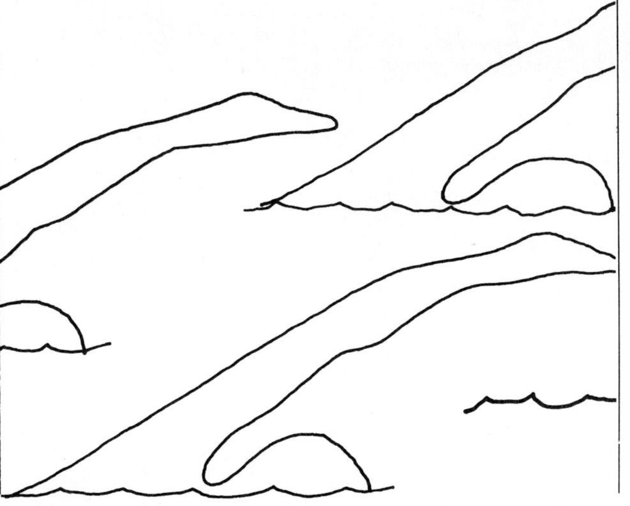

Aqua Dynamics—For Whom

The activities in this aquatic program are designed for the individual in sound health. A yearly medical examination is advisable for every adult. Such an examination should be taken before beginning a conditioning program.

How to Work

Exercise programs should be adapted to each person's tolerance level—the level at which he can perform comfortably and without undue distress. In order for workouts to be comfortable and continuous, and to achieve maximum potential, a combination system of training should be employed, using both "change of pace" and "interval training." Change of pace consists of the shifting from one activity to another involving a different set of muscles or type of stress and the changing of the intensity of the work. Interval training is interspersing repeated periods of physical work with recovery periods during which activity of a reduced intensity is performed.

Warming Up

During a workout the body should be warmed up by light conditioning and stretching exercises before heavier activities are attempted. Deck exercises including flexibility and strength activities with heavy breathing are appropriate. Various strokes may be simulated. Participants should begin with light rhythmical work at a slow pace. A tempo should be gradually accelerated, alternating slow with faster work, until one nears perspiration.

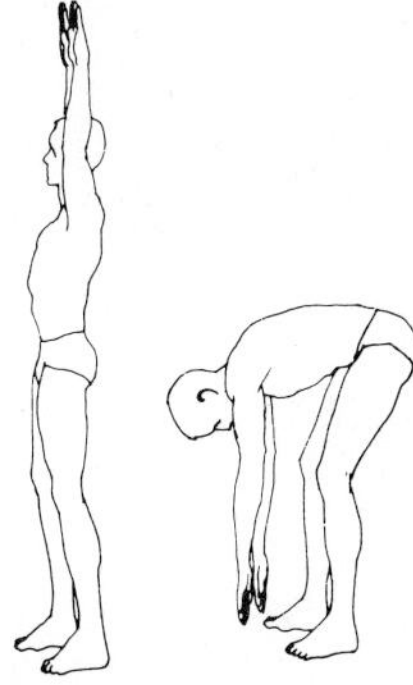

Most swimming activities cause the back to be in hyperextended position, thus specific back stretching exercises should be completed both at the beginning and end of the workout. For maximum benefit, the individual should stand with legs apart, extending the hands high over head and reaching as high as is possible. After approximately 5–10 seconds in the arms-over-head reaching position, one should bend the trunk forward and down, flexing the knees, and the bending and stretching position should be held for approximately 20–30 seconds, then the high reaching followed by the bending and stretching action should be repeated.

Through proper warm-up the body's deep muscle temperature will be raised and the ligaments and connecting tissues stretched, thereby preparing the body for vigorous work. This will help avoid injury and discomfort.

The following is Aqua Dynamics, a regimen of high-potential physical activities which can be used in a small pool or in a limited area of a crowded institutional pool.

STANDING WATER DRILLS

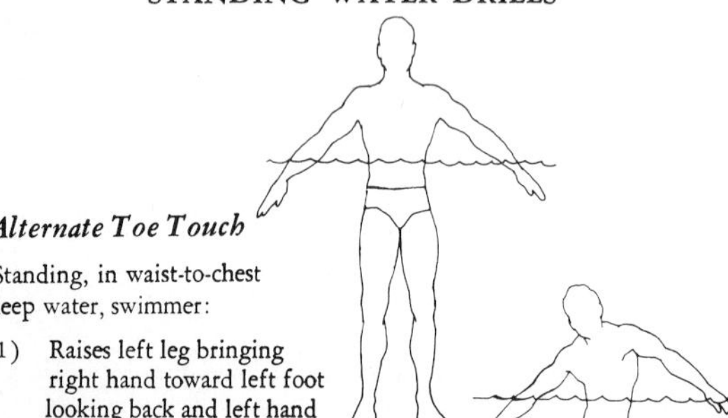

Alternate Toe Touch

Standing, in waist-to-chest deep water, swimmer:

(1) Raises left leg bringing right hand toward left foot looking back and left hand extended rearward.
(2) Recover to starting position.
Repeat.
Reverse.

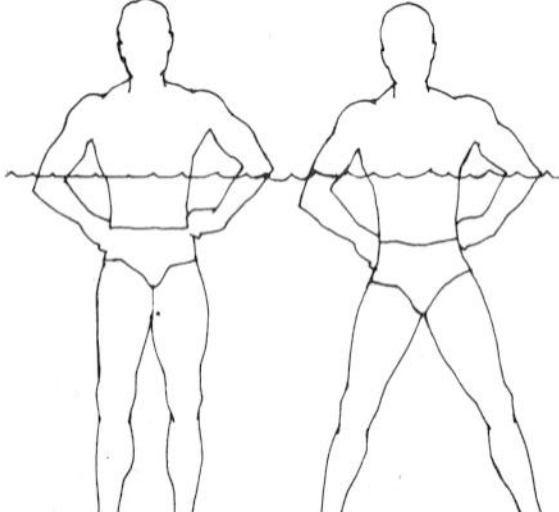

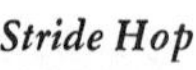

Side Straddle Hop

Standing in waist-to-chest deep water with hands on hips, swimmer:

(1) Jumps sideward to position with feet approximately two feet apart.
(2) Recovers.

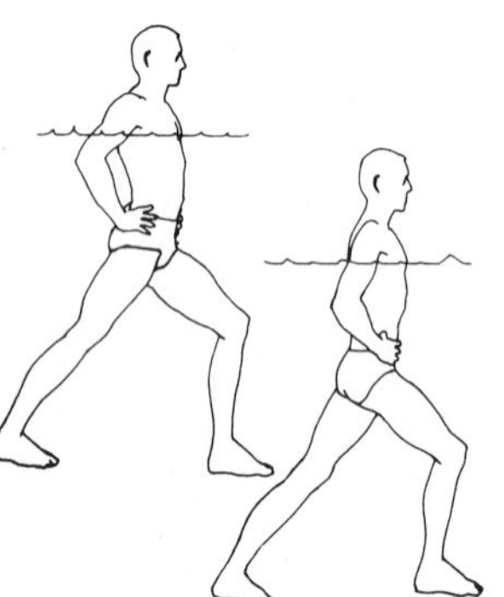

Stride Hop

Standing in waist-to-chest deep water with hands on hips, swimmer:

(1) Jumps, with left leg forward and right leg back.
(2) Jumps, changing to right leg forward and left leg back.
Repeat.

Toe Bounce

Standing in waist-to-chest deep water with hands on hips, swimmer:

(1) Jumps high with feet together through a bouncing movement of the feet.
Repeat.

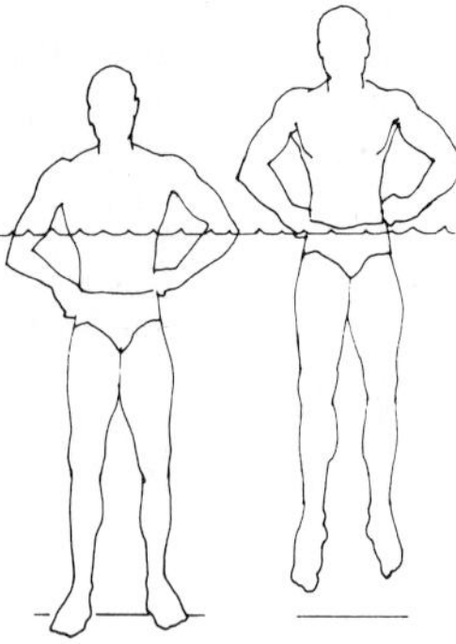

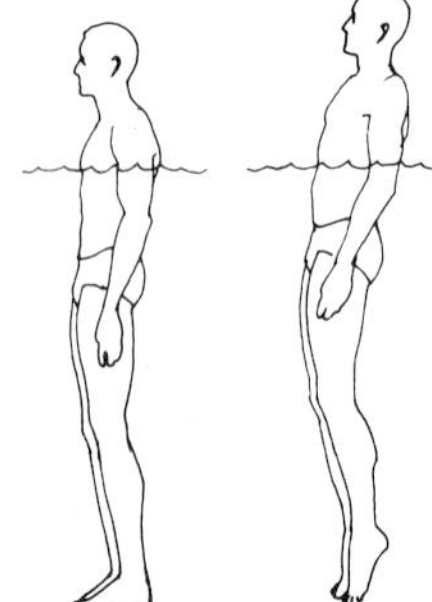

Raise on Toes

Standing in chest-deep water, swimmer:

(1) Raises on toes.
(2) Lowers to starting position.
Repeat.
Accelerate.

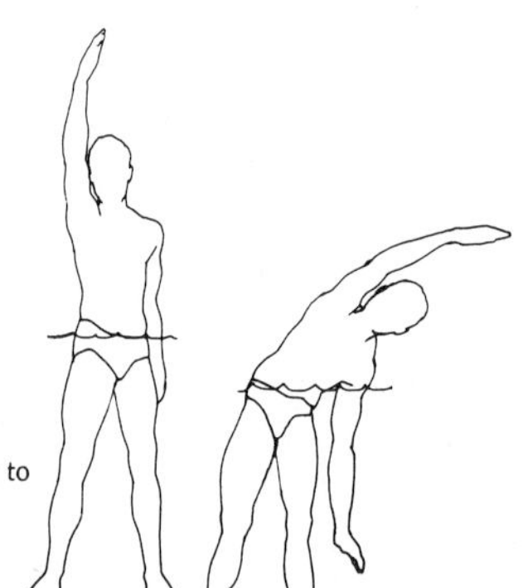

Side Bender

Standing in waist-deep water with left arm at side and right arm over head, swimmer:

(1) Stretches, slowly bending to the left.
(2) Recovers to the starting position.
Repeat.
Reverse to right arm at side and left arm overhead.

Standing Crawl

Standing in waist-to-chest deep water, swimmer:

(1) Simulates the overhand crawl stroke by:
  (a) Reaching out with the left hand, getting a grip on the water, pressing downward and pulling, bringing the left hand through to the thigh.
  (b) Reaching out with the right hand, etc.
  Repeat.

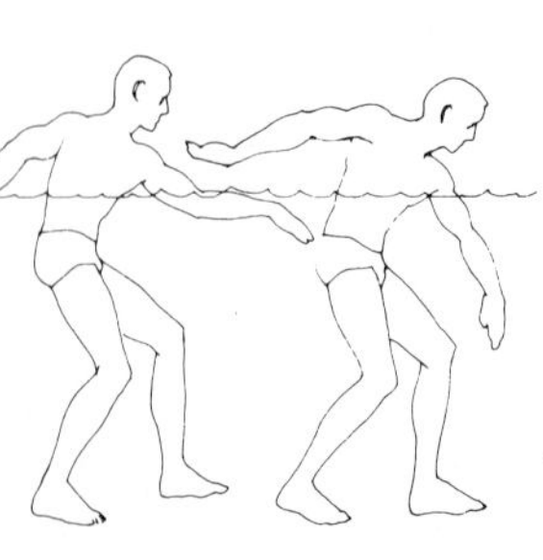

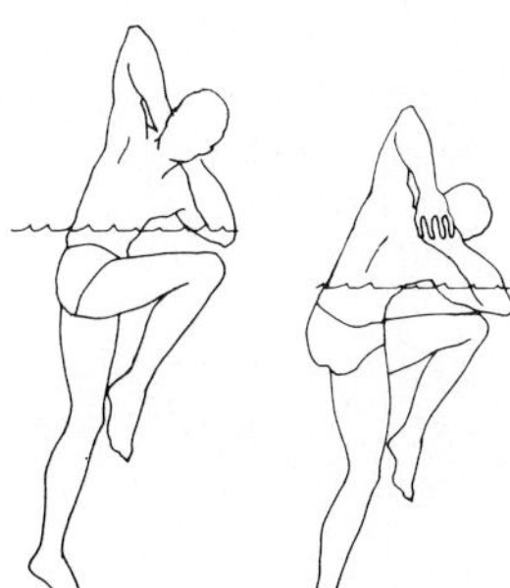

Walking Twists

With fingers laced behind neck, swimmer:

(1) Walks forward bringing up alternate legs twisting body to touch knee with opposite elbow.
Repeat.

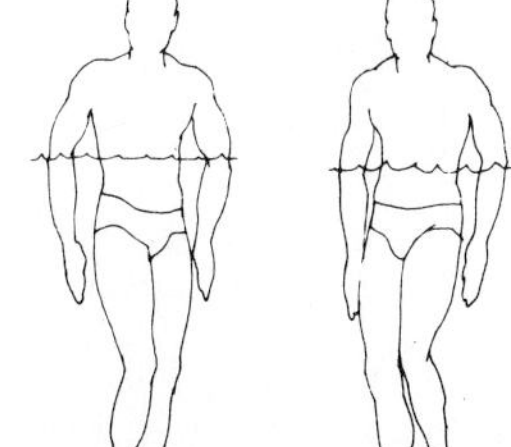

Bouncing

Standing in chest-deep water, swimmer:

(1) Bounces on left foot at the same time pushing down vigorously with both hands causing the upper body to rise, and
(2) Bounces similarly on right foot pushing down with both hands, etc.
Repeat.

Bounding in Place With Alternate Arm Stretch Forward

Standing in waist-deep water, swimmer:

(1) Bounds in place with high knee action; right arm outstretched far forward when left knee is high, and the left arm and hand stretched rearward.
(2) When right knee is high, outstretches the left arm and hand forward, with the right arm and hand stretched rearward.
Special Note: When the position of the arm and hand are reversed, pull down and through with hand simulating the propulsion of the crawl stroke.
Repeat.

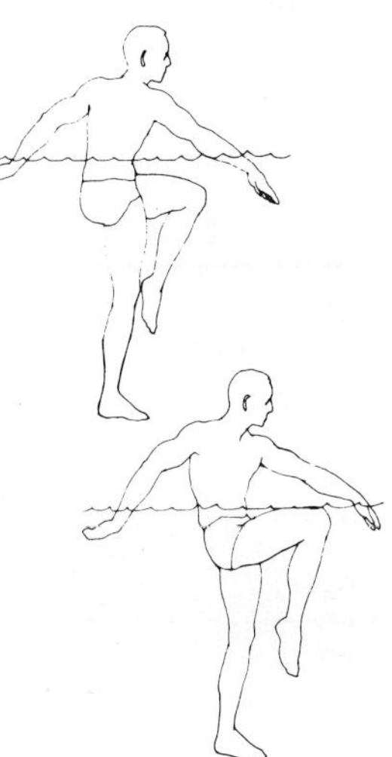

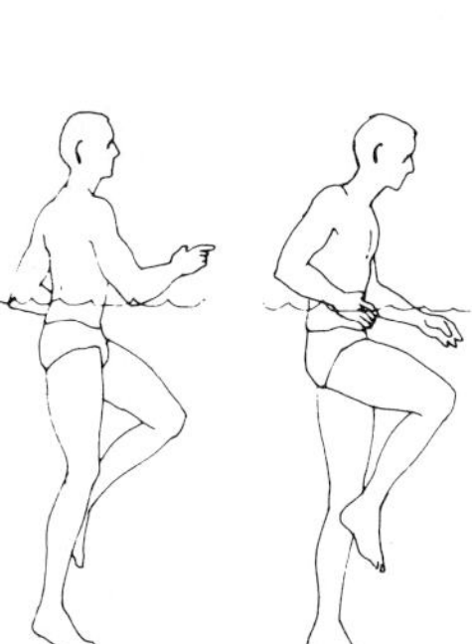

Jogging in Place

Standing with arms bent in running position, swimmer:

(1) Jogs in place.

POOL-SIDE STANDING DRILLS

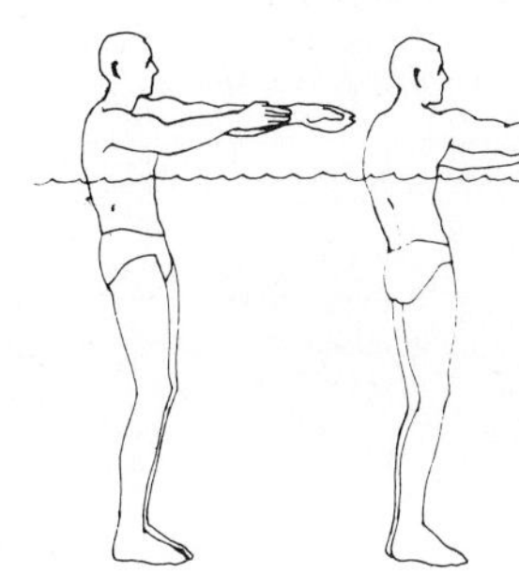

Stretch and Touch

Standing, facing wall with arms extended and fingertips approximately 12" from wall, swimmer:

(1) With shoulders under water, twists left and tries to touch wall with both hands.
(2) Twists right and tries to touch wall with both hands.
Repeat.

Flat Back

Standing at side of pool in waist-to-chest deep water, swimmer:

(1) Presses back against wall, holding for six counts.
(2) Relaxes to starting position.
Repeat.

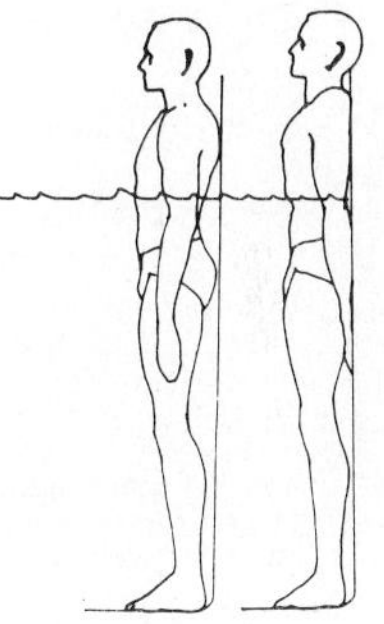

Leg Out

Standing at side of pool with back against wall, swimmer:

(1) Raises left knee to chest.
(2) Extends left leg straight out.
(3) Stretches leg.
(4) Drops leg to starting position.
Repeat.
Reverse to right leg

Pull and Stretch

Standing at side of pool with back against wall, swimmer:

(1) Raises left leg and clasps calf with both arms pulling leg vigorously to the chest.
(2) Recovers to starting position.
(3) Raises right leg and clasps calf with both arms pulling leg vigorously to the chest.
(4) Recovers to the starting position.

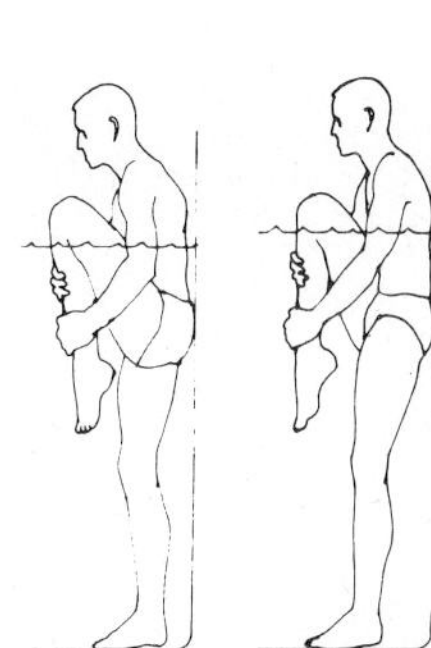

GUTTER-HOLDING DRILLS

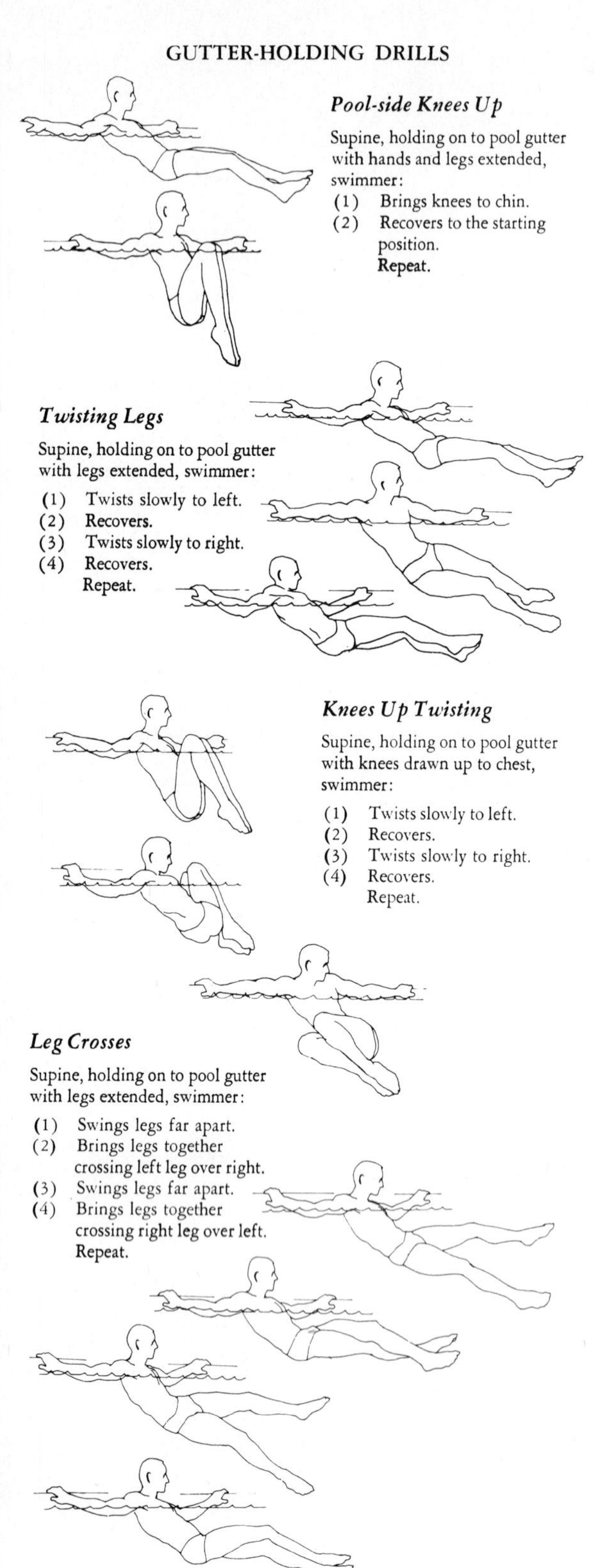

Pool-side Knees Up

Supine, holding on to pool gutter with hands and legs extended, swimmer:

(1) Brings knees to chin.
(2) Recovers to the starting position.
Repeat.

Twisting Legs

Supine, holding on to pool gutter with legs extended, swimmer:

(1) Twists slowly to left.
(2) Recovers.
(3) Twists slowly to right.
(4) Recovers.
Repeat.

Knees Up Twisting

Supine, holding on to pool gutter with knees drawn up to chest, swimmer:

(1) Twists slowly to left.
(2) Recovers.
(3) Twists slowly to right.
(4) Recovers.
Repeat.

Leg Crosses

Supine, holding on to pool gutter with legs extended, swimmer:

(1) Swings legs far apart.
(2) Brings legs together crossing left leg over right.
(3) Swings legs far apart.
(4) Brings legs together crossing right leg over left.
Repeat.

Twist Hips

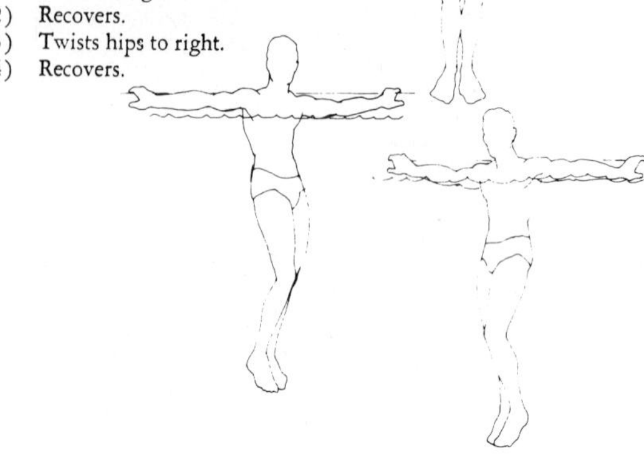

Standing, holding on to pool gutter with hands, with back to wall, swimmer:

(1) Twists hips to left as far as possible, keeping the upper trunk facing forward.
(2) Recovers.
(3) Twists hips to right.
(4) Recovers.

Alternate Raised Knee Crossovers

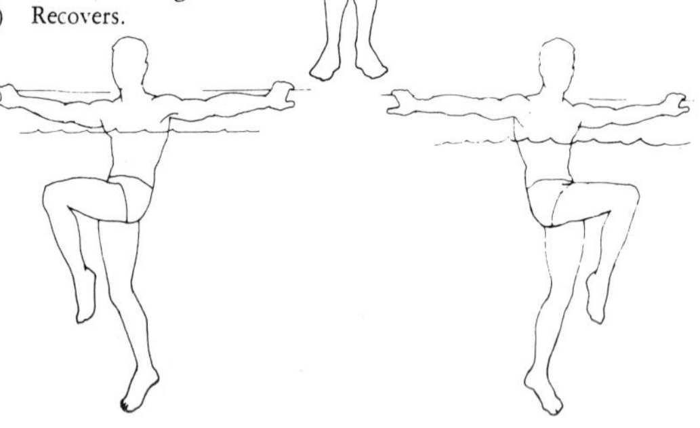

Standing, holding on to pool gutter with hands, back to wall:

(1) Lifts left knee and crosses it over. Twists to the right.
(2) Recovers.
(3) Lifts right knee and crosses it over, twisting to left.
(4) Recovers.

Legs Together on Back

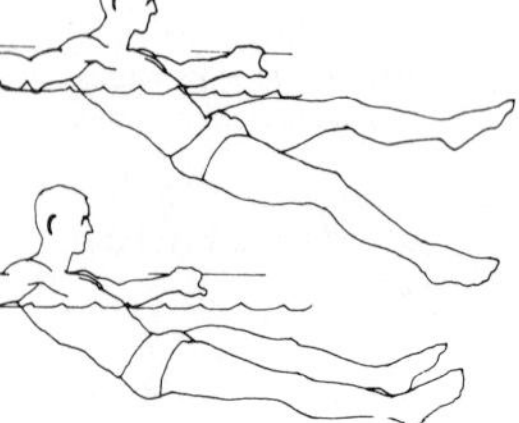

Supine, holding on to pool gutter with hands. Legs together and extended with feet about 6″ under the water:

(1) Spreads legs apart as far as as possible.
(2) Pulls feet and legs vigorously together.
Repeat.

Legs Together on Front

Prone, holding on to pool gutter with one hand flat on wall to push legs out, with feet together, swimmer:

(1) Spreads legs apart as far as possible.
(2) Pulls feet and legs vigorously together.
Repeat.

Raising Hips

Prone, holding on to pool gutter with one hand flat on wall to push legs out, swimmer:

(1) Raises hips, holding for four counts.
(2) Relaxes.
Repeat.

Circle Legs

Prone, holding on to pool gutter, with one hand flat on pool wall to push legs out, swimmer:

(1) Circles legs outward left.
(2) Repeat.
(3) Reverses to right.
Repeat.

Leg Swing Outward

Standing with back against poolside, and hands sideward holding gutter, swimmer:

(1) Raises left foot as high as possible with leg straight.
(2) Swings foot and leg to left side.
(3) Recovers to starting position by pulling left leg vigorously to right.
Repeat.
Reverses to right leg.
Repeat.

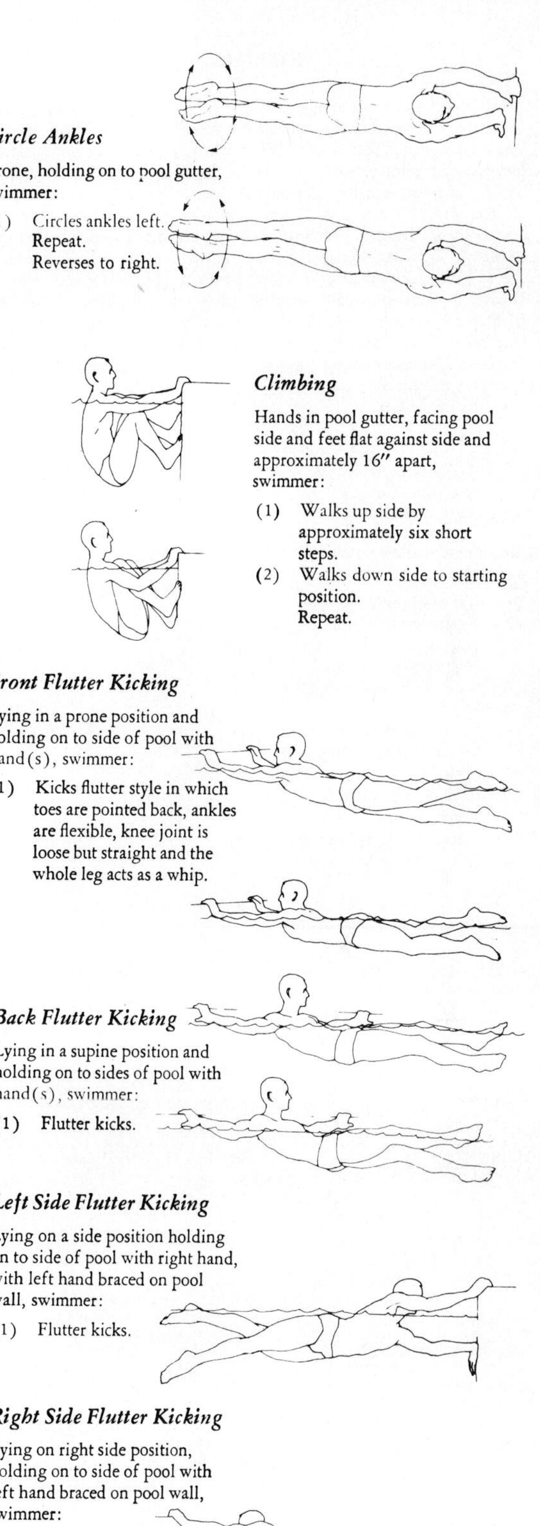

Circle Ankles

Prone, holding on to pool gutter, swimmer:

(1) Circles ankles left.
Repeat.
Reverses to right.

Climbing

Hands in pool gutter, facing pool side and feet flat against side and approximately 16″ apart, swimmer:

(1) Walks up side by approximately six short steps.
(2) Walks down side to starting position.
Repeat.

Front Flutter Kicking

Lying in a prone position and holding on to side of pool with hand(s), swimmer:

(1) Kicks flutter style in which toes are pointed back, ankles are flexible, knee joint is loose but straight and the whole leg acts as a whip.

Back Flutter Kicking

Lying in a supine position and holding on to sides of pool with hand(s), swimmer:

(1) Flutter kicks.

Left Side Flutter Kicking

Lying on a side position holding on to side of pool with right hand, with left hand braced on pool wall, swimmer:

(1) Flutter kicks.

Right Side Flutter Kicking

Lying on right side position, holding on to side of pool with left hand braced on pool wall, swimmer:

(1) Flutter kicks.

BOBBING

An excellent conditioning activity in water is "bobbing." In "bobbing," the head and shoulders are pushed out of the water much like a cork held under water "bobs" when released. "Bobbing" is a feet-first surface dive. Some experts say that if one had only five minutes for exercise each day, it would be best to spend that time in one of four ways: 1) running, 2) trampolining, 3) rope skipping, or 4) high bobbing. During "bobbing" activities, the demands for breathing are great. "Bobbing" forces the breathing. Breathing itself is an exercise and the quick inhaling and forced exhaling requires greater effort. Maximum exertion usually demands maximum respiration. This is facilitated by regular practice of deep respirations during "bobbing". One realizes the stimulus of forced, heavy breathing after advanced "bobbing" for five minutes (approximately 100–125 times). Approximately 20 percent of Aqua Dynamics is devoted to "bobbing."

Elementary Bobbing

Standing in shallow water, swimmer:

(1) Takes a breath.
(2) Submerges in a tuck position with feet on the pool bottom in shallow water. Exhales during (2) and (3).
(3) Shoves up off the bottom and regains a standing position.
(4) Inhales with head out of water.
(5) Repeat (2), (3), (4), etc.

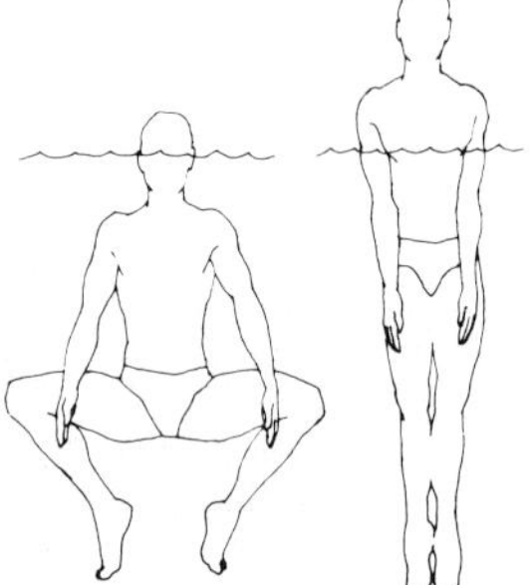

Alternate Leg Rearward Bobbing

Standing in shallow water, swimmer:

(1) Takes a breath.
(2) Submerges in shallow water with left leg in a squatting position with left foot on the pool bottom and right leg extended rearward. Exhales during (2) and (3).
(3) Shoves up off the bottom reversing the position of the legs, inhaling when the head is out of water.
(4) Submerges with right leg in a squatting position with right foot on pool bottom and left leg extended rearward. Exhales during the action.
(5) Repeat 1, 2, 3, and 4.

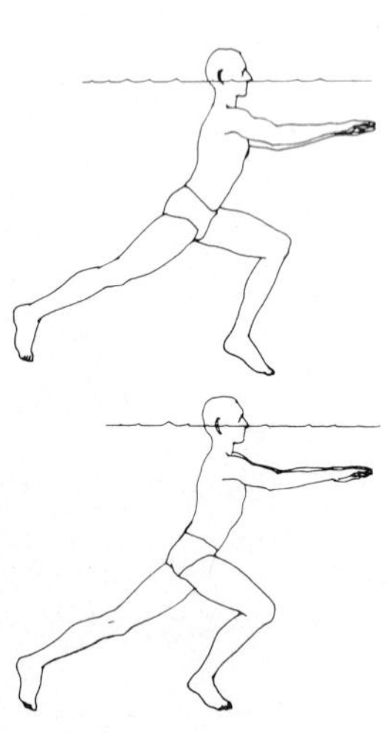

Alternate Leg Sideward Bobbing

Standing in waist-to-chest deep water, swimmer:

(1) Takes a breath.
(2) Submerges with left leg in a full squatting position, left foot on pool bottom and right leg extended sideward, (exhales during (2) and (3)).
(3) Shoves up off bottom reversing the position of the legs and inhaling when the head is out of water.
(4) Submerges with the right leg in a full squatting position with the right foot on pool bottom and the left leg extended sideward (exhales during the action). Repeat.

Legs Astride Bobbing

Standing in waist-to-chest deep water, swimmer:

(1) Takes a breath.
(2) Submerges with legs astride, left leg forward and right leg rearward, (exhales on (2) and (3)).
(3) Shoves off bottom, inhaling when head is out of water.
(4) Submerges with legs astride.
Repeat.

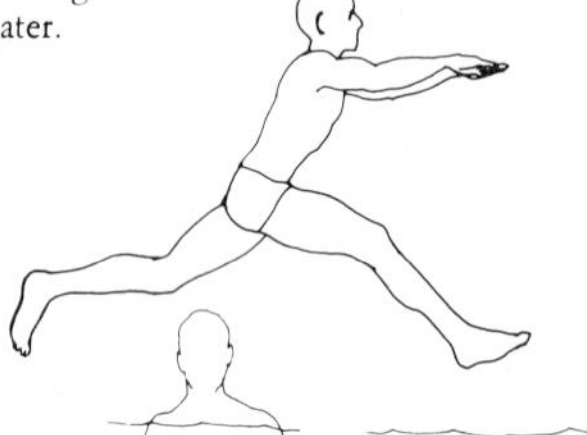

Advanced Bobbing

Treading in deep water, swimmer:

(1) Assumes a vertical position with hands extended outward from the sides, just under the surface of the water, with palms turned downward. Legs are drawn in a position of readiness for a frog or scissors kick.
(2) Executes kick as hands are pulled sharply to thighs and legs. (As a result of this action, the head and shoulders rise out of the water and a deep breath is taken at the highest point reached).
(3) As the body sinks, the arms are outstretched overhead and swimmer exhales.
Repeats (1), (2), and (3).

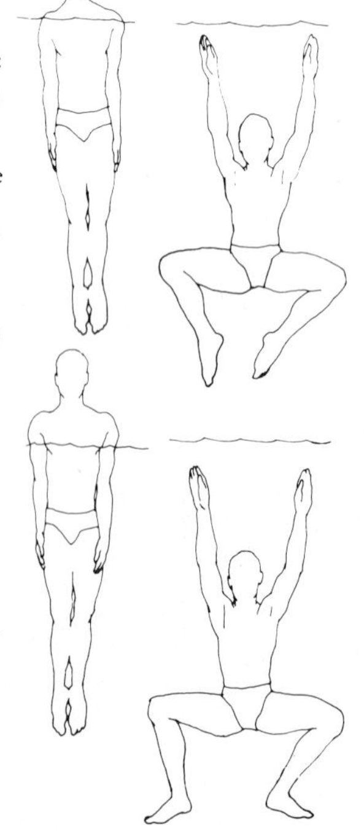

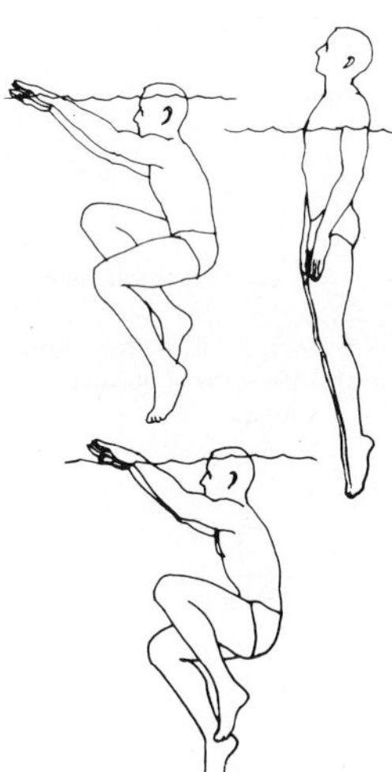

Left/Right Leg Bobbing

Standing or treading in deep water, swimmer:

(1) Takes a breath.
(2) Submerges in a tuck with right leg drawn up with left foot on pool bottom.
(3) Pushes upward off left leg thrust, exhaling during (1) and (2).
(4) Inhales with head out of water.
(5) Repeat.
Reverse to right leg.

Progressive Alternate Leg Forward Bobbing

Standing, swimmer:

(1) Performs action described in Alternate Leg Rearward Bobbing (page 9), alternating legs, bobbing progressively, and moving forward the length of the pool or a specified distance.

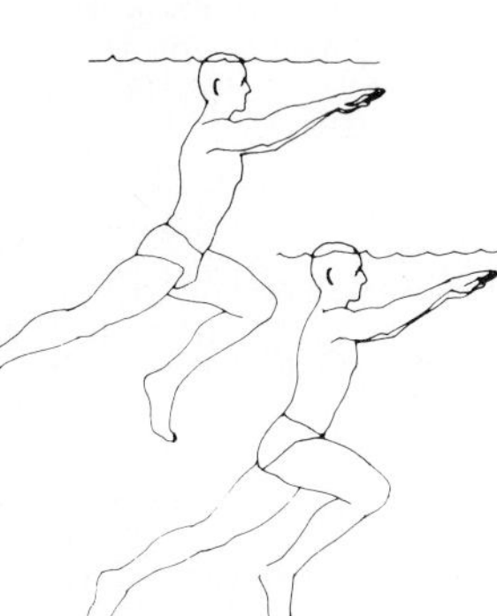

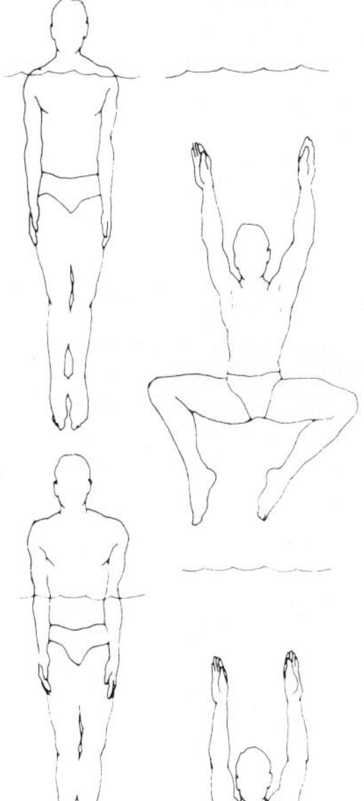

High Bobbing

In water approximately one to three feet over the swimmer's head, swimmer:

(1) Takes a vertical position, hands extended outward from the sides with palms turned downward. Legs are drawn in position for frog kick.
(2) Simultaneously pulls hands sharply to thighs with legs executing frog kick.
(3) Inhales at peak of height.
(4) Drops with thrust of arms downward with palms turned upward until feet reach bottom of the pool and tucks to a squat position. Exhales throughout this action.
(5) Jumps upward with power leg thrust at the same time pulling arms in in a breast stroke position downward, causing the head and shoulders to rise high out of water. Exhales during (4) and (5).
(6) Inhales and repeats cycles (4) and (5), etc.

Progressive "Bunny Hop" Bobbing

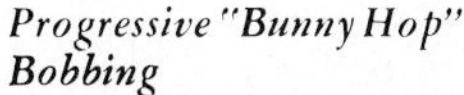

Standing, swimmer:

(1) Takes a breath.
(2) Submerges in a tuck or full squatting position with feet on the pool bottom.
(3) Pushes up and forward off bottom of the pool, exhaling during (2) and (3).
(4) Inhales with head out of water.
(5) Repeat, pushing forward the length of the pool or a specified distance.

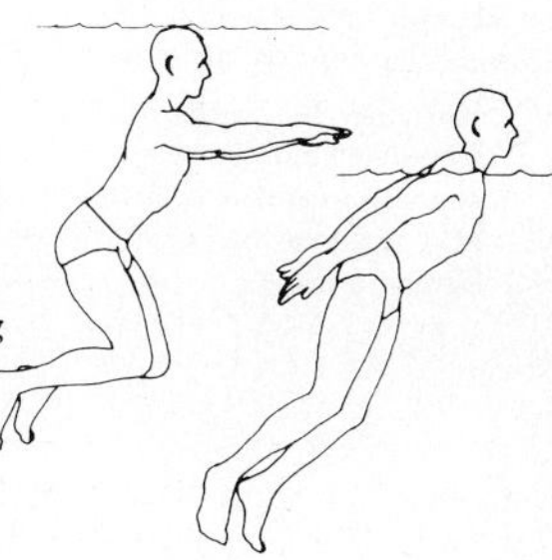

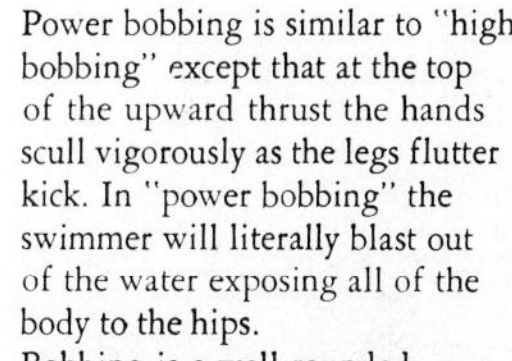

Power Bobbing

Power bobbing is similar to "high bobbing" except that at the top of the upward thrust the hands scull vigorously as the legs flutter kick. In "power bobbing" the swimmer will literally blast out of the water exposing all of the body to the hips.
Bobbing is a well-rounded workout involving leg power, arm and shoulder work, heavy forced breathing, and rhythmical vigorous action.

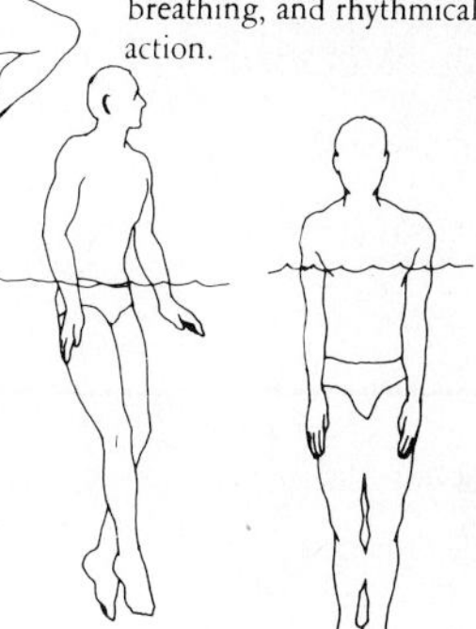

TREADING WATER

Elementary Treading

In water deep enough that toes will not touch bottom, in a perpendicular position, swimmer:

(1) Sculls or fins as he kicks bicycle, scissors, or frog style.

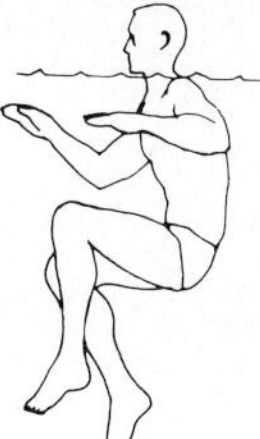

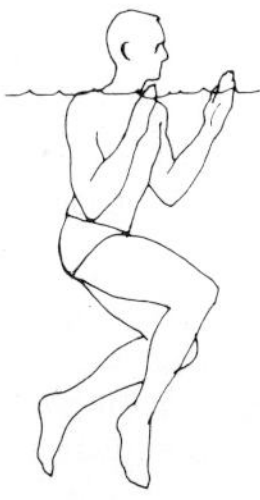

Advanced Treading

In water over head in a perpendicular position, swimmer:

(1) Kicks bicycle, scissors, or frog style with hands held shoulder high and body in a perpendicular position.

One Hand High Treading

In water over head in a perpendicular position, swimmer:

(1) Kicks bicycle, scissors, or frog style holding one arm straight up and other hand held shoulder high. Reverse arms.

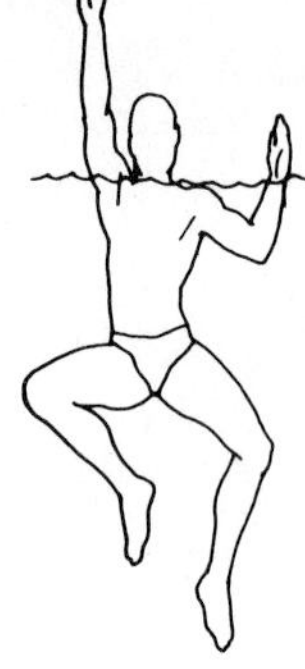

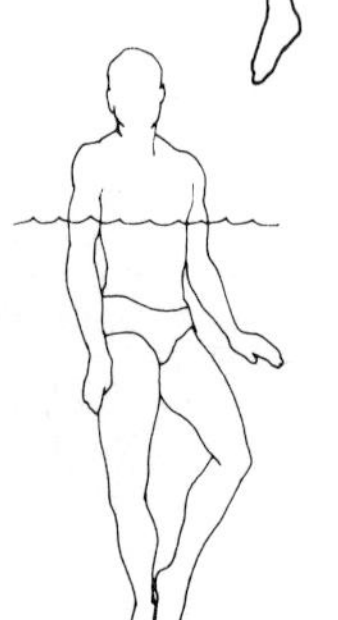

Two Hands High Treading

In water over head in a perpendicular position, swimmer:

(1) Kicks bicycle, scissors, or frog style holding both arms straight up out of water.

Look-Out Treading

In deep water in a perpendicular position, swimmer:

(1) Kicks vigorously at the same time thrashing the water by sculling, thereby raising the shoulders and chest high out of the water.

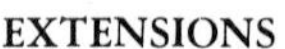

EXTENSIONS

Breathing

Controlled breathing is essential for the activities which follow. The swimmer should inhale through the mouth and exhale through the nose. One should be exhaling through the nose at any time the head is under water.

Sculling

"Extension" activities are largely dependent upon sculling ability. Sculling is done by arm and hand action. The use of the hands in sculling is the same basic maneuver regardless of the position of the body or the direction one wishes to go. Sculling can provide lifting power or combined lifting and propulsion power. Action usually begins by pushing down on palms, with arms sideward. Hands are flat, fingers together, and thumbs close to forefingers. With thumbs up, rotate wrists, bringing palms forward, then turn palms downward and backward. Downward pressure should be held constant on both the sideward and forward movements. Lifting power is provided as the hand is drawn to the front and side and parallel to the water surface.

Special Note: On all "extension" activities which follow, *swimmer should stay in the same place in the pool.*

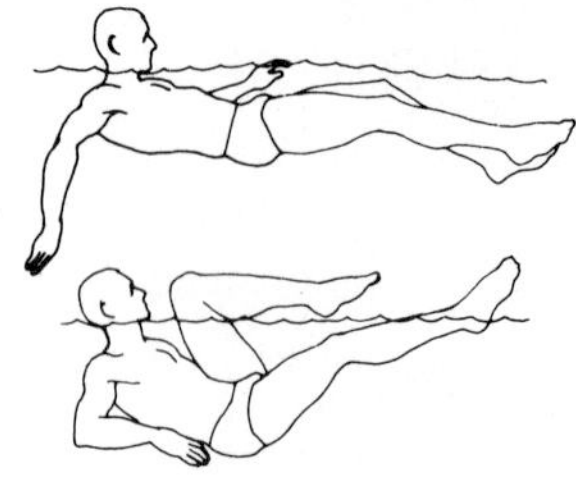

Left Knee Up, Back

Assuming a supine position, swimmer:

(1) Sculls, drawing left knee up to chest with right leg extended and toes on the right foot out of water.

(2) Sculls, straightening the left leg thus returning to the starting position. Repeat.

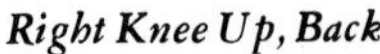

Right Knee Up, Back

Assuming a supine position, swimmer:

(1) Sculls, drawing right leg up to chest with left leg extended and toes on the left foot out of water.

(2) Sculls, straightening the right leg thus returning to the starting position. Repeat.

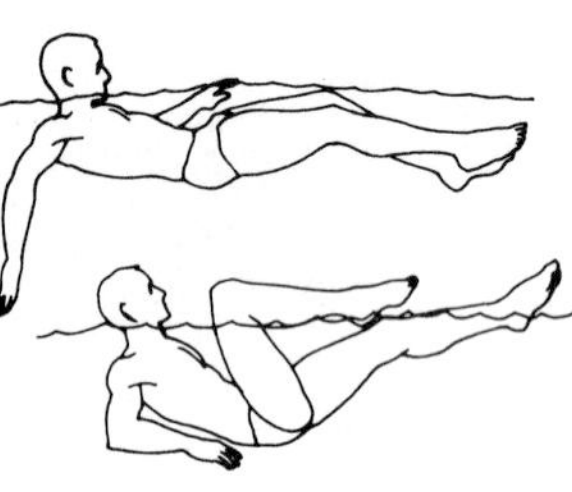

Knees Up, Back

Starting from a back-lying position, swimmer:

(1) Sculls, drawing knees up to chest.

(2) Sculls, shoving legs forward returning to a back-lying position. Repeat.

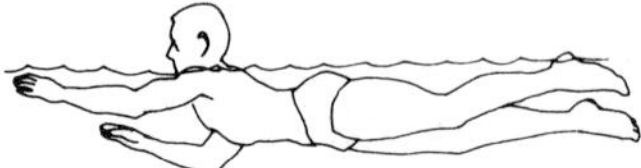

Knees Up, Front

Starting from a front-lying position, swimmer:

(1) Sculls, drawing knees up to chest.

(2) Sculls, shoving legs backward returning to the front-lying position. Repeat.

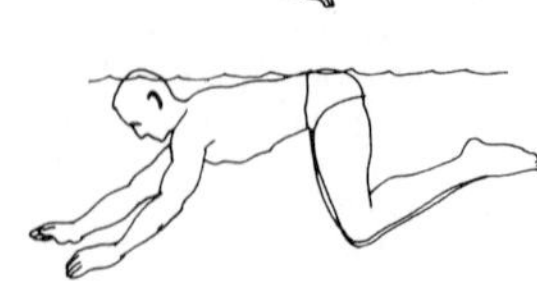

Knees Up, Left Side

Starting from a left side stroke position, swimmer:

(1) Sculls, drawing knees up to chest.

(2) Sculls, shoving legs to the right side causing the body to be in a left side stroke position. Repeat.

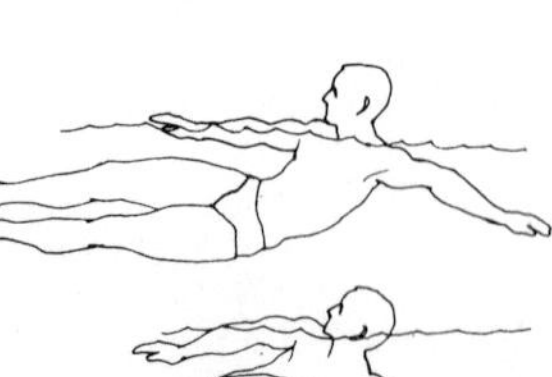

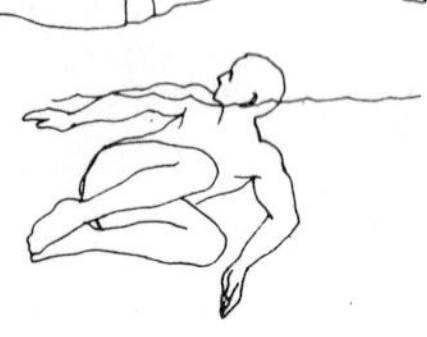

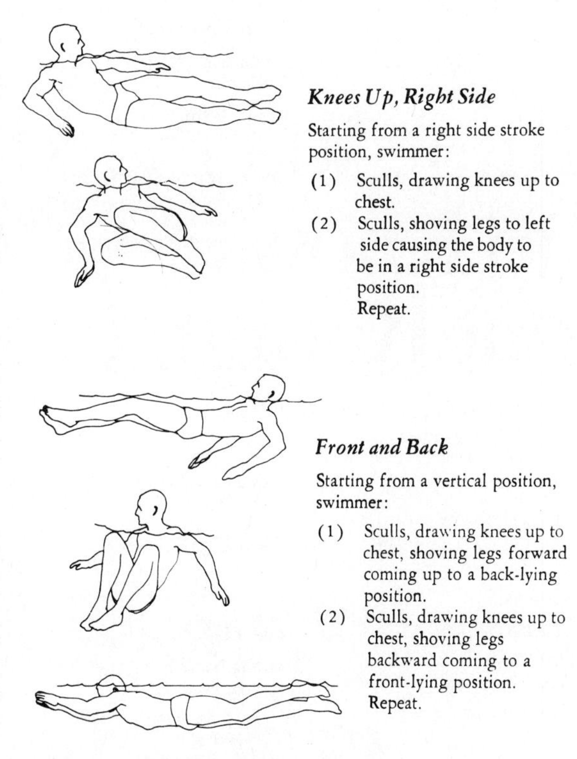

Knees Up, Right Side

Starting from a right side stroke position, swimmer:

(1) Sculls, drawing knees up to chest.
(2) Sculls, shoving legs to left side causing the body to be in a right side stroke position.
Repeat.

Front and Back

Starting from a vertical position, swimmer:

(1) Sculls, drawing knees up to chest, shoving legs forward coming up to a back-lying position.
(2) Sculls, drawing knees up to chest, shoving legs backward coming to a front-lying position.
Repeat.

Reverse Sides Extension

Starting from a vertical position, swimmer:

(1) Sculls, drawing knees up to chest, shoving legs to left side causing body to be in a right side stroke position.
(2) Sculls vigorously, drawing knees up to chest and reversing position, shoving legs to the right side, shifting body to a left side stroke position.
Repeat.

LAP SWIMMING

Despite the small distance covered after shove-off the side and glide in the residential pool, lap swimming is still an excellent activity. If the pool is clear, take off and enjoy swimming hard until you begin to feel winded. Ease off by loafing with a lazy breast or side stroke until you feel recovered, then go again. Another way to begin the interval training program in the swimming pool is to swim one length of the pool, get out, walk back, and repeat a number of times. For an individual in poor physical condition, a regimen of 5 to 10 lengths, walking back after each length may be necessary for several weeks or months. As endurance improves the number of lengths should be increased progressively.

WORKOUTS

In order to illustrate how the aforementioned water exercises could be combined in different workouts, the following examples are provided:

Very Low Gear 15 minutes

Side Straddle Hop	15 seconds
Standing Crawl	30 seconds
Walking Twists	15 seconds
Toe Bounce	15 seconds
Flat Back	15 seconds
Pull and Stretch	30 seconds
Leg Out	30 seconds
Front Flutter	30 seconds
Back Flutter	30 seconds
Alternate Leg Rearward Bobbing	1 minute
Leg Swing Outward	30 seconds
Bounding in Place with Arm Stretch	30 seconds
Elementary Treading	30 seconds
Lap Swimming—Interval	9 minutes

Low Gear 20 minutes

Stride Hop	15 seconds
Standing Crawl	30 seconds
Front Flutter	1 minute
Back Flutter	1 minute
Front Flutter	1 minute
Pull and Stretch	30 seconds
Leg Swing Outward	1 minute
Advanced Bobbing	1 minute
Left Knee Up, Back	30 seconds
Right Knee Up, Back	30 seconds
Alternate Leg Rearward Bobbing	30 seconds
Knees Up, Back	30 seconds
Alternate Leg Sideward Bobbing	30 seconds
Bounding in Place with Arm Stretch	45 seconds
Knees Up, Front	30 seconds
Advanced Bobbing	1 minute
Knees Up, Left	30 seconds
Knees Up, Right	30 seconds
Advanced Bobbing	1 minute
Reverse Sides Extension	30 seconds
Lap Swimming—Interval	6½ minutes

Middle Gear 30 minutes

Front Flutter	2 minutes
Back Flutter	2 minutes
Front Flutter	1 minute
Alternate Leg Rearward Bobbing	1 minute
Knees Up, Front	1 minute
Knees Up, Back	1 minute
Alternate Leg Sideward Bobbing	1 minute
Front and Back Extensions	1 minute
High Bobbing	3 minutes
Reverse Sides Extension	1 minute
Progressive Bobbing	2 minutes
Rub-A-Dub-Dub	2 minutes
Left Leg Raiser	15 seconds
Right Leg Raiser	15 seconds
Alternate Leg Raisers	30 seconds
High Bobbing	1 minute
Lap Swimming—Interval	10 minutes

High Gear 60 minutes

Front Flutter	3 minutes
Back Flutter	3 minutes
Advanced Bobbing	3 minutes
Left Knee Up, Back	1 minute
Right Knee Up, Back	1 minute
Knees Up, Back	1 minute
High Bobbing	3 minutes
Knees Up, Front	1 minute
Alternate Leg Rearward Bobbing	2 minutes
Front and Back Extensions	2 minutes
Alternate Leg Sideward Bobbing	2 minutes
Reverse Sides Extensions	2 minutes
Bounding in Place with Arm Stretch	3 minutes
Progressive Alternate Leg Forward Bobbing	3 minutes
Rub-A-Dub-Dub	3 minutes
Left Leg Raiser	30 seconds
Right Leg Raiser	30 seconds
Power Bobbing	1 minute
Alternate Leg Raiser	30 seconds
Bounding in Place with Arm Stretch	3 minutes
Toe Bounce	1½ minutes
Leg Swing Outward	2 minutes
Lap Swimming—Interval	Remainder

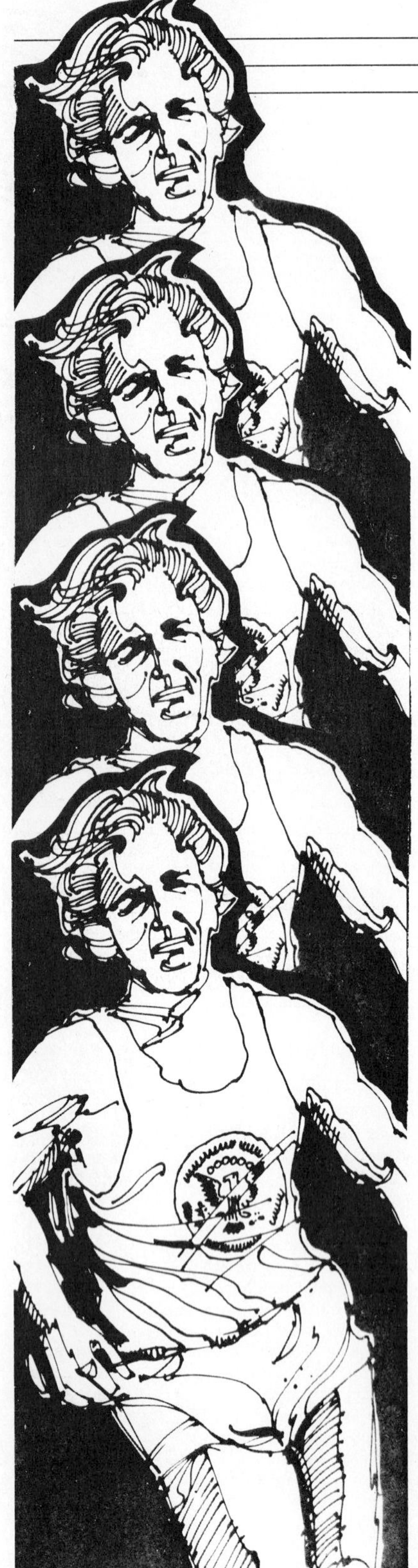

Everything You Need to Know About Running

THE RUNNING REVOLUTION

Millions of Americans are running. Young, old, and in-between, male and female, plodders and speedsters, you see them everywhere: loping through parks, pounding city pavements, chugging along suburban streets, and doggedly circling school running tracks.

Surveys show that more than 17 million adult Americans are running regularly. Most run a mile or two at a time, two or three times a week, but many run several miles a day. Consider these facts: some 50,000 Americans have completed at least one marathon race (26 miles, 385 yards), and nearly 4,000 of them have done it in less than three hours.

Running as a mass participation sport and fitness activity in America is approximately 15 years old and still growing. The number of runners has doubled in the past five years and is increasing faster than ever.

THE REASONS FOR RUNNING

Health clearly is the No. 1 reason why so many Americans are running. Studies have shown that regular, vigorous exercise can improve the body's ability to consume oxygen during exertion, lower the resting heart rate, reduce blood pressure, and increase the efficiency of the heart and lungs. It also helps burn excess calories.

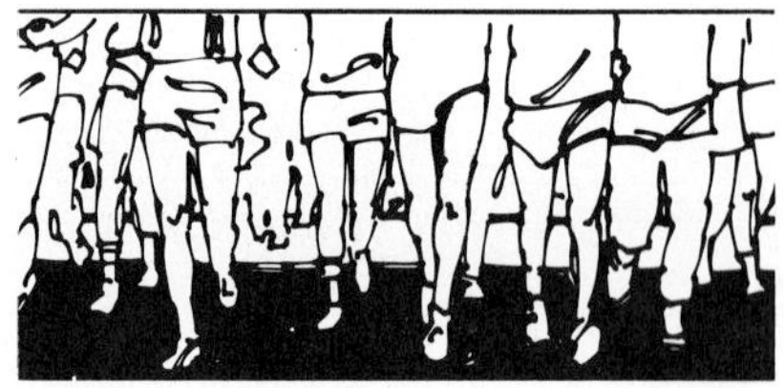

Since obesity and high blood pressure are among the leading risk factors for heart attack and stroke, exercise offers protection against two of our major killers.

Possibly more important for motivational purposes are the immediate benefits that beginning runners experience. They almost invariably report that they feel better, tire less easily, and have fewer illnesses.

There are other reasons to run. Some do it because they enjoy it, or because it helps them get rid of tensions. Others do it for the competition, or to prove something to themselves. Many do it to shed pounds and tone flabby muscles.

Experienced runners say they develop a "positive addiction" to running and don't feel right if they don't do it. Ask almost any runner why he or she began and you will get an answer something like this: "To get in shape and lose weight." Ask them why they continue and you will be struck by a subtle difference in the reply: "Because I enjoy it." "I feel I'm cheating myself when I don't do it." "I like knowing that I'm capable of running five or six miles."

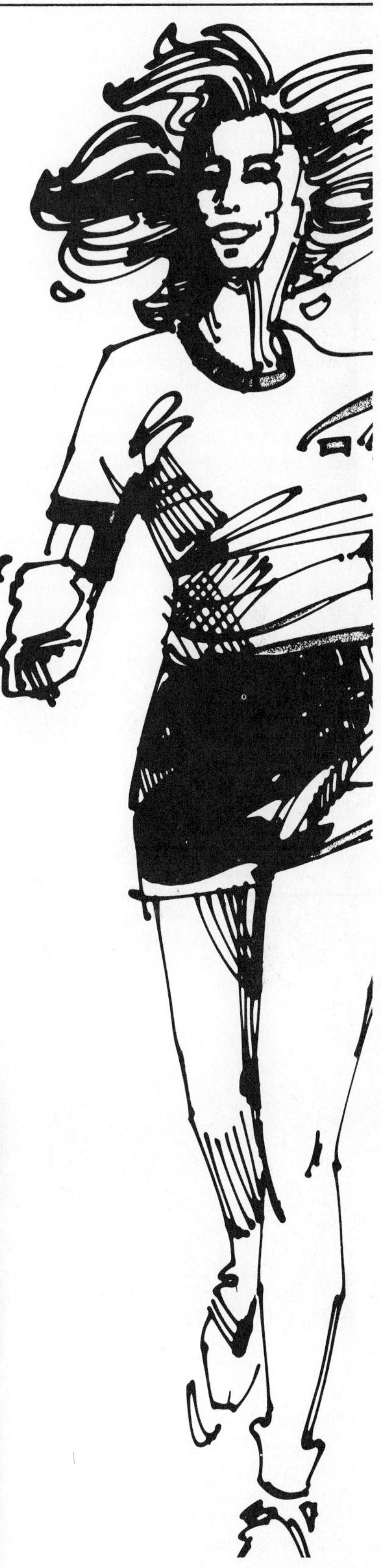

Running also exerts a favorable influence on personal habits. For example, smokers who begin running often cut down or quit. There appear to be two reasons for this. One, it's difficult to run if you smoke, and two, improved physical condition encourages a desire to improve other aspects of your life.

Several forms of endurance exercise – cycling, swimming, and cross-country skiing among them – are as effective as running, but running's immense popularity is due to its unique advantages. Some of these are:

Almost everyone can do it.
You don't have to take expensive lessons to be a runner. If you can walk, you probably can work up to running. You can learn what you need to know from magazines, books, and acquaintances who are runners.

You can do it almost anywhere.
Running doesn't require expensive facilities. You can run in parks, on streets or country roads, in gymnasiums, or on the tracks and running trails found in almost every community. (If you run on roads or streets, stay on the shoulder or close to the curb and run facing traffic. A few localities have banned runners from roadways, so you should check to see if yours is one of them.)

You can do it almost anytime.
You don't have to get a team together to run, so you can set your own schedule. Weather doesn't present the same problems and uncertainties that it does in many sports. Running is not a seasonal activity, except in the most extreme climates, and you can do it in daylight or darkness. (Wear light-colored or reflective clothing and exercise extreme care if you run at night. Several runners are struck and killed each year by autos.)

It's inexpensive.
You don't have to pay to do it, and the only special equipment required is a good pair of running shoes.

RUNNING STYLE

In most sports we are taught to run for speed and power. In running for fitness the objectives are different and so is the form. Here are some suggestions to help you develop a comfortable, economical running style:

- Run in an upright position, avoiding excessive forward lean. Keep back as straight as you comfortably can and keep head up. Don't look at your feet.
- Carry arms slightly away from the body, with elbows bent so that forearms are roughly parallel to the ground. Occasionally shake and relax arms to prevent tightness in shoulders.
- Land on the heel of the foot and rock forward to drive off the ball of the foot. If this proves difficult, try a more flat-footed style. Running only on the balls of your feet will tire you quickly and make the legs sore.
- Keep stride relatively short. Don't force your pace by reaching for extra distance.
- Breathe deeply with mouth open.

WHAT TO WEAR

The most important item of apparel for the runner is a pair of sturdy, properly-fitting running shoes. Training shoes with heavy, cushioned soles and arch supports are preferable to flimsy sneakers and racing flats. (Several running magazines annually rate the major brands and popular models.)

Weather will dictate the rest of your attire. As a general rule, you will want to wear lighter clothing than temperatures might seem to indicate. Running generates lots of body heat.

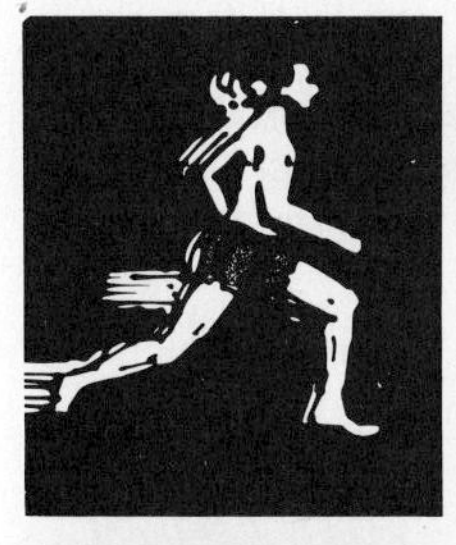
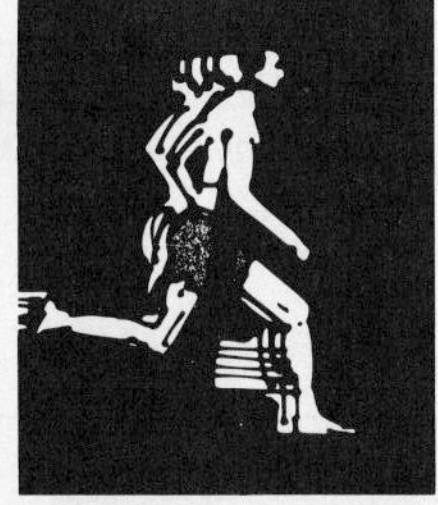
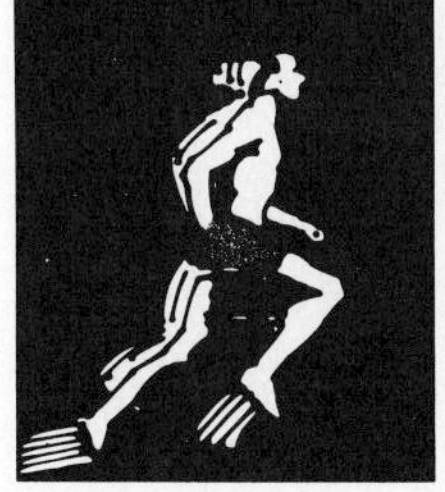
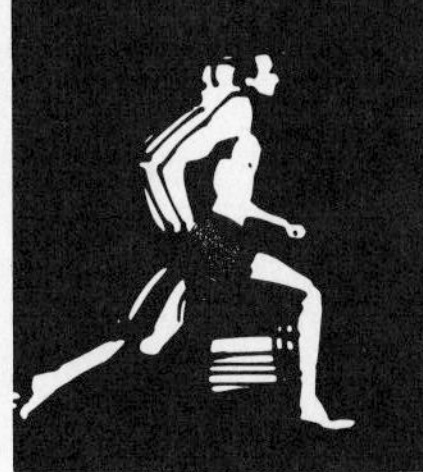

Light-colored clothing that reflects the sun's rays is cooler in the summer, and dark clothes are warmer in the winter. When the weather is very cold, it's better to wear several layers of light clothing than one or two heavy layers. The extra layers help trap heat, and it's easy to shed one of them if you become too warm.

You should wear something on your head when it's cold, or when it's hot and sunny. Wool watch caps or ski caps are recommended for winter wear, and some form of tennis or sailor's hat that provides shade and can be soaked in water is good for summer.

Don't wear rubberized or plastic clothing. Such garments interfere with the evaporation of perspiration and cause body temperature to rise to dangerous levels.

If you dress properly, you can run in almost any weather, but it's advisable not to run when it's extremely hot and humid. On such days, plan to run early in the morning or in the evening.

GETTING A 'GREEN LIGHT'

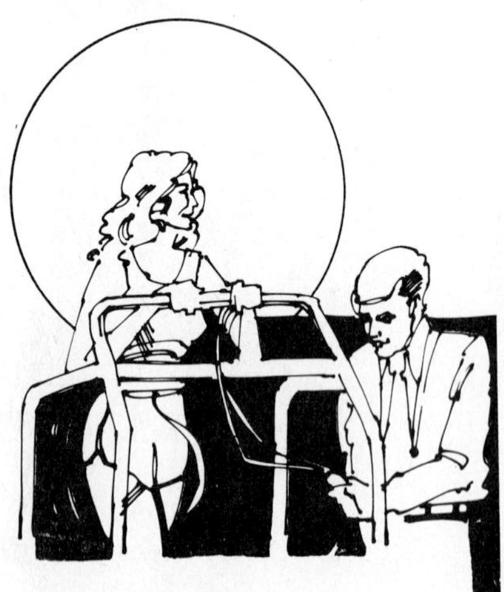

Before you begin running you should have a complete medical examination. Chances are that your physician will give you a go-ahead. Even persons with serious organic disorders, including many heart attack victims, are able to run under carefully prescribed conditions.

If you have a history of cardiovascular problems, or if you have reason to suspect the existence of such problems, it's a good idea to have an exercise, or stress, electrocardiogram (ECG). It will help your physician detect any complications that might be provoked by prolonged, strenuous exertion.

'WARMING UP' AND 'COOLING DOWN'

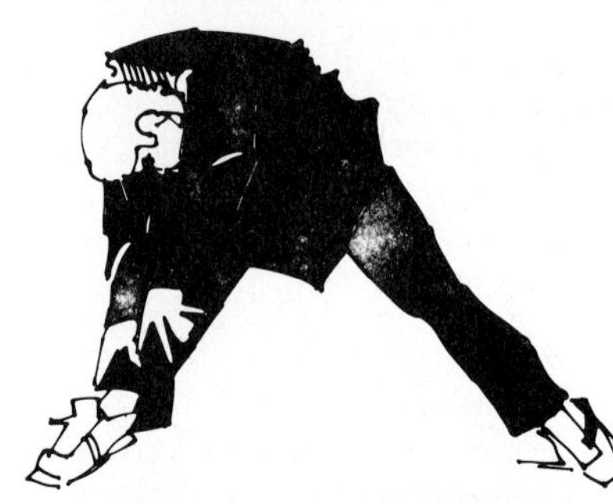

Now you're ready to begin running – or almost. Elsewhere in this booklet you will find a set of six stretching exercises. These should **always** be done before running. They will stretch the muscles you use in running and prepare the joints for movement through a full range of motion.

The six stretching exercises should be repeated during a "cooling down" period following each run. When you have finished running, walk until breathing returns to pre-exercise levels and then do the exercises. This will help prevent muscle soreness and also aid the return of the blood from the extremities to the heart.

RUNNING

Now that you really are ready to run, you may find that you have to begin by walking. If so, don't be discouraged. Few beginners are capable of running continuously for any distance. It probably took you several years to get in the shape you're in, and it will take awhile to repair the neglect. Patience is the key to success.

The "walk test" will help you determine where to begin. If you can comfortably walk three miles in 45 minutes, it's okay to start running. Or, more precisely, alternately running and walking. If you can't pass the test, walk three miles a day until you can.

In the beginning you should alternately run and walk continuously for 20 minutes. Speed is not important, but the amount of time is. It takes about 20 minutes for your body to begin realizing the "training effects" of sustained, vigorous exercise.

No one can tell you exactly how far you should run/walk at the beginning. Exercise capacity varies widely, even in individuals of similar age and build. Here's a rule of thumb to follow:

> After your warmup, walk briskly until you are moving easily. Run at a comfortable pace until you begin to become winded or tired or both. Walk until you're ready to run again. Repeat the cycle until your 20 minutes are up.

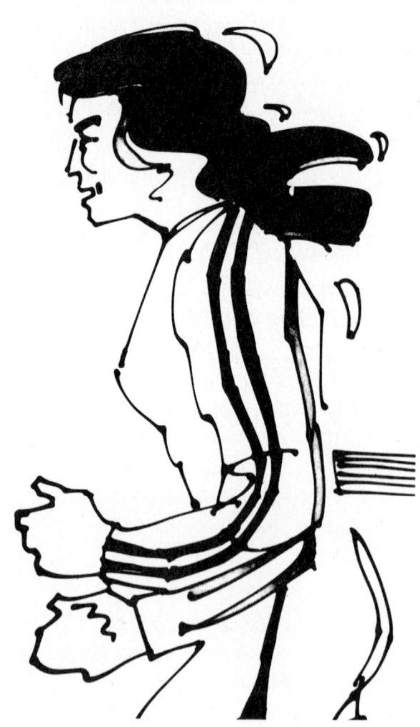

The more often you run, the faster you will improve. At least five workouts a week are recommended for persons trying to raise their level of fitness. Three workouts a week generally are considered to be the minimum number needed to maintain a desirable state of fitness.

The "talk test" can help you find the right pace. You should be able to talk while running, or while alternately running and walking. If you're too breathless to talk, you're going too fast.

When you first begin running, progress will seem slow, but gradually in the weeks ahead you will become aware that your strength and staying power are increasing. After eight or 10 weeks, if you work out faithfully, you should be able to run the full 20 minutes at a reasonable pace, although this process may take somewhat longer for older persons.

After you have completed the reconditioning phase, you should extend your run to 30 minutes. Remember, the amount of time you invest is more important than your time for a specific distance.

STRETCHING EXERCISES

To minimize the chances of injury or soreness, the following exercises should be done **before** and **after** running. If you find the exercises difficult to perform, you may want to do them twice when warming up to increase flexibility. Stretch slowly and do not bounce to attain prescribed positions.

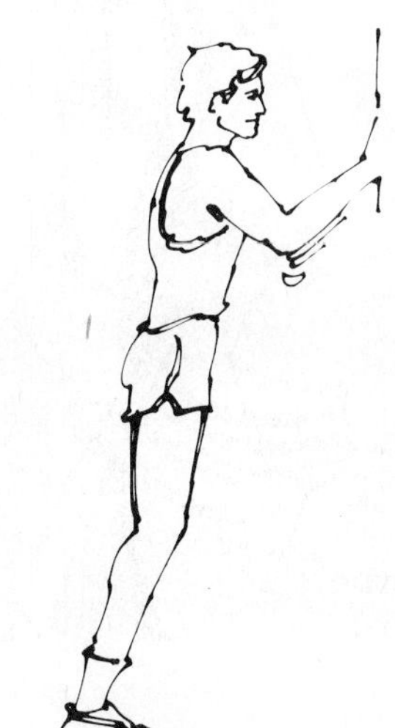

Achilles Tendon and Calf Stretcher

Stand facing wall approximately three feet away. Lean forward and place palms of hands flat against wall. Keep back straight, heels firmly on floor, and slowly bend elbows to hands, and tuck hips toward wall. Hold position for 30 seconds.

Repeat exercise with knees slightly flexed.

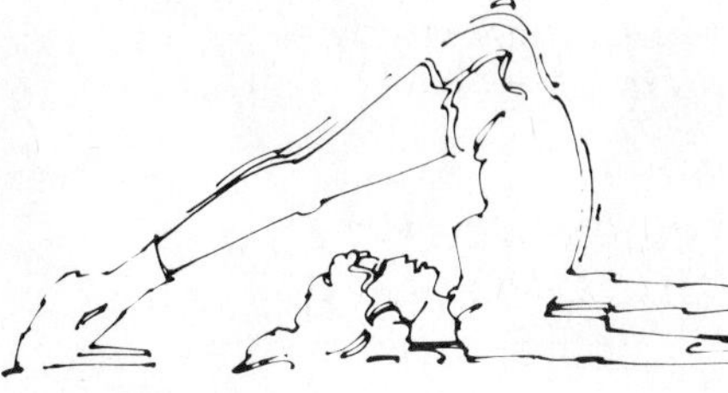

Back Stretcher

Lie on back with legs straight and arms at sides with palms down. Slowly lift legs, hips, and lower part of back and attempt to touch toes to floor behind head. Keep legs straight and hold position for 30 seconds.

Thigh Stretcher

Stand arm's length from wall with left side toward wall. Place left hand on wall for support. Grasp right ankle with right hand and pull foot back and up until heel touches buttocks. Lean forward from waist as you lift. Hold for 30 seconds.

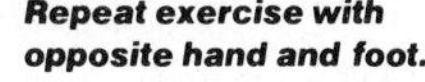

Repeat exercise with opposite hand and foot.

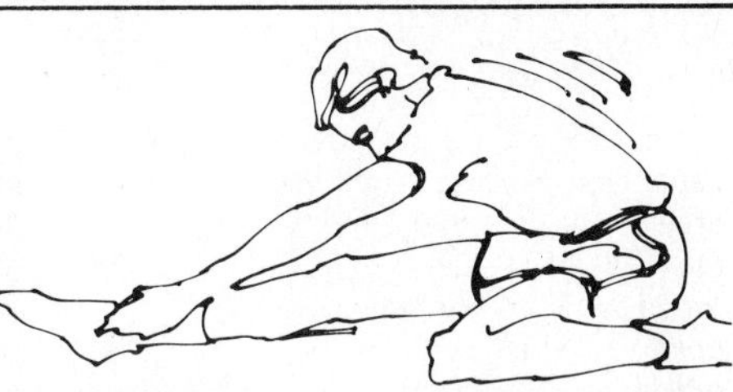

Hurdler's Stretch

Sit on floor with one leg extended straight ahead. Upper part of other leg should be at right angle to body, with heel close to buttocks. Slowly slide hands down extended leg and touch foot. Hold position for 30 seconds. Keeping legs in same position, slowly lean back and rest elbows on floor. Hold for 30 seconds.

Reverse position and repeat both stages of exercise.

Straddle Stretch

Sit on floor and spread straight legs about twice shoulder width. Slowly lean forward from waist, sliding hands along floor, as far forward as you can. Hold for 30 seconds.

Return to starting position. Slowly stretch forward over right leg, sliding both hands down

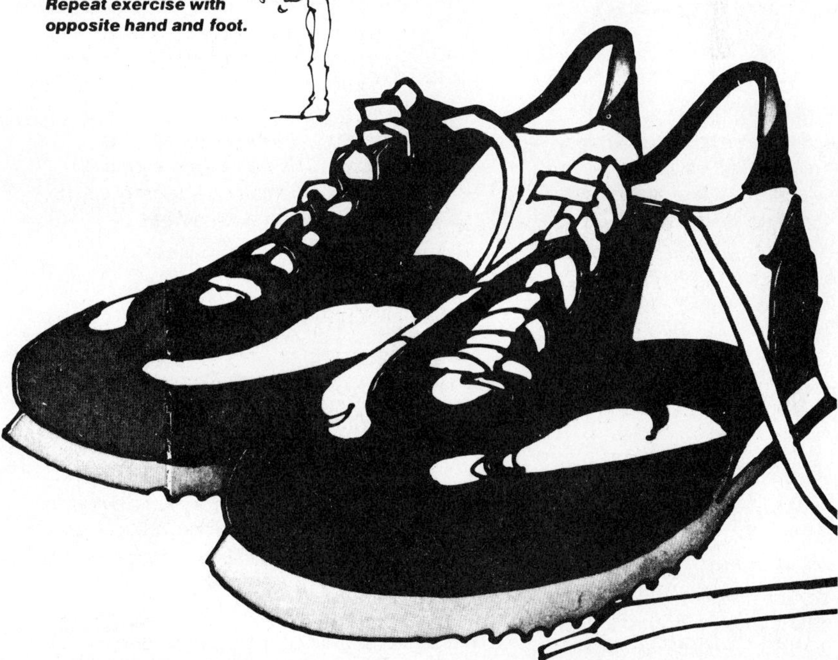

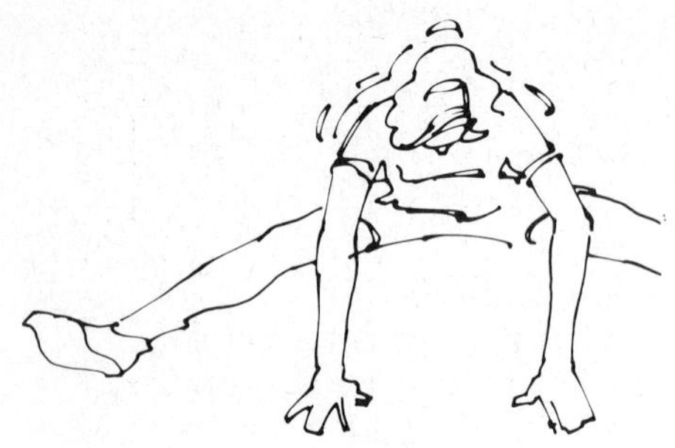

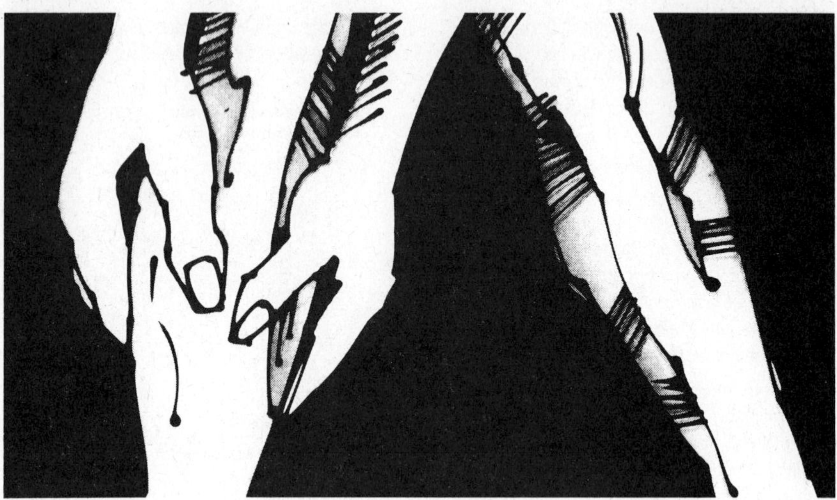

to right ankle. Try to keep knee straight and touch chin to right knee cap. Hold for 30 seconds.

Return to starting position. Repeat second step of exercise to left side.

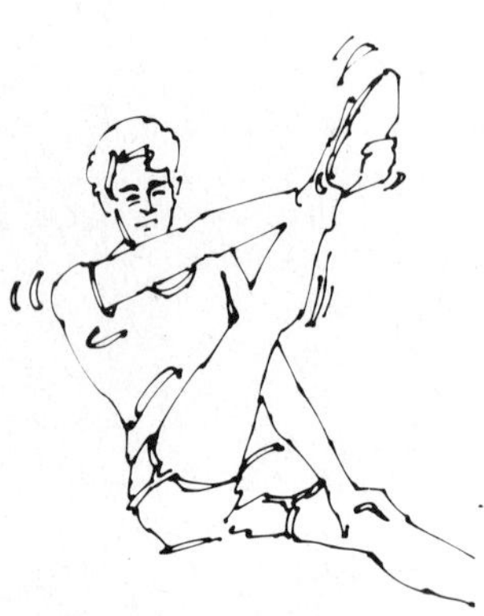

Leg Stretcher

Sit in same position as in preceding exercise. Rest left hand on left thigh and grasp inside of right foot with right hand. Keep back straight and slowly straighten right leg, letting it raise to about a 45 degree angle. Hold position for 30 seconds.

Repeat exercise with other leg.

A FEW WORDS OF CAUTION

Listen to your body when you run. If you develop pain, or any other unusual symptom, slow down or stop. If the problem persists, see your physician before running again.

Don't compete with others until you are an experienced, well-conditioned runner. Your objective in the beginning should be to steadily improve your own performance, not to run faster than someone else.

Running is a great endurance exercise, but it is not a complete exercise program. Persons who limit themselves to running tend to become stiff and inflexible, with short, tight muscles in the back and in the backs of the legs. They also may lack muscle tone and strength in the trunk and upper body. These conditions can lead to poor posture and chronic lower-back pain, a condition that partially cripples or disables thousands of middle-aged and older Americans.

The stretching exercises you do before and after running will give you needed flexibility. In addition, you should do some strength exercises, such as pushups and bent-knee situps, to give your fitness regimen proper balance.

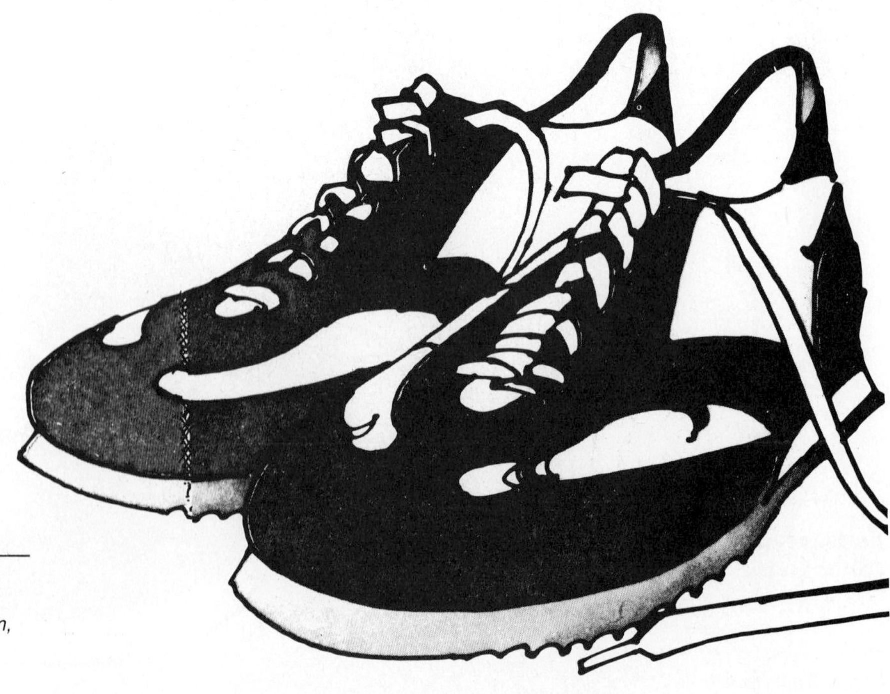